THE ENCYCLOPEDIA OF

THE BACK AND SPINE SYSTEMS AND DISORDERS

Mary Harwell Sayler
with
Arya Nick Shamie, M.D.
Director, UCLA Comprehensive Spine Center
VA Wadsworth Medical Center
Assistant Professor of Orthopaedic Surgery and Neurosurgery
UCLA School of Medicine

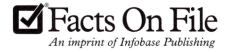
Facts On File
An imprint of Infobase Publishing

The Encyclopedia of the Back and Spine Systems and Disorders

Copyright © 2007 by Mary Harwell Sayler

Facts On File, Inc.
An imprint of Infobase Publishing
132 West 31st Street
New York NY 10001

Library of Congress Cataloging-in-Publication Data

Sayler, Mary Harwell.
The encyclopedia of the back and spine systems and disorders /
Mary Harwell Sayler with Arya Nick Shamie.
p. cm.
Includes bibliographical references and index.
ISBN 978-0-8160-6678-0 (hc : alk. paper) 1. Back—Diseases—Encyclopedias.
2. Spine—Diseases—Encyclopedias. I. Shamie, Arya Nick. II. Title.
III. Title: Back and spine systems and disorders.
RD768.S6277 2007
617.5′64—dc22   2006035678

Text and cover design by Cathy Rincon

Printed in the United States of America

VB Hermitage 10 9 8 7 6 5 4 3 2 1

This book is printed on acid-free paper.

Dedicated to Backbone
for Bob

The spine defines us:
fish, amphibian,
reptile, bird,
or mammal
crawling,
crouching,
reaching
toward upright.

Uptight or loosely
woven, we struggle
to correct each
complication
of age or accident
we've fallen
heir to
in this relentless art
of balancing our act.

CONTENTS

Foreword   v

Preface   viii

Acknowledgments   xi

Introduction   xii

Entries A–Z   1

Appendix I: National and International Organizations
for the Back and Spine   321

Appendix II: Related Organizations   323

Appendix III: Other Relevant Web Sites   327

Appendix IV: Internet Journals and Magazines   328

Bibliography   329

Index   331

About the Authors   354

FOREWORD

Back pain and neck pain are very common disorders that affect 90 percent of the adult population sometime in their life span. The good news is that only 10 percent of these disorders require any treatment, and most will get better spontaneously within weeks after the onset of symptoms. Of the patients who need treatment, only 10 percent will require surgical treatment (1 percent of all patients). Most will be treated with medications, physical therapy, and/or injections.

Despite the generally good outcome after the onset of back and neck pain, the disorder can be quite debilitating. When severe pain occurs, patients desperately seek any treatment that may help, but many of the advertised treatments lack any sound evidence that they work. The patient takes herbal medications, gets a massage to relieve "knots of muscles," or uses traction that promises to get rid of pain. The interesting fact is that, in most cases, if patients just waited four to six weeks, the pain would disappear on its own! Unproven treatments also take money out of a patient's pocket because insurance companies do not cover the costs. Some treatments can even be harmful to patients or worsen their symptoms. The bottom line is, use common sense or ask a professional to help you decide which treatments to invest in.

The most common initial treatments offered to patients are bed rest for a maximum of one to two days, anti-inflammatory medications or injections including steroids, some form of exercise or physical therapy, and/or pain medication including narcotics like codeine. Bed rest for more than one to two days is not advised, because it can cause atrophy of the muscles and other problems associated with immobility.

Typically, pain in the spine is caused by inflammation that stimulates pain receptors in the area. Therefore, medications that block inflammation will also help pain. For instance, the class of medication called NSAIDs, or nonsteroidal anti-inflammatory drugs, are generally safe and not habit-forming but should be taken with food to minimize risks of gastrointestinal upset. In some cases, especially with larger doses and prolonged use, these medications can cause a peptic ulcer. The first sign of this condition is pain in the stomach area that may or may not be relieved by ingesting food. If these symptoms develop, you should immediately stop the medication and consult your physician.

Steroids (a form of hormone) can also be prescribed to cut down inflammation. Steroids are generally more effective than NSAIDs in treating inflammation but have more side effects. The steroids can be given either by mouth (with more systemic effects) or via direct injection of a small amount at the site of the inflammation or injury.

Physical therapy offers another treatment prescribed during the acute phase of the disease. This therapy may include exercise, ultrasound heating of sore muscles, and/or massage treatments to ease muscles "knotted" by contraction. There is controversy over whether this treatment modality actually works, probably because of non-standardized treatments or variations in the success rate. Physical therapy theoretically helps patients by stretching then strengthening muscles around the spine, which ultimately takes the pressure off the spinal joints. Not to be regarded as a quick fix, physical therapy should be continued in a regimented fashion even after the pain has subsided to prevent a recurrence of symptoms.

If none of the above treatments helps to alleviate symptoms, then surgical intervention is considered. A subgroup of patients do need some form of treatment, but before talking about that, a review of spine anatomy will help to explain the three main categories of spine disease: degenerative disc disease (DDD), stenosis, and instability.

The spinal column consists of bony vertebrae stacked on top of each other from the neck to the tail bone. Between each of these vertebrae there is a cushion known as the intervertebral "disc." These discs have a jelly core, much like a jelly doughnut, and the jelly withstands much of the force that is transmitted through the vertebrae. The jelly dries up as we age, and this leads to normal aging or degeneration in the spine, a process known as DDD.

As this cushion dries up and the vertebrae settle on top of one another, pain ensues. This is much like the degeneration of the hips and knees that we have been treating for years with hip and knee replacement. The treatment of the degeneration in the spine, however, is more complex. First of all, the spine has many discs that can degenerate together, and the challenge comes in treating the correct level that is the source of the pain. Secondly, we did not have a good way to replace degenerative discs safely until recently. Fusion has been the mainstay of treatment for degenerative discs. The logic behind this treatment is that, if the degenerated cushion causes pain in adjacent vertebrae, fusing the two vertebrae together should get rid of the patient's pain. The fusion treatment has been only partially successful though, because after two vertebrae are fused together, the stresses are transferred to the levels above and below this fused level, and this may result in more rapid degeneration of those adjacent levels. In rare cases, the degeneration or other disease processes can cause instability of the spine. When this occurs, one vertebra slides on top of another, putting the nerves passing through them at risk. In the case of instability, we have no choice but to fuse the vertebrae.

Disc replacement is a new alternative to fusion for DDD. A disc replacement device is implanted in the disc space that is degenerated. Since the device has a built-in mechanical joint, it theoretically preserves the motion in the disc space. This prevents the extra stress that may occur in adjacent discs so may prevent adjacent level disease. However, disc replacement devices require a stable spine, so spinal instability precludes their use. Currently, disc replacement is approved only for the lumbar spine, but cervical spine disc replacement is under clinical trials and will soon be available.

Since the discs in the spine are in front of the nerves, disc replacement does not adequately address stenosis or narrowing around the nerves, especially if stenosis is caused by structures in the back of the spine. Stenosis causes pressure on the nerves and, hence, can result in nerve pain (radiculopathy or sciatica.) DDD often causes stenosis in its late form. As the discs degenerate, the joints in the back of the spine called the facet joints see more stress and enlarge or hypertrophy. Nerves exit through holes (foramina) in front of the facet joints at every level of the spinal column. Enlarged facets can cause stenosis in these holes and, hence, cause nerve pain. When facet disease is prominent, just addressing the disc in the front with a disc replacement will not treat the symptoms. Therefore, stenosis is typically addressed from the back of the spine to free up nerves in the foramina. The exception to this rule is in the cervical spine (neck) where most of the early stenosis occurs from a disc herniation or bone spurs in front of the spine. If a facet is much enlarged and part of it has to be removed to decompress the nerves, the patient's spine also has to be fused. The two facets act as the posterior (back) stabilizers of the spine, while the disc is the anterior (front) stabilizer. This configuration is present in most levels of the spinal column.

Traditionally, stenosis is treated with a laminectomy (and partial facet removal). Lamina form the posterior arch of the spine, which is removed in order to decompress the nerves in the center of the spinal column. Through this posterior opening the foramina are also accessed and decompressed using special tools. Laminectomy is a safe procedure and can significantly improve a debilitating condition. Laminectomy is not, however, without its potential limitations and complications.

A new alternative to a laminectomy is a procedure performed while the patient is awake. This procedure does not require bone removal but accomplishes decompression indirectly by implantation of a device called the X Stop. When the stenotic patient bends forward, the foramina in the back of the spine enlarge and free the nerve from pressure. X Stop is implanted in the back of the spine between the spinous processes at the level where the problem exists, thus functionally opening the foramina.

The field of spine surgery is evolving rapidly. With the advent of new technology and surgical techniques, patients are being treated more effectively and safely. This advancement is possible only through continued efforts of scientists in various disciplines and their interdisciplinary collaboration. MRI has tremendously advanced the diagnosis of spinal disease in the last 20 years. With live X-ray now available in the operating room, we are able to perform surgeries through small skin incisions. This translates to more accurate surgeries and quicker recovery for patients.

With the rapid advancement in technology, it is imperative that physicians and patients alike are educated in the best treatment (not necessarily always the newest) modality for their condition. This textbook is an attempt to help readers understand the often complex spinal conditions. Understanding the nomenclature will possibly aid in understanding the processes and treatments available for the common condition of spine-related pain.

—Arya Nick Shamie, M.D.
Director, UCLA Comprehensive Spine Center
VA Wadsworth Medical Center
Assistant Professor of Orthopaedic Surgery
and Neurosurgery
UCLA School of Medicine
www.espinecare.com

PREFACE

Almost anywhere you go, you will find a country overly populated with aching backs. Undoubtedly, this sad fact helped the Bone and Joint Decade (2000–10) become an international event. Yet, despite the global momentum toward universal back pain, books on the subject often focus on such specialized treatments as trigger point therapy or microsurgery. Or the spine of a book might cover the aging spine.

Although my own back heatedly objects to the inflammation typically associated with aging, I wanted a book to consider a wide range of spine-related topics, including ample options for treating various levels of pain. I also wanted a broader view of the back to help me and, I hope, you to avoid preventable problems, make informed decisions about our vertebral health, and remain upright inhabitants of our own bodies.

What, for example, should be considered before you flex muscles that have begun to conform to an ergonomic chair? Would certain exercises strengthen your spine without weakening a disc? Could information about the anatomy and function of your neck and back help to show you what has happened and, thereby, clarify what to do?

Do all natural treatments naturally assure safe usage? Are herbal remedies strong enough to assuage your night-time pain? Will anything restore collagen, rebuild bone, or keep your cartilage from wearing out? What medical tests might provide you with a clearer picture? And how much should you heed ongoing word fights over food? With conflicting advice to confuse this very personal issue, do you need more calcium or less?

Remembering the adage, "You are what you eat," I like to think there is more to me than mozzarella, but a one-ounce slice of my favorite part-skim brand gives 20 percent of the daily requirement of calcium needed by most adults. The question is whether *I* need that much or more. Do you, even if the calcium comes with 8 percent fat and 5 percent cholesterol squeezing through the creamery? Would 6 percent calcium in two tablespoons of fat-free, cholesterol-free sour cream be a better choice for you, or would 0 percent fat and 2 percent cholesterol warrant a cup of fat-free yogurt with 40 percent of your daily calcium need?

Such mathematical questions might be directed to a cardiologist or other specialist who assesses your level of cholesterol and its effects on your heart and veins. To evaluate your overall food patterns, however, a nutritionist can address your individual tastes, habits, weight, activities, family history, symptoms, and unique nutritional needs before planning the best course of meals and snacks for you. As a registered dietitian, a nutritionist can also separate the fat everyone needs from the amount you personally require to store fat-soluble vitamins, lubricate joints, and transport hormones throughout your body. Too much fat, of course, is literally overkill, but, in moderation, a fatty layer of protection can shield and cushion your bones in wintry weather—or in a fall.

To help you keep your balance, a healthful diet includes energizing carbohydrates and muscle-building protein. As a general rule, well-balanced meals tip the scales toward fresh fruit, vegetables, and whole grains with dairy and meat products dished lightly on the side. Since the optimum amounts of proteins, carbohydrates, and fats fluctuate from person to person, a nutritionist can determine the percentages appropriate for you. If any changes occur in your health or habits though, your nutritional needs will change too.

As yet another variable, the level of stress you experience today will seldom be the same a week or a month from now. If tension builds, so will muscle tightness, thereby restricting blood flow and causing muscle cramps. Back pain may then arise with a new slew of questions. For example, would a good massage help your muscles to relax and, if so, what type would be best for you? Do you need kneading? Or would pressing pressure points release those bundles of nerves? A licensed massage therapist can explain the styles and purpose of each stroke, but if you're worried about having a stroke, ask your doctor about the elevation in blood pressure a massage conceivably could cause.

Questions about the minimal risks of a stroke might also go to your osteopath or chiropractor, especially if your cervical spine needs to be realigned. Both specialists have been trained to manipulate neck and back vertebrae to treat musculoskeletal complaints. However, differences between these medical professionals occur not only in their training but also in the theory behind each approach to treatment. A chiropractor, for example, may focus on the nerves involved in adjusting your tendons and joints. After taking your medical history and, possibly, X-rays, a chiropractor might treat your neck or backache with spinal manipulation, massage, ultrasound, acupressure, trigger point therapy, or a combination of those options. An instrument such as an Activator might also be used, but more likely, you will be given hands-on treatment. If poor postural habits, stress, or injury have caused your spine to lose its natural curves, your vertebrae may need a well-planned series of adjustments to get back in shape.

A doctor of osteopathy (D.O., or osteopath) performs similar treatments but with the understanding that proper alignment of the spine allows a body to function better. Because your spinal column houses the nervous system that controls your bodily functions, the condition and position of your vertebrae can affect your entire body. This viewpoint may lead an osteopath to educate you about self-care and disease prevention.

A D.O. might also choose a medical specialty similar to the ones pursued by a medical doctor (M.D.). Although a D.O. and an M.D. both adhere to the Hippocratic oath, "First, do no harm," they may have slightly different interpretations of what this rule means. For example, a D.O. may see your symptoms as an indication of some disorder in your defense system, which, when set right, could evoke a natural response of healing. Despite a belief in the healing mechanisms inherent in the body, a D.O. can still prescribe medication as, of course, an M.D. can. Prior to writing prescriptions or practicing medicine though, both types of physicians must pass their state licensing exams. Both can then opt to continue their studies to obtain certification in such specialized areas as pediatrics, or the spinal care of infants, children, and teens.

As another specialist of the musculoskeletal system, a rheumatologist treats autoimmune disorders and conditions of the spine, such as juvenile arthritis, ankylosing spondylitis, or rheumatoid arthritis. Similarly, an orthopedic specialist treats disorders of muscles, bones, joints, and connective tissue, such as tendons and ligaments. However, a rheumatologist generally concentrates on soft tissue as an underlying indicator of back pain, whereas an orthopedist often focuses on the hard matter in matters of bone fracture, injuries, and abnormalities in bone growth.

To treat spinal cord injuries and spinal nerve involvement, a D.O. or M.D. may decide to specialize in neurology, or, to repair structural problems, a physician may elect surgery. With numerous procedures available, surgeons usually avoid any invasive course of action unless an identifiable condition shows a particular procedure to be the best choice. If so, minimally invasive surgery can often be used to speed recovery, thereby enabling you to resume your normal activities or begin therapy more quickly.

The type of therapy depends, of course, on what you need. For instance, physical therapy usually addresses larger groups of muscles to get you mobile again. Occupational therapy aids smaller motor movements and gives you creative tools and training to regain your independence in completing daily routines, such as dressing yourself or bathing.

With or without surgery, questions may continue to arise about what is best for you. For example, do you need cold therapy to alleviate vertebral swelling or heat therapy to increase the circulation in your back? Would water therapy ease pain in your arthritic joints, or would a specific exercise work best for your particular condition? Is someone in your area trained to treat the pain of arthritis or postoperative nausea with acupuncture? Would increasing your intake of filtered water and natural nutrients help your body to heal faster?

Successful treatments depend, in part, on the type of treatment you give yourself, but success may also reflect the quality and extent of training a therapist or other specialist has received. An Internet search may provide important information about the credentials, experience, and success rate of a health-care practitioner. For more details about a specific condition of the back or spine, Appendixes I, II, and III list relevant Web sites sponsored by reputable hospitals, universities, organizations, and government agencies. For an overview of anatomy and function, the Introduction may give you a clearer picture of your vertebrae and, perhaps, a better idea of what to ask your therapist or physician as you continue to seek solutions and question almost everything.

ACKNOWLEDGMENTS

Special thanks go to my dear friend of many years, Lynda Anderson Edwards, for her help in gathering the resources for this book. Her work within the library system of Kentucky gave her access to a wealth of publications, which she generously shared and which led me to discover the extensive resources available to almost anyone with a library card. In my own state, for example, I had only to go to the Florida State Library system Web site, check-in via the numbers on the back of my local library card, and check-out hundreds of recently published articles on the back and spine. Living, as I do, in a small community on a sand road where the only honking traffic comes from a family of sandhill cranes, I had not anticipated such instant access to up-to-date findings on the spine.

I also want to thank my talented and supportive siblings, especially my sister, Marcia A. Harwell, an occupational therapist in Tennessee, who provided me with materials she uses in her work and gave me valuable insight into occupational and physical therapies. I am also grateful to my brother, Mark A. Harwell, an academic scientist who served on the Science Advisory Board of the Environmental Protection Agency for many years and, for two terms, chaired the Ecological Processes and Effects Committee. By giving me a glimpse into the complexities of environmental factors, he helped me to find direction in researching an entry for this book.

Thanks also go to Dana Cassell, another writer for the Health and Living series published by Facts On File and the director of the national organization Cassell Network of Writers. Not only did Dana introduce me to medical writing in general, she has often contributed articles and ideas on my topics of interest.

Once again, I am delighted to say how much I appreciate the excellent staff at Facts On File. Their responsiveness, guidelines, and commitment to high publishing standards make my work with editor in chief James Chambers, associate editor Vanessa Nittoli, and editorial assistant Matthew Anderson a pleasure and privilege. I also appreciate greatly the time Nick Shamie took to proofread this manuscript and write an informative foreword. Literally and literarily, I could not have done this book without their assistance.

Last in word, but first in thought, I thank my husband, Bob, for his confidence in me and his ongoing enthusiasm for my work as a medical writer and poet. When I feel discouraged, he helps me to recall courage. When my back aches, he massages knotted muscles and releases trigger points. Although he has not completely cooked his way around the kitchen, he has custom-built cabinets to my height, so I do not have to bend over a standard-sized counter. Then he regularly washes dishes! How much I have to be thankful for and acknowledge.

Mary Harwell Sayler
Lake Como, Florida

INTRODUCTION

At this very moment, 31 million people in the United States have a backache. Throughout the year, half of our working population will have some type of spinal concern. Within five years, 33 percent of Americans over 18 will seek medical attention to alleviate back pain. Indeed, 90 percent of our citizens will encounter back pain at some point in their lives. If similar statistics occurred with a manufactured product, we would probably investigate the misuse of the merchandise or the defects in design.

The Spine's Design

From a posterior or back view, an inside look at a healthy spinal column gives the impression of stacked petals of bone whose beauty lies in the strength of its construction. Fitted together in a three-dimensional puzzle, 32 to 33 vertebrae extend from the neck to the tailbone, not as a rigid pole, but as a sequence of curves. This intricate design brings flexibility in movement, while the interlocking bones also provide vertebral strength. As seen from a lateral or side view, the natural curves of the neck and spine distribute weight evenly while holding the head and body upright.

Besides this amazingly efficient design, 19 of the 33 vertebral bones comprise the spinous process you feel as your fingers bump along the bony projections down the middle of your back. If you could see inside that protective column of bone, your spinal cord might look like a finger-thick stem, flowering into your brain. Or you might see it as an electric cord, fraying at one end. With either visual to aid your glimpse, the lower portion of this 17- to 18-inch-long stem terminates in a picture of root-like nerves sinking into the lumbar region. A more humorous comparison arose in Latin-speaking times as people noticed hair-like nerves fanning above the pelvic bones like a horse's tail, then appropriately named this area the *cauda* (horse) *equina* (tail.)

Stripped of other metaphors, and also of body matter, spinal nerves up and down the back look like the elongated skeleton of a fish or a long, skinny caterpillar legging in all directions. The latter simile comes with a creepy connotation of easily being squished, but a slight shift in focus shows each vertebra, viewed from above, looking like Brunhilda's helmet. As any Viking warrior could see, those irregularly shaped rings of vertebral bone protect the spinal nerves, spinal fluid, and arteries encased inside.

Literally speaking, every little vertebra is not, of course, the same. Some vary by design, depending on their function. For example, the first cervical vertebra, known as the atlas, looks like a small but stout yoke or collar of bone on which the skull rests. The second ring of cervical bone, the axis, includes a rounded "tooth" known as the dens (Latin for tooth) that fits in a space notched into the atlas. When the atlas and axis work well together, this unique pair of bones eases movement and allows rotation of the head.

The remaining cervical bones look similar to other vertebrae of the spine. Because neck vertebrae support the head and not the weight of the body, these cervical bones remain smaller than the vertebrae of the upper and lower back. Those larger back bones graduate in size to protect your internal organs and support your body weight. The back vertebrae also connect to your ribs that are shaped like the bottom of a boat, except for the lowest ribs, which seem to be afloat.

To locate a specific bone with greater accuracy, each vertebra has been assigned a sort of area code according to its region. For example, C1 through C7 specify the seven cervical bones of the neck, including the atlas (C1) and axis (C2.) The twelve thoracic vertebrae of the upper back or thorax have numerical codes of T1 through T12, whereas L1 through L5 indicate the five vertebrae of the lumbar or lower back. Several small bones then fuse together for strength in the sacral region, which, in keeping with the Latin word, *sacrum,* may be somewhat sacred to some.

Back Pain Potential

Assuming no accident, injury, or genetic flaw rearranges the design, a healthy spine supports the body's weight and pain-free movement. Sometimes, however, tension creates pain as tightened muscles twist the spine, or an underlying medical condition causes an otherwise healthy back to ache. For example, a problem with either kidney may generate pain since those organs reside in the middle of the back beneath the lower ribs. More commonly, backaches result from improper maintenance, poor posture, overuse, repetitive use, misuse, or general wear and tear.

With advancing age or frequent friction, movable joints generally do not wear too well. In addition to this problem, the spine has even more possibilities for discomfort since each vertebra connects with the one above and below, creating various types of joints. To cushion those joints, soft-centered discs of fibrous cartilage separate individual vertebral bones from C2 through L5, but these protective pads can rupture, subsequently compressing or irritating the nerve tissue in that area. Usually, strong fibrous ligaments help to protect the spinal discs by acting as strapping devices that secure one vertebra to another, but those ligaments can themselves cause pain if torn or pulled. In good working order, the sturdy spinal system has remarkable

strength and flexibility. Yet, the spine does have its nerve.

Through a large hole in the center of each vertebral bone, millions of nerve fibers travel through the spinal canal. Housed in the protective membrane (dura mater) of the spinal cord and surrounded by spinal fluids, this nervous system connects your brain to the rest of your body. Between the vertebrae, small spaces (neural foramina) in the bones allow nerve roots to exit. These pairs of nerves then act like tiny extension cords, connecting the spinal cord to related parts of your body. For example, nerves extending from the cervical spine affect your upper chest and arms. Nerves in the thoracic region connect to your chest and abdomen, whereas the lumbar nerves affect your legs, bladder, and bowels.

Besides controlling body movement and organ function, spinal nerves send electrical impulses to your brain, giving sensations, including pain, in the associated area. When nerves themselves suffer damage, you might experience tingling or numbness instead of pain. If nerve compression occurs, which happens most often in the weight-bearing lumbar region, the nerves may scream in proportion to the pressure felt.

Unhindered, spinal nerves quietly await your every thought of getting up and moving. Fortunately, you do not have to remember to set your heart or other organs into motion, but your body will not move unless your muscles receive instructions to that effect from your central nervous system. Then movement will likely involve your spine because of its unique attachment to the paraspinal muscles of your back. On either side of each thoracic and lumbar vertebra, muscles affix to little protrusions of bone called transverse processes. As the brain stimulates nerves in the area, muscles contract and relax, moving bones and enabling your body to bend, flex, sit, stand, walk, or run. Too much movement too quickly, though, can prod muscles and connective tendons into pain or muscle spasm. That problem has an obvious means of prevention, but with so many connections and so much going on throughout the spine, numerous factors can converge to produce back pain. Addressing every possibility or preventative could take a lifetime or, perhaps, a lifestyle. The question is, what signs of the spine signal a need for change?

Back in Style

As you evaluate the effects your lifestyle has on your back and spine, begin by covering the basics. For instance, everyone needs to drink adequate water, eat nutritious foods, get enough sleep, and exercise regularly. As a mnemonic device for those pain-reducing basics, just remember to defuse with FEWS: Food, Exercise, Water, Sleep. Natural foods, sensible activities, fresh water, and restful sleep naturally help you to maintain your health. Such steps will not cure a neurological disorder, spinal cord injury, or other severe conditions of the back, but a healthy lifestyle generally does no harm. Therefore, the following pages will include natural aids whenever possible.

Meanwhile, the FEWS in your lifestyle can offer clues about back pain. If other symptoms, such as fatigue, tension, or dryness in your joints and skin, add to your discomfort, those warning signs may suggest solutions or preventatives too. For example, if you notice a pad of tummy fat pulling your lower back into a painful position, you can see such options as losing weight or beginning an exercise program to tighten the stomach and strengthen your back muscles. By paying attention to pain and any other symptoms, your body alerts you to potential problems. So, as you question what works wellness for you, consider your basic needs and the kind of accommodation with which you treat your aching back.

References

American Chiropractic Association. "Back Pain Statistics." Available online. URL: http://www.amerchiro.org/media/whatis/benefits.shtml. Downloaded on June 13, 2005.

Back.com. "Anatomy - Lumbar Spine." Available online. URL: http://www.back.com/stripcontent.php?parent_file=/anatomy-lumbar.html. Downloaded on August 30, 2005

Bridwell, Keith, M.D. "Vertebral Column," SpineUniverse. Available online. URL: http://www.spineuniverse.com/print.php/article1286.html. Last updated June 30, 2005.

Shiel, William C. Jr., M.D. "Lower Back Pain," MedicineNet.com. Available online. URL: http://www.medicinenet.com/script/main/art.asp?articlekey=289&pf=3&page=1. Downloaded on August 31, 2005.

Southern California Orthopedic Institute. "Anatomy of the Spine." Available online. URL: http://www.scoi.com/spinanat.htm. Downloaded on August 30, 2005.

Spine University. "Introduction." Available online. URL: http://www.spineuniversity.com/public/print.asp?id=71. Downloaded August 30, 2005.

abatacept   This drug literally belongs in a class by itself. As the first of a new class of agents known as selective costimulation modulators, abatacept blocks a key signal the body awaits before activating T-cells. Figuratively speaking, that signal opens a gate for T-cells to search and destroy the invasion of foreign agents, such as bacteria or a virus. In an autoimmune disease such as RHEUMATOID ARTHRITIS (RA), the gate stays open, confusing T-cells into attacking healthy cells. To stop this reaction, abatacept intercepts and unscrambles mixed signals, thus causing T-cells to cease firing on friendly targets.

As explained in the *Briefing Document For Abatacept,* "it selectively modulates T-cell activation, and secondarily affects key mechanisms of inflammation and progressive joint destruction in RA." For patients who have had an inadequate response to a DISEASE MODIFYING ANTI-RHEUMATIC DRUG (DMARD), "abatacept is indicated for reducing signs and symptoms, inducing major clinical response, inhibiting the progression of structural damage, and improving physical function in adult patients with moderately to severely active rheumatoid arthritis. . . ."

Dosage and Potential Side Effects

Lauded as "generally safe and well-tolerated" at doses of 2 mg/kg and 10 mg/kg, the briefing document also described the most common adverse event (AE) as headache. However, "no specific AE led to discontinuation in more than 0.2% of patients, with the exception of back pain in 0.3% of placebo-treated patients," but "infections were the most common reason for study discontinuation. . . ."

Statistics and Studies

Since abatacept acts on the immune system, the manufacturing company, Bristol-Myers Squibb (BMS), anticipated incidents of infection. Indeed, the researchers found "the overall frequency of infections was slightly increased in abatacept-treated patients, but the severity, treatment, and outcome was similar to that in placebo-treated patients. Serious viral, fungal, or mycobacterial infections were uncommon." To better define the risks, the manufacturer announced "a post-marketing pharmacovigilance plan" to last at least until the year 2010.

Bristol-Myers Squibb Company, *Briefing Document for Abatacept (BMS-188667) Biological License Application 125118,* Food and Drug Administration, Arthritis Advisory Committee, September 6, 2005, pages 14, 15, 19, 97, 145, 147, 148. Available online. URL: http://www. fda.gov/ohrms/dockets/ac/05/briefing/2005-4170B1_ 01_01-BMS-Abatacept.pdf. Downloaded November 11, 2005.

absorptiometry   This type of BONE MINERAL DENSITY TEST uses protons or X-RAY to reveal spinal strengths and weakness. If bones thin too much, a person's own body weight can cause breakage, such as occurs in a VERTEBRAL COMPRESSION FRACTURE. That type of deterioration often happened without warning until the development of single proton absorptiometry (SPA) in the 1960s. Radiologists later used dual proton absorptiometry (DPA) to assess spine health and the risk of fractures, but high costs and technical limitations made DPA less popular after dual energy X-ray absorptiometry (DEXA or DXA) arrived in the late 1980s.

Although other types of bone tests have since been developed, DEXA presently provides the most commonly used diagnostic tool to detect OSTEOPOROSIS and other conditions causing bone loss. DEXA monitors those conditions, too, by establishing a baseline. To do this, a peripheral DEXA measures the bone density in the arms, legs, or wrist, while a central DEXA assesses bones in the hips and spine. Once a baseline has been established, follow-up tests note further deterioration as well as the strengthening effects of BONE BUILDING treatments. Comparisons also occur as DEXA scores are themselves graded on a curve. For example, the T-score compares a person's bone density to that of a healthy young adult of the same sex. Normal bone rates a -1 while a score of -1 to -2.5 indicates the first stage of bone loss or OSTEOPENIA. T-scores below -2.5 suggest osteoporosis. Similarly, the Z-score compares bone density to that of other people of the same age, size, and gender.

Procedure

Cramming for a DEXA test must exclude CALCIUM supplements for at least 24 hours. Besides that dietary change, a week must lapse between DEXA and other tests involving barium or contrast dye, so absorptiometry usually comes first.

Prior to DEXA, a radiologist or radiologic technician explains the procedure, answers questions, and also asks a few. Those questions concern recent tests, current medications, and previous treatments for bone loss, such as HORMONE REPLACEMENT THERAPY. A medical history will be taken, too, with particular emphasis on metal implants or anything that could affect bone density measurements. Metal-free street attire, such as sweat pants and a plain T-shirt, can be worn for this outpatient procedure, but a poor wardrobe choice may necessitate changing into a hospital gown or scrubs. With no shoes, belt, or jewelry to mar the readings, clothes need to be loose enough and comfortable enough to accommodate a few minutes of lying still.

A scan table about three feet high allows most people to get on and off easily. Table padding generally increases comfort, but patients with KYPHOSIS, SCOLIOSIS, or other problems with POSTURE may require additional accommodation. Instead of the patient lying flat on the back as typically occurs, such devices as rice bags, rolled towels, or firm sponges may be used to assist patient positioning. If so, that information needs to be recorded to ensure use of the same aids and angles in follow-up DEXA tests.

Even small variations can mar the results, so the X-RAY angle also bears noting. Some DEXA tests acquire data from a small angle beam or pencil beam of X-ray that moves over the spine in a linear fashion. With its wider angle, a fan beam DEXA sweeps the body more rapidly, using less time but more radiation. Often, new equipment incorporates both angles, combining the lower dose of radiation with a faster scan. Regardless of the equipment, the same type of X-ray should be used for the next test to ensure the most accurate readings of patient progress or decline.

Risks and Complications

Painless, noninvasive, and fairly quick, absorptiometry demands no exertion but the effort of remaining motionless for 20 minutes or less, depending on the equipment. Misdiagnosis is rare. Nevertheless, collected data can mislead doctors and patients into inappropriate treatments, especially if bone density readings have been obtained from different types of machines or taken from too small an area. The latter seldom affects tests of the LUMBAR SPINE, but other variations can occur because of differences in computer software, incorrect positioning, or inconsistencies in reading DEXA data. Other types of scans, such as QUANTITATIVE COMPUTED TOMOGRAPHY (QCT), may be more accurate in assessing bone density, but QCT costs more and uses 10 times the radiation.

Although researchers continue to work toward standardizing measurements and techniques, variables increase for young patients, mainly because DEXA was devised to determine bone density in adults. Everything from the equipment to the T-scores to the distance between the X-ray source and the bones being measured has been calibrated with full-grown bones in mind. Pediatric software can overcome this problem by enabling the technician to adjust readings to evaluate smaller bones. Often, though, CHILDREN with chronic spinal conditions experience slower bone growth, so that potential variable must also be considered.

Outlook and Lifestyle Modifications

Within a few days, the primary physician will receive a report and consider DEXA data in conjunction with general observation, medical history, current symptoms, and results of other diagnostic tests. This information shapes suggestions for any changes to be made. For example, a reading slightly below normal may indicate a need to increase calcium intake or reassess any medications and supplements known to interfere with calcium absorption. The addition of WEIGHT-BEARING EXERCISE, such as walking or dancing, may be recommended to strengthen the spine. Other lifestyle modifications may include changes in daily ACTIVITY, NUTRITION, PAIN MANAGEMENT, the type of therapy, or medication, such as ANTIRESORPTIVE DRUGS. To allow newly initiated treatments time to take effect, a follow-up DEXA may be scheduled in one to two years. For growing children, new readings may be needed every six to 12 months.

Brigham and Women's Hospital. "Dual Energy X-ray Absorptiometry (DEXA or DXA)." Available online. URL: http://healthgate.partners.org/browsing/browse Content.asp?fileName=22174.xml&title=Dual%20 Energy%20X-ray%20Absorptiometry%20(DEXA%2 0or%20DXA) Downloaded October 1, 2005.

Fewtrell, M. S. "Bone Densitometry in Children Assessed by Dual X-ray Absorptiometry: Uses and Pitfalls," *Archives of Disease in Childhood* 88, no. 9 (September 2003): 795–799.

Johnson, Kate. "Do Careful Reading of DEXA Reports for BMD Assessment," *Family Practice News* 30, no. 8 (April 15, 2000): 33.

Reynolds, Jim. "Dual Energy X-Ray Absorptiometry/ Densitometry (DEXA)," Nuclear Medicine at NIH. Available online. URL: http://clinicalcenter.nih.gov/ imaging/nucmed/. Last modified October 1, 2005.

Staff. "Bone Densitometry," Patient Page, *Radiologic Technology* 73, no. 2 (November–December 2001): 200.

Trevino, Merlina. "Site Selection, Measurement Strategies Could Reduce Variability in Densitometry Readings— DXA Evaluation Moves toward Standardization," *Diagnostic Imaging* vol., no. NA (April 1, 2002): 12.

acetaminophen Sold under brand names, such as Tylenol and Liquiprin, or combined with other analgesics, as occurs in Excedrin and Percocet, acetaminophen reduces fever and peaks pain relief within an hour or two. True to advertising claims, this popular PAIN RELIEVER seldom affects the stomach as can ASPIRIN and other types of NONSTEROIDAL ANTI-INFLAMMATORY DRUG (NSAID) THERAPY. However, acetaminophen lacks the anti-inflammatory benefits of an NSAID, so the medication may not be as effective in easing ARTHRITIS or other inflammatory conditions that affect the back and spine.

In some situations, inflammation can be welcomed. For example, quick recovery from back SURGERY relies on natural inflammation to assist healing and aid BONE BUILDING. To keep from interfering with that normal healing process, an injectable form of acetaminophen can deliver high-speed relief directly into a pain site.

Dosage and Potential Side Effects
Even an infant can be given liquid drops of acetaminophen within the recommended dosage. For children, choices include chewable tablets and suppositories in smaller doses than the regular strength (325 mg) and extra strength (500 mg) tablets, caplets, or gel-caps available for adults. Each dosage must comply with the instructions on the label, because an excess can cause liver damage or even death. Alcohol consumption adds to the risk as does taking acetaminophen with other drugs or herbs known to affect the liver.

Unless a doctor prescribes otherwise, acetaminophen should not be used for back pain lasting longer than ten days. Rare side effects include lightheadedness and a rash, the latter of which may indicate a potentially serious allergic reaction requiring emergency medical attention. Regular users of acetaminophen may be more likely to aggravate or acquire a respiratory problem such as asthma. However, symptoms of nausea, sweating, or loss of consciousness indicate an overdose that can lead to liver failure and death unless emergency treatment begins within a few hours. If the presence of toxicity seems unclear or emergency facilities too far, the National Poison Control center offers advice on a toll-free hotline: 1-800-222-1212.

Statistics and Studies
According to the Food and Drug Administration (FDA), 100 deaths and 56,000 visits to the emergency room each year can be attributed to acetaminophen poisoning. To reduce the risk of liver failure, the FDA approved an injectable antidote,

Acetadote, to be administered within eight hours of overdose. N-acetylcysteine (NAC) also counteracts toxicity. Despite these emergency efforts, acetaminophen poisoning causes more deaths from overdose than any other drug in America, but then it is the most widely used drug in America too.

Often, OVER-THE-COUNTER PRODUCTS for children favor this pain reliever and fever reducer, which can be toxic at a single dose of 150 mg. Since young children metabolize acetaminophen at a higher rate than adults, parents should err on the side of caution. Unfortunately, parents and also adult patients sometimes ignore label instructions and warnings, expecting a higher dosage to work better or faster. They may be unaware, too, that approximately 600 other medicines, such as cough syrup, contain acetaminophen, thus increasing potential for an inadvertent overdose. People can also confuse the times and amounts of a dosage, especially when alternating acetaminophen with other pain relievers such as IBUPROFEN. Unless a physician prescribes a specific combination as a means of PAIN MANAGEMENT, various types of analgesics, including HERBAL THERAPY for pain, should not be combined or interchanged.

A.D.A.M., U.S. National Library of Medicine, NIH. "Acetaminophen Overdose," MedlinePlus. Available online. URL: http://www.nlm.nih.gov/medlineplus/ency/article/002598.htm. Updated on February 15, 2005.

MayoClinic.com. "Acetaminophen: Watch Dosage for Children," Mayo Clinic Medical Services. Available online. URL: http://www.mayoclinic.com/invoke.cfm?id=HO00002. Posted September 21, 2005.

Staff. "First Injectable Treatment for Acetaminophen Toxicity," *Consultant* 44, no. 4 (April 1, 2004): 531.

Staff. "New Rules for Pain Relief Guard Against Overuse of Acetaminophen," *Prevention* 54, no. 4 (April 2002): 54.

Staff. "Safer Drugs Reduce Need for Narcotics," *USA Today Magazine* 130, no. 2681 (February 2002): 10–11.

Tenenbein, Milton. "Acetaminophen: The 150 mg/kg Myth," *Journal of Toxicology: Clinical Toxicology* 42, no. 2 (March 2004): 145–149.

Tucker, Jeffrey, M. D. "Toxicity, Acetaminophen," eMedicine.com, inc. Available online. URL: http://www.emedicine.com/ped/topic7.htm. Last updated December 12, 2003.

ache   See BACKACHE; FIBROMYALGIA.

achondroplasia   See DWARFISM.

acromegaly   See GROWTH HORMONE DISORDERS.

activity, daily   Unlike the precise movements that usually accompany EXERCISE, an activity can be anything that gets a person up and moving. This motion may be less than a workout but more of an accomplishment as people retain their ability to remain mobile, maintain independence, and decrease the risks of a fall. Besides improving overall health, daily activity lowers the risk of a VERTEBRAL COMPRESSION FRACTURE due to OSTEOPOROSIS or other conditions involving bone loss in the SPINE.

Many decades divide CHILDREN from ELDERLY persons, but the heightened activity typical of childhood maximizes bone mass acquired at full growth and minimizes the bone loss that occurs during aging. One energetic hour each day for children and a half-hour for adults will be well-spent time on the spine. WEIGHT-BEARING EXERCISE can especially be bone-strengthening, but recreational activities have been proven more effective in reducing LOW BACK PAIN than exercises with that goal. Studies do not say why, but moving around and having fun apparently has an advantage.

Risks and Complications

The biggest risk in daily activity seems to be avoiding it. According to sources cited by the Centers for Disease Control and Prevention (CDC), common barriers to a physically active lifestyle include physiological, behavioral, and psychological influences that patients view as a personal deficit. Also, lack of time, energy, skill, companionship, motivation, resources, and good weather discourage sedentary people from enjoying activities, but just identifying a barrier can often bring a workable solution. Many people, for example, express fears about taking a walk in their own neighborhoods. However, an enclosed mall can be ideal for walking breezily beyond obstacles of unsafe surroundings or inclement weather. Indoor gyms, dance studios, multistoried buildings with stairs, and social events involving activities offer options too.

Statistics and Studies

More than half of the adults and one-third of the adolescents in America do less physical activities than needed to maintain optimal health. According to the American Academy of Orthopaedic Surgeons (AAOS), only one in four school-aged children spends the 35 to 60 minutes recommended for daily activity. Yet childhood offers the best opportunity for BONE BUILDING the bone mass that a person draws from throughout life.

In April 2004, researchers from the University of California, San Diego (UCSD) School of Medicine reported on their study of the effects of NUTRITION and exercise on 878 young people, ages 11 to 15. To record physical activity accurately, each student wore a measuring device continuously for one week. The device showed that boys and girls of normal weight spent only two to four minutes more per day in vigorous activity than did students who were overweight, but those small increments of energy made a discernible difference. By contrast, moderate increases in activity produced little change.

In June 2005, the President's Council on Physical Fitness and Sports reported that 33.4 percent of students in grades nine through 12 do not join in enough activities, particularly as their attendance in physical education (PE) classes steadily declines. In general, "non-Hispanic Black and Mexican American children were less likely to participate in vigorous physical activity than non-Hispanic Whites. Girls consistently tended to participate less in vigorous activities than boys. More troublesome is the fact that as girls get older there is a steady decline in physical activity; however, as boys get older the percent who participate in vigorous active pursuits increases." The report also said, "Environmental variables included perceived physical activity, behavior of parents and peers, access to sporting and/or fitness equipment at home, involvement in community physical activity organizations . . . and self-reported hours spent watching television or playing video games. Results showed that active African American boys exhibited higher levels of self-efficacy toward physical activity and reported

greater involvement in community-based, physical activity organizations than low-active boys. Active African American girls were more likely to have higher levels of self-efficacy and higher scores on beliefs regarding physical activity outcomes (e.g., keep me in shape, make me more attractive, be fun) than less active African American girls. Self-efficacy—the belief that a person possesses the ability to perform a particular behavior—is consistently an important predictor of physical activity in children and adults regardless of race."

Special Aids and Adaptations

Generally, studies of children rely on various types of devices to record movement, whereas adult participants often just fill out a questionnaire. However, Dixie Thompson, Director of the Center for Physical Activity and Health at the University of Tennessee, distributed pedometers to two groups of women between the ages of 33 and 55 to use four days a week while they walked a pet or took a ten-minute stroll during lunch break. Instructing one group to walk for a half-hour and the other to take a total of 10,000 steps throughout a day, Thompson discovered the 30-minute walkers took about 9,505 steps whereas the 10,000-step group averaged 11,775.

For most people, physical activity requires no measuring device or special equipment except a reasonably sound body and a mind set on moving it. However, excellent aids come through simple devices, such as a lawn mower, garden rake, vacuum cleaner, dust cloth, or broom. Many occupations offer an outlet for physical activity, too, as construction workers, maintenance staff, hospital personnel, cable installers, stay-at-home moms, and others get a hard workout by working hard. Prior to industrialization, employment often involved physical activity, and before the two-car garage, children typically walked or rode bicycles to school. Cultural changes discourage such activities now. However, parents, teachers, and other educators can help children to become more active by providing adequate PE classes, safe playground equipment, ample time for recess, and encouragement of intramural sports or before-and-after school activities.

Just being aware of the fun and benefits of physical activity helps too. In 2002, for example, the CDC launched a national, multiethnic VERB ™ campaign targeting youth aged nine to 13. Using successful marketing principles, the government agency widely advertised the advantages of healthy play. A year later, 74 percent of the nine- to 10-year-olds surveyed had heard of the program. Of those, 34 percent spent more of their free time in physical activity than did children who remained unaware of the ads. At this writing, ideas from VERB ™ can be found on http://www.verbnow.com, moving readers toward action as any good verb will do.

American Academy of Orthopaedic Surgeons (AAOS). "Kids Need To Get Up, Get Out and Get Moving," AAOS. Available online. URL: http://orthoinfo.aaos.org/fact/thr_report.cfm?Thread_ID=344&topcategory=Children. Downloaded October 26, 2005.

Bloomfield, Susan A. "Contributions of Physical Activity to Bone Health Over the Lifespan," *Topics in Geriatric Rehabilitation* 21, no. 1 (January–March 2005): 68–76.

CDC. "Physical Activity for Everyone: Making Physical Activity Part of Your Life: Overcoming Barriers to Physical Activity," Division of Nutrition and Physical Activity, National Center for Chronic Disease Prevention and Health Promotion. Available online. URL: http://www.cdc.gov/nccdphp/dnpa/physical/life/overcome.htm. Last reviewed September 28, 2005.

Crespo, Carlos J. "Physical Activity in Minority Populations: Overcoming a Public Health Challenge," President's Council on Physical Fitness and Sports, *Research Digest* 6, no. 2 (June 2005): 1–8.

Huhman, Marian, Lance D. Potter, Faye L. Wong, Stephen W. Banspach, Jennifer C. Duke, and Carrie D. Heitzler. "Effects of a Mass Media Campaign to Increase Physical Activity among Children: Year-1 Results of the VERB Campaign," *Pediatrics* 116, no. 2 (August 2005): 487–488.

Hurwitz, Eric L., Hal Morgenstern, and Chi Chiao. "Effects of Recreational Physical Activity and Back Exercises on Low Back Pain and Psychological Distress: Findings from the UCLA Low Back Pain Study," *The American Journal of Public Health* 95, no. 10 (October 2005): 1817–1824.

Potera, Carol. "30 Minutes or 10,000 Steps?" *Shape* 25, no. 1 (September 2005): 152–153.

acupressure   In using many of the same principles and paths as ACUPUNCTURE, this type of COMPLEMENTARY AND ALTERNATIVE MEDICINE involves no invasive technique. Instead a practitioner uses a thumb, finger, fingernail, and, sometimes, elbow to apply pressure to a very specific body site. In traditional Asian medicine, those sites may be referred to as meridian points or channels through which *qi* (energy) flows. If something blocks the energy, such symptoms as LOWER BACK PAIN, inflammation, muscle spasm, or tingling will occur. In Western medicine, similar symptoms suggest causes other than blocked *qi,* yet some people see acupressure as a beneficial means of releasing natural chemicals such as the endorphins a body produces in response to pain.

Procedure

Regardless of the underlying principle, acupressure usually involves a circular motion, a slight in-out push, or a combination of those two types of pressure for two to 10 seconds at a time. These sets of brief pressure followed by release may occur repeatedly for several minutes with a full session lasting up to an hour. Depending on the relevant meridian site, a patient may sit, fully clothed, or lie comfortably on a table, covered with a blanket or towel.

Although often confused with TRIGGER POINT THERAPY or other types of MASSAGE, acupressure is actually a form of acupuncture without needles. Both rely on precisely mapped meridians that may be far from the site of discomfort. For example, pressing a fingernail into the space between the upper lip and nose has been said to ease back pain. Nailing that spot with precision, though, may require more expertise.

Risks and Complications

Acupressure safely treats most people with BACKACHE and TENSION, but adverse effects can occur in patients with circulatory problems and high blood pressure. Also, acupressure should not be directly applied to lymph nodes, open wounds, bruises, areas of inflammation or swelling, scar tissue, weakened bones, or a bone FRACTURE. Pregnant women especially should avoid acupressure, as the treatment could cause a miscarriage.

After back surgery, acupressure may help to prevent complications. In 30 percent of all types of surgeries, postoperative nausea increases hospital time and the need for additional medication. For high-risk patients, numbers dramatically increase with up to 70 percent experiencing postoperative vomiting. However, researchers have found that acupressure of a specific meridian on the wrist may alleviate nausea. As Dr. Mary Hardy reported, "Most studies have used a specific point, pericardium 6 (P6), in therapeutic trials. The P6 point, also called the Nieguan point, is located on the flexor surface of the wrist, 4 cm proximal to the wrist crease between the palmaris longus and flexor carpii radialis tendons." At that site, "acupressure stimulation of the P6 point can be achieved either by direct pressure or by use of a special wrist band." Interestingly, an over-the-counter capsicum patch at the P6 site produced similar results with postoperative nausea "significantly lower . . . at 24 hours after surgery."

Outlook and Lifestyle Modifications

In China and other countries where this ancient medical art has been practiced for many thousands of years, people apply acupressure to themselves and their families as a form of PAIN MANAGEMENT or first aid. Even so, they seek help from a professional for persistent conditions such as CHRONIC BACK PAIN. Therefore, people with no experience do well to seek hands-on instruction from a trained practitioner and obtain carefully devised charts to locate specific meridians. For example, pressing the Sea of Energy located two finger-widths below the navel will reportedly alleviate a lower back problem, assuming, of course, one knows just where to press.

Hardy, Mary L., M.D. "Giving a Helping Hand to Postoperative Nausea and Vomiting," *Alternative Therapies in Women's Health* 5, no. 10 (October 2003): 78–80.

Spinasanta, Susan. "Acupressure: A Safe, Alternate Therapy," SpineUniverse. Available online. URL: http://www.spineuniverse.com/displayarticle.php/article785.html. Downloaded October 27, 2005.

WholeHealthMD. "acupressure." Available online. URL: http://www.wholehealthmd.com/refshelf/substances_view/1,1525,662,00.html. Downloaded October 27, 2005.

acupuncture Thousands of years ago, Chinese medicine developed techniques to accommodate the body's natural flow of energy or *qi* (pronounced *chee.*) Gradually, practitioners of ACUPRESSURE identified and recorded many hundreds of sites that responded to a fingernail or other small instrument rubbed in a circular motion or pressed quickly and released. At some point, acupuncturists inserted needles into these meridian pathways or channels as a stronger means of stimulating an area, freeing *qi,* and restoring energy to the body.

Procedure

To treat back problems and other conditions, an acupuncturist commonly uses six to nine needles but may go up to 20. Each needle slants toward the appropriate meridian at a 15- to 90-degree angle to the skin. As the thin instrument penetrates a depth of ½ to two inches, a sensation will be felt but should be painless. Immediately, the acupuncturist moves the needle, using one of several techniques, such as raising and thrusting, twirling and rotating, trembling (vibrating), or a combination of these and similar movements.

Depending on the condition, acupuncture may include other therapeutic options, such as the use of HEAT THERAPY to alleviate the pain of ARTHRITIS. For LOWER BACK PAIN caused by an underlying medical condition, acupressure releases energy into the affected organ. However, a BACKACHE or back SPRAIN may be treated with cupping, a procedure that relies on suction to stimulate an appropriate site.

Risks and Complications

Acupuncturists must follow the same safety standards and biohazard regulations as other medical professionals in the United States, so practitioners may opt for disposable needles to eliminate the risk of infection. Since gold needles remain a favorite, the risk of contamination depends on how well those reusable needles have been sterilized.

Another common concern involves needle placement. The choice of meridian sites can vary from one practitioner to another, even if they treat the same type of pain or backache. Questions also arise as to the size of a chosen site, which, by standards in Japanese acupuncture, may be quite small. Other acupuncturists, however, see each site as encompassing a few inches of workable space, which leaves more room for error.

Outlook and Lifestyle Modifications

Western medical sciences usually prefer results that can be predicted, verified, and reproduced. In the West, then, researchers attempt to redefine ancient understandings of *qi* energy in current terms. For instance, they might use ULTRASOUND or imaging devices to see if nerve pathways and connective points correspond to long-established meridians. New applications of old methods may be investigated too. For example, some patients cannot be given an EPIDURAL INJECTION for anesthesia prior to SURGERY for a HERNIATED DISC. In such cases, acupuncture provides an old option in a new setting with the added potential of subsequent PAIN MANAGEMENT. New applications of acupuncture principles also include such developments as the use of wrist bands to treat postoperative nausea by stimulating an established meridian site.

Most Americans consider acupuncture a form of COMPLEMENTARY AND ALTERNATIVE MEDICINE rather than primary care. Nevertheless, primary care physicians, chiropractors, osteopaths, and surgeons occasionally add acupuncture to their regular medical procedures. In an article discussing the phenomenon of doctors' combining ancient arts with current practices, Stephen J. Kaufman wrote, "Instead of mystical, vague and energetic theories, they have focused on pragmatic, results-oriented techniques. This has resulted in new styles of acupuncture that are much simpler, scientifically defensible, and highly effective. They are also practically painless." In his own practice as a chiropractic physician and acupuncturist, Kaufman has developed techniques, such as Eight Needle acupuncture which reportedly gives "superlative results in any musculoskeletal disorder. . . ." In assessing the possibilities, Kaufman summarized, "Benefits of this 21st century acupuncture include more rapid results, shorter treatment times, a higher degree of effectiveness, much greater patient comfort and acceptance, and a greater ability to scientifically apply treatment."

Jedeikin, Robert, Brian Fredman, Bernardo Goldstein, M.D., Edna Zohar, M.D., Tuvia Scott, et al. "The Efficacy of Acupuncture Analgesia versus Epidural Steroids in the Treatment of Acute Low Back Pain," *Anesthesiology* 95 (2001): A951. Available online. URL: http://www.asaabstracts.com/strands/asaabstracts/abstract.htm;jsessionid=6756415C0ED0F91FE36A01702AA81ACB?year=2001&index=11&absnum=256. Downloaded on October 28, 2005.

Kaufman, Stephen J. "Trigger Point Acupuncture and Sports Injuries—Exciting New Developments!" *Townsend Letter for Doctors and Patients* (July 2003) 68–70.

Singer, Jeffrey A. "Acupuncture, A Brief Introduction," Acupuncture.com. Available online. URL: http://www.acupuncture.com/education/theory/acuintro.htm. Downloaded October 28, 2005.

acute back pain   The primary distinction between CHRONIC BACK PAIN and acute back pain does not refer to intensity but to time. While chronic pain persists three months or more, acute back pain typically resolves itself within a few weeks. An ongoing condition, such as ARTHRITIS, may produce sudden flare-ups for a day or two, but if the back pain does not improve in 72 hours, professional treatment may help. The presence of additional symptoms, such as fever, abdominal pain, nausea, numbness in the limbs, or a sharp rise in pain, indicates an immediate need for medical attention.

Symptoms and Diagnostic Path

Although most cases of acute back pain come on quickly, the type of pain reflects the probable cause. For instance, stabbing or burning pain typically indicates spinal nerve involvement, whereas dull pain or pressure often results from an injury, such as a back SPRAIN or associated muscle STRAIN. Mechanical back pain from a HERNIATED DISC or a VERTEBRAL COMPRESSION FRACTURE will worsen with coughing, sneezing, or moving around, but a fever suggests a SPINAL INFECTION or other underlying medical condition, such as a SPINAL TUMOR. When SCIATICA produces sudden back pain, radiating pain may affect the legs and lower body, but SPINAL STENOSIS may cause numbness or tingling of the limbs.

An accurate description of symptoms aids a diagnosis as does a medical history. The physician also needs to know about recent activities, mishaps, and changes in diet, routines, or medication. A physical examination may include evaluating POSTURE and RANGE OF MOTION as the doctor instructs the patient to sit, stand, walk, or move in a particular manner. If the findings or additional symptoms suggest an underlying medical condition or neurological involvement, the physician will prescribe an X-RAY or other imaging tests, such as COMPUTED TOMOGRAPHY (CT) SCAN or MAGNETIC RESONANCE IMAGING (MRI). Blood tests may also be needed.

Treatment Options and Outlook

On rare occasions, acute back pain may reveal a serious medical problem such as CAUDA EQUINA SYNDROME. That medical emergency needs to be evaluated by a neurologist or orthopedic surgeon as soon as possible. If chronic leg pain equals or exceeds the back pain, SURGERY may be needed.

Since most cases of acute back pain are temporary, conservative treatments will be used. For example, discomfort may be alleviated with PAIN RELIEVERS, such as NONSTEROIDAL ANTI-INFLAMMATORY DRUG (NSAID) THERAPY or ACETAMINOPHEN. If inflammation increases the discomfort of an injury, COLD THERAPY or ice packs applied for 20 minutes at a time can help to reduce swelling. For various types of back pain, COMPLEMENTARY AND ALTERNATIVE MEDICINE treatments may include ACUPRESSURE, ACUPUNCTURE, MASSAGE THERAPY, or SPINAL MANIPULATION.

If the patient experiences relief when lying flat on the back, bed rest may be prescribed for a day or two. Too much bed rest, however, can be counterproductive as circulation slows and muscles weaken from lack of use. Therefore, doctors often recommend curtailing activities or resting the site of pain while exercising unaffected areas of the body.

With or without treatment, 90 percent of the instances of acute back pain resolve in four to six weeks. About half of the patients, however, need to make changes in their lifestyles to keep back pain from coming back or becoming chronic.

Risk Factors and Preventive Measures

According to the National Institute of Neurological Disorders and Stroke (NINDS), acute back pain can often be prevented. "Engaging in exercises that don't jolt or strain the back, maintaining correct posture, and lifting objects properly can help prevent injuries. Many work-related injuries are caused or aggravated by stressors such as heavy lifting, vibration, repetitive motion, and awkward posture. Applying ergonomic principles—designing furniture and tools to protect the body from injury—at home and in the workplace can greatly reduce the risk of back injury and help maintain a healthy back."

Besides ERGONOMIC FACTORS, posture, and proper LIFTING, people of all ages and body types can help their backs by building PARASPINAL MUSCLES with appropriate EXERCISE. Usually, though, sit-ups, toe-touches, back-arches, and hip-twists should be avoided, since those movements often aggravate vertebral pain and inflammation. A primary care physician or therapist can recommend specific exercises for an individual, but most people benefit from noncontact sports or activities. For instance, swimming, walking, dancing, skiing, or biking can add strength to back muscles, enjoyment to life, and greater ease to those episodes of pain.

Atlas, Steven J., M.D. and Richard A. Deyo, M.D. "Evaluating and Managing Acute Low Back Pain in the Primary Care Setting," *Journal of General Intern Medicine* 16, no. 2 (February 2001): 120–131.

Medtronic Sofamar Danek. "Symptoms: Pain," Back.com. Available online. URL: http://www.back.com/symptoms-pain.html. Updated March 7, 2005.

National Institute of Neurological Disorders and Stroke (NINDS). "NINDS Back Pain and Information Page," NINDS, National Institutes of Health. Available online. URL: http://www.ninds.nih.gov/disorders/backpain/backpain.htm. Last updated October 13, 2005.

Patel, A. T., M.D. and A. A. Ogle, M.D. "Diagnosis and Management of Acute Low Back Pain," *American Family Physician* 62, no. 11 (December 1, 2000): 2,414–2,415.

Patient UK. "Acute Back Pain in Adults—A Summary." Available online. URL: http://www.patient.co.uk/showdoc/23069182/. Updated April 2005.

University of Michigan Health System (UMHS). "Acute Low Back Pain: Patient Education Handout Associated with UMHS Clinical Care Guideline." Available online. URL: http://www.med.umich.edu/1libr/guides/lowback.htm. Downloaded October 31, 2005.

adhesive arachnoiditis   See ARACHNOIDITIS.

adolescent scoliosis   See IDIOPATHIC SCOLIOSIS.

adolescents, spinal concerns for   CHILDREN and teenagers have remarkable resiliency that often protects them from back problems. Therefore, even the smallest complaint of a BACKACHE or wince of ACUTE BACK PAIN warrants investigation of the symptoms and also of the child's habits. For example, an ATHLETE who hopes for a scholarship may become aggressive in sports, whereas an academically inclined teen may bend over books too long, developing a problem with POSTURE. Other factors, such as BACKPACK SAFETY or the effects of WEIGHT on the SPINE, also bear consideration, as does a family's medical history. For example, GENETIC FACTORS may reveal an underlying medical condition, such as early onset scoliosis (IDIOPATHIC SCOLIOSIS), that affects growing VERTEBRAE.

For most teens, proper growth and bone strength depend on well-balanced NUTRITION, including CALCIUM from dairy products and natural food sources. For youth nine to 18, the recommended daily intake is 1,300 mg. Yet, right when the need for calcium increases during active spurts of growth, consumption often falls to a precarious low. Right when teenagers need more ACTIVITY, daily participation in sports and other events frequently declines. If adolescents perceive themselves as nonathletic, unpopular, or overweight, the poor choices that affect future SPINE health may become more likely.

Risks and Complications

After surveying 4,100 adolescents, researchers from the University of Minnesota found that almost one-third of the boys and over one-half of the girls relied on "unhealthy tactics for dropping unwanted pounds." As reported in *Prevention*, "To lose weight, the teens skipped meals, smoked, used laxatives, and induced vomiting. The girls also ate fewer fruits, vegetables, and whole-wheat grains and took in fewer vitamins and minerals when compared with those who didn't diet or used only healthy means, such as exercise and smart eating. Surprisingly, dieting boys ate more fruit than their peers." That last

clue gives parents cause for pause. Uncharacteristic dietary habits may suggest EATING DISORDERS with far-reaching effects, such as the bone loss resulting in OSTEOPENIA or OSTEOPOROSIS. If parents observe sudden changes in an adolescent's eating habits or other behavioral patterns, though, they can seek professional advice with greater speed.

Statistics and Studies

According to the Centers for Disease Control and Prevention (CDC), only 15 percent of adolescent girls in the United States get enough calcium each day but exceed the healthy limit for saturated fat. Such dietary habits adversely affect the back since growing bones lack the calcium needed for strength, while the increased body weight caused by a fatty diet puts undue stress on the vertebrae. As the CDC said, "Most young people are not following the recommendations set forth in the Dietary Guidelines for Americans: of U.S. youth aged 6–19, 67% exceed dietary guideline recommendations for fat intake, 72% exceed recommendations for saturated fat intake. In 2003, only 22% of high school students reported eating the recommended five daily servings of fruits and vegetables (when fried potatoes and potato chips are excluded) during the past 7 days."

Besides this lack of nutrition, many adolescents lack adequate EXERCISE. In a report on the physical activity of youth, the CDC warned, "In 2003, more than one-third of high school students did not regularly engage in vigorous physical activity and only 28% of high school students attended physical education class daily. Participation in physical activity declines strikingly as children age."

With the same phenomenon occurring in other countries, researchers in Sweden investigated common factors affecting the level of physical activity among 16-year-olds. In studying students of both sexes, researchers noted lower levels of activity among adolescents with fewer socio-economic advantages, less parental support, and lower perceptions of their own health. Additionally, inactive students expressed negative attitudes toward physical activities. As the study also pointed out, these findings suggest the importance of developing positive school-based programs.

The CDC would likely applaud such efforts. As stated in their "Physical Activity" report, "Regular physical activity in childhood and adolescence improves strength and endurance, helps build healthy bones and muscles, helps control weight, reduces anxiety and stress, increases self-esteem, and may improve blood pressure and cholesterol levels. Positive experiences with physical activity at a young age help lay the basis for being regularly active throughout life."

Special Aids and Adaptations

Many adolescents remain unaware of the effects their present physical activities and dietary choices have on long-term bone health. However, information may be only a mobile phone call away. In an effort to inform youth in the United Kingdom about health options and preventive care, registered nurse Sharon Utting wrote of "a text messaging service where young people could text their question and get a reply within a week from a nurse. This would provide anonymity, be confidential and be accessible," particularly since 94 percent of the teens surveyed had access to a mobile phone.

Providing adolescents with information, answers, and opportunities may involve innovative adaptations on the part of parents and educators, but taking a new tack can help spinal health too. For example, researchers in Australia followed 79 high school students into adulthood, conducting over 500 interviews with a goal of understanding "the place and meaning of health and physical activity in young people's lives." By using this sociological approach, researchers found that commitment to physical activity did not "fit with the unpredictable times of casual and part-time work, nor the evening and weekend work that must be fitted around study. In addition, long hours of work often leave the participants exhausted with little energy for 'purposive activity,' casual or organised." As adolescents entered their twenties, some returned to sports. In general though, researchers concluded, "Strategies to attempt to increase the physical activity of this group at this point in time, particularly when that physical activity is understood as an additional component of their lives, may be irrelevant and misdirected." In other words, the physical and emotional stress of studying and/or earning an income often keep young people from getting the exercise they need for spinal health. There-

fore, workable solutions to these concerns remain a highly individualized matter.

Centers for Disease Control and Prevention (CDC). "Nutrition," Healthy Youth! National Center for Chronic Disease Prevention and Health Promotion. Available online. URL: http://www.cdc.gov/Healthy Youth/nutrition/index.htm. Last reviewed October 12, 2005.

Centers for Disease Control and Prevention (CDC). "Physical Activity," Healthy Youth! National Center for Chronic Disease Prevention and Health Promotion. Available online. URL: http://www.cdc.gov/HealthyYouth/physicalactivity/index.htm. Last reviewed October 12, 2005.

Spine-health.com. "Back Pain in Kids and Teens." Available online. URL: http://www.spine-health.com/topics/cd/kids/kids01.html. Downloaded November 1, 2005.

Staff. "Hazards of Kids' Diets," *Prevention* 56, no. 12 (December 2004): 36.

Utting, Sharon. "How Teenagers Got the Health Message: Sharon Utting Gives a Personal Account How Health Text-in, a Text Messaging Service for Teenagers, Has Drastically Improved Response Rates from the Young," *Primary Health Care* 14, no. 2 (March 2004): 12–15.

Westerstahl, M., M. Barnekow-Bergkvist, and E. Jansson. "Low Physical Activity among Adolescents in Practical Education," *Scandinavian Journal of Medicine & Science in Sports* 15, no. 5 (October 2005): 287–298.

Wright, Jan, Doune Macdonald, Johanna Wyn, and Lynda Kriflik. "Becoming Somebody: Changing Priorities and Physical Activity," *Young Studies Australia* 24, no. 1 (March 2005): 16–21.

aging vertebrae See ELDERLY, SPINAL CONCERNS OF THE.

alendronate A type of BISPHOSPHONATE, this ANTIRESORPTIVE DRUG works in conjunction with the body's natural bone remodeling cycle. Normally, osteoblasts lay down new cells, and osteoclasts remove old ones, but imbalances in that arrangement can cause such conditions as OSTEOPOROSIS and OSTEOGENESIS IMPERFECTA (brittle bone disease) that weaken VERTEBRAE and other bones. To restrain osteoclasts from removing cells that can still be useful, an antiresorptive drug may be prescribed.

Dosage and Potential Side Effects

Available in generic form and under various brand names, alendronate may best be known as Fosamax. This may be prescribed as 10 mg tablets taken daily or a 70 mg dosage taken weekly, but taking alendronate any time can be tricky. Unlike many medications, a bisphosphonate should *not* be ingested with food but must be quickly swallowed and immediately washed down with a full glass of water first thing in the morning. No other beverages, no food, and no other medication, including herbs and vitamins, can be consumed for at least 30 minutes. The person must remain upright for that half hour too. If sitting and swallowing prove too difficult, bisphosphonates must be avoided since damage to the esophagus or other soft tissue will be likely to occur.

Other potential side effects include headache, muscle ache, and stomachache, which, reportedly, are mild. For most people, alendronate provides a safe means of strengthening bones. However, safety has not yet been established for CHILDREN or pregnant women, perhaps because of the conflict between this drug and the CALCIUM required by changing bodies and bones. Since decreases in calcium and phosphate can occur with the use of alendronate, natural food sources or supplements may be needed.

Statistics and Studies

CLINICAL TRIALS of people with osteoporosis indicate that alendronate alone can increase bone density about 50 percent in the SPINE. In addition, two articles in the August 11, 2005 issue of *The New England Journal of Medicine* (NEJM) discussed the effectiveness of alendronate in conjunction with PARATHYROID HORMONE (PTH). In the first report, PTH had been given for one year to increase calcium absorption. Since PTH can be prescribed for only two years, researchers wanted to see how effective alendronate would be in maintaining the improvements PTH had made in the bone density of patients with osteoporosis. During the second year, PTH treatment continued with a placebo added for one group and alendronate for the other. Subsequent BONE MINERAL DENSITY (BMD) TESTS showed that spinal bone strength had been maintained and even increased with the addition of alendronate but had substantially decreased in the placebo group.

In the second NEJM article, 126 women with osteoporosis had taken alendronate for a year or longer. One group received a daily addition of PTH while another took PTH in cycles of three months. In the cyclical group, BMD levels dropped slightly during the three months without PTH, but in both groups, bone density increased in the spine.

Black, Dennis M., John P. Bilezikian, M.D., Kristine E. Ensrud, M. D., Susan L. Greenspan, M.D., Lisa Palermo, Trisha Hue, Thomas F. Lang, Joan A. McGowan, and Clifford J. Rosen, M.D., for the PaTH Study Investigators. "One Year of Alendronate after One Year of Parathyroid Hormone (1-84) for Osteoporosis," *The New England Journal of Medicine* 353, no. 6 (August 11, 2005): 555–565.

Cosman, Felicia, M.D., Jeri Nieves, Marsha Zion, Lillian Woelfert, Marjorie Luckey, M.D., and Robert Lindsay, M.D. "Daily and Cyclic Parathyroid Hormone in Women Receiving Alendronate," *The New England Journal of Medicine* 353, no. 6 (August 11, 2005): 566–575.

MedicineNet.com. "Alendronate," Written by Pharmacists, Reviewed by Doctors. Available online. URL: http://www.medicinenet.com/alendronate/article.htm. Downloaded November 2, 2005.

allograft bone graft   See BONE GRAFT.

alternative medicine   See COMPLEMENTARY AND ALTERNATIVE MEDICINE (CAM).

anabolic therapy   See PARATHYROID HORMONE (PTH).

anaerobic spondylodiscitis   See SPINAL INFECTION.

analgesic   See PAIN RELIEVERS.

ankylosing spondylitis Also known as Marie-Strumpell disease and rheumatoid spondylitis, this rheumatic disease gives a person a bent look as extreme inflammation and ARTHRITIS fuse together spinal VERTEBRAE.

Symptoms and Diagnostic Path

Besides symptoms of rigidity and inflammation in the SPINE, ankylosing spondylitis (AS) causes morning stiffness and evening PAIN. Mild to severe discomfort in the lower back and SACROILIAC JOINT often eases with activity, but the vertebrae may become dramatically less flexible, limiting RANGE OF MOTION. Also, ankylosed or fused joints in the mid and upper back can keep the chest from expanding enough for the person to take in deep breaths.

As a member of the spondyloarthropathy family, AS shares the genetic marker HLA-B27, which can be detected by blood testing. However, approximately 80 percent of the children who inherit this GENETIC FACTOR will not develop AS. Besides a medical history and physical examination, X-RAY may confirm a diagnosis. Also, imaging tools, such as COMPUTED TOMOGRAPHY or MAGNETIC RESONANCE IMAGING, may be used to establish a baseline. With that information, a rheumatologist or other physician can note the progression of the disease and any changes that occur in the back, such as spontaneous spinal fusion.

Treatment Options and Outlook

With no known cure, AS treatments primarily aim to alleviate symptoms. For example, NONSTEROIDAL ANTI-INFLAMMATORY DRUG (NSAID) THERAPY or other medications may keep inflammation and pain under control, or a CORTICOSTEROID INJECTION may be given. A rheumatologist or primary physician may also recommend STRENGTH TRAINING or a therapeutic EXERCISE, such as swimming, to assist POSTURE and build up PARASPINAL MUSCLES.

As the disease progresses, inflammation can affect the eyes and internal organs. For ankylosed joints or other spinal deformities, SURGERY may help to ease pain, improve range of motion, and restore mobility. AS patients might also want to consider participating in government-sponsored studies, such as those posted at http://www.ClinicalTrials.gov.

Risk Factors and Preventive Measures

In the United States, an estimated 129 of 100,000 people have AS. Highest risks occur for Caucasian and Native American men, ages 17 to 35. People with an HLA-B27 genetic marker or a family history of AS encounter a higher risk too. Since a specific cause has not yet been identified, preventive measures have not been established. However, early diagnosis and prompt treatment can delay and, in some cases, prevent spinal deformities or other complications from arising.

Although physical activity will not cure AS, specific exercises help to manage the symptoms. For example, before getting out of bed, the person lies flat on the back with knees bent and feet on the mattress. The hips are then raised as high as possible without straining the CERVICAL SPINE. After holding that position for about five seconds, the person slowly lowers his or her hips back onto the bed for a few more seconds then repeats the exercise for a total of five sets. Turning over, the person kneels on hands and knees, keeping the arms straight, the head tucked, and the back arched like a stretching cat. Then, reversing the position, the head goes up as the back dips into a hollow. After the person gets up, a warm-up of light stretches with the body kept straight, the chin tucked in, and the arms raised straight overhead, one at a time, may ease morning stiffness and aid posture too.

American College of Rheumatology. "Ankylosing Spondylitis," Fact Sheet. Available online. URL: http://www.rheumatology.org/public/factsheets/as.asp?aud=pat. Downloaded November 3, 2005.

ClinicalTrials.gov. "Spondylitis, Ankylosing," National Institutes of Health information about ongoing AS-related trials still recruiting patients. Available online. URL: http://clinicaltrials.gov/ct/gui/action/FindCondition?ui=D013167&recruiting=true.

Genetics Home Reference. "Ankylosing Spondylitis," U.S. National Library of Medicine. Available online. URL: http://ghr.nlm.nih.gov/condition=ankylosingspondylitis. Published October 28, 2005.

Holy Cross Hospital. "Diseases, Conditions and Injuries: Ankylosing Spondylitis (Marie-Strumpell Disease)," EBSCO Publishing consumer health and medical information. Available online. URL: http://healthychoice.epnet.com/GetContent.asp?siteid=holycross&docid=/

dci/ankylosingspondylitis. Downloaded November 3, 2005.

MayoClinic.com. "Ankylosing Spondylitis," Mayo Clinic Health Information. Available online. URL: http://www.mayoclinic.com/health/ankylosing-spondylitis/DS00483. Updated June 3, 2004.

National Ankylosing Spondylitis Society (NASS). "Useful Exercises." Available online. URL: http://www.nass.co.uk/exercises.htm. Downloaded November 3, 2005.

Spondylitis Association of America (SAA). "Ankylosing Spondylitis (AS)," SAA overview. Available online. URL: http://www.spondylitis.org/About/as.aspx. Downloaded November 3, 2005.

anorexia See EATING DISORDERS, BONE LOSS CAUSED BY.

anterior cervical discectomy As the name indicates, this surgical procedure enters the front of the neck. A DISCECTOMY in the CERVICAL SPINE may then be used to remove a HERNIATED DISC damaged by a SPINAL INJURY or caused by DEGENERATIVE DISC DISEASE. With the rupture of one or more discs, the VERTEBRAE lose the protective cushion between the neck bones, which, in turn, causes inflammation and sometimes bony overgrowth. In addition, a ruptured DISC can press the spinal nerves, generating neck pain. Or arms may feel numb, and fingers may tingle. Similar symptoms can also occur if an OSTEOPHYTE pushes on nerves of the SPINE, so the same surgical procedure may be used to eliminate that bone spur.

Procedure

As the sedated patient lies flat on the back, the surgeon makes an incision toward the front of the neck, slightly to one side to avoid the larynx and esophagus. After soft tissue has been drawn aside, the disc and any bony overgrowth can be removed to relieve nerve compression. If the cervical spine needs stabilization, a small metal plate or other type of implant may be inserted through the surgical opening. To restore or maintain vertebral height, a BONE GRAFT may be needed too. If so, a tiny piece of bone will usually be obtained from the patient's hip, which requires another small incision.

Risks and Complications

As with any SURGERY, complications of a blood clot, infection, damage to surrounding areas, or an adverse reaction to medication can occur. Occasionally, a discectomy causes swelling in neck tissue, which then presses against the windpipe and hinders breathing. If this happens, steroids may be given through an IV before the patient can be discharged from the hospital. Additional surgery may be required if the bone graft or implant shifts, but that slippage may not be apparent until the patient returns to normal daily ACTIVITY. For 99 percent of patients, however, no complications occur.

Outlook and Lifestyle Modifications

After a cervical discectomy, patients may be hoarse but still be up and walking around by evening. Difficulty in swallowing can prolong a hospital stay, but most people go home in a day or two. General activities must be curtailed for about two weeks with a cervical collar often prescribed to support the neck and restrict cervical movement.

Restricting movement gives the graft time to produce natural fusion and rebuild bone at the surgical site. That healing can be hindered, however, by such adverse factors as poor NUTRITION, poor POSTURE, nicotine usage, or too much WEIGHT. Besides addressing those issues, lifestyle modifications often include an appropriate course of therapy or EXERCISE to stretch and strengthen the neck. For most patients, cervical pain subsides noticeably after surgery with a full recovery expected in two months or less.

Mayfield Clinic. "Anterior Cervical Discectomy and Fusion," reviewed by Robert Bohinski, M.D. , The Neuroscience Institute at University Hospital in Cincinnati, Ohio. Available online. URL: http://www.mayfieldclinic.com/PE-ACDF.htm. Downloaded November 5, 2005.

Medtronic Sofamor Danek. "Surgical: Anterior Cervical Discectomy with Fusion," NeckSurgery.com. Available online. URL: http://www.neckreference.com/treatment-surgical-fusion.html. Downloaded November 5, 2005.

NeuroSurgery InfoNet. "Risks and Complications: Cervical Discectomy Anterior." Available online. URL: http://uscneurosurgery.com/infonet/surgery/understand/risks/procedure/ACD.htm. Downloaded November 5, 2005.

Zigler, Jack, M.D. "Patient Information Sheet on Cervical Fusion Materials," Cervical Spine Research Society. Available online. URL: http://www.csrs.org/patientinfo/cervicalfusion.htm. Downloaded November 5, 2005.

anti-inflammatory medication See NONSTEROIDAL ANTI-INFLAMMATORY DRUG (NSAID) THERAPY.

antiresorptive drugs This category of drugs includes BISPHOSPHONATES, CALCITONIN, estrogen, and SELECTIVE ESTROGEN RECEPTOR MODULATORS, which may be used alone, in various combinations, or with PARATHYROID HORMONE (PTH). Whether testosterone also functions well as an antiresorptive has yet to be adequately studied.

In the natural process of bone remodeling, osteoclasts release bone cells for resorption into the body, making a place for osteoblasts to stimulate new formation. That growth accelerates in childhood and dwindles in later years, but for most of an adult's life, bone resorption and formation stay in fairly even balance. If, however, new cells mineralize faster than the old ones can be removed, conditions of bone overgrowth, such as OSTEOPETROSIS, can occur. Conversely, normal aging and common disorders, such as OSTEOPENIA and OSTEOPOROSIS, increase the bone deficit by releasing old cells faster than new ones arrive. To retain old cells, particularly in ELDERLY patients or those at risk for a VERTEBRAL COMPRESSION FRACTURE, an antiresorptive drug may be prescribed to slow the loss of bone density.

Dosage and Potential Side Effects

Each antiresorptive has a similar goal, yet each affects patients differently. For example, HORMONE REPLACEMENT THERAPY can help to prevent bone loss with little risk of side effects in younger women who have had a hysterectomy or gone through early menopause. Patients at risk for FRACTURE may be especially helped by a combination of estrogen and another antiresorptive drug. However, effectiveness often declines and side effects increase if estrogen is taken long-term or begun well after menopause. Estrogen may also be contraindicated for women at risk for breast tumors since hormonal

treatments increase those risks. In addition, some women just cannot tolerate estrogen.

As another option, a bisphosphonate may be prescribed to slow bone loss and decrease fracture risks. With various choices available, this type of drug can also be prescribed for CHILDREN, ADOLESCENTS, and men. For proper absorption, a bisphosphonate must be taken on an empty stomach, but this can be hard to stomach for sensitive children or people with digestive problems. The drug can irritate the esophagus too, especially if directions from the pharmacist have not been meticulously followed.

For women, selective estrogen receptor modulators (SERMs) provide another choice. Although estrogen and bisphosphonates have a stronger effect on bone, SERMs have fewer side effects. Calcitonin has even fewer but usually offers a less effective treatment. Nevertheless, this naturally occurring hormone has been prescribed for years to prevent and treat osteoporosis.

As a relatively gentle choice, calcitonin regulates calcium and bone metabolism in the body. Since the substance is also a type of digestible protein, calcitonin must not be taken orally, mainly because digestion would begin before the medication has time to work. Instead, typical treatment comes through a daily skin injection of 50–100 IU or a nasal spray of 200 IU, either of which can irritate the soft tissue surrounding a site. Reportedly though, both the spray and the injection reduce the risk of vertebral fracture.

Coupled with bone-building CALCIUM, VITAMIN D, and EXERCISE, calcitonin and other antiresorptive drugs labor against bone loss. However, a newer drug, STRONTIUM RANELATE, can be employed for both tasks of bone remodeling. The first such prospect to meet the approval of the Food and Drug Administration (FDA), this compound works to decrease bone resorption while stimulating formation of new bone.

Statistics and Studies

An editorial in *The Journal of Clinical Endocrinology & Metabolism* discussed the use of the bisphosphonate ALENDRONATE with the SERM raloxifene. According to the article, "the combined use of these two drugs is associated with increased bone density and lower bone turnover markers than one can achieve with either drug alone." The editorial went on to state, "It remains to be seen whether any of the combination antiresorptive approaches will be associated with reductions in fracture incidence that are greater than what can be achieved with monotherapy." Besides that still-open question and the cost of added medication, "a second potential disadvantage to combination antiresorptive therapy is that bone turnover could be reduced to levels that adversely affect skeletal mineralization. Under usual therapeutic circumstances, the percentage of bone that is mineralized . . . is increased when bone turnover is reduced," which, potentially, "causes bones to become more and more brittle."

What happens in one patient may not occur in another. An article in *The Journal of Bone and Mineral Research* pointed out, "In clinical trials, patients enrolled typically are not a homogenous population and have different baseline characteristics." However, "when conducting meta-analysis using summary statistics, all patients from the same treatment group within a study are treated exactly the same. As a consequence, the information from each individual patient is not fully or accurately used in the analysis." For example, "several studies have indicated that the short-term decrease of bone turnover markers, especially those of resorption, is significantly associated with the subsequent risk of vertebral and nonvertebral fractures in patients treated with antiresorptive drugs. As pointed out recently, the mechanisms by which these therapies reduce skeletal fragility are probably more complex than initially thought. They induce a marginal increase in bone mass, which is overestimated by the apparent increase in BMD."

Questions about bone mineral density (BMD) and bone quality continue to arise. In an article for *Mayo Clinic Proceedings*, Dr. Solomon Epstein of Mount Sinai School of Medicine in New York wrote, "Properties related to bone strength include rate of bone turnover, bone mineral density, . . . microarchitecture, and . . . mineralization. These properties (with or without bone density) are sometimes collectively referred to as bone quality. Antiresorptive agents may reduce fracture risk by several separate but interrelated effects on these individual properties. For example, antiresorptive agents have been

reported to reduce bone turnover, stabilize or increase bone density, . . . reduce the number or size of resorption sites, and improve mineralization." As Dr. Epstein summarized, "Reductions in fracture risk are the most convincing evidence of good bone quality. Data from well-designed randomized clinical trials with up to 10 years of continuous antiresorptive therapy have shown that certain antiresorptive agents effectively reduce fracture risk and (together with extensive preclinical data) suggest no deleterious effects on bone quality."

AMA. "Treatment of Osteoporosis in Men," American Medical Association. Available online. URL: http://www.ama-cmeonline.com/osteo_mgmt/module07/06trea/04.htm#. Downloaded November 8, 2005.

Delmas, P.D., Li Zhengqing, and Cyrus Cooper. "Relationship Between Changes in Bone Mineral Density and Fracture Risk Reduction With Antiresorptive Drugs: Some Issues With Meta-Analysis," *The Journal of Bone and Mineral Research* 19, no. 2 (February 2004): 330–337.

Epstein, Solomon, M.D. "The Roles of Bone Mineral Density, Bone Turnover, and Other Properties in Reducing Fracture Risk During Antiresorptive Therapy," *Mayo Clinic Proceedings* 80, no. 3 (March 2005): 379–388.

Ettinger, Bruce and John P. Bilezikian. "Editorial: For Osteoporosis, Are Two Antiresorptive Drugs Better Than One?" *The Journal of Clinical Endocrinology & Metabolism* 87, no. 3 (March 2002): 983–984.

Harvard Health Publications. "Update on Osteoporosis Drugs," Harvard Medical School. Available online. URL: http://www.health.harvard.edu/newsweek/Update_on_osteoporosis_drugs.htm. Downloaded November 9, 2005.

Merck.com. "Osteoporosis, Prognosis and Treatment," The Merck Manual of Geriatrics. Available online. URL: http://www.merck.com/mrkshared/mmg/sec7/ch49/ch49b.jsp. Downloaded November 8, 2005.

National Osteoporosis Foundation. "Medications to Prevent & Treat Osteoporosis," NOF. Available online. URL: http://www.nof.org/patientinfo/medications.htm. Downloaded November 8, 2005.

arachnoiditis   As one of three coverings around the spinal cord and nerves, the arachnoid membrane is normally thin and pliable. When inflammation causes the delicate tissue to thicken and swell, arachnoiditis compresses the spinal nerves, producing CHRONIC BACK PAIN, leg pain, or SCIATICA. If the condition worsens, scarring and stickiness can bind the spinal nerves and the sheath around the spinal cord, producing the debilitating disorder known as adhesive arachnoiditis.

Symptoms and Diagnostic Path

Initially, inflammation can begin for various reasons. For example, arachnoiditis can result from a trauma to the SPINE, a side effect of SURGERY, or SPINAL INFECTION brought on by a virus, a fungus, or a complication of SPINAL TUBERCULOSIS. More commonly, an allergic reaction to a medication, preservative, or dye introduced through a SPINAL INJECTION can inflame the sensitive arachnoid membrane.

As inflammation continues, back pain becomes the strongest complaint. Other symptoms vary, depending on the location and severity of the spinal nerve involvement. For example, stabbing pain may plunge deeply into the lower back. Joints may ache. PARASPINAL MUSCLES may twitch or cramp. Skin may crawl or itch, making clothing feel burdensome or annoying. In some people, shooting pain darts down both legs. Others feel tingling or numbness in the limbs with less control of the lower part of the body. In rare instances, patients with severe cases of adhesive arachnoiditis may become paralyzed. Diverse causalities make the disorder difficult to detect, especially in the presence of a pre-existent spinal condition. Nevertheless, spinal injections or other invasions of the sensitive area beneath the delicate arachnoid membrane provide a strong diagnostic clue.

Treatment Options and Outlook

Since no cure exists, primary care aims for PAIN MANAGEMENT. Surgical repair seldom provides long-term relief, since the surgery itself may cause additional scarring. However, EXERCISE and other types of therapy, such as COLD THERAPY, HEAT THERAPY, HYDROTHERAPY, and MASSAGE, may help a patient to manage daily ACTIVITY with greater ease. Steroid injections, electrical stimulation, and treatment with TRANSCUTANEOUS ELECTRONIC NERVE STIMULATION (TENS) may be useful, but more CLINICAL TRIALS are needed to investigate the pos-

sibilities and establish protocol. For information about current studies recruiting patients, ClinicalTrials.gov offers updates on http://clinicaltrials. gov/search/term=Arachnoiditis.

Risk Factors and Preventive Measures

Within the human body, the most delicate balance exists just below the arachnoid membrane. Yet this space has become a virtual subway system for medical transport. In the 1950s, for example, medical personnel washed reusable needles with detergent before injecting anesthesia into the spine of a surgical patient. Unfortunately, traces of cleanser shot into the spine too, causing many patients to develop permanent paralysis. Disposable needles washed away that causative factor, but other problems surfaced. For instance, the dyes developed to enhance X-RAY images often damaged spinal nerves. Although water-soluble agents now greatly reduce that particular risk, *The Burton Report* cautioned,

> "When water-soluble dyes are used appropriately their risk is low and the benefit to the patient can be high. When they are used inappropriately (wrong agent, wrong concentration, etc.) they continue to have the potential of being highly toxic to the tissues of the nervous system. The unknown factor in all cases of introducing a foreign body substance into the subarachnoid space is the nature of any given individual's auto immune response to it."

Since areas of sensitivity vary from one person to the next, each should be aware of his or her level of tolerance to preservatives, dyes, and medications. Such information should also be provided to a primary physician, surgeon, gynecologist, and others who may need emergency access to the spine.

Burton Report®, "The Anatomy of Adhesive Arachnoiditis." Available online. URL: http://www.burtonreport. com/InfSpine/AdhesArachAnatomy.htm. Downloaded November 10, 2005.

Circle Of Friends With Arachnoiditis, COFWA. "Arachnoiditis Information and Support." Available online. URL: http://www.cofwa.org/. Downloaded November 10, 2005.

Dawson, Edgar G., M.D. "Arachnoiditis," SpineUniverse. Available online. URL: http://www.spineuniverse.

com/displayarticle.php/article180.html. Last updated August 12, 2005.

National Institute of Neurological Disorders and Stroke. "NINDS Arachnoiditis Information Page," National Institutes of Health. Available online. URL: http://www.ninds.nih.gov/disorders/arachnoiditis/arachnoiditis.htm. Last updated May 6, 2005.

arthritis   As its Greek name denotes, arthritis refers to joint inflammation, which, for about 43 million Americans, spells PAIN. Of those diagnosed, nearly 300,000 patients are CHILDREN with JUVENILE ARTHRITIS, JUVENILE RHEUMATOID ARTHRITIS, or other conditions that affect the BACK or joints of the VERTEBRAE. Another 20 million or more people of all ages, sex, and ethnic backgrounds have arthritis but do not know it.

Symptoms and Diagnostic Path

Since this rheumatic condition appears in over 100 forms, the symptoms vary widely. For most people with arthritis, joints characteristically inflame, producing swelling that impedes flexibility. Stiffness often occurs in fingers, weight-bearing joints, and vertebral joints, resulting in mild to severe discomfort. Occasionally, other symptoms arise too. For example, the RANGE OF MOTION may decrease as OSTEOARTHRITIS affects the SPINE. With the progression of ANKYLOSING SPONDYLITIS, bones in the back fuse together, producing rigid POSTURE. If an auto-immune disease such as RHEUMATOID ARTHRITIS (RA) affects the internal organs, symptoms may include fever and pain in corresponding areas of soft tissue.

If a rheumatologist suspects RA, blood tests and a urinalysis can aid a diagnosis. For most types of arthritis, an X-RAY or other imaging device may be needed to examine the vertebral joints. In mild cases, a family history and physical examination may provide enough information for the rheumatologist, pediatrician, or other physician to determine which type of arthritis to treat.

Treatment Options and Outlook

With more investigation needed, researchers in Australia have discovered that the ADAMTS5 enzyme, present in all persons, can become over-active, thus provoking an attack on the cartilage molecule known as aggrecan. Reportedly, this phenomenon activates arthritis and may also activate future research in developing appropriate drugs.

At present, conservative medication usually begins with NONSTEROIDAL ANTI-INFLAMMATORY DRUG (NSAID) THERAPY, which includes ASPIRIN, NAPROXEN, and IBUPROFEN but not ACETAMINOPHEN. Since the latter has no impact on inflammation, acetaminophen does not belong in the NSAID category but may be preferred for pain and fever in patients with gastrointestinal sensitivity. Unlike an NSAID, acetaminophen does not restrain the inflammation-producing cyclooxygenase (COX) that protects the stomach from bleeding and also reduces tissue swelling.

Eventually, researchers identified and isolated COX-2, which has little influence on bleeding but still provokes inflammation. This discovery led to the development of COX-2 inhibitors, such as Vioxx and Celebrex, which soon became the norm for arthritis treatment. Over time though, serious adverse events, such as heart attack and stroke, were noted in some patients, which resulted in voluntary recall of Vioxx and warnings about Celebrex. Around the same time, the Food and Drug Administration (FDA) also issued a public health advisory for NSAIDs, which left arthritis patients wondering what to do.

Since no two patients are the same, a rheumatologist or primary physician can advise each patient, individually, on the most appropriate treatment. Patients whose family history and medical tests show no inclination toward cardiovascular conditions may be prescribed a COX-2 inhibitor. PAIN MANAGEMENT may also rely on various forms of COMPLEMENTARY AND ALTERNATIVE MEDICINE, such as HERBAL THERAPY or HOMEOPATHIC MEDICINE. Indeed, so many arthritis patients have opted for herbal alternatives that, in November 2005, the FDA issued a warning letter to manufacturers who claim their products offer curative benefits not substantiated by research.

Studies of alternative treatments, of course, had already begun. In an article for *Clinical Psychiatry News*, Doug Brunk recounted the findings of Dr. Robert Bonakdar, the director of pain management at the Scripps Center for Integrative Medicine in

La Jolla, California. Reportedly, willow bark, the forerunner of aspirin, reduced pain scores in osteoarthritis patients by 40 percent. Another favorite herb, devil's claw, was given to patients with osteoarthritis and low back pain for three to eight weeks in dosages of 50–100 mg. With only minimal side effects, "the treatments significantly improved the pain level and joint mobility in study participants." Other natural herbs such as ginger and turmeric "also demonstrated anti-inflammatory activity in preliminary basic research of human trials."

Similarly, Kerry Bone reported in the *Townsend Letter for Doctors and Patients* that a trial showed "standardized willow bark compared well with a conventional treatment for arthritis." After considering "evaluation of functional capacity, evaluation of pain intensity during different activities, impairment of daily activity, estimation whether pain was localized or diffuse, . . . and time of stiffness of the observed joint," the trial indicated a 48 percent pain reduction in participants who received NSAIDs. Two other groups experienced a 31.3 to 39.5 percent reduction in pain after taking the lower to higher recommended dosages of willow bark.

Some may wonder though, if arthritis treatments have been barking up the wrong tree. Finnish researchers, for example, located groups of anti-inflammatory compounds (phonemics) in the Scotch pine commonly known as the Christmas tree. Apparently its bark gives forth an extract with strong anti-inflammatory properties. Although studies still need to establish the optimal dose and identify potential side effects, the bark of Christmas or other pines brighten prospects for body tissue wrapped in inflammation.

Meanwhile, COLD THERAPY offers relief when inflammation flares, while HEAT THERAPY, a warm bath, or a MASSAGE with warmed oil may ease stiffness. TOPICAL ANALGESICS often relieve mild discomfort, but a CORTICOSTEROID INJECTION may be needed for severe or chronic joint pain. To ease spinal nerve pain, a physician or therapist may recommend electrical treatment with TRANSCUTANEOUS ELECTRONIC NERVE STIMULATION (TENS).

For spinal instability, a back brace, neck brace, or other ORTHOTIC may help temporarily. Some arthritis patients also respond well to ACUPUNCTURE or SPINAL MANIPULATION. If the condition progresses into DEGENERATIVE DISC DISEASE, the patient may need ARTHRODESIS or other type of SURGERY on one or more vertebrae in the neck or back.

Risk Factors and Preventive Measures

According to current statistics, women acquire arthritis more often than men. Indeed, 25 million women but fewer than 17 million men in the United States have been diagnosed by a physician. Reportedly, however, another 20 million patients have not asked a doctor for directions in locating the source of their pain, so one might wonder if men predominantly comprise that group. Regardless, half of the people who have been medically diagnosed think nothing can be done to help.

Language also presents a barrier in obtaining a prompt diagnosis and beginning effective treatment. According to a report in *The Journal of Musculoskeletal Medicine,* "Early intervention in patients with arthritis is crucial to slowing or halting disease progression . . . , but Hispanic patients often do not talk about pain and may not visit a physician when it occurs." While the same might be said for patients from other cultures, information in Spanish has recently become available, notably from the Arthritis Foundation.

For peoples of all languages and body types, preventive strategies include EXERCISE, ample fresh water, adequate SLEEP, and wholesome NUTRITION. For example, the omega-3 fatty acids in such cold water fish as salmon, cod, and mackerel have anti-inflammatory properties not found in the saturated fats of other meat products. Whether for cooking or massaging, olive oil or oils with VITAMIN E can lubricate and soothe dry skin, parched cells, and achy joints. Drinking several glasses of filtered water a day can cleanse the body of toxins and hydrate cells. Strengthening PARASPINAL MUSCLES, flexing joints, and stretching vertebrae can also help, even if just to get a sedentary body up and moving toward feeling better overall.

Arthritis Foundation. "The Facts About Arthritis." Available online. URL: http://www.arthritis.org/resources/gettingstarted. Downloaded November 10, 2005.

Bone, Kerry. "Willow Bark versus NSAID," *Townsend Letter for Doctors and Patients* 265–266 (August–September 2005): 46–47.

Brunk, Doug. "Patients Seek Natural Alternatives to NSAIDs," *Clinical Psychiatry News* 33, no. 7 (July 2005): 52–53.

CDC. "Arthritis: Data and Statistics," Centers for Disease Control and Prevention (CDC), National Center for Chronic Disease Prevention and Health Promotion. Available online. URL: http://www.cdc.gov/arthritis/data_statistics. Last reviewed August 22, 2005.

Mooney, Vert, M.D. "Spinal Arthritis Complete Treatment Guide," Spine-health.com. Available online. URL: http://www.spine-health.com/topics/conserv/osteo arthtreat/osteoarthtreat01.html. Downloaded November 12, 2005.

Nader, Carol. "All Smiles at Arthritis Find for Young and Old," *Australasian Business Intelligence* (March 31, 2005).

Rados, Carol. "Helpful Treatments Keep People with Arthritis Moving," *FDA Consumer* 39, no. 2 (March–April 2005).

Shiel, William C. Jr., M.D. "Arthritis," MedicineNet.com. Available online. URL: http://www.medicinenet.com/arthritis/article.htm. Last reviewed June 4, 2005.

Staff. "Bark Has Bite," *Better Nutrition* 67, no. 3 (March 2005): 22–23.

Staff. "The Arthritis Foundation Addresses a Growing Need for Better Information—Helping Hispanic Patients Manage Arthritis," *The Journal of Musculoskeletal Medicine* (September 1, 2005): 430.

arthrodesis Commonly known as spinal fusion, arthrodesis surgically joins two or more VERTEBRAE to stabilize, repair, or straighten joints marred by injury, deformity, or disease. If a DISCECTOMY or DISC REPLACEMENT does not offer a viable option for a patient with a HERNIATED DISC or DEGENERATIVE DISC DISEASE, arthrodesis may be performed. This procedure fuses the vertebrae together, strengthens that area of the SPINE, and avoids the pain that inevitably follows whenever bones rub against bones.

Arthrodesis can fuse joints in the neck or CERVICAL SPINE, but more often the procedure performs LUMBAR SPINAL FUSION in the lower back. To redirect or align bone growth throughout the spine, arthrodesis can also be used to surgically treat patients with KYPHOSIS, SCOLIOSIS, or other vertebral disorder affecting POSTURE. Damage from a vertebral FRACTURE may benefit from the procedure too.

Procedure

In making an incision, the surgeon uses either an anterior (front) or posterior (back) approach. For MINIMALLY INVASIVE SURGERY, the opening may be no longer than an inch. Regardless of size, the opening then makes way for a stabilizing metal device to be implanted. Traditionally, a surgeon would insert a BONE GRAFT to promote bone growth during healing, but now BONE MORPHOGENETIC PROTEIN (BMP) may be used in place of or in conjunction with a graft. Either way, BMP introduces a synthetic form of a naturally-produced body chemical into the surgical site. When used alone, BMP avoids the pain associated with a graft, yet this procedure has been shown to be as effective as using a patient's own bone to heal a fusion site. With effects similar to a bone graft, BMP stimulates cells into making new bone to complete the spinal fusion in a healing process that continues long after the hospital stay.

The length of hospitalization depends, in part, on the location of the SURGERY since each area has specific needs. If, for example, anterior arthrodesis fuses joints in the THORACIC SPINE, a drainage tube will be inserted into the chest and left in place for one to three days. Patients having surgery on the LUMBAR SPINE may require a urinary catheter and, possibly, intravenous feeding until the lower body functions normally again. Because of this, fusion in the lower back may require two or three days in the hospital.

Risks and Complications

After arthrodesis, most patients experience pain severe enough to require medication for the first few days. Some respond poorly to that medication or preoperative anesthesia, and all patients risk infection and bleeding after surgery of any type.

If a bone graft comes from the patient's hip or other area, that site also requires an incision, which can produce lingering discomfort. However, patients receiving bone grafts from their own bodies have a more successful recovery than occurs when a donor graft has been used. If multiple joints require fusion, the rate of success declines.

Outlook and Lifestyle Modifications

During hospitalization, the patient will be taught to move and turn the body as a unit to avoid spinal twisting. Depending on the location of surgery, a neck brace, back brace, or other type of ORTHOTIC may be prescribed during the recovery period to stabilize the site and allow new bone time to form. This ongoing process of bone growth completes the spinal fusion in about six to nine months.

Fusing a vertebral joint can straighten and strengthen an area but also reduce the RANGE OF MOTION in that section of the spine. Since most bending occurs in the hip and not the spine, flexibility will be limited only if several joints need fusion. Regardless, most patients prefer to sacrifice some litheness in favor of less pain.

American Academy of Orthopaedic Surgeons (AAOS.) "Spinal Fusion," AAOS. Available online. URL: http://orthoinfo.aaos.org/fact/thr_report.cfm?Thread_ID=1 56&topcategory=Spine. Downloaded November 14, 2005.

Chen, Andrew L., M.D. "Spinal Fusion," MedlinePlus, National Institutes of Health. Available online. URL: http://www.nlm.nih.gov/medlineplus/ency/article/002968.htm. Updated July 4, 2004.

Medtronic Sofamor Danek. "Modern Spinal Fusion," Back.com. Available online. URL: http://www.back.com/articles-modern_spinal_fusion.html. Updated July 7, 2005.

Spine Institute of New York. "Spinal Fusion," Beth Israel Medical Center. Available online. URL: http://www.spineinstituteny.com/treatments/spinalfusion.html. Downloaded November 14, 2005.

arthroplasty   See DISC REPLACEMENT.

artificial disc   See DISC REPLACEMENT.

ascorbic acid   See VITAMIN C.

aspirin   Technically known as acetylsalicylic acid or salicylate, this NONSTEROIDAL ANTI-INFLAMMATORY DRUG (NSAID) not only thwarts inflammation but acts as a PAIN RELIEVER and fever reducer. All NSAIDs have similar actions, but, unlike the others, aspirin hinders blood platelets from clotting.

This reduced clotting action has an adverse effect in patients with bleeding problems, but it can save lives, especially of those in danger of a clot-induced event such as a heart attack or stroke.

The effects of this century-old drug may vary dramatically from one person to the next. In everybody's body, however, hormone-like substances signal PAIN to the brain. That alarm system triggers production of cyclooxygenase (COX) and prostaglandins that cause pain, inflammation, and fever. Despite the bad press, such symptoms do not always produce ill effects. For instance, pain indicates something is wrong. Fever burns off infection. Inflammation assists the body's circulatory efforts toward healing. Each of those natural reactions has curative value until that individually-derived moment when too much just becomes too much. When that happens, aspirin intercepts the pain, calms the inflammation, reduces the fever, and thins blood clots within minutes.

Dosage and Potential Side Effects

Aspirin slows inflammation caused by prostaglandins, but this can be a problem if those same substances need to be left alone to do their other jobs of shielding the stomach and keeping down gastric acid. By hindering the protective action of prostaglandins, aspirin irritates a sensitive digestive track. Although this happens most often in CHILDREN or ELDERLY patients, too much aspirin can cause stomach bleeding in anyone.

To avoid stomach irritation, buffered aspirin can be taken with milk or food. Taking a lower dose also helps, especially since a maintenance dosage of only 81 mg provides the amount usually recommended to avoid blood clots. However, up to 1,000 mg a day may be prescribed for patients at high risk for a cardiovascular event. A doctor may prescribe even higher doses to inhibit ARTHRITIS pain, but at any dosage, aspirin should not be taken with a HOMEOPATHIC MEDICINE, pharmaceutical drug, or herb that thins the blood unless a physician says otherwise.

Taken by itself, a toxic dose of aspirin depends on the person's body weight, but depending on sensitivity, toxicity can occur above 150 mg/kg to 300 mg/kg. In the event of an overdose, symptoms can vary widely. For instance, the ears may ring, the mouth get dry, and the pulse rate increase. The person may also feel nauseated or drowsy. Large quantities of water, milk, or other beverage may dilute the toxic effect, but a sharp drop in respiration or blood pressure signals a medical emergency.

Statistics and Studies

An April 2005 health advisory from the Food and Drug Administration (FDA) warned of the dangerous side effect of cardiovascular events that NSAIDs can produce. As the only NSAID able to reduce blood clotting, however, aspirin was omitted from the list, which came as good news for patients with arthritis and CHRONIC BACK PAIN.

More good news arrived in 2005 from Brigham and Women's Hospital in Boston. As reported in the *AORN Journal* published by the Association of Operating Room Nurses, "Researchers have demonstrated in a randomized clinical trial that low-dose aspirin (i.e., 81 mg) triggers the human body to generate its own anti-inflammatory compounds that help fight unwanted inflammation. . . . The finding has implications for people with heart disease, arthritis, and many other diseases that are known to be associated with inflammation. The study demonstrated that unlike COX-2 inhibitors, aspirin—a COX-1 inhibitor—also generates 'good' anti-inflammatory compounds necessary to fight disease."

Also in 2005, Dr. Victor L. Serebruany reported the results of a study involving over 192,000 patients. As quoted in *Family Practice News,* Dr. Serebruany told attendees at the American College of Cardiology annual meeting in Orlando, "We do not know if 75 mg/day of aspirin is better or worse than 325 mg in terms of efficacy, because there has been no direct comparative trial. However, now we know for sure that the lower the dose, the less the bleeding risk." Dr. Serebruany also said, "If you give 25 mg of aspirin, you have complete platelet inhibition within 10 minutes. This is a fact."

In some instances, patients may need more aspirin to address severe back pain or rheumatologic issues such as gout. Others may be relieved to hear of studies on willow bark, the forerunner of aspirin, that has provided successful treatment for ARTHRITIS. Recent findings emphasize the importance of an individual assessment for each patient. Nevertheless, no one concerned about health should exceed the dose recommended on the label without the say-so of a personal care physician.

Center for Drug Evaluation and Research. "FDA Public Health Advisory," U.S. Food and Drug Administration. Available online. URL: http://www.fda.gov/cder/drug/advisory/COX2.htm. Downloaded November 15, 2005.

Jancin, Bruce. "Aspirin Below 100 mg/day Is Safest, Metaanalysis Shows." *Family Practice News* 35, no. 10 (May 1, 2005): 8.

MedlinePlus. "Aspirin Overdose," U.S. Library of Medicine. Available online. URL: http://www.nlm.nih.gov/medlineplus/ency/article/002542.htm. Updated November 9, 2005.

MedlinePlus. "Drug Information: Aspirin," U.S. Library of Medicine. Available online. URL: http://www.nlm.nih.gov/medlineplus/print/druginfo/medmaster/a682878.html. Downloaded on November 15, 2005.

Staff, Association of Operating Room Nurses, Inc. "Low-dose Aspirin Offers Adults Inflammation Protection," *AORN Journal* 81, no. 2 (February 2005): 428.

athletes, spinal concerns of   With or without contact and competition, a chosen sport can strengthen the VERTEBRAE and PARASPINAL MUSCLES or add undue stress. Although usually thought of as recreational, an athletic activity can be occupational too. Regardless of the goal, sports generally gain positive support for the BACK and SPINE.

Risks and Complications

An article posted on the Spine-health.com Web site reported that up to 20 percent of all sports injuries involve either the neck or the lower back. As the article explained, "Sports that use repetitive impact (e.g., running) or weight loading at the end of a range-of-motion (e.g., weight lifting) commonly cause damage to the lumbar spine (lower back). Sports that involve contact (e.g., football) place the cervical spine (neck) at risk of injury. The thoracic spine (mid portion of the spine at the level of the rib cage) is less likely to be injured in sports because it is relatively immobile due to the rib cage." Failing to warm up, exceeding physical limits, and using poor equipment, such as improperly fitted shoes, increase the risk of back injury, as can too much loading.

An article in the *Journal of Athletic Training* focused on neck injuries caused by overloading the CERVICAL SPINE: "Because of the potentially catastrophic and life-altering nature of cervical spine injury (CSI), much concern exists regarding the prehospital management of the cervical spine-injured athlete. This is evidenced by a multiprofessional task force effort initiated by the National Athletic Trainers' Association to establish general guidelines for the acute care of the spine-injured athlete. Major CSIs, although rare compared with sprain and strain injuries to the extremities, are troubling because of mortality rates, and the potential permanent loss of neural function. A CSI requires an immediate and deliberate, yet sensitive, response. The highest rate of severe neck injuries has occurred in American football and rugby. Other sports and activities that contribute to a high rate of CSI are wrestling, diving, recreational diving, ice hockey, gymnastics, and horseback riding." For example, "when contact is applied to the crown of the head or helmet in the football player, the cervical spine experiences a compressive load from the torso. As the padding provided by the helmet reaches its absorptive limits, the head then reverses direction, resulting in an increased compressive load as the cervical spine is compressed between the head and torso. When this compressive force exceeds the spine's absorption capabilities, soft and hard tissue components fail." Besides the possibility of a broken bone, that type of injury often results in a wryneck (TORTICOLLIS) or a FLEXION-EXTENSION INJURY similar to a whiplash.

An article in *American Family Physician* discussed stingers as the most common cervical spine-related injury in football. Over half of the players who experience one such injury will have another, but previous conditions such as SPINAL STENOSIS increase the likelihood. As the article said, "In older athletes, about 94 percent of persistent stingers are associated with disc degeneration or other pathology." Since the injury must be taken seriously, "full evaluation and exclusion from play are indicated if stingers persist longer than 24 hours or recur. Any evidence of neurologic deficit, persistent pain, loss of motion, or cervical myelopathy requires full investigation for cervical pathology."

Statistics and Studies

The article "Preventing Severe Head and Neck Injuries in High School and Collegiate Athletes," posted online by the American Academy of Orthopaedic Surgeons (AAOS), stated that college athletes experience more injuries than do high school students. In both groups, "the number-one sport responsible for female direct catastrophic injuries" is cheerleading, "with approximately two direct catastrophic injuries per year." The sport increasingly includes gymnastic stunts, with the greatest threats occurring in the pyramid and in the basket toss. Often, the frequency and extent of injuries depend on the number of cheerleaders involved and the height attained. Adverse conditions, such as a wet floor or the lack of floor mats and spotters, have a dramatic impact too. The AAOS added, "However, the physical, mental and social benefits of team sports significantly outweigh the risks involved: only one out of every 100,000 athletes suffers from a direct catastrophic injury."

In another online report, "A Guide to Safety for Young Athletes," the AAOS provided statistics on the number of annual injuries in children under 15: basketball, 574,000; football, 448,200; baseball, 252,665; soccer, 227,100; hockey, 80,700; gymnastics, 75,000; volleyball, 50,100. These injuries involve various bones, muscles, ligaments, and tendons, commonly resulting in a SPRAIN, STRAIN, or FRACTURE. Such injuries may only temporarily remove athletes from play, but others can cause permanent damage to growing bones.

For ELDERLY athletes, another AAOS report stated, "The most common injuries among aging athletes are chronic, overuse injuries such as muscle strains and tendinitis. These types of injuries result from a decrease in musculoskeletal flexibility and participation in endurance sports, such as long-distance running, which promote muscle fatigue and predisposition to injury. Chronic and overuse injuries account for approximately 70 percent of injuries in veteran athletes age 60 and older, whereas only 41 percent of younger athletes ages 21–25 are affected by these same injuries." Such injuries aside, the AAOS also reported positive outcomes for older participants in sports. For instance, "with regular, intensive muscle training, aging athletes well into their 80s can minimize or reverse age-related declines in muscle mass."

Athletes of all ages may be more concerned about muscle spasm. As Dr. Norman L. Epstein reported in the *Canadian Medical Association Journal,* "Many patients arrive in the emergency department with acute lumbar and cervical muscle spasm . . . that occurs either spontaneously or secondary to nonimpact axial injuries (i.e., lifting and twisting)." Although these injuries can happen to anyone, athletes encounter such problems with greater frequency. When this happens, "current treatment options, such as opioids, NSAIDs and anxiolytics, provide either minimal or no relief or precipitate undesirable side effects." However, Dr. Epstein decided to study the effects of Benztropine, a drug used to treat Parkinson's, in relieving muscle spasm and providing pain relief. While more studies will be needed to corroborate the findings and their application for athletes, this particular study showed, "Every patient experienced substantial relief and improved range of motion."

Special Aids and Adaptations

The American Academy of Orthopaedic Surgeons warned that over half of golfers twist their lower backs when they make contact with the ball or follow through with high velocity. In reporting on these AAOS findings, the American Council on Exercise (ACE) explained, "Unfortunately, while your stance may be beneficial to your golf score, it could result in the wearing of the disc in the spine. An alternative stance, such as standing up straighter on the follow-through, could help eliminate the back pain, but send your handicap skyrocketing."

What constitutes a handicap remains a matter of perception, as shown each year by young athletes who compete in the Special Olympics (SO). This international nonprofit organization offers year-round training and events in 25 sports for athletes eight and older who have been diagnosed with varying degrees of mental retardation. Many of the athletes also have physical disabilities that make a sport more challenging. For example, the person may have poor muscle tone, SCOLIOSIS, a musculoskeletal condition, or a problem affected by WEIGHT, making properly fitted equipment and shoes especially important in preventing injuries.

As an added precaution, the Special Olympics requires medical approval for each participant. According to an article by Linda Platt, "Athletes who have abnormal radiographs are eliminated from contact sports such as diving, gymnastics, floor hockey, and soccer and are limited to non-contact competition such as bowling, swimming, cross-country skiing, figure skating, and distance running. Swimmers who have abnormal radiographs are restricted from starting on the blocks and required to start in the pool." Besides these special concerns, the Special Olympics offered sensible instructions for bone health in general. For instance, "athletes need to be reminded often to continue to hydrate before, during, and after competition and practice."

ACE, acefitness.org. "Golf Is a Pain in the Back for Some," American Council on Exercise. Available online. URL: http://www.acefitness.org/fitfacts/fitbits_display.aspx?itemid=115. Updated November 15, 2005.

American Academy of Orthopaedic Surgeons. "Aging Athletes Require Tailored Exercise Regimen to Avoid Overuse Injuries: Orthopaedic Surgeons Study Most Common Bone, Joint and Muscle Problems in Mature Athletes," Newsroom. Available online. URL: http://www6.aaos.org/pemr/news/press_release.cfm?PRNumber=402. Downloaded November 16, 2005.

American Academy of Orthopaedic Surgeons. "A Guide to Safety for Young Athletes," AAOS, Sports/Exercise. Available online. URL: http://orthoinfo.aaos.org/brochure/thr_report.cfm?ThreadID=34&topcategory=Sports%20%2F%20Exercise. Downloaded November 16, 2005.

American Academy of Orthopaedic Surgeons. "Preventing Severe Head and Neck Injuries in High School and Collegiate Athletes: Orthopaedic Research Reveals Benefits of Enhanced Protective Gear, Preventive Strategies, Rule Revisions," Newsroom. Available online. URL: http://www6.aaos.org/pemr/news/press_release.cfm?PRNumber=408. Downloaded November 16, 2005.

Epstein, Norman L., M.D. "Benztropine for Acute Muscle Spasm in the Emergency Department," *Canadian Medical Association Journal* 164, no. 2 (January 23, 2001): 203–204.

Hyde, Thomas E. "Sports Injuries and Back Pain," Spine-health.com. Available online. URL: http://www.

atlantoaxial instability 25

spine-health.com/topics/cd/sports/spsp/spsp01.html. Downloaded November 15, 2005.

Platt, Linda S. "Medical and Orthopaedic Conditions in Special Olympics Athletes," *Journal of Athletic Training* 36, no. 1 (March 2001): 74–80.

Swartz, Erick E., R. T. Floyd, and Mike Cendoma. "Cervical Spine Functional Anatomy and the Biomechanics of Injury Due to Compressive Loading," *Journal of Athletic Training* 40, no. 3 (July 2005): 155–161.

Walling, Anne D., M.D. "Cervical Spine Conditions in Athletes," *American Family Physician* 71, no. 11 (June 1, 2005): 2,194.

atlantoaxial instability The Greek god Atlas did not actually carry the weight of the world on his shoulders, but the first bone of the CERVICAL SPINE carries his name and the weight of a globe-shaped head. Just below the atlas or C1 vertebra sits the axis (C2) on which the head rotates. Connecting those two VERTEBRAE, a tooth-shaped bone known as the dens acts as a pivotal device. However, a trauma such as a FLEXION-EXTENSION INJURY (whiplash) can dislodge the vertebrae, jiggle the "tooth," or loosen the supportive ligaments. In addition, atlantoaxial instability can result from spinal conditions or disorders, such as ANKYLOSING SPONDYLITIS, OSTEOGENESIS IMPERFECTA, RHEUMATOID ARTHRITIS, or SCOLIOSIS. SPINAL INFECTION and SPINAL TUMOR can be causative factors too.

Symptoms and Diagnostic Path

Instability in the neck commonly produces pain, occasionally with CERVICAL RADICULOPATHY, often indicating a pinched nerve. If symptoms include TORTICOLLIS, the head tilts to one side, which can increase pain or cause muscle spasm. Some patients also experience vertigo and, in severe cases, may have trouble with movement and mobility.

If vertebrae have shifted out of alignment, X-RAY may show this VERTEBRAL SUBLUXATION. However, an article in *Postgraduate Medicine* warned, "Radiographs obtained in neutral position may fail to show the instability." To provide a clearer diagnosis and also assess any soft tissue involvement, a MAGNETIC RESONANCE IMAGING (MRI) or a COMPUTED TOMOGRAPHY (CT) SCAN may be needed.

Treatment Options and Outlook

A *Southern Medical Journal* (SMJ) article said, "It is well known that the atlantoaxial segment is the most mobile region of the entire vertebral column. Approximately 50% of the rotation of the cervical spine occurs at the C1-C2 joint. The average rotation at the C1-C2 joint has been calculated to be 43 degrees (range, 32 to 50 degrees). When destabilized, its range of motion increases significantly, with consequent risk of severe neurological damage." If neurological damage does occur, the person may have difficulty walking or lose bladder or bowel control over the lower part of the body. In such cases, prompt SURGERY will usually be needed.

Regarding surgery, the *SMJ* article discussed the use of a device known as a transarticular screw to stabilize the area. According to the article, "C1–C2 posterior transarticular screw fixation is a biomechanically superior fixation technique that provides immediate rigid stability without the use of rigid external orthosis." However, "meticulous preoperative planning and precise operative techniques are required for successful transarticular screw fixation, because the tolerance for error in this region of the spine is very limited. Ultimately . . . it is up to the surgeon to weight the advantages of this technique against the possible risk of screw malposition and neural or vascular injury, and to choose the technique most appropriate for each patient."

In discussing atlantoaxial instability among CHILDREN, a group of doctors from the Department of Neurosurgery at the Medical College of Georgia reported in *Neurosurgical Focus*, "Atlantooccipital injuries are commonly seen among pediatric spine injuries. When surgical intervention is indicated, we have used different fusion methods—all with excellent outcomes." If patients present a wry neck or torticollis, "diagnosis is controversial, however, most cases resolve with the use of cervical bracing for time periods shorter than 6 weeks." With trauma causing 83 percent of the cases of atlantoaxial instability in children and infection 17 percent, the article further stated, "Most cases . . . reduced spontaneously with the use of a rigid cervical collar (50%) or with 48 to 72 hours of traction followed by the use of a collar (33%)." Regardless of whether an ORTHOTIC device or SURGERY provides the best option, "dynamic imaging is critical to properly assessing patients with continued complaints of neck pain." In other words, the treating physician needs a good picture of what is happening to determine the optimal options.

Risk Factors and Preventive Measures

Childhood trauma, aging, and diseases such as RHEUMATOID ARTHRITIS sometimes cause atlanto-axial instability. As the *Postgraduate Medicine* article stated, "Neck pain in a patient with rheumatoid arthritis can be an important clue to serious cervical spine involvement." Then loss of bone cartilage, laxity of ligaments, "and bone erosion can lead to potentially fatal spinal cord instability in these patients." To prevent fatality, "indications for surgery to correct rheumatoid atlantoaxial instability include neurologic deterioration and intractable pain. In patients with severe atlantoaxial instability and a stable or no neurologic deficit, the indications for surgery are less clear."

An online article from eMedicine.com stated, "In traumatic situations, approximately 10% of cervical fractures involve some injuries to the atlantoaxial level. Of injuries to the atlantoaxial complex, only 16% produce neurologic deficits secondary to the wide spinal canal at this level." Although paralysis and death rarely occur, "symptomatic patients are at risk for progressive neurologic symptoms." In addition, patients with BIRTH DEFECTS OF THE SPINE may be at greater risk after age 30. Risks increase, too, for individuals with Downs syndrome. Although some patients may not need any treatment, "spinal cord compression can arise or worsen if susceptible patients are subjected to extreme ranges of motion. Special care should be taken to avoid excessive flexion or extension of the neck."

Alberstone, Cary D., M.D. and Edward C. Benzel, M.D. "Cervical Spine Complications in Rheumatoid Arthritis Patients," *Postgraduate Medicine* 107, no.1 (January 2000). Available online. URL: http://www.postgradmed.com/issues/2000/01_00/alberstone.htm. Downloaded December 9, 2005.

Banit, Daxes, M.D., Daniel Murray, M.D., and Bruce Darden II, M.D. "Atlantoaxial Instability," eMedicine.com. Available online. URL: http://www.emedicine.com/orthoped/topic503.htm. Downloaded December 9, 2005.

Fountas, K. N., E. Z. Kapsalaki, I. Karampelas, V. G. Dimopoulos, C. H. Feltes, M. A. Kassam, A. N. Boev, K. W. Johnston, H. F. Smisson, E. C. Troup, and J. S. Robinson Jr. "C1–C2 Transarticular Screw Fixation for Atlantoaxial Instability," *Southern Medical Journal* 97, no. 11 (November 2004): 1,042–1,048.

Rahimi, Scott Y., M.D., E. Andrew Stevens, David John Yeh, M.D., Ann Marie Flannery, M.D., Haroon Fiaz Choudhri, M.D., and Mark R. Lee, M.D. "Treatment of Atlantoaxial Instability in Pediatric Patients," *Neurosurgical Focus: Clinical Pearl* 15, no. 6 (December 2003).

autologous bone graft   See BONE GRAFT.

back The posterior region between the neck and hips has a lot riding on it, including all sorts of lively commands: stand back, double back, knock back, hang back, back away, back up, back down, back in, back out. Although those familiar phrases express some type of choice or action, many people sit back with no ACTIVITY or EXERCISE to strengthen PARASPINAL MUSCLES or assist the body in BONE BUILDING. When those laid-back persons happen to be CHILDREN or ADOLESCENTS, their bone growth and future bone strength may be set back, especially if CALCIUM and other elements of good NUTRITION have been pushed back as priorities.

To glimpse other potential causes of ACUTE BACK PAIN, CHRONIC BACK PAIN, LOW BACK PAIN, and the common BACKACHE, the flipside of the backside provides an interesting view. For example, the effects of WEIGHT may be apparent in slack abdominal muscles that pull the VERTEBRAE in the LUMBAR SPINE. Also, GENETIC FACTORS, ENVIRONMENTAL INFLUENCES, and ERGONOMIC FACTORS bring back-to-back distress. For instance, a poorly designed mattress may compromise the SLEEP needed to rid the body of toxins and renew cellular strength. Back up again, a person's POSTURE may indicate SCOLIOSIS or another structural problem in the THORACIC SPINE, whereas general slumping implies the felt weight of the world. For the latter, MASSAGE THERAPY offers a particularly curative touch, and almost everybody seems to appreciate an occasional pat on the back.

Risks and Complications

Back pain can bring temporary discomfort after too much activity or too little, but additional symptoms usually indicate something else going on. For example, leg pain that increases with movement can signal SPINAL STENOSIS, a HERNIATED DISC, or DEGENERATIVE DISC DISEASE. Vertebral stiffness that does not ease with activity can mean ANKYLOSING SPONDYLITIS, but joint stiffness throughout the body or in weight-bearing joints may indicate OSTEOARTHRITIS.

If sudden movement precipitated back pain, a muscle STRAIN or SPRAIN may have occurred, but numbness and tingling suggest spinal nerve involvement such as occurs in SCIATICA. Symptoms of fatigue or weight loss can point to a SPINAL TUMOR, whereas a fever may indicate DISCITIS or a SPINAL INFECTION of some kind. In any case, the risk comes in ignoring unexplained back pain beyond a day or two.

Statistics and Studies

According to WorkSafeBC of British Columbia, up to 40 percent of absences from work in Canada are back-related with an average of 45 days lost per incident. Of back strains in general, about two-thirds result from physical exertion such as pushing, pulling, or LIFTING improperly. Over 90 percent of back pain in the lumbar region, however, has no explicable cause.

In the United States, the American Academy of Orthopaedic Surgeons reported that back problems instigated around 31 million doctor visits in 2003. That same year, over 8 million were hospitalized because of musculoskeletal conditions, which not only affect the back but getting back to work.

Researchers in Norway investigated influential factors, such as the level of fear, confidence, disability, and cardiovascular fitness, that help to predict if people will return to work after back pain has kept them home. According to an abstract of the report in the *Journal of Rehabilitation Medicine,* "The predictors identified in the present study may reflect personal risk factors in a patient who gets acute low back pain. On the other hand, they may support that fear of pain and injury may be more disabling than pain itself."

Special Aids and Adaptations

According to the therapists writing for the American Physical Therapy Association (APTA) Web site, "Most bad backs respond well to rest and conservative treatment." To prevent back pain, the APTA recommended being aware of posture, lifting with the legs instead of the back, sitting with care, and keeping body weight at an optimal level. Since people spend about a third of life in bed, the APTA suggested safe sleep with vertebrae in a straight or neutral position, whether on the side or on the back. If the bed sags, a board beneath the mattress may keep a good back from going bad.

AAOS. "Orthopaedic Fast Facts," American Academy of Orthopaedic Surgeons. Available online. URL: http://orthoinfo.aaos.org/fact/thr_report.cfm?Thread_ID=93 &topcategory=General%20Information. Downloaded November 17, 2005.

Edgelow, Peter, Glenda Key, Stanley Paris, and Lamont Smith. "Taking Care of Your Back," APTA, American Physical Therapy Association. Available online. URL: http://www.apta.org/AM/Template.cfm?Section=Search&template=/CM/HTMLDisplay.cfm&ContentID=20406. Downloaded November 17, 2005.

Medtronic Sofamor Danek. "Causes," Back.com. Available online. URL: http://www.back.com/causes.html. Downloaded November 17, 2005.

Storheim, K., Brox J. Ivar, I. Holm, and K. Bo. "Predictors of Return to Work in Patients Sick Listed for Sub-acute Low Back Pain: a 12-month Follow-up Study," *Journal of Rehabilitation Medicine,* 37, no. 6 (November 2005): 365–371.

WorkSafebc.com. "Back pain statistics," WorkSafeBC. Available online. URL: http://www2.worksafebc.com/Topics/Ergonomics/BackPainBasics.asp. Downloaded November 17, 2005.

backache   Unlike nerve pain, the muscle pain of a backache often involves soft tissue. Sometimes a sudden twist or abrupt movement tightens the PARASPINAL MUSCLES, resulting in ACUTE BACK PAIN that may be intense but, nevertheless, temporary. Faulty POSTURE can cause CHRONIC BACK PAIN, par-

ticularly in growing CHILDREN and ADOLESCENTS. Young people may also exceed their limits of LOAD TOLERANCE or be generally unaware of BACKPACK SAFETY, thus causing muscle STRAIN or vertebral shifting such as occurs in SPONDYLOLISTHESIS.

In adults or ELDERLY patients, certain medications, such as cholesterol-lowering drugs, may cause a backache with muscle pain or weakness. Anyone experiencing those side effects should talk to a primary care physician immediately to avoid progression into a serious condition, such as RHABDOMYOLYSIS.

Symptoms and Diagnostic Path

Most backaches disappear with light EXERCISE and ACTIVITY followed by restful SLEEP. For children, the American Academy of Orthopaedic Surgeons (AAOS) said, "Most often, musculoskeletal strain is responsible for childhood and adolescent back discomfort. The pain frequently responds to rest, anti-inflammatory medications and an exercise program." However, "other more serious diagnoses must always be given consideration." As the AAOS warned, backaches in children may indicate an underlying medical condition, especially in the presence of additional symptoms, such as fever, weight loss, or leg pain. In such instances, persons of any age should seek the advice of a doctor, who will take a medical history, perform a physical examination, and recommend appropriate tests and treatments.

Treatment Options and Outlook

With the first line of treatment being rest, The National Pain Foundation also suggests alternating COLD THERAPY and HEAT THERAPY. For about 10 minutes at a time, "apply cold packs to the affected area in the first few days (up to 72 hours), then switch to applying heat for 20 to 30 minutes, three to four times a day. This may help ease pain by relieving muscle spasm or cramping. Cold stimulation, such as icing, can also activate the body's mechanisms that shut down pain signals as they enter the spinal cord. Applied warmth also decreases stiffness and prepares muscles for stretching." If pain continues with no underlying cause, ULTRASOUND THERAPY may ease an achy back.

Meanwhile, back in the herb garden, an article for Holisticonline.com frankly stated, "Many of the herbs used for pain relief use the same biochemical pathways as the non-opiate pain-relieving drugs, but they are not as effective. However, on the positive side, many of these herbs have multiple effects. Their antispasmodic and circulation-promoting constituents may make up for what these plants lack." For example, chamomile tea may calm smooth muscle tissue, while bromelain (pineapple extract) eases inflammation. A long soak in a warm bath of Epsom salts may soften skin and ease a backache, but this centuries-old treatment is not recommended for patients with high blood pressure or circulatory problems.

For a TOPICAL ANALGESIC, a very tiny sprinkle of capsicum (cayenne pepper) in a base of vegetable oil may relieve mild pain, but this fiery ointment can irritate sensitive skin. According to *The People's Pharmacy Guide To Home And Herbal Remedies,* "Capsaicin is so strong that people can detect it at a concentration as low as just one part in eleven million." Fortunately, many OVER-THE-COUNTER PRODUCTS contain capsicum, thus taking out the guess work. Also, one might consider wintergreen instead of red pepper rubs. "One of the oldest remedies for muscle aches and pains was originally made from the wintergreen shrub. The compound that was distilled from the leaves was methyl salicylate, a chemical relative of aspirin (though it is not swallowed the way aspirin is). Virtually the same compound could be extracted from the bark of sweet birch (also known as cherry birch)." Today, oil of wintergreen may be synthetically produced and added to various types of ointments that can be applied to the skin.

Unless an underlying medical condition exists, most backaches disappear within a day or two. Until then, the conservative RICE METHOD of rest, ice, compression, and elevation may ease minor discomfort. For pain relief and preventatives, patients might also try ACUPUNCTURE, HOMEOPATHIC MEDICINE, MASSAGE THERAPY, SPINAL MANIPULATION, and a fitting pair of shoes. (Low heels come highly recommended.)

Risk Factors and Preventive Measures

In the online article "How To Prevent Back Pain," the AAOS listed people at risk if their responsibilities necessitate LIFTING, bending, or carrying objects. Caretakers at work or home may be particularly at risk for backaches and BACK INJURY. To avoid this, the AAOS recommended, "Avoid twisting your body; instead, point your toes in the direction you want to move and pivot in that direction." Other suggestions included planning ahead, slowing down, tightening stomach muscles, and asking for help when needed. The AAOS also advised, "Keep a positive attitude about your job and home life; studies show that persons who are unhappy at work or home tend to have more back problems and take longer to recover than persons who have a positive attitude."

American Academy of Orthopaedic Surgeons. "Back Pain in Children," AAOS. Available online. URL: http://orthoinfo.aaos.org/fact/thr_report.cfm?Thread_ID=329&topcategory=Spine. Downloaded November 18, 2005.

American Academy of Orthopaedic Surgeons. "How to Prevent Back Pain," AAOS. Available online. URL: http://orthoinfo.aaos.org/fact/thr_report.cfm?Thread_ID=90&topcategory=Spine. Downloaded November 18, 2005.

Graedon, Joe and Teresa Graedon. *The Peoples Pharmacy Guide to Home and Herbal Remedies.* New York: St. Martin's Press, 2001, pages 57, 59.

Holisticonline.com. "Back Pain, Herbs," ICBS, Inc. Available online. URL: http://holistic-online.com/Remedies/Backpain/back_herbs.htm. Downloaded November 18, 2005.

Huang, Julian, M.D. "Potential Causes of Back Pain in Children and Teens," Spine-health.com. Available online. URL: http://www.spine-health.com/topics/cd/kids/kids2.html. Downloaded November 18, 2005.

National Pain Foundation, The. "My Treatment: Back and Neck Pain Overview." Available online. URL: http://www.nationalpainfoundation.org/MyTreatment/articles/Back_Overview.asp. Updated August 1, 2005.

back brace   See ORTHOTICS.

back injury   With a fall, a twist, or sudden movement, a vulnerable spot can stretch, squeeze, or buckle into ACUTE BACK PAIN. Back injuries occur among ATHLETES participating in sports, CHILDREN playing, or ELDERLY people enjoying a daily ACTIV-ITY. A back injury can happen to anyone anytime at home, at leisure, or at work.

According to The National Institute for Occupational Safety and Health (NIOSH), "One out of every four injuries in general industry are due to back sprain and strain. Yet back and shoulder injuries are responsible for 54 percent—over half—of all injuries and illnesses among nursing assistants. While the number of back injuries is going down in manufacturing, the number has gone up among nursing assistants over the last 10 years."

The U.S. Bureau of Labor Statistics reported back injuries and disorders as being responsible for 23.1 percent of the days lost from work in 2003. That same year, most of the days lost among construction workers, manufacturing crews, and miners resulted from injurious encounters with equipment. For those in health services, fatigue and overexertion caused injuries and cost the most days from work. Employees aged 35 to 44 had the highest number of incidents, with time away from work increasing proportionately with age. On average, workers in all categories lost seven workdays because of injuries and backaches.

Symptoms and Diagnostic Path

With pain as the common denominator, some back injuries can send PARASPINAL MUSCLES into muscle spasm. Others cause a HERNIATED DISC with SCIATICA occurring as pain radiates down the legs. That shooting pain or, conversely, no pain but numbness and tingling, may indicate pressure on the spinal nerves. If back pain severely worsens in a reclining position, X-RAY may be required to investigate the possibility of FRACTURE. Other imaging devices, such as a COMPUTED TOMOGRAPHY (CT) SCAN or MAGNETIC RESONANCE IMAGING (MRI), will seldom be used except to confirm suspected nerve involvement or a need for SURGERY.

Treatment Options and Outlook

In the online article "Chronic Back Injury," The Arthritis Society stated, "Back pain will often go away on its own." For pain and stiffness after an injury, a physician may recommend ACETAMINO-PHEN unless inflammation makes a NONSTEROIDAL ANTI-INFLAMMATORY DRUG (NSAID) more advisable.

Swelling and inflammation may also respond well to an ice pack or other form of COLD THERAPY. For stiffness, however, a hot shower or other type of HEAT THERAPY can relax achy muscles and relieve soreness in spinal joints. The Arthritis Society further stated, "Seventy percent of people with back pain recover within a month. Back pain that persists for more than six months occurs in only 1% to 5% of the chronic back injury cases. About half of the people with long-term back injury return to work."

Risk Factors and Preventive Measures

In a booklet published by The American Occupational Therapy Association, Inc., Michael Melnik described the normal recovery process as occurring in three stages: acute, subacute, and recovered. Since the body attempts to protect itself during the first stage, "activities during this time should be limited only to those that cannot be avoided, and they should be done in a manner that minimizes the demands on your back." As pain subsides in the subacute stage and movement increases, "activities will need to be chosen carefully to maximize the healing process." During recovery, the risk of reinjury increases with too much movement too soon. Also, most patients should lift no more than 20 pounds. "Yet if you bend over to pick up your shoes, which probably weigh just a couple of pounds, you actually put 200 to 300 pounds of pressure on your spine through the weight of your upper body." That body may be lightweight, but the principles of body mechanics are not. To reduce pressure on the back, Melnik suggested visualizing a bridge. "Building a bridge connects your body to stationary objects that provide support. A bridge is connected to solid ground on two sides." This means, "by simply placing one arm down on the counter, or even leaning your body weight into the counter, you connect the bridge and reduce the pressure on your back." So, "any time you must bend, think of your lower back as one end of a bridge and look for a place to 'connect' the other side."

To connect to preventive measures, a Health-Link article listed key components as proper POS-TURE, conditioning, and body mechanics. Regarding posture, the article advised, "If possible, get in the habit of holding in the belly to keep it from protruding and putting excess force on the spine. When standing, bend your knees slightly." For overall conditioning, walking, swimming, and biking were suggested. In addition, "stretching to increase back and abdomen flexibility should be done 5–7 days per week, and strengthening exercises should be done at least 4–5 days per week. Because back conditions vary, strengthening and stretching the muscles of the spine and abdomen should be done under the direction of a physician or physical therapist. These stabilizing exercises improve support for the spine itself, but proper technique is essential."

Addressing body mechanics, the article suggested that workers take frequent breaks and shift into varied positions. "When sitting at a desk, think in terms of right angles (90°, or the shape of an L). Knees should be at 90° angles when the soles of the feet are touching the floor. The back and thighs should form 90° angles when the body is sitting properly in a chair. Wrists should be straight and elbows at 90° angles when the hands are on the desk or keyboard." For standing, a cushioned floor may help, and, "when lifting, avoid reaching too far out for the object to be moved; instead, stand close and grasp the object close to the body."

Since many jobs involve LIFTING, some employers supply workers with back belts in hope of avoiding work-related back injuries. While the device does not inhibit forward bending, a belt can restrain RANGE OF MOTION side to side and also act as a simple reminder. However, an article on the NIOSH Web site cautioned that, "Workers wearing back belts may attempt to lift more weight than they would have without a belt. A false sense of security may subject workers to greater risk of injury." Therefore, the NIOSH recommended, "Rather than relying solely on back belts, companies should begin to implement a comprehensive ergonomics program that strives to protect all workers. The most effective way to prevent back injury is to redesign the work environment and work tasks to reduce the hazards of lifting. Training in identifying lifting hazards and using safe lifting techniques and methods should improve program effectiveness."

Arthritis Society, The. "Chronic Back Injury." Available online. URL: http://www.arthritis.ca/types%20of%20arthritis/chronicback/default.asp?s=1. Updated March 29, 2005.

Bureau of Labor Statistics. "Occupations with the Most Injuries and Illnesses with Days Away from Work, 2003," U.S. Department of Labor, pages 7, 8, 11, 13, 17. Available online. URL: http://www.bls.gov/iif/oshwc/osh/case/osch0029.pdf. Downloaded November 18, 2005.

HealthLink. "Three Key Components in Back Injury Prevention," Medical College of Wisconsin Spine Care Clinic. Available online. URL: http://healthlink.mcw.edu/article/1012425715.html. Downloaded November 18, 2005.

Melnik, Michael. *Understanding Your Back Injury.* Rockville, Maryland: The American Occupational Therapy Association, Inc., 1994, pages 2–4.

Milne, Chris, M.D. "Back Injuries—a Patient's Guide," Medic8 ® Family Health Guide. Available online. URL: http://www.medic8.com/healthguide/articles/backinjury.html. Downloaded November 18, 2005.

National Institute for Occupational Safety and Health, The. "Back Belts: Do They Prevent Injury?" NIOSH. Available online. URL: http://www.cdc.gov/niosh/backbelt.html. Downloaded November 18, 2005.

Occupational Safety & Health Administration. "Activity 1: Can Nursing Home Work Be Hazardous to Your Health?" OSHA Healthcare Facilities, Back Facts. Available online. URL: http://www.osha.gov/SLTC/healthcarefacilities/training/activity_1.html. Downloaded November 18, 2005.

backpack safety Over 40 million CHILDREN and ADOLESCENTS lug a backpack during the school year. According to the North American Spine Society (NASS), about half that number carry twice the weight recommended for their age and size. To determine a safe LOAD TOLERANCE, the NASS and other experts on the subject advise that backpacks should not exceed 10 to 15 percent of a person's body weight.

Risks and Complications

Overloading a backpack could cause growing bones to become misshapen, but that risk increases when a child slings a backpack over one shoulder, distributing weight unevenly. Besides this potential for POSTURE problems, other risks include muscle STRAIN, LOW BACK PAIN, pain in the upper back or THORACIC SPINE, BACK INJURY, spinal shifting, and a HERNIATED DISC.

Statistics and Studies

In a survey of 200 chiropractors, Backpack Safety America discovered that 89 percent had treated patients aged five to 18 for back, neck, and shoulder PAIN brought on by heavy backpacks. Among these young patients, the survey reported 126 cases of VERTEBRAL SUBLUXATION and 44 of back SPRAIN or strain. Four patients also exhibited backpack-induced bruising.

Similarly, a fact sheet on the National Safety Council (NSC) Web site reported, "According to the U.S. Consumer Product Safety Commission there were more than 21,000 backpack-related injuries treated at hospital emergency rooms, doctors' offices, and clinics in the year 2003. Injuries ranged from contusions, to sprains and strains to the back and shoulder, and fractures."

Special Aids and Adaptations

How can a child, teen, or parent know when packing too much backpack weight has become too much? The NSC and others concerned about backpack safety noted the importance of noticing postural changes. For instance, a too-heavy pack usually tilts the whole body forward at a 45-degree angle to the ground. Other visual warnings include a student's struggle to put on a backpack or red marks that remain after taking off the pack.

The online article "Backpack Safety," published by KidsHealth, explained, "Your child's spine is made of 33 bones called vertebrae, and between the vertebrae are discs that act as natural shock absorbers. When a heavy weight, such as a backpack filled with books, is incorrectly placed on your child's shoulders, the weight's force can pull your child backward. To compensate, your child may bend forward at the hips or arch his or her back, which can cause your child's spine to compress unnaturally. Because of the heavy weight, your child might begin to develop shoulder, neck, and back pain." In addition, narrow straps can dig into the shoulders, interfering with circulation or causing spinal nerves to tingle. To avoid this, wide padded straps help to distribute weight evenly on both shoulders. Also, properly securing a backpack belt around the waist helps to distribute weight around the whole body.

The American Occupational Therapy Association (AOTA) reminded parents, "School backpacks come in different sizes for different ages. Choose the right size pack for your child's back as well as one with enough room for necessary school items." To determine the correct size, AOTA said, "The bottom of the pack should rest in the curve of the lower back. It should never rest more than four inches below the child's waistline."

The American Academy of Orthopaedic Surgeons (AAOS) advises adjusting the straps to keep the backpack evenly balanced at two inches above the waist and close to the body. Heavier items should be placed closest to the back with compartments used for other objects to avoid shifting weight as the person moves. No matter how well-organized and well-fitted the equipment may be though, no one should bend at the waist when wearing a backpack.

Rolling packs offer a solution for some students, but corridor crowding, unwieldy stairways, or other logistical concerns often prohibit packs on wheels. Regardless, parents and school authorities can find ways to take a load off their child's growing bones. For example, paperback books, compact disks, and computerized texts lighten a burdensome backpack. Adequate time between classes and assurances of safety in the locker room might also encourage students to carry only what they need for the next class. To keep students from carting a library back and forth from home to school, a second set of books may be more affordable when used books can be purchased. Otherwise, photocopying or computer scanning the pages needed for a reading assignment can turn a hefty backpack into a manageable paper weight.

American Academy of Orthopaedic Surgeons. "Backpack Safety," AAOS. Available online. URL: http://www.orthoinfo.org/fact/thr_report.cfm?Thread_ID=105&topcategory=Children. Downloaded November 18, 2005.

American Occupational Therapy Association, The. "Backpack Strategies for Parents and Children, National School Backpack Awareness Day 2005," AOTA. Available online. URL: http://www.promoteot.org/AI_BackpackStrategies.html. Downloaded November 18, 2005.

Backpack Safety America. "Backpack Safety America/International™ North American Chiropractic Survey," September 16, 2002. Available online. URL: http://www.backpacksafe.com/news/doctorsurvey.htm.

Gavin, Mary L., M.D. "Backpack Safety," KidsHealth, Nemours Foundation. Available online. URL: http://kidshealth.org/parent/firstaid_safe/home/backpack.html. Last reviewed August 2004.

North American Spine Society. "The ABCs of Backpacks," NASS. Available online. URL: http://www.spine.org/fsp/backpacking_abc.cfm. Downloaded November 21, 2005.

NSC.org. "Backpack-related Injuries in Children," National Safety Council. Available online. URL: http://www.nsc.org/library/facts/backpack.htm. Updated August 23, 2004.

back pain See ACUTE BACK PAIN, BACKACHE, CHRONIC BACK PAIN, LOW BACK PAIN, SCIATICA.

biofeedback This type of PAIN MANAGEMENT uses various devices to measure physical responses as practitioners guide patients into thoughts and images of restful then stressful situations. With a monitor to display the changes in breathing, blood pressure, heart rate, body temperature, and muscle TENSION, patients can soon see for themselves how quickly their thoughts and feelings affect them, physically.

Procedure

For this noninvasive treatment, a therapist places sensors or electrodes on the skin to obtain readings that help patients recognize and respond to signals from their own bodies. As the Biofeedback Certification Institute of America (BCIA) explained, "Individuals with stress-related disorders learn to relax and improve their overall health. . . . Typically, biofeedback treatment involves a regular series of sessions over a period of several weeks. Some courses of treatment may involve as few as 10 or 15 sessions; other disorders may require 40 or 50. The good news is that biofeedback teaches individuals self regulation. Once the techniques are learned, the patient may never again require biofeedback therapy or only a 'refresher' session now and then."

An online article from the American Academy of Orthopaedic Surgeons (AAOS) Web site mentions biofeedback as a COMPLEMENTARY AND ALTERNATIVE MEDICINE for treating RHEUMATOID ARTHRITIS. To illustrate how the technique works, the article said, "For example, an electromyogram (EMG) machine measures muscle tension. . . . As the muscle tenses, a light flashes or a beep sounds. The intensity of the light or sound varies with the degree of tension in the muscle. To relax the muscle, a patient must first become aware of the body's signals. Then, by using mental processes, the patient can try to slow the flashing or beeping."

Risks and Complications

A MayoClinic.com article advised patients to obtain approval from a doctor before beginning biofeedback. The article also suggested keeping a journal to note symptoms before, during, and after each treatment. Since biofeedback offers a form of mind-body therapy, the article warned that this treatment may not be appropriate for patients with mental problems. Also, biofeedback can interfere with some medications, but then, the treatment can decrease the need for some medications too.

Outlook and Lifestyle Modifications

An article in *Chemist & Druggist* stated, "Biofeedback helps reduce drug dose." This can be particularly important in ELDERLY patients who inappropriately receive medications such as antipsychotic and antispasmodic drugs. Biofeedback may also prove more useful than pharmaceuticals routinely given as a MUSCLE RELAXANT.

Dr. Robert Anderson recounted beneficial effects biofeedback has on the immune system as shown by a study of 41 adults. As he reported, "Biofeedback has little to no downside and facilitates the process of change at profound levels which medications can never do." In another article, "Low back pain and biofeedback," Dr. Anderson discussed a ten-year study of 44 patients. "Initially," he said, "benefits are seen only while biofeedback or any relaxational approach to therapy is actually being practiced. Once they have been practiced long enough to be habitual, the benefits generalize to most of the waking hours. An essential part of the benefits derive from the higher threshold at which subjects respond to stressful stimuli. The training time required varies greatly but usually takes several weeks to several months." Although no one can guarantee success, biofeedback "offers potentially permanent benefits."

American Academy of Orthopaedic Surgeons. "Complementary Therapies: Biofeedback," AAOS. Available online. URL: http://orthoinfo.aaos.org/fact/thr_report.cfm?Thread_ID=272&topcategory=General%20Information. Downloaded November 18, 2005.

Anderson, Robert A., M.D. "Benefits of biofeedback," *Townsend Letter for Doctors and Patients* 265–266 (August–September 2005): 102.

———. "Low Back Pain and Biofeedback," *Townsend Letter for Doctors and Patients* 259–260 (February–March 2005): 48.

Biofeedback Certification Institute of America. "What is Biofeedback?" BCIA. Available online. URL: http://www.bcia.org/pages/index.cfm?pageid=76. Downloaded November 18, 2005.

Hart, Jacqueline A., M.D. "Biofeedback," MedlinePlus, National Institutes of Health. Available online. URL: http://www.nlm.nih.gov/medlineplus/ency/article/002241.htm. Updated December 5, 2003.

MayoClinic.com. "Biofeedback: Using the Power of Your Mind to Improve Your Health," Mayo Clinic Medical Services. Available online. URL: http://www.mayoclinic.com/invoke.cfm?id=SA00083. Updated October 7, 2005.

Staff. "Many Elderly on Inappropriate Medicines," *Chemist & Druggist* (August 14, 2004): 24.

birth defects of the spine   One in every 33 babies born in the United States has a birth defect. The Centers for Disease Control and Prevention (CDC) also state that birth anomalies account for over 20 percent of infant mortalities. To better understand what happens and why, Congress passed the Birth Defects Prevention Act of 1998, which became Public Law 105–168. As the CDC explained, "This bill authorized CDC to (1) collect, analyze, and make available data on birth defects; (2) operate regional centers for applied epidemiologic research on the prevention of birth defects; and (3) inform and educate the public about the prevention of birth defects." By collecting such information in earlier years, the CDC discovered that "mothers who are obese when they become pregnant have a higher risk of serious birth defects of the brain and spine."

Besides the effects of WEIGHT during PREGNANCY, other risk factors for birth defects include womb crowding, lack of FOLIC ACID, poor NUTRITION, GENETIC FACTORS, ENVIRONMENTAL INFLUENCES, and BIRTH INJURY. In addition, newborn INFANTS who show no evidence of spinal problems may exhibit symptoms of GROWTH HORMONE DISORDERS or early onset scoliosis within the first few weeks to the first few years of life.

Risks and Complications

Without adequate information, awareness, and prenatal care, the risk of birth defects increases. For example, teenage girls and young women may not know to abstain from alcohol, drugs, cigarettes, artificial sweeteners, and other synthetic additives, such as food coloring and preservatives. During child-bearing years, nutrients, such as VITAMIN B-COMPLEX, become especially important in preventing such birth defects as SPINA BIFIDA. Fresh water, natural food sources, EXERCISE, and SLEEP have a profound influence on fetal development too. However, this type of prenatal care may be more accurately called pre-pregnancy care since an embryo feels the effects of a lifestyle before most pregnancies have been confirmed.

Within thirty days of conception or less, the SPINE of a fetus begins to form, first as a notochord then as the spinal cord and individual VERTEBRAE. In an online article "Pediatric Spinal Anomalies," a group of doctors from the University of California, San Diego, explained, "Most developmental disorders of the spine occur in either the upper cervical or lower thoracic and lumbar regions. . . . They are found as isolated entities or in combination with one another." As cells multiply rapidly, deviations can occur. For example, the spinal cord may split. Nerves may bind, and adhesions, tumors, fibrous cysts, or spurs may develop instead of vertebral bone.

An eMedicine.com article "Congenital Spinal Deformity" said, "Molecular and cellular tissue interaction and increasing organ complexity characterize the fundamental features of the embryonic developmental process." On a minuscule level, "alteration in the molecular and macromolecular process may lead to structural defects involving the spine and spinal cord. Such defects may occur prenatally, postnatally, or both. These may be divided into 3 categories from the standpoint of basic developmental pathogenesis: malformation, disruption, and deformation." While malformation occurs during the development of the embryo, "disruption is a structural defect resulting from destruction of a part that formed normally during the embryonic period. This mechanism involves the limbs . . . more frequently than the spine during the fetal stage." Finally, "deformation is an alteration in the shape or structure of an individual vertebra or of the entire spine during the fetal and/or postnatal periods," which differs somewhat from congenital SCOLIOSIS. In womb-crowding, for example, "late gestational deformations have an excellent prognosis. Approximately 90% of such deformations noted at birth correct spontaneously." Also, "the earlier a deformation is recognized, the greater the likelihood of correcting it or at least preventing further deformation."

Statistics and Studies

According to the fact sheet "Birth Defects" on the March of Dimes Web site, "About 150,000 babies are born each year with birth defects." Several thousand anomalies have been identified, but causes for 60 to 70 percent remain unknown. As the March of Dimes explained, "Every human being has 20,000 to 25,000 genes that determine traits like eye and hair color, as well as direct the growth and development of every part of our physical and biochemical systems. Genes are packaged into each of the 46 chromosomes inside our cells." Yet, "a single abnormal gene can cause birth defects."

Pre-pregnancy visits and prenatal care may reduce birth defects as doctors offer genetic screening, nutritional counseling, and vaccinating against measles or other illnesses known to cause birth anomalies. Fetal disorders detected through amniocentesis can sometimes be treated prenatally with medications, blood transfusions, or surgery. As the March of Dimes reported, "More than 100 babies have undergone experimental prenatal surgery to repair spina bifida before birth."

Special Aids and Adaptations

Some conditions cannot be adequately treated until a child has reached full growth. However, children born with vertebrae missing from the lumbosacral spine may become ambulatory with early operative treatment. To study this possibility, a group of doctors writing for *The Journal of Bone and Joint Surgery* "reviewed the records and radiographs of eighteen patients with total or partial absence of the lumbar spine and total absence of the sacrum." As the doctors concluded, "patients should have correction of lower extremity deformities as they have a very good potential to walk. The other patients should have operations on the lower extremities only if the deformities preclude sitting or wearing shoes or braces."

X-RAYS and other imaging devices such as MAGNETIC RESONANCE IMAGING (MRI) help to determine a specific diagnosis and also monitor development of spinal misalignment during periods of bone growth. As babies reach the first stages of mobility, devices may be needed to assist crawling and walking. At home, adaptations can usually be made to accommodate a walker, wheelchair, or other aid to mobility.

As WorldOrtho.com reported in "Paediatric Spinal Disorders," ORTHOTIC devices such as a back brace may also assist development. In early onset scoliosis, "bracing does not rectify the problem but does halt rapid progression." Although ARTHRODESIS must often be delayed until teen years, spinal fusion may help 50 percent of the ADOLESCENTS who exhibited scoliosis at birth or shortly thereafter. With congenital KYPHOSIS, however, "posterior fusion is the most effective in children under 5 years with curves less than 50 degrees."

Advances in reconstructive surgery and in research continue to offer possibilities. Since defects rarely replicate themselves from one child to another, unique anomalies have yet to be studied. However, several states have implemented birth defect programs in conjunction with the Centers for Birth Defects Research and Prevention and National Birth Defects Prevention Study. The CDC posted information on those centers at http://www.cdc.gov/ncbddd/bd/nbdps.htm. In addition, information about clinical trials still recruiting patients can be found at http://www.clinicaltrials.gov.

Centers for Disease Control and Prevention. "Birth Defects," CDC, Department of Health and Human Services. Available online. URL: http://www.cdc.gov/node.do/id/0900f3ec8000dffe. Downloaded November 22, 2005.

Guille, James T., M.D., Ricardo Benevides, M.D., Carlos Cuevas DeAlba, M.D., Vijay Siriram, M.D., and S. Jay Kumar, M.D. "Lumbosacral Agenesis: A New Classification Correlating Spinal Deformity and Ambulatory Potential," *The Journal of Bone and Joint Surgery* 84 (2002): 32–38.

Huckstep, R. L. and Eugene Sherry. "Paediatric Spinal Disorders," WorldOrtho.com. Available online. URL: http://www.worldortho.com/database/etext/spinal_disorders.html. Downloaded November 22, 2005.

Letts, Robert Mervyn, M.D. and Ayman Hussein Jawadi. "Congenital Spinal Deformity," eMedicine. Available online. URL: http://www.emedicine.com/orthoped/topic618.htm. Updated September 16, 2004.

March of Dimes. "Birth Defects," Quick References and Fact Sheets, Pregnancy & Newborn Health Education Center, March of Dimes. Available online. URL: http://www.marchofdimes.com/pnhec/4439_1206.asp. Downloaded November 22, 2005.

Peck, Wallace W., M.D., John R. Hesselink, M.D., and A. James Barkovich, M.D., University of California, San Diego. "Pediatric Spinal Anomalies," UCSD, NeuroWeb. Available online. URL: http://spinwarp.ucsd.edu/NeuroWeb/Text/sp-140.htm. Downloaded November 22, 2005.

birth injury to the spine   A difficult labor or the use of such devices as forceps can cause a perfectly healthy newborn to experience a birth injury. Damage most commonly affects a shoulder, but on rare occasions, a FRACTURE or other spinal injury may occur.

Symptoms and Diagnostic Path

If a fracture involves the CERVICAL SPINE, symptoms may include swelling, abnormal movement, and evidence of PAIN. A diagnosis may rely on an X-RAY or other test, such as a COMPUTED TOMOGRAPHY SCAN, to offer detailed imagery of the injured area.

Although rare, a birth injury can affect the SPINAL CORD. In the online article "Spinal Cord Injury," Children's Hospital Boston described typical symptoms: "Initially, the child may experience spinal shock, which causes loss of feeling, muscle movement, and reflexes. As swelling subsides, other symptoms appear depending on the location of the injury. Generally, the higher up the level of the injury to the spinal cord, the more severe the symptoms. For example, an injury on the neck, at C1 or C2 (the first and second vertebrae in the spinal column), affects the respiratory muscles and the ability to breathe, as well as the ability of both the upper and lower extremities to move. A lower injury, in the lumbar vertebrae, may affect the nerve and muscle control to the bladder, bowel, and legs."

Treatment Options and Outlook

If a birth injury causes a cervical fracture, a stabilizing ORTHOTIC brace may be required and, in rare instances, SURGERY. With proper immobilization and prompt treatment, full recovery usually occurs, but the outlook may be less hopeful if a birth injury damages the spinal cord.

In the online article "Spinal Fracture," the Children's Hospital Boston reported, "Most compression fractures are stable (remain in normal alignment) and can be treated without surgery, as long as there is no damage to the spinal cord, by immobilization of the affected area until the fracture heals. Spinal cord injury is a far more complex problem that can cause permanent disability and death in children." More often, however, birth trauma affects the nervous system without lasting impairment.

In the journal article "Healing Birth Trauma: Spinal Misalignment and Your Child," Jennifer Harris discussed VERTEBRAL SUBLUXATION complex (VSC), stating, "VSC occurs when the communication link between the brain and the body has been interfered with. The brain communicates with the body by sending out nerve impulses that flow down the spinal cord and its nerve roots, and a millisecond later, these impulses travel back up again to the brain." If a difficult birth caused vertebrae to shift out of alignment, injured joints may press the spinal nerves, causing muscle spasm or weakened movements in the limbs. However, SPINAL MANIPULATION by a pediatric chiropractor or children's osteopath may relieve or even cure this condition, assuming, of course, that the newborn sustained no fractures during birth.

Risk Factors and Preventive Measures

At Johns Hopkins University, a team of biomedical engineers designed a birthing simulator to find the least forceful way to handle problem deliveries. As *Ascribe Newswire: Health* reported, about five percent of births have injury potential when the baby lodges in the birth canal. "Of these, up to a quarter of deliveries may result in an injury to the baby's brachial plexus, the nerves that control movement and sensation in the arm. As many as 10 percent of infants may sustain some permanent damage." To see what increases that risk, study leader Dr. Edith Gurewitsch performed 30 mock deliveries with a birthing simulator to replicate different obstetrical maneuvers. The first maneuver turned the baby's spine toward the mother's belly. The second placed the baby's spine toward the mother's spine, and the third repositioned the mother's legs. To summarize, *Ascribe Newswire: Health* reported, "The first maneuver was associated with the least amount of force, at 6.5 pounds, to the baby's head necessary to achieve delivery. The other techniques applied 8.5 pounds and 16 pounds, respectively." As this insight arrives in the medical community, more newborns may be delivered from birth injuries.

Children's Hospital Boston. "Spinal Cord Injury," Harvard Medical School. Available online. URL: http://www.childrenshospital.org/az/Site1150/mainpageS1150P0.html. Downloaded November 22, 2005.

———. "Spinal Fracture," Harvard Medical School. Available online. URL: http://www.childrenshospital.org/az/Site1114/mainpageS1114P0.html. Downloaded November 22, 2005.

Harris, Jennifer. "Healing Birth Trauma: Spinal Misalignment and Your Child," *New Life Journal: Carolina Edition* 5, no. 1 (August–September 2004): 8–9.

Staff. "Hopkins-Designed Birth Simulator Helps Physicians Identify Least Forceful Way to Manage Problem Deliveries," *Ascribe Newswire: Health,* (December 22, 2004): 1–3.

bisphosphonates Used to treat OSTEOPENIA, OSTEOPOROSIS, CANCER, and other bone-weakening conditions, this drug category includes ALENDRONATE (Fosamax), IBANDRONATE (Boniva), and RISEDRONATE (Actonel.) As a type of ANTIRESORPTIVE DRUG therapy, bisphosphonates slow bone resorption, thereby reducing bone loss and lessening the risk of FRACTURE.

Risks and Complications

To be effective, bisphosphonate therapy must continue for at least one year, but medical and pharmaceutical databases of 6,825 patients showed irregular usage. With that data in mind, a Roche Laboratories advertisement in *Consultant* and other journals said, "Even with weekly dosing, almost half of all patients on bisphosphonates stop therapy within 12 months." Short-term use not only thwarts the treatment but has the opposite effect intended. As the company warned, "Suboptimal long-term compliance puts patients at increased risk of fracture; in fact, data indicate a 25% greater fracture risk in patients using bisphosphonates [less than or equal to] 75% of the time."

Besides problems caused by sporadic usage, others arose from failure to follow specific instructions. For example, the stomach must be empty. Patients must have a full glass of water with a bisphosphonate. They must wait at least a half hour after taking alendronate or risedronate and at least one hour after taking ibandronate before having any food. During that wait, patients must also remain upright. Anyone who can not adhere to those precise instructions should not take a bisphosphonate, since the risk of gastrointestinal problems or damage to the esophagus increases radically. In addition to those concerns, the National Osteoporosis Foundation reported complications involving visual disturbances and bone problems in or around the jaw.

Statistics and Studies

The July 19, 2005, Medical Study News on News-Medical.Net recounted an analysis of cancer patients involved in "randomized controlled trials that evaluated oral or intravenous bisphosphonates in addition to hormone therapy or chemotherapy." Of these, "all 12 studies that evaluated the rate of bone problems revealed reductions ranging from 14 to 48 percent with bisphosphonate treatment. The study treatment also led to significant lessening of bone pain." If cancer metastasizes in bone, "bisphosphonates can reduce skeletal damage. . . . While the new treatment approach does not improve survival rates, it can minimize disabling fractures, spinal cord compression and pain."

In ELDERLY persons or patients with weakened bone, a disabling VERTEBRAL COMPRESSION FRACTURE can also break the quality of life and length of survival. However, a BONE MINERAL DENSITY (BMD) TEST may help to ascertain the level of risk and appropriate treatment. For example, an article in the *Canadian Medical Association Journal (CMAJ)* said, "It is now well established that taking bisphosphonates leads to consistent increases in . . . BMD, irrespective of the severity of the underlying osteoporosis. Randomized controlled clinical trials . . . demonstrated BMD gains of 4.5%–8.3% at the lumbar spine . . . for patients treated for 3–4 years." By contrast, "patients in the control groups, who are usually treated with calcium and vitamin D supplements, show no clinically significant changes in measured BMD."

Special Aids and Adaptations

CALCIUM, VITAMIN D, and other elements of NUTRITION may not have the desired effect when taken alone after a fracture, but their BONE BUILDING efforts can increase when combined with medication. For example, *Drug Topics* reported, "Alendronate . . . 70 mg/2800 IU (Fosamax Plus D, Merck) tablets have been cleared for the treatment of osteoporosis in postmenopausal women and to increase bone mass in men with osteoporosis." Now available in U.S. pharmacies, "Fosamax Plus D is the only bisphosphonate with a weekly dose of vitamin D."

In Canada, adaptations of another sort may be underway as bisphosphonates become OVER-THE-COUNTER (OTC) PRODUCTS. This has already happened in the United Kingdom. Nevertheless, a group of Canadian doctors considered the pros and cons in an essay for *CMAJ*, commenting, "Within the drug reimbursement policies of most provincial drug plans and private insurance plans, the result of a change in the status of a substantial number of prescription drugs to OTC could mean that a considerable portion of drug costs would be passed on to patients, with reduced costs for private and public insurers. Conversely, because patients with drug plans are more likely to be prescribed a medication that is covered by their plan, the granting of OTC status could promote changes in therapy from older, less expensive drugs that have been granted OTC status (and subsequently become uninsured) to newer, more costly drugs that are available by prescription only." Another possibility warned that "deciding whether to initiate or continue treatment will make patients' nonmedical characteristics (e.g., expected quality of life and health expectations, level of education, and health insurance coverage) much more salient in the decision-making progress." If the U.S. changes the status of bisphosphonates from prescription drugs to OTC products, one might hope this book would speedily reach patients who must decide for themselves which medications would be appropriate for their own BACK and SPINE.

Hodsman, Anthony B., M.D., David A. Hanley, and Robert Josse. "Do Bisphosphonates Reduce the Risk of Osteoporotic Fracture? An Evaluation of the Evidence to Date," *Canadian Medical Association Journal* 166, no. 11 (May 28, 2002): 1,426–1,430.

Lynd, Larry D., M.D., Jeffrey Taylor, Roy Dobson, and Donald J. Willison. "Prescription to Over-the-counter Deregulation in Canada: Are We Ready for It, or Do We Need to Be?" *Canadian Medical Association Journal* 173, no. 7 (September 27, 2005): 775–777.

News-Medical.net. "New Protective Drugs Called Bisphosphonates Reduce Pain and Fractures in Metastatic Breast Cancer, " Medical Study News, published July 19, 2005. Available online. URL: http://www.news-medical.net/?id=11842. Downloaded November 26, 2005.

NOF.org. "Medications to Prevent & Treat Osteoporosis," National Osteoporosis Foundation. Available online. URL: http://www.nof.org/patientinfo/medications.htm. Downloaded November 25, 2005.

Roche Laboratories, Inc., advertisement. "Either Way You Look at It, There's a Persistence Problem with Bisphosphonate Therapy," *Consultant* 45, no. 8 (July 2005): 837.

Staff. "New Fosamax Formulation also Contains Vitamin D," *Drug Topics* 149, no. 9 (May 2, 2005): 10.

bone break   See FRACTURES.

bone building   Bone strength begins as CHILDREN build a bone bank their bodies will ultimately draw from throughout life. For instance, bone building NUTRITION emphasizes natural sources of CALCIUM, VITAMIN D, and OMEGA-3 fatty acids. Although dietary needs differ among INFANTS, ADOLESCENTS, and ELDERLY persons, age-appropriate foods and daily ACTIVITY continue to strengthen bone mass and, later, slow the loss of bone density that occurs over time. As explained by the article "Bone Health" posted by the Centers for Disease Control and Prevention, "Peak bone mass refers to the genetic potential for bone density" that can be maximized with good nutrition and WEIGHT-BEARING EXERCISE. Conversely, "inadequate calcium consumption and physical activity early on could result in a failure to achieve peak bone mass in adulthood."

Risks and Complications

According to the article "Tips on Maintaining a Healthy Bone Mass" posted on the Back.com Web site, "Approximately 99 percent of the calcium in the body is stored in the bones and teeth. The other one percent is used to help carry out other essential bodily functions, such as enabling the heart and other muscles to contract. A deficient level of calcium in the blood causes the body to take the calcium it needs for these bodily functions from our bones in order to keep a constant level in the blood stream." When the body has what it needs, new bone cells replace old ones in ongoing cycles of about 90 days. However, Back.com reminded readers, "A decrease in the intake of sodium can also help maintain healthy bone mass." Otherwise, "sodium can strip bones of their calcium," thereby causing bone loss instead of the bone building desired.

With a disruption in MINERAL BALANCE, loss of calcium, and eventually, loss of bone, the risks increase for a VERTEBRAL COMPRESSION FRACTURE. Yet no symptoms may occur until a bone actually breaks. To keep that potentially serious problem from going undetected, a BONE MINERAL DENSITY (BMD) TEST can show if bone loss has occurred and, if so, to what degree. When needed, ANTIRESORPTIVE DRUGS, HORMONE REPLACEMENT THERAPY (HRT), or PARATHYROID HORMONE (PTH) may be prescribed to slow bone loss and aid bone rebuilding.

Every drug carries potential side effects, but a larger risk may come in letting bone loss con-

tinue without treatment. Unchecked, ENVIRONMENTAL INFLUENCES, SPINAL INFECTIONS, CANCER, and other conditions, such as OSTEOGENESIS IMPERFECTA, OSTEOARTHRITIS, OSTEOPENIA, or OSTEOPOROSIS, reduce bone strength in the BACK and SPINE. Smoking and alcohol consumption adversely affect vertebral bone mass, too, as can menopause, normal aging, poor POSTURE, and a sedentary lifestyle. Growing teenagers and children with bone loss caused by EATING DISORDERS remain at especially high risk, not only in the present but in the future condition of their bones.

Statistics and Studies

Cultural and socio-economic factors also affect bone density. In an article for *BMC Family Practice,* medical faculty from Dicle University in Turkey addressed "the relationship between educational level and bone mineral density in postmenopausal women." For the study, "a total of 569 postmenopausal women, at 45 to 86 years of age . . . were considered," along with the results of a standardized interview "to obtain information on demographic, life-style, reproductive and menstrual histories" Reportedly, "the findings of this study imply that osteoporosis which is related to bone mineral density, may be related to the educational level and the risks due to higher birth rate, excessive breast-feeding and insufficient calcium intake, and may be controlled through an improvement in educational level." As the study concluded, "Losses in BMD for women of lower educational level tend to be relatively high, and losses in spine . . . BMD showed a decrease with increasing educational level."

Age may be a factor, too, as most teenagers do not consume enough calcium during peak periods of bone growth. An online article from the National Institutes of Health Osteoporosis and Related Bone Disease warned, "Calcium deficiencies in young people can account for a 5 to 10 percent difference in peak bone mass and can increase the risk for hip fracture later in life. Surveys indicate that teenage girls in the United States are less likely than teenage boys to get enough calcium. In fact, less than 10 percent of girls ages 9 to 17 are actually getting the calcium they need each day." This has particular significance, since "up to 90 percent of peak bone mass is acquired by age 18 in girls and age 20 in boys, which makes youth the best time to 'invest' in your bone health."

Studies from the United Kingdom concurred. As the MRC Human Research Center explained, "After peak bone mass is reached, bone mass starts to decline." However, "60–70% of the variation in peak bone mass between individuals is related to genetics and about 30–40% to environmental factors during fetal life, childhood and/or adolescence such as diet and physical activity."

Special Aids and Adaptations

An article in *The Journal of Musculoskeletal Medicine* reported, "Physical activity is the only known intervention that has the potential to increase bone mass and strength in younger persons and reduce the risk of falling in older persons, according to a position stand released by the American College of Sports Medicine (ACSM)." The article also stated, "High-intensity, high-impact activities are recommended for children to build bone. Moderate to high-intensity weight-bearing activities are recommended for adults to maintain bone mass." In addition, the ACSM position "notes that bone health is important for men as well as women, because the predicted increase in falls and osteoporotic fractures in men is even greater than in women. Weight-bearing physical activities are recommended for even the most frail and elderly persons, as long as they can perform them safely."

Besides the natural aids of exercise and nutrition, two primary types of drugs assist bone building. To summarize, Internet information from the American Medical Association (AMA) said, "Antiresorptive drugs reduce bone loss, while anabolic agents stimulate new bone formation." As the AMA explained, "Antiresorptive therapies include bisphosphonates, estrogen, selective estrogen receptor modulators (SERMs), and calcitonin. These agents act to lessen the risk of bone fracture by decreasing bone turnover, reducing bone loss, and stabilizing bone microarchitecture."

Additional treatment options may be forthcoming as an aging population adapts to a longer life expectancy. Meanwhile, the U.S. Department of Health and Human Services has assessed a communal need for bone building. As stated in the Executive Summary of *Bone Health and Osteoporosis: A Report from the Surgeon General,* "There are four distinct systems-based activities that collectively encompass the overall goal of improving bone health status of Americans: ~ Identifying and developing intervention strategies for various risk levels of the population. ~ Educating and raising awareness among clinicians and the public about bone disease. ~ Ensuring that individuals receive appropriate preventative, diagnostic, and treatment services based upon their level of risk. ~ Monitoring and evaluating bone health outcomes within populations and the community." As governmental agencies, medical professionals, and international groups work to increase public awareness, most people can naturally rely on meeting their own basic needs and establishing a healthy lifestyle to support their bone building efforts.

American Medical Association. "Summary, Osteoporosis Management: Pharmacologic Prevention and Treatment of Osteoporosis," AMA. Available online. URL: http://www.ama-cmeonline.com/osteo_mgmt/module05/09sum/. Downloaded November 28, 2005.

Centers for Disease Control and Prevention. "Bone Health: Home," CDC, Department of Health and Human Resources. Available online. URL: http://www.cdc.gov/nccdphp/dnpa/bonehealth/. Downloaded November 28, 2005.

Gur, Ali, Ayşegül Jale Sarac, Kemal Nas, and Remzi Cevik. "The Relationship Between Educational Level and Bone Mineral Density in Postmenopausal Women," *BMC Family Practice* 5, no. 18 (September 2004).

MCR, Human Nutrition Research, U.K. "Peak Bone Mass." Available online. URL: http://www.mrc-hnr.cam.ac.uk/research/bone_health/pbm.html. Downloaded November 28, 2005.

Medtronic Sofamor Danek. "Tips on Maintaining a Healthy Bone Mass," Back.com. Available online. URL: http://www.back.com/articles-tips.html. Updated February 17, 2005.

National Institutes of Health Osteoporosis and Related Bone Diseases. "Osteoporosis—Peak Bone Mass in Women," NIH National Resource Center. Available online. URL: http://www.osteo.org/newfile.asp?doc=r701i&doctitle=Peak+Bone+Mass+in+Women&doctype=HTML+Fact+Sheet. Last revised March 2005.

Staff, Clinical Update, in Musculoskeletal Medicine. "Physical Activity for Lifelong Bone Health," *The Journal of Musculoskeletal Medicine* 22 (January 2005): 6.

U.S. Department of Health and Human Services. *Bone Health and Osteoporosis: A Report from the Surgeon General.* Rockville, Md.: U.S. Department of Health and Human Services, Office of the Surgeon General (2004): 17.

bone cancer   See CANCER; SPINAL TUMOR.

bone density   See BONE BUILDING.

bone graft   This procedure typically assigns an autograft (bone from one's own body) or allograft (bone from a donor) to an awaiting space. For instance, a bone FRACTURE or SPINAL INJURY may need a graft to mend a gap in or around a bone. To strengthen and hold a joint, real bone or a synthetic version may be grafted during a surgical procedure such as ARTHRODESIS or LUMBAR SPINAL FUSION. As an article in the *Mayo Clinic Health Letter* explained, "Bone and other materials used in bone grafts either serve as structural scaffolding on which bone cells can form bone or act to stimulate cells to form bone." According to the article, "more than 2 million bone grafts are done each year in America."

Procedure

With a minimally invasive bone graft, the procedure begins not with a scalpel but a needle. As the article "Minimally Invasive Bone Grafting" explained, "The goals and principles of bone grafting is the same, in the conventional bone grafting procedures, and these new minimally invasive procedures. Only the way in which the graft is delivered to the site differs. There are currently only three injectable graft materials available: bone marrow, setting calcium phosphate cements, and . . . allograft bone matrix gel. . . . Bone marrow cells can . . . be used to supplement the healing in a new fresh fracture." To this, bone matrix gel may be added for support. Also, "several formulations of injectable pastes of calcium and phosphate are now available. After injection, these pastes will set firmly, like a cast, but inside the body. The calcium and phosphate in the paste form a hard mass of calcium phosphate ceramic, which is very similar to the mineral found in bone."

Unfortunately, minimally invasive grafts do not work on every patient. For example, scar tissue may invade the space and prevent healing. Therefore, most bone grafts or transplants require a larger surgical incision to expose the defective or injured site. When the size and shape of the damaged area has been ascertained, the graft is shaped accordingly then inserted into or around the awaiting space. Often, pins, plates, or screws of appropriate materials will be inserted, too, to keep the graft from slipping and to hold the area steady until the bone graft heals and fuses the surgical area.

Risks and Complications

Sometimes a graft slips during recovery as the person becomes more active, in which case additional SURGERY may be needed. As with any surgical procedure, risks commonly include bleeding, infection, or reaction to medication. If an allograft has been used, rejection of the donor bone can also occur, although this, too, is rare.

Stringent guidelines prevent potential problems with the new bone itself. In discussing the risk of inserting a virus or bacteria along with an allograft, an article from the American Academy of Orthopaedic Surgeons (AAOS) explained, "The information collected on potential donors is compared against criteria established by the United States Public Health Service to identify and exclude individuals with high-risk behaviors. Furthermore, all tissue is held in quarantine until microbiological and blood tests are completed. . . . The allograft is then soaked in various solutions to prevent the transmission of bacteria and viruses." Low dose radiation may also be used to assure sterilization. Another article on the AAOS Web site thoroughly addressed an "overview of allograft soft tissue processing" and provided a list of centers accredited by the American Association of Tissue Banks.

Sometimes an allograft must be obtained because the age or poor health of the patient makes an autograft too risky. For example, an infection anywhere in the body may rule out safe use of the person's own bone. If an autograft can be used, the procedure requires an additional incision. Dr. Jeffrey C. Wang and Mary Clare Walsh explained that a patient may then experience "pain and soreness which often last well after the surgery is healed, as well as possible complications such as increased blood loss and prolonged time in the operating room. Complications such as these occur in about 10%–35% of patients and vary in their severity."

Outlook and Lifestyle Modifications

As scientists continue to research alternatives to bone grafts, an article on the North American Spine Society Web site mentioned demineralized bone matrix which "contains collagen, proteins and growth factors . . . extracted from the allograft bone." Extensive processing assures "little risk for disease transmission," but the material does not yet maintain optimal strength. However, "a newer area of bone graft substitutes, graft composites use combinations of other bone grafting materials and/or bone growth factors to gain the benefits of a variety of substances. Among the combinations in use are a collagen/ceramic composite, which closely reproduces the composition of natural bone." Also, "bone morphogenetic proteins (BMPs) are produced in our bodies and regulate bone formation and healing. Scientists have discovered that these proteins can speed up healing as well as limit the negative reaction some people have to donor bone and the nonbone substitutes." BONE MORPHOGENETIC PROTEINS offer a promising outlook for improving the success of fusions, particularly in small areas of the neck or spine.

For areas that need a larger bone transplant, innovative researchers applied a harmless but active virus to bone from cadaver donors. As explained in an online article posted by the University of Rochester Medical Center, this "method triggers the tissue surrounding the graft to produce . . . proteins continuously for up to three weeks, long enough for the body to trigger the perpetual bone remodeling response." Subsequently, "New blood vessels begin to grow around and into the bone splint, stripping it down in times when the body needs the calcium, and rebuilding it when calcium levels rise. The bone that is rebuilt is now fully the patient's own, as if the dead bone were a house being renovated by replacing a single brick at a time without tearing the whole structure apart."

With or without the latest procedures in bone grafts, most patients recover within several weeks. Energetic EXERCISE may be limited for up to four months, with long-term improvement depending on the quality of bone graft and type of defect or injury. Up-to-date methods undoubtedly affect the success of a graft. However, patients aid their healing by refraining from smoking, modifying lifestyles as needed, and maintaining the BONE BUILDING balance of NUTRITION and daily ACTIVITY.

American Academy of Orthopaedic Surgeons. "What Can You Tell Me About Bone and Tissue Transplantation?" AAOS. Available online. URL: http://orthoinfo.aaos.org/brochure/thr_report.cfm?Thread_ID=53&topcategory=Gene ral% 20Information. Downloaded November 29, 2005.

Cleveland Clinic Health Information Center, The. "Minimally Invasive Bone Grafting," SpineUniverse.com. Available online. URL: http://www.spineuniverse.com/displayarticle.php/article2019.html. Last updated April 26, 2005.

North American Spine Society. "Bone Graft Alternatives," NASS. Available online. URL: http://www.spine.org/articles/bone_grafts.cfm. Downloaded November 29, 2005.

Staff. "Bone Transplants," *Mayo Clinic Health Letter* 23, no. 12 (December 2005): 4–5.

University of Rochester Medical Center. "Gene Therapy Converts Dead Bone Graft to New, Living Tissue," News Archives, Friday, February 18, 2005. Available online. URL: http://www.urmc.rochester.edu/pr/news/story.cfm?id=734. Updated November 2, 2005.

Vangsness, C. Thomas Jr., M.D. "Overview of Allograft Soft Tissue Processing," American Academy of Orthopaedic Surgeons (AAOS) Bulletin. Available online. URL: http://www2.aaos.org/aaos/archives/bulletin/feb04/feature1.htm.

Wang, Jeffrey C., M.D. and Mary Clare Walsh. "Bone Grafts: No Longer Just a Chip Off the Ol' Hip," Spine Universe.com. Available online. URL: http://www.spineuniverse.com/displayarticle.php/article1766.html. Last updated April 20, 2004.

bone mass   See BONE BUILDING.

bone mineral density (BMD) tests   Noninvasive and painless, bone mineral density tests use QUANTITATIVE COMPUTED TOMOGRAPHY (QCT) or various types of ABSORPTIOMETRY to assess bone mass and ascertain the likelihood of FRACTURE. For example, QCT measures the SPINE and, sometimes, other sites. Quantitative ultrasound uses sound waves to measure small areas such as the heel, whereas dual energy X-ray absorptiometry (DEXA) assesses BMD in the spine or total body. Although seldom used, dual photon absorptiometry can confirm or contest bone weakening in the spine.

Risks and Complications

BMD tests using radiation present only a minimal risk of exposure. A greater risk comes in not detecting OSTEOPENIA, OSTEOPOROSIS, or other condition of bone loss, thus increasing the likelihood of a VERTEBRAL COMPRESSION FRACTURE. ELDERLY or other patients who have easily broken a bone may be at particularly high risk, as are those with circulatory problems, kidney conditions, and RHEUMATOID ARTHRITIS. Steroid use can also thin bones. In addition, postmenopausal women who do not take estrogen but have a family history of bone frailty may be at greater risk for fractures.

Patients with SCOLIOSIS or skeletal deformity risk getting false test results as do CHILDREN or adults who are small in stature. This occurs partly because the equipment may not adapt to special needs and also because the test results depend on comparative analysis. For example, a BMD reading gives a Z-score that compares bone density to that of other people the same age, while a T-score shows a standard deviation (SD) above or below the peak bone mass acquired in youth. To explain this concern, the article "Osteoporosis Tests" on the American Academy of Orthopaedic Surgeons (AAOS) Web site said, "As a general rule, for every SD below normal the fracture risk doubles. Thus, a patient with a BMD of 1 SD below normal (a T-score of -1) has 2 times the risk of fracture as a person with a normal BMD. If the T-score is -2 the risk of fracture is 4 times normal. A T-score of -3 is 8 times the normal fracture risk." However, differences in comparatives, manufacturers, and software produce varying conclusions.

Differences also arise because of the site tested. As the AAOS article explained, "One of the problems with peripheral testing is that only one site is tested and low bone density in the hip or spine may be missed." Furthermore, "discordance in BMD among various skeletal sites is more common in the years just following menopause. BMD may be normal at one site and low at another site. In these early postmenopausal years, bone density in the spine decreases first because the turnover in this . . . bone is higher than other skeletal sites. Bone density at various skeletal sites begins to coincide at about age 70." Therefore, "in early post menopausal women . . . up to the age of about 65, the most accurate site to measure is probably the spine. In older women over the age of 65, the concordance of skeletal sites is much closer and it may not make much difference which site is measured." However, "caution must be used in interpreting spine scans in elderly patients because of degenerative changes falsely elevating the BMD values."

With any patient, variations in readings can occur. For example, a comprehensive article entitled "Bone Mass Measurement Techniques in Clinical Practice" in *Topics in Geriatric Rehabilitation* said that three "lumbar spine bone density studies performed within minutes of each other on the same patient will not produce identical results no matter how carefully the studies were performed." This could notably affect comparisons between a baseline reading and a follow-up BMD test done a year or two later.

Complication of irregularities in BMD readings may soon change. For example, a staff article in the *Southern Medical Journal* announced a high-resolution spinal imaging modality called RVA, an acronym for Radiologic Vertebral Assessment. For those assessing a patient's osteoporotic fracture risk, "RVA also aids physicians in better differentiating benign degenerative changes in the spine, from osteoporotic fractures caused by fragility." As the news release pointed out, "The radiograph is the established tool to visualize vertebral deformations. However, higher dose, and the need to perform a separate procedure, has resulted in two out of three fractures being undiagnosed."

Statistics and Studies

With fracture prevention as the primary goal of BMD tests, new equipment or methods measure bone mass with greater accuracy, but researchers from Georgetown University took another tack. Instead of typical bone mineral density tests, they used the same equipment on 26 participants to measure bone marrow fat. According to their report in the *American Journal of Roentgenology,* correlations can be found between increased bone marrow fat and increases in bone loss.

At present, people seldom equate bone marrow with bone narrowing. Regardless of the method used, an article in the *Current Women's Health Reports* reported some alarming statistics by saying, "Unfortunately, an estimated 18 million women with low bone mass have yet to be diagnosed or treated." However, "it has been estimated that 50% of white women older than 50 will experience an osteoporosis-related fracture in their lifetime. Overall, the disorder is responsible for 1.5 million fractures annually, including 700,000 at the vertebral site."

Special Aids and Adaptations

"Surprisingly, there is still debate about what constitutes a vertebral fracture," according to an article in *Radiology.* The same article thoroughly discussed BMD tests, including adaptations that must be made from one machine, one test, one patient, and, yes, one season to the next. "Such small differences become important when it is realized that physiologic and therapeutic changes in mineralization may amount to no more than 0.5% per year. Likewise, there are winter losses and summer gains in BMD, especially in more northerly latitudes, of about 1%." Because of those minimal changes, a follow-up BMD will seldom be warranted before two years. Even then, "it is also important to recognize that reporting of T scores in patients undergoing treatment to build bone mass is not entirely valid and may mislead about the scale of fracture risk." For example, "the data from several trials indicate that drugs such as the bisphosphonates and selective estrogen receptor modulators produce a drop in fracture rates in excess of that expected on the basis of any increase in BMD that results from treatment." After expressing hope for the aid of diagnostic tools that examine bone architecture in greater detail, the article summarized the importance of basing individual adaptations and lifestyle modifications "on the patient's history and physical, radiologic, and biochemical examination results . . . synthesized into a comprehensive index of risk."

Bonnick, S. L. "Bone Mass Measurement Techniques in Clinical Practice: Methods, Applications, and Interpretation," *Topics in Geriatric Rehabilitation* 21, no. 1 (January–March 2005): 30–41.

Kaufman, John D., M.D. "Osteoporosis Tests," American Academy of Orthopaedic Surgeons. Available online. URL: http://orthoinfo.aaos.org/fact/thr_report.cfm?Thread_ID=176&topcategory=Osteoporosis. Downloaded November 29, 2005.

Lentle, Brian C., M.D. and Jerilynn C. Prior, M.D. "Osteoporosis: What a Clinician Expects to Learn from a Patient's Bone Density Examination," *Radiology* 228, no. 3 (September 2003): 620–628.

Placide, Jon, M.D. and Mark G. Martens, M.D. "Comparing Screening Methods for Osteoporosis," *Current Women's Health Reports* 3, no. 3 (May–June 2003): 207–210.

Schellinger, D., C. S. Lin, J. Lim, H. G. Hatipoglu, J. C. Pezzullo, and A. J. Singer. "Bone Marrow Fat and Bone Mineral Density on Proton MR Spectroscopy and Dual-Energy X-Ray Absorptiometry: Their Ratio as a New Indicator of Bone Weakening," *American Journal of Roentgenology* 183, no. 6 (December 2004): 1,761–1,765.

Staff. "Hologic Introduces RVA, a New High-resolution Spinal Imaging Modality Available Exclusively on Discovery Series Bone Densitometers," *Southern Medical Journal* 98, no. 2 (February 2005): 260.

bone morphogenetic protein (BMP)   Found in trace amounts in human bone, this specific protein has been clinically proven to assist bone growth and healing. Although retrieval from living bone was tedious and costly, this was the only accessible method for over twenty years as the discoverer of the protein, Dr. Marshall Urist, labored in the Bone Research Lab at UCLA Medical School. Eventually, the work he began in 1965 advanced into the operating rooms of every up-to-date orthopedic surgeon. Before the use of bone morphogenetic protein (BMP) could become readily available though, it had to be synthetically produced.

"To solve this problem of finite supply," the Spine Institute of New York explained that a version of naturally occurring BMP can be manufactured as recombinant human bone morphogenetic protein 2 or rhBMP-2. "Instead of using bone harvested from other parts of the patient's body to generate bone growth in the spine, doctors insert rhBMP-2 between two or more vertebrae. This insertion induces bone growth and causes the vertebrae to fuse together, re-establishing spinal stability and alleviating pain caused by pressure on the nerves."

Not only does BMP induce fusion in the implanted site, this unique protein completes natural healing in less time than does autograft bone taken from a patient's own body. According to an article by Dr. Setti S. Rengachary, "In humans, healing is complete by 8 to 10 weeks as opposed to 12 to 16 weeks when autograft is used." Furthermore, "the quality of BMP-induced bone is comparable with and is indistinguishable from the natural bone." There is a difference though. As Dr. Rengachary explained, "Under normal conditions in the absence of BMP the bone growth occurs from the bone margins of the gap to be filled and progressively creeps from the ends toward the center." Conversely, BMP-induced bone transforms inflammatory cells into bone-making cells that "freely cross the gap in a concurrent fashion and lay down bone simultaneously to close the gap."

Risks and Complications

This unique, water-soluble protein diffuses easily in body fluids, which makes it highly adaptable, but some type of carrier must contain BMP in order to confine it to the desired site. As Dr. Rengachary explained, "Uncontrollable bone growth in the vicinity of the neural structures, especially nerve roots and cauda equina, is a potential problem. This can only be solved using efficient carriers that bind the protein tightly." However, the carrier must not trigger an immune reaction and must be absorbable with no residue after the site has healed. In addition, Dr. Rengachary noted the unknown risk to a developing embryo, which may exclude pregnant women from BMP treatment.

Statistics and Studies

Clinical trials on the synthetic form of BMP have begun to study such matters as the best carrier devices to use and the optimal amount of BMP to be delivered to a site. The North American Spine Society reported, "Although the Food and Drug Administration has not fully approved the use of BMPs, many clinical trials have found the substance to be effective in generating bone in the spine. Current research is also focusing on the most effective method of introducing the substance into the spine, such as collagen sponges. . . . The research is ongoing and the spine community is encouraged by BMPs and hopes they may someday reduce postsurgical pain and improve the effectiveness of spinal surgeries." At such time, statistical data will undoubtedly become available.

Special Aids and Adaptations

BMP is itself an adaptation of a natural process. As an article on the Back.com Web site said, "Bone is made up of about 65–70% mineral and 30–35% organic matrix." Once Urist discovered that bone could be demineralized and the remaining organic matrix used to promote bone formation, further RESEARCH began to consider appropriate applications. For example, "new bone formation is required to achieve a successful spinal fusion. Without bone growth, a patient will not obtain a solid fusion and the pain that was the main reason behind having the surgery in the first place will not be relieved." However, the Back.com article concluded on this encouraging note, "A huge amount of resources are currently being devoted to developing a BMP alternative to patient harvested bone as part of a spinal fusion surgery." At present, many fusion surgeries of the spine using BMP have an excellent rate of success.

Medtronic Sofamor Danek. "Bone Morphogenetic Proteins (BMP)," Back.com. Available online. URL: http://www.back.com/articles-bmp.html. Updated February 17, 2005.

North American Spine Society. "Bone Morphogenetic Protein," NASS. Available online. URL: http://www.spine.org/articles/NT_Bone_Morph_Protein.cfm. Downloaded November 29, 2005.

Rengachary, Setti S., M.D. "Bone Morphogenetic Proteins: Basic Concepts," *Neurosurgery Focus* 13, no. 6 (December 2002).

Spine Institute of New York. "BMP (Bone Graft)," Beth Israel Medical Center. Available online. URL: http://www.spineinstituteny.com/research/bmp.html. Downloaded November 29, 2005.

bone scan To assess SPINAL TUMORS, SPINAL INFECTIONS, FRACTURES, CANCER, or other bone conditions of the SPINE, this type of radionuclide imaging offers a more accurate image than an X-RAY usually provides. A scan can also detect OSTEITIS DEFORMANS, ARTHRITIS, RICKETS, and other sources of bone PAIN.

Procedure

With no preparation but the removal of jewelry and other metals, a patient undergoes a procedure as described on the Spine Institute of New York Web site: "during a bone scan, a radioactive chemical is injected into the bloodstream." In about three hours, "this chemical adheres to parts of the bone which are undergoing rapid changes. After a gamma camera scans the area, these parts show up as dark areas on the film."

A full body scan takes less than an hour. Once the affected area has been located, additional tests may be recommended. For example, Spine-health.com said, "Bone scans . . . cannot distinguish what a lesion represents, and therefore cannot differentiate between a tumor, an infection or a fracture. Therefore, this type of imaging study usually needs to be followed by a CT scan and/or MRI scan to better characterize the lesion."

Risks and Complications

With radiation lower than the amount in an X-ray, a bone scan carries a minimal risk of exposure. This does, however, present risks to an unborn child, so women must avoid this test during PREGNANCY. Also, some patients may experience an allergic reaction to use of the dye.

Outlook and Lifestyle Modifications

To wash the unused radioactive material from the system, patients should drink several glasses of water after the test. According to MayoClinic.com, radioactivity disappears in one to three days, during which time new mothers should refrain from nursing their INFANTS. Otherwise, most patients experience no side effects nor need for additional care except individual treatment of the condition.

MayoClinic.com. "Bone Scan: Using Nuclear Medicine to Look for Bone Abnormalities," Mayo Clinic Health Information. Available online. URL: http://www. mayoclinic.com/health/bone-scan/CA00020. Updated October 27, 2005.

Spinasanta, Susan. "Bone Scan," SpineUniverse.com. Available online. URL: http://www.spineuniverse. com/displayarticle.php/article245.html. Last updated June 2, 2004.

Spine-health.com. "Bone Scan." Available online. URL: http://www.spine-health.com/topics/diag/diag09. html. Downloaded December 2, 2005.

Spine Institute of New York. "Bone Scan," Beth Israel Medical Center. Available online. URL: http://www. spineinstituteny.com/conditions/bonescan.html. Downloaded November 29, 2005.

bone spur See OSTEOPHYTE.

brace, back See ORTHOTICS.

brace, neck See ORTHOTICS.

brachial plexus injury The seven bones of the CERVICAL SPINE accommodate the brachial plexus nerves that travel down the neck and into the shoulder. If an injury occurs in that area, the condition may be referred to as a burner or stinger, mainly because that describes the type of pain typically felt.

Symptoms and Diagnostic Path

When the head has been shoved or the neck pushed aside too quickly, burning or stinging pain may shoot down the arms. After performing a physical examination, a physician may request an X-RAY, COMPUTED TOMOGRAPHY (CT) SCAN, or MAGNETIC RESONANCE IMAGING (MRI) to rule out a FRACTURE. If the arms or hands feel weak or numb, an ELECTROMYOGRAM (EMG) or a NERVE CONDUCTION STUDY may be needed to detect any damage to the muscles or nerves.

Treatment Options and Outlook

Until a doctor has confirmed a brachial plexus injury, the area should be immobilized and precautions taken as for a suspected SPINAL INJURY. After a diagnosis, an ice pack can be applied for about

20 minutes every three to four hours. When pain subsides in two to three days, HEAT THERAPY generally replaces COLD THERAPY, especially if the neck muscles feel stiff and achy. A physician may also prescribe NONSTEROIDAL ANTI-INFLAMMATORY DRUG (NSAID) THERAPY or other PAIN RELIEVER. If the injury caused VERTEBRAL SUBLUXATION with no bone fracture, a chiropractor or osteopath may perform SPINAL MANIPULATION to ease neck VERTEBRAE into place. MASSAGE THERAPY may lessen the discomfort too.

Risk Factors and Preventive Measures

STRENGTH TRAINING acts as a preventive and addresses the spinal concerns of ATHLETES who engage in contact sports. EXERCISE designed to strengthen the neck can reduce the risk of a brachial plexus injury, but a helmet will not prevent one when contact comes head-on. If a stinger does occur, rest and prompt treatment score the quickest goal of recovery.

Rouzier, Pierre, M.D., for McKesson Provider Technologies. "Brachial Plexus Injury (Stinger/Burner)," University of Michigan Health System. Available online. URL: http://www.med.umich.edu/1libr/sma/sma_stinger_sma.htm. Last modified April 19, 2005.

Smith, Carrie Myers. "Burner or Stinger (Brachial Plexus Injury)," Holy Cross Hospital. Available online. URL: http://healthychoice.epnet.com/GetContent.asp?siteid=holycross&docid=/dci/burner. Last reviewed September 2005. Downloaded December 2, 2005.

brittle bone disease   See OSTEOGENESIS IMPERFECTA.

bulimia   See EATING DISORDERS, BONE LOSS CAUSED BY.

calcitonin This naturally occurring hormone regulates bone metabolism and CALCIUM absorption throughout the body. The manufactured form of calcitonin offers a type of ANTIRESORPTIVE DRUG therapy and provides an older alternative to the BISPHOSPHONATE drugs commonly prescribed to treat bone loss.

An article on the Web site of the American Medical Association (AMA) explained, "Continuous use of calcitonin is associated with a persistent decrease in the rate of bone resorption," thus reducing the loss of bone mass. "Calcitonin is also thought to have an analgesic effect on bone pain associated with vertebral fractures. For this reason, calcitonin is often used to treat the pain associated with acute vertebral fragility fractures."

Dosage and Potential Side Effects

Doses vary, depending on the form of calcitonin and the age of the patient. Originally designed as an injection, approval later arrived for a nasal spray of salmon calcitonin to treat OSTEOPOROSIS and prevent VERTEBRAL COMPRESSION FRACTURE. While the spray can irritate sensitive sinus passages, an injection brings potential side effects of an upset stomach or nausea. Rare side effects of a severe nosebleed, chills, fever, weakness, or respiratory problems should be reported to a doctor right away.

Statistics and Studies

According to the AMA article, "the largest randomized controlled trial of nasal calcitonin . . . demonstrated a reduction in vertebral fractures for those individuals taking 200 IU/d, but there was no significant decline for those receiving 100 or 400 IU" per day. Although the drug may lessen the risk of bone FRACTURES in general, the AMA reported, "Intranasal calcitonin has not been shown to sig-

nificantly decrease nonvertebral fracture rates after 5 years."

ELDERLY patients often receive calcitonin, but specific studies of that age group have not been made, nor have studies of CHILDREN or unborn INFANTS. If studies of animals provide an indicator though, an infant's birth weight may be slightly lower when the mother takes calcitonin. Nevertheless, pregnant women with conditions such as OSTEITIS DEFORMANS or patients who cannot take bisphosphonates or HORMONE REPLACEMENT THERAPY may need calcitonin to strengthen bones and assist BONE BUILDING.

American Medical Association. "Antiresorptive Therapy: Calcitonin," AMA. Available online. URL: http://www.ama-cmeonline.com/osteo_mgmt/module05/06anti/index.htm. Downloaded December 2, 2005.

Thompson MICROMEDEX. "Calcitonin (Systemic)," MedlinePlus Drugs, National Institutes of Health. Available online. URL: http://www.nlm.nih.gov/medlineplus/druginfo/uspdi/202106.html. Last updated October 27, 2005.

calcium Can milk give a person backbone? Maybe. Whether from milk or other natural sources, calcium builds bones that, in turn, store the mineral for use throughout the body. In the BACK, SPINE, or elsewhere, bones do not provide a warehouse so much as a "where-housed?" In other words, bone calcium acts as a distribution center to provide whatever the body consumes. As with any item a consumer needs, the demands can be high.

Besides bone formation, a body needs calcium to maintain a regular heartbeat, appropriately clot the blood, prevent muscle cramps, and activate nerves for movement. Calcium also offers a calming effect that soothes aching joints and enables a body to SLEEP, unless something disrupts the process. For example, caffeine, alcohol, table salt, and white flour can cause calcium loss, while sugars, fat, and protein interfere with calcium absorption. With too many disruptions or too low a calcium intake, the body robs calcium from wherever it is housed, which, about 99 percent of the time, will be in bones.

Dosage and Potential Side Effects

Adequate calcium intake has particular importance during the BONE BUILDING years of childhood. For CHILDREN, the Milk Matters Web site from the National Institute of Child Health and Human Development listed these requirements: From birth to six months, 210 mg; six months to one year, 270 mg; one- to three-year-olds, 500 mg; four- to eight-year-olds, 800 mg; and children nine to 18, 1,300 mg. With dairy products a primary source of calcium, one cup of milk or three slices of American cheese have 300 mg. A cup of child-favored macaroni and cheese holds about 100 mg of calcium, and a nice slice of cheese pizza, 200.

A dietary fact sheet from the National Institutes of Health (NIH) recommended 1,000 mg of calcium for adults, 19 to 50, with 1,300 mg for pregnant women and 1,200 mg for adults over 50. People who do not tolerate milk may do fine with a cup of yogurt, which has the same calcium as a cup of milk, but a cup of calcium-fortified orange juice has even more. Other food sources to rival a cup of milk include one and a half cups of kale, two and a quarter cups of cooked broccoli, or four ounces of canned salmon with the soft bones crushed into the fish. Although most people would not object to three cups of ice cream, calcium does not have to come in one food at one time. Each milligram counts, whether milk goes into pudding, pancakes, mashed potatoes, or cereal. Cheese chunks atop chili or grated over pasta add flavor, color, and calcium too.

Natural sources of calcium usually incur no side effects other than food allergies or lactose intolerance. Often, the latter can be remedied by using soured dairy products, such as sour cream, yogurt, and the buttermilk great for plumping biscuits, but other foods can thwart calcium use. For instance, VITAMIN D increases absorption, whereas the oxalic acid found in beans, greens, and sweet potatoes hinders calcium uptake. Foods high in phytate, such as fiber or wheat bran, also interfere with calcium absorption. "However, the effect of fiber on calcium absorption is more of a concern for individuals with low calcium intakes," according to NIH information, because "the average American tends to consume much less fiber per day than the level that would be needed to affect calcium absorption." Similarly, "the effect of dietary phosphorus on calcium is minimal. Some researchers speculate that the detrimental effects of consuming foods high in phosphate such as carbonated soft drinks is due to the replacement of milk with soda rather than the phosphate level itself." In addition, food and beverages low in calcium but high in protein, potassium, sodium, and caffeine can affect MINERAL BALANCE.

Statistics and Studies

In *Food Chemical Toxicology*, R. P. Heaney reported, "Human physiological studies and controlled balance studies show a clear but only a very small depressant effect of caffeine itself on intestinal calcium absorption," with no effect on calcium excretion during a 24-hour period. If a person ingests the recommended daily dose of calcium, caffeine usually has no harmful effects on bone status. However, "low calcium intake is clearly linked to skeletal fragility, and it is likely that a high caffeine intake is often a marker for a low calcium intake." The solution? For coffee-drinkers concerned about bone health, "the negative effect of caffeine on calcium absorption is small enough to be fully offset by as little as 1–2 tablespoons of milk."

Heaney, R. P. "Effects of Caffeine on Bone and the Calcium Economy," *Food Chemical Toxicology* 40, no. 9 (September 2002): 1,263–1,270.

Milk Matters. "Tweens and Teens Need Calcium Now More Than Ever," National Institutes of Health, National Institute of Child Health and Human Development. Available online. URL: http://www.nichd.nih.gov/milk/milk.cfm. Downloaded December 2, 2005.

Office of Dietary Supplements. "Dietary Supplement Fact Sheet: Calcium," National Institutes of Health. Available online. URL: http://ods.od.nih.gov/factsheets/calcium.asp. Updated September 23, 2005.

cancer   Healthy growth in INFANTS, CHILDREN, and ADOLESCENTS counts on cells' dividing in an orderly fashion and staying within the boundaries of a functional design. In all age groups, normal repairs throughout the body depend on systematic cellular division. If cells rampantly divide, however, disorderly growths or tumors appear, eventually displacing healthy bone and tissue. These benign growths may not be life-threatening, but they can cause PAIN by invading vertebral spaces and pressing spinal nerves. If malignant cells begin to form anywhere in the body, cancer can spread to the VERTEBRAE and other bones.

Less often, cancerous cells originate in bone or as SPINAL TUMORS. As the American Cancer Society (ACS) said, "In 2005, about 2,570 new cases of cancer of the bones and joints will be diagnosed, and about 1,200 deaths from these cancers are expected," but, "primary cancers of bones account for less than 0.2% of all cancers."

Symptoms and Diagnostic Path

For early detection, the ACS recommended routine testing and regular physical examinations. Prompt attention must be given to such signs as gradually increased pain, swelling, or the presence of a lump or knot. A spontaneous or easily occurring FRACTURE can be a symptom, too, but this usually happens in a limb that has been achy or painful for weeks. More often, patients experience weight loss and fatigue, especially if cancerous cells have spread into bones or body organs.

To expose cancer in a bone, an X-RAY may detect a hole-like appearance or other irregular shape. An oncologist or other physician will also recommend a urinalysis, blood test, and needle biopsy to confirm or rule out a malignancy. Additional tests may include a BONE SCAN, COMPUTED TOMOGRAPHY (CT) SCAN, MAGNETIC RESONANCE IMAGING (MRI), or POSITIVE EMISSION TOMOGRAPHY (PET) SCAN to determine the site of origin and see if spreading has occurred.

Treatment Options and Outlook

The article "Metastatic Bone Disease" posted by the American Academy of Orthopaedic Surgeons (AAOS) summarized: "The skeleton is the third most common site of spread of cancers that arise from organs or carcinomas. Metastases to the lung and liver are often not detected until late in the course of disease because patients experience no symptoms. On the contrary, bone metastases are generally painful when they occur. The vast majority of bone metastases originate from cancers of the breast, lung, and prostate, followed by the thyroid and kidney. The most common sites of spread in the skeleton include the spine, pelvis, ribs, skull, upper arm and leg long bones. Interestingly, these sites correspond to areas of bone marrow that demonstrate high levels of red blood cell production, the cells responsible for carrying oxygen to tissues in the body."

Treatment depends on the patient and the type and stage of cancer, but questions can be asked and specific information found on numerous Web sites. For example, http://www.curesearch.org/ offers help on Ewing's sarcoma and other cancers that affect the BACK and SPINE. The U.S.A. Children's Cancer Resource Directory is located on http://www.cancerindex.org/ccw/guide2us.htm. For PAIN MANAGEMENT in children, the Texas Cancer Council offers suggestions on http://www.childcancerpain.org/. For information about dealing with pain, mood swings, medications, and side effects experienced in all age groups, The National Pain Foundation provides helps on http://www.nationalpainfoundation.org. Also, the U.S. Government hosts a Cancer Information Service with hotline (800) 4–CANCER (6237) and Web site http://cis.nci.nih.gov/. Contacts for other relevant and reliable organizations appear in the appendixes of this book.

With the diagnosis of a tumor, the most common outlook is fear. However, facts often overcome fears and feelings of hopelessness. For example, information from the AAOS said that most bone tumors are benign and may just need to be watched, whereas others may disappear with medication. If a tumor becomes invasive or develops cancer cells, SURGERY can generally remove the growth. Surgical procedures may also be combined with radiation therapy, which uses high levels of X-rays to kill cancer cells. To explain another option, the AAOS said, "Systemic treatment (chemotherapy) is often used to kill tumor cells when they have spread into the blood stream but cannot yet be detected on tests and scans. Chemotherapy is generally used when cancerous tumors have a very high chance of spreading."

If medical treatment does not prove effective, some patients elect various types of COMPLEMENTARY AND ALTERNATIVE MEDICINE to delay progression, manage CHRONIC PAIN, or improve mental outlook. Many patients also have the option of participating in CLINICAL TRIALS to contribute to future resources and receive the latest treatments. Often, cancer centers, universities, and pharmaceutical companies sponsor relevant RESEARCH too, sometimes with significant results.

For example, a study headed by J. R. Ross evaluated BISPHOSPHONATES as a treatment option. Reporting on that study in "Bisphosphonates and Skeletal Morbidity in Patients with Metastatic Cancer," Mohit Bhandari explained, "Cancer patients with bone metastases can suffer from hypercalcemia," an excess of calcium released from the bones into the blood, and also experience "fractures, spinal cord compression, reduced mobility and pain." Although "a completely satisfactory therapeutic option has yet to be found . . . analyses confirm the efficacy of bisphosphonates—potent medications that inhibit bone resorption—in increasing bone mineral density and reducing fracture rates." The treatment does not extend rate of survival but does increase quality of life by delaying the "first skeletal event," such as a VERTEBRAL COMPRESSION FRACTURE. Therefore, "bisphosphonate therapy should be initiated when skeletal metastases are identified and continued for at least 6 months for clinical benefit."

Since those findings first appeared, however, The International Myeloma Foundation (IMF) warned, "Be alert and aware that bisphosphonate use can be associated with jaw or dental problems, including pain, bone loss, and poor healing. Problems are more likely with longer periods of bisphosphonate use (e.g., several years) and possibly more potent bisphosphonates." To avoid complications, the IMF suggested taking "conservative measures such as antibiotic treatment and mouth rinses" and having regular dental checkups. Despite potential side effects, the IMF said, "Bisphosphonates remain a critical element of care to reduce bone destruction." Therefore, each patient must be assessed by both a doctor and a dentist to avoid the impact of a dental crisis. Difficulties with chewing and eating not only affect the outlook and quality of life, but the length of life, particularly if weight has begun to decline.

Risk Factors and Preventive Measures

NUTRITION has a vital role for every individual, not only to sustain life but to reduce the risk of bone cancer and improve the survival rate for those who have been diagnosed. In the *Nutrition Journal*, research scientist Michael S. Donaldson reported, "It has been estimated by the American Institute for Cancer Research and the World Cancer Research Fund that 30–40 percent of all cancers can be prevented by appropriate diets, physical activity, and maintenance of appropriate body weight." For example, "obesity accounted for 14 percent of all cancer deaths in men and 20 percent of those in women."

Besides the effects of WEIGHT, other risk factors include alcohol consumption, cigarette smoking, and low intake of FOLIC ACID. Donaldson further reported, "The 'western' dietary pattern, with its higher intakes of red meat and processed meats, sweets, and desserts, French fries, and refined grains, was associated with a 46% increase relative risk of colon cancer in the Nurses' Health Study." Conversely, "one of the most important messages of modern nutrition research is that a diet rich in fruits and vegetables protects against cancer" of all types as well as cardiovascular and other life-threatening diseases. "For most cancers, people in the lower quartile (¼ of the population) who ate the least amount of fruits and vegetables had about twice the risk of cancer compared to those in the upper quartile who ate the most fruits and vegetables. Even in lung cancer, after accounting for smoking, increasing fruits and vegetables reduces lung cancer" by 20 to 33 percent. Similarly, "85% of the studies that queried raw vegetable consumption found a protective effect," especially in carrots, green vegetables, garlic, onions, tomatoes, and cruciferous vegetables, such as broccoli, cauliflower, cabbage, and Brussels sprouts.

Various anticarcinogenic properties have also been identified in other natural sources, such as flavanol in green tea and proanthocyanidin in grape seed extract. For cancer prevention, VITAMIN A, VITAMIN C, and VITAMIN E may be particularly helpful, with supplements supplying the daily requirement if needed. As a general principle, though, the closer a food remains to its natural state, the more healthful it will be in preventing cancer, building bone, and strengthening the whole body.

American Academy of Orthopaedic Surgeons. "Bone Tumor," AAOS. Available online. URL: http://orthoinfo. aaos.org/fact/thr_report.cfm?Thread_ID=278&topcate gory=Tumors. Downloaded December 5, 2005.

————. "Metastatic Bone Disease," AAOS. Available online. URL: http://orthoinfo.aaos.org/indepth/thr_ report.cfm?Thread_ID=13&topcategory=Tumors. Downloaded December 3, 2005.

American Cancer Society. "Detailed Guide: Bone Cancer," ACS, Cancer Reference Information. Available online. URL: http://www.cancer.org/docroot/CRI/CRI_2_3x. asp?rnav=cridg&dt=2. Last revised May 27, 2005.

Bhandari, Mohit. "Bisphosphonates and Skeletal Morbidity in Patients with Metastatic Cancer," *Canadian Medical Association Journal* 169, no. 10 (November 11, 2003): 1,053.

Donaldson, Michael S. "Nutrition and Cancer: A Review of the Evidence for an Anti-cancer Diet," *Nutrition Journal* 3, no. 19 (October 20, 2004).

International Myeloma Foundation. "Myeloma Minute: Special Advisory on Osteonecrosis of the Jaws," IMF. Available online. URL: http://www.myeloma.org/ main.jsp?type=article&id=1223. Downloaded December 3, 2005.

capsaicin   See TOPICAL ANALGESIC.

carcinoma   See CANCER.

CAT scan or CT scan   See COMPUTED TOMOGRAPHY SCAN.

cauda equina syndrome (CES)   The bundle of spinal nerves fanning into the image of a horse's tail gave cauda (horse) equina (tail) its amusing name. However, the syndrome involving those nerves brings no humor but, instead, shows a probability of emergency surgery. As an online fact sheet from the American Academy of Orthopaedic Surgeons (AAOS) explained, "Cauda equina syndrome (CES) occurs when the nerve roots are compressed and paralyzed, cutting off sensation and movement. Nerve roots that control the function of the bladder and bowel are especially vulnerable to damage."

Probable causes of CES include a HERNIATED DISC, SPINAL INFECTION, SPINAL TUMOR, SPINAL STENOSIS, OSTEOPHYTE, or a trauma, such as a severe blow to the lower back. BIRTH DEFECTS of the LUMBAR SPINE can also obstruct cauda equina nerves, as can the formation of a blood clot following lumbar SURGERY.

Symptoms and Diagnostic Path

Severe LOW BACK PAIN radiating into the legs usually indicates SCIATICA. If the lower body suddenly loses the ability to function, however, CES may be more likely. Specific symptoms include motor weakness, loss of reflexes in the legs, and abrupt onset of dysfunction in the bladder and bowels. MAGNETIC RESONANCE IMAGING of the SPINE may indicate nerve involvement, while a MYELOGRAM shows the location and type of obstruction that must be surgically tended.

Treatment Options and Outlook

The best outlook comes when surgery can be performed within 48 hours of onset of CES. As a general rule, the longer the time lapse, the greater the likelihood of permanent nerve damage. If nerve impairment continues, the American Association of Neurological Surgeons (AANS) warned, "CES can affect people both physically and emotionally, in particular if it is chronic. People with CES may no longer be able to work, either because of severe pain, socially unacceptable incontinence problems, motor weakness and sensory loss, or a combination of these problems." Sexual dysfunction and urinary tract infections may become commonplace, while weakness in the lower body can make walking difficult. Even so, the AANS said, "There are several medications prescribed to address pain, bladder and bowel problems. In addition, some patients find that physical therapy and psychological counseling help them cope with CES."

Risk Factors and Preventative Measures

Staff from the Department of Orthopaedic Surgery at Johns Hopkins University addressed CES in patients with ANKYLOSING SPONDYLITIS as having "a high index of suspicion for this problem," especially if a history of incontinence exists. Although NONSTEROIDAL ANTI-INFLAMMATORY DRUGS (NSAID) offer some degree of PAIN MANAGEMENT, a PAIN RELIEVER will not remove a neurologic problem caused by pressure on the spinal nerves. Prompt surgical intervention, however, will often correct a causal factor before the nerves sustain permanent damage.

In an article for *Neurosurgery Focus,* Dr. John P. Kostuik addressed the postoperative occurrence of CES as, "a totally preventable complication." To keep CES from happening after spinal surgery, patients should have a full neurological examination. However, Dr. Kostuik suggested, "It is recommended that every patient, regardless of the spinal surgery undergone, have a postoperative rectal examination . . . to establish a baseline. If the patient complains of increasing back pain . . . or increasing numbness, subsequent follow-up data can be compared with the baseline data."

Ahn, N. U., U. M. Ahn, L. Nallamshetty, B. D. Springer, J. M. Buchowski, L. Funches, E. S. Garrett, J. P. Kostuik, K. M. Kebaish, and P. D. Sponseller. "Cauda Equina Syndrome in Ankylosing Spondylitis (the CES-AS Syndrome): Meta-analysis of Outcomes after Medical and Surgical Treatments," *Journal of Spinal Disorders* 14, no. 5 (October 2001): 427–433.

American Academy of Orthopaedic Surgeons. "Cauda Equina Syndrome," AAOS. Available online. URL: http://orthoinfo.aaos.org/fact/thr_report.cfm?thread_id=285&topcategory=spine. Downloaded December 7, 2005.

Kostuik, John P., M.D. "Cauda Equina Syndrome," *Neurosurgery Focus* 16, no. 6 (June 2004).

NeurosurgeryToday.org. "Cauda Equina Syndrome (CES)," American Association of Neurological Surgeons. Available online. URL: http://www.neurosurgerytoday.org/what/patient_e/cauda.asp. Downloaded December 7, 2005.

cervical brace   See ORTHOTICS.

cervical disc disease   See HERNIATED DISC.

cervical foraminal stenosis   Spinal nerves exit the spinal cord through tiny spaces or foramen between the VERTEBRAE then connect into muscles to provide the area with movement. Sometimes, though, narrowing or stenosis makes a tiny foraminal opening even smaller, thereby producing this condition.

Symptoms and Diagnostic Path

Foraminal stenosis of the CERVICAL SPINE commonly occurs between the C5 and C6 neck vertebrae or between the C6 and C7 level. As spinal nerves become irritated, pain radiates from the neck into the shoulders and down the arms. To diagnose the condition, a physician will usually request MAGNETIC RESONANCE IMAGING or a COMPUTED TOMOGRAPHY (CT) SCAN with a MYELOGRAM.

Treatment Options and Outlook

The type of treatment varies with the underlying problem as well as with the specialty of the physician or therapist. If joint inflammation causes foraminal constriction, a doctor may recommend the RICE METHOD of rest, ice, compression, and elevation with NONSTEROIDAL ANTI-INFLAMMATORY DRUGS (NSAIDs) to relieve the pain. A chiropractor or osteopath may perform SPINAL MANIPULATION and suggest therapeutic EXERCISE, whereas an orthopedist may recommend an EPIDURAL INJECTION, NERVE BLOCK, or TRACTION. In severe instances of unremitting pain, SURGERY, such as an ANTERIOR CERVICAL DISCECTOMY, cervical FORAMINOTOMY, CERVICAL LAMINAPLASTY, or insertion of a BONE GRAFT, may be needed to relieve chronic pressure on spinal nerves.

Risk Factors and Preventive Measures

As a person stands or walks, spinal vertebrae settle somewhat, reducing the foraminal space even more. Since stretching has the opposite effect, patients with cervical foraminal stenosis can sometimes prevent painful episodes by becoming aware of their movements. For example, most people turn their heads to one side during a conversation, yet they can avoid pain by facing the other person and maintaining a neutral position in the vertebral joints. Cradling a phone with the neck triggers pain and inflammation, but using a headset or speaker phone can prevent that problem. Good POSTURE, daily ACTIVITY, and simply moving around instead of sitting like an unused appliance can get spinal fluids flowing. If the neck begins to ache or stiffen, resting on a flat surface with a rolled hand towel or small pillow cradled into the neck curve may relieve the pressure enough to prevent a mild discomfort from becoming an imperial pain.

Ullrich, Peter F. Jr., M.D. "Cervical Foraminal Stenosis," Spine-health.com. Available online. URL: http://www. spine-health.com/topics/cd/overview/cervical/cerv02. htm. Downloaded December 8, 2005.

Walker, Richard S., M.D. "Sciatic and Brachalgia," Coventry Pain Clinic. Available online. URL: http://www.coven-trypainclinic.org.uk/spinalpain-sciaticaandbrachalgia. htm. Downloaded December 8, 2005.

cervical laminaplasty   By taking the pressure off the spinal cord and spinal nerves, this surgical procedure may be referred to as spinal decompression. Initially, the pressure may come from a HERNIATED DISC, FRACTURE, or some type of DEGENERATIVE DISC DISEASE that affects the lamina or flat bones on the backs of the VERTEBRAE.

Procedure

Unlike the frontal access of an ANTERIOR CERVICAL DIS-CECTOMY, laminaplasty takes a posterior approach. In an article posted by SpineSource, Dr. John J. Regan described the procedure: "An incision is made down the back of the neck to expose the cervical vertebrae. On one side of the vertebral column, the lamina are cut through just far enough to create a hinge-like movement, much like a door. Then the lamina on the other side are cut all the way through to, in effect, open the door." Once the incision has been made, "The back portion of the vertebrae, the spinous processes (bumps you feel on the back) are removed to make more room for the 'door' to open. After gently opening the 'door' of each vertebra to create more room for the spinal cord and nerve roots behind it, bone wedges are inserted to keep the 'door' from totally closing. Then the 'door' is closed securely onto the wedges, resulting in an expanded 'doorway' for the nerves."

Risks and Complications

As occurs with any surgery, risks include damage to a surrounding area, which, in this case, would be the larynx, esophagus, or spinal cord. Dr. Brian R. Subach of The Virginia Spine Institute discussed other risks of laminaplasty, saying, "Disadvantages include a slightly reduced range-of-motion and increased risk of neck pain, as well as potential injury to the C5 nerve root during the procedure. This is thought to occur as a result of traction on the nerve root as the spinal bones shift."

A study from Japan indicated that RANGE OF MOTION may continue to decrease between the third and fifth postoperative years. To assess "curvature and range of motion of the cervical spine after laminaplasty," researchers from the Institute of Clinical Medicine at the University of Tsukuba in Ibaraki took radiographs of 26 patients before laminaplasty and again at one, three, and five years later. The surgery somewhat reduced vertebral flexibility, but reportedly, LORDOSIS diminished too.

Outlook and Lifestyle Modifications

Overall, laminaplasty effectively treats SPINAL STE-NOSIS with less loss of flexibility than occurs with a cervical fusion. While the procedure may prevent spinal deformity and preserve neck stability, the long-term outlook depends on addressing the initial cause of a neck problem. To do this, lifestyle changes may be required, including therapeutic EXERCISE, supportive NUTRITION, MASSAGE THERAPY, adequate SLEEP, ORTHOTICS, and SHOES chosen to aid POSTURE. Also, ERGONOMIC FACTORS have particular importance in providing ongoing support for the SPINE.

Aita, I., Y. Wadano, and T. Yabuki. "Curvature and Range of Motion of the Cervical Spine after Laminaplasty," *Journal of Bone & Joint Surgery,* American volume 82-A, no. 12 (December 2000): 1,743–1,750.

Regan, John J., M.D. "Cervical Disc Herniation," Spine-Source. Available online. URL: http://www.spinesource. com/Back-Pain-Disorders/cervical-disc-herniation. html. Downloaded December 8, 2005.

Subach, Brian R., M.D. "Cervical Laminaplasty: An Option for Some Patients with Cervical Myelopathy," The Virginia Spine Institute. Available online. URL: http://www.spinemd.com/laminaplasty.htm. Downloaded December 9, 2005.

cervical laminectomy   See LAMINECTOMY.

cervical radiculopathy Commonly known as a pinched nerve, cervical radiculopathy is a pain in the neck. In the CERVICAL SPINE, nerves exit the spinal cord through tiny holes or neuroforamen. When everything works well, those nerves aid movement in the neck, shoulders, arms, and hands. If pressure on the VERTEBRAE occurs because of CERVICAL FORAMINAL STENOSIS, SPINAL STENOSIS, a HERNIATED DISC, DEGENERATIVE DISC DISEASE, or an OSTEOPHYTE (bone spur), the compressed spinal nerves may get irritated enough to complain.

Symptoms and Diagnostic Path

With cervical radiculopathy, the most common complaints are PAIN, tingling, numbness, or weakness. To be more specific, Dr. Charles Tuen, a neurologist at Methodist Medical Center in Dallas, pointed to the C7 neck vertebra as the most likely suspect if numbness affects the middle finger, with the probable cause being a herniated DISC. If pain shoots down the middle finger, a disc lesion of some kind may be pressing the C6 to C7 area. If pain extends into the thumb and index finger, a lesion or CERVICAL SPONDYLOSIS may be affecting C5 or C6. However, pain radiating down the back of the arm into the little finger may be coming from a problem at C8 or between C7 and the T1 vertebra of the THORACIC SPINE.

Besides inquiring about symptoms, a physician will evaluate a medical history and RANGE OF MOTION in the neck and arms. While X-RAY will assess vertebral bones, MAGNETIC RESONANCE IMAGING or a COMPUTED TOMOGRAPHY SCAN may be needed to evaluate spinal nerves and soft tissue involvement.

Treatment Options and Outlook

An article posted online by the American Academy of Orthopaedic Surgeons (AAOS) said, "Initial treatment is usually conservative and aims to reduce the pain by easing the pressure on the nerves. The treatment consists of three parts: rest, medication and physical therapy." The doctor may also prescribe NONSTEROIDAL ANTI-INFLAMMATORY DRUG (NSAID) THERAPY to relieve pain and swelling. COLD THERAPY may be recommended for a swollen neck and HEAT THERAPY for stiffness with stretching EXERCISES helpful to both. However, "if conservative treatment doesn't relieve your pain over the course of 6 to 12 weeks . . . surgery may be an option."

Regarding the potential need for surgery, information from the DynoMed.com Web site stated, "If significant compression on the nerve exists to the extent that motor weakness results, surgery may be necessary to relieve the pressure by either removing the offending disk material or enlarging the space where the nerve root exits the vertebrae. This may be called a laminectomy, because the lamina, which is a portion of the bone in the vertebra, is often removed in order to make more room for the exiting nerve root. If the pressure is more severe and disc space narrowed more, an anterior discectomy and fusion can be done."

Risk Factors and Preventive Measures

The type of SURGERY determines the risks. For example, an ANTERIOR CERVICAL DISCECTOMY can affect swallowing, whereas failed ARTHRODESIS can cause vertebral instability. A BONE GRAFT with donor bone could be rejected or simply not heal. A posterior spinal fusion may have a higher rate of success than an anterior (front) approach, but pain during recovery can be more intense. In any case, an orthopaedic surgeon will discuss specific risks and prescribe appropriate treatments to assist BONE BUILDING and healing.

American Academy of Orthopaedic Surgeons. "Cervical Radiculopathy," AAOS. Available online. URL: http://orthoinfo.aaos.org/fact/thr_report.cfm?Thread_ID=179&topcategory=Neck. Downloaded December 9, 2005.

Bolesta, Michael J., M.D. "Patient Information Sheet on Surgical Indications and Procedures for Cervical Myelopathy, Radiculopathy, and Axial Neck Pain," Cervical Spine Research Society. Available online. URL: http://www.csrs.org/patientinfo/surgicalindications.htm. Downloaded December 9, 2005.

DynoMed.com. "Cervical Radiculopathy," Patient Encyclopedia. Available online. URL: http://www.dynomed.com/encyclopedia/encyclopedia/spine/Cervical_Radiculopathy.htm. Downloaded December 9, 2005.

Tuen, Charles, M.D. "Cervical Radiculopathy," Neuroland. Available online. URL: http://neuroland.com/spine/c_radi.htm. Downloaded December 9, 2005.

cervical spinal fusion See ARTHRODESIS.

cervical spine In the upper SPINE, seven little neck bones come together as the C1 through C7 VERTEBRAE to uphold the head, direct the eyes and ears, and offer a way for the brain to connect the senses and good sense with action. For the connection, tiny foramine open on either side of each neck bone to give numerous spinal nerves a place to exit the spinal cord and burrow into the muscles to which they are assigned.

To connect neck vertebrae, small pedicles in the front (anterior) and back (posterior) fasten each bone to the one above and the one below. Thus joined, the cervical spine aligns not in a straight line, but in a gentle forward curve. To secure the area more and yet provide RANGE OF MOTION, facet joints join one vertebra to another on the posterior side of the spinal column, forming a row of bony projections that can be felt down the BACK. Those connective bones can make way for FACET JOINT DISORDER problems, but bigger problems come if anything hinders a neck from doing its many jobs.

Risks and Complications

In writing for the Cervical Research Society, Dr. Jamie Baisden identified three potential factors for complications in the neck: mechanical problems, nerve root problems, and spinal cord problems. Mechanical problems involve the bones and DISCS, for instance, in DEGENERATIVE DISC DISEASE, bone FRACTURE, HERNIATED DISC, or problems with POSTURE as occur in KYPHOSIS, LORDOSIS, and SCOLIOSIS. Regarding nerve root problems, Dr. Baisden said, "When a disc herniation, bone spur, or tumor press on a nerve root, it produces what is called a radiculopathy. Since each nerve root supplies a specific muscle group and sensory area, a physician can often interpret the patient's symptoms and physical findings and determine which nerve root is irritated. Irritation of a nerve root (radiculopathy) typically produces pain, weakness, numbness, tingling and possibly decreased reflexes, depending on which nerve root is irritated." Dr. Baisden further explained, "If disc or bone push on the spinal cord, the symptoms are called myelopathy. The signs of myelopathy are variable, but typically are also associated with decreased motor and sensory functions, sometimes involving arms and legs, and sometimes altering bowel and bladder control. There may also

be increased reflexes or potentially absent reflexes if the cord injury is severe."

Treatment Options and Outlook

Treatments for neck pain often begin with home remedies, such as the RICE METHOD of rest, ice, compression, and elevation. NONSTEROIDAL ANTI-INFLAMMATORY DRUG (NSAID) THERAPY and other OVER-THE-COUNTER PRODUCTS, such as HOMEOPATHIC MEDICINE, may prove useful too. When home treatments do not ease a cervical spine problem, ACUPRESSURE, ACUPUNCTURE, or MASSAGE THERAPY may be performed by a licensed therapist. If the neck has lost its curve, an osteopath or chiropractor can often reestablish this natural position within a few weeks through SPINAL MANIPULATION. To manage ACUTE PAIN or CHRONIC PAIN, a physician may prescribe medication. Later, the doctor may recommend X-RAY to assess bones or discs and MRI (MAGNETIC RESONANCE IMAGING) or COMPUTED TOMOGRAPHY SCAN to get a clearer picture of soft tissue, tendons, and ligaments. If a doctor suspects disc herniation, a DISCOGRAM may be needed, but for spinal nerve involvement, a neurologist may be called to review results of a NERVE CONDUCTION STUDY. With SURGERY, a neurosurgeon or orthopedic surgeon may relieve spinal compression and other conditions affecting spinal nerves with procedures such as ANTERIOR CERVICAL DISCECTOMY, CERVICAL LAMINAPLASTY, or various types of MINIMALLY INVASIVE SURGERY that may or may not require a BONE GRAFT.

Statistics and Studies

Writing for the Hospital Practice Web site, Dr. David G. Borenstein of The George Washington University Medical Center in Washington, D. C., said, "A common complaint evaluated by primary care physicians, neck pain affects about 10% of the population of the United States every year." With causes ranging from neck STRAIN to CERVICAL SPONDYLOSIS, "most biomechanical disorders of the cervical spine have a natural history of improvement. More than 50% of patients will have decreased pain in two to four weeks; 80% will be asymptomatic in two to three months, and most will improve without requiring diagnostic x-rays or laboratory tests. Such studies are reserved for patients with histories or physical findings that suggest cord or nerve root compression or systemic illness. These disorders are uncommon causes of neck pain but require thorough evaluation and immediate treatment."

Immediate evaluation is also needed after an accident or injury. As an eMedicine.com article said, "Cervical spine injuries cause an estimated 6000 deaths and 5000 new cases of quadriplegia each year." With a ratio of four males to one female injured, "approximately 80% of patients are aged 18–25 years." About 5 to 10 percent of the unconscious patients who receive emergency care "as the result of a motor vehicle accident or fall have a major injury to the cervical spine." To be more precise, "most cervical spine fractures occur predominantly at 2 levels. One third of injuries occur at the level of C2, and one half of injuries occur at the level of C6 or C7. Most fatal cervical spine injuries occur in upper cervical levels, either at craniocervical junction C1 or C2."

Unfortunately, not every neck injury will be readily apparent. As reported in a ScienceDaily article, "Study authors found that x-rays failed to detect secondary injuries in 81 of the 224 patients identified with cervical spine injuries or 36 percent."

Special Aids and Adaptations

An injury in the upper cervical vertebrae can result in paralysis or even death. Therefore, a SPINAL INJURY must be treated promptly with care taken to immobilize the victim until a medical specialist can evaluate the trauma and provide appropriate treatment. Often, severe injuries can be prevented with the aid of properly fitted athletic equipment and other safety devices, such as a seat belt or sturdy car seat to protect the spines of INFANTS and CHILDREN. A thin little bathing cap, however, does nothing to protect a swimmer who dives into rock-infested waters or the shallow end of a pool.

If a head trauma occurs for any reason, a neck injury should be suspected. In the book *Health At Home*, presented in part on the Internet, Don R. Powell suggested, "Tell the victim to lie still and not move his or her head, neck, back, etc." Then, "place rolled towels, articles of clothing, etc. on both sides of the neck and/or body. Tie and wrap in place, but don't interfere with the victim's breathing. If necessary, use both of your hands, one on each side of the victim's head, to keep the head from moving." If a victim must be moved before the ambulance

arrives, the flat surface of a board or door can be used as a transporting device, but "several people should carefully lift and move the person onto the board, being very careful to align the head and neck in a straight line with the spine. The head should not rotate or bend forward or backward."

Rotating, bending, and stretching the neck of someone with a cervical spine injury can be fatal. In everyday life though, that same range of motion allows a healthy neck to function well and remain flexible. Everyday assistance also comes through foods rich in CALCIUM and other elements of good NUTRITION. Although vitamin and mineral supplements can be added for special needs, sunlight aids a body in producing VITAMIN D, while daily ACTIVITY and EXERCISE assist BONE BUILDING.

Usually, people think of STRENGTH TRAINING as a means of pumping arm muscles. However, specific exercises strengthen the neck and, sometimes, relieve pain. For example, an article in *Harvard Women's Health Watch* offered this exercise: "1. Sit in a neutral position and look straight ahead. Allow your head to protrude slightly forward. 2. Slowly glide your head backward, tucking in your chin until you have pulled your head and chin as far back as they will go. Keep your head level. Move your head slowly back and forth 10 times between this position and the neutral position. 3. For a stronger stretch, gently apply pressure to your chin with your fingers and release. Repeat every two hours as needed." However, the article cautioned, "if this exercise increases your pain, try it lying on your back with your head on a pillow. If pain increases or numbness develops, stop and contact your clinician." This particular article did not say so, of course, but anyone with cervical spine problems might also refrain from sticking out their necks, racing neck-to-neck, hanging the head, or adhering to the often-lauded advice of holding a chronic "chin up" position.

Baisden, Jamie, M.D. "Patient Information Sheet on Introduction to the Cervical Spine," Cervical Spine Research Society. Available online. URL: http://www.csrs.org/patientinfo/introtocspine.htm. Downloaded December 6, 2005.

Barrett, Tyler W., M.D., Jerome R. Hoffman, M.D., and Michael I. Zucker, M.D. "UCLA Study Helps ER

Physicians Identify Previously Undetectable Spinal Injuries," Science*Daily.* Available online. URL: http://www.sciencedaily.com/releases/2005/09/050907100756.htm.

Belaval, Emilio, M.D. and Simon Roy, M.D. "Fractures, Cervical Spine," eMedicine.com. Available online. URL: http://www.emedicine.com/emerg/topic189.htm. Last updated January 19, 2005.

Borenstein, David G. "Management of Neck Pain: A Primary Care Approach," Hospital Practice. Available online. URL: http://www.hosppract.com/issues/1998/10/boren.htm. Downloaded December 10, 2005.

Ghanayem, Alexander, M.D. "Patient Information Sheet on Conservative Care for Cervical Spine Disorders," Cervical Spine Research Society. Available online. URL: http://www.csrs.org/patientinfo/conservativecare.htm. Downloaded December 10, 2005.

Powell, Don R. *Health At Home,* ©1999, American Institute for Preventive Medicine. "Neck/Spine Injuries, Chapter 23. Emergency Conditions," Saints Self-Care Medical Library. Available online. URL: http://www.saintsok.com/pages/medicallibrary/NECKSPIN.HTM. Downloaded December 10, 2005.

Staff. "Oh, My Aching Neck," *Harvard Women's Health Watch* 12, no. 3 (November 2004): 7.

cervical spondylosis   Normal wear and tear eventually wear down vertebral DISCS and BACK bones, causing this condition. Also, aging and ARTHRITIS can deposit hardened minerals where cushy discs should be. Adding insult to that non-injury, OSTEOPHYTES (bone spurs) can also form. According to National Institutes of Health statistics reported on the MedlinePlus Web site, "By age 60, 70% of women and 85% of men show changes consistent with cervical spondylosis on X-ray."

Symptoms and Diagnostic Path

Typical symptoms include neck pain radiating into the arms and shoulders, neck stiffness, or a CERVICOGENIC HEADACHE stemming from the CERVICAL SPINE. The RANGE OF MOTION may decrease, but less frequently, pressure on the spinal nerves affects balance and movement of the lower body. X-RAYS can show evidence of this degenerative condition, but a COMPUTED TOMOGRAPHY SCAN will usually be needed to clarify the extent of damage.

Treatment Options and Outlook

Besides NONSTEROIDAL ANTI-INFLAMMATORY DRUG (NSAID) THERAPY or other types of PAIN MANAGEMENT, typical treatments include TRACTION, SPINAL MANIPULATION, HEAT THERAPY, COLD THERAPY, cortisone injection, and, temporarily, an ORTHOTIC device or neck brace. For neck spasm, a MUSCLE RELAXANT may be prescribed. If, however, bone overgrowth or pressure on the VERTEBRAE affect the spinal cord, prompt SURGERY may be needed to prevent nerve damage and permanent disability.

Risk Factors and Preventive Measures

A previous neck injury puts a person at higher risk for cervical spondylosis. According to an article in *The Practitioner,* "Men are affected as often as women overall, though they seem to be affected at a slightly younger age." To prevent the condition from worsening, "most patients who have recurrent episodes of pain can be managed successfully with gentle physiotherapy and NSAIDs." In addition, neck and shoulder EXERCISES can be strengthening.

Spinal manipulation can relieve pressure on spinal nerves that travel through tiny openings between the vertebrae, but an article for *The Journal of Manual & Manipulative Therapy* lamented that, "the majority of articles published related to serious anatomical injury seen in association with cervical manipulation." Minimal risks of vertebral damage or a stroke do exist, but as a preventive measure, "the therapist . . . verbally directs how a particular spinal movement is to take place. Performed in this fashion, active cervical movement testing allows the patient to do what he feels able to."

Regarding surgical risks, a team of doctors from the Department of Orthopaedic Surgery at Yale University joined with a group of physicians from Germany to research the results of cervical disc replacement in treating spondylosis. As reported in the *Journal of Neurosurgery: Spine,* adverse outcomes included less range of motion (ROM), BONE GRAFT failure, and complications with the stabilizing devices surgically inserted into the neck. The researchers said, however, "Recent advances in material and implant design have enabled the development of a novel implant design . . . , which follows the principles of providing immediate implant stability, ease and safety of insertion . . . and optimization of functional ROM."

A.D.A.M., MedlinePlus. "Cervical Spondylosis," U.S. National Library of Medicine, National Institutes of Health. Available online. URL: http://www.nlm.nih.gov/medlineplus/ency/article/000436.htm. Last updated November 9, 2005.

Bertagnoli, Rudolf, M.D., James J. Yue, M.D., Frank Pfeiffer, M.D., Andrea Fenk-Mayer, M.D., James P. Lawrence, M.D., Trace Kershaw, and Regina Nanieva. "Early Results after ProDisc-C Cervical Disc Replacement," *Journal of Neurosurgery: Spine,* no. 2 (April 2005): 403–410.

Creighton, Douglas S., James Viti, and John Krauss. "Use of Translatoric Mobilization in a Patient with Cervical Spondylotic Degeneration: A Case Report," *The Journal of Manual & Manipulative Therapy* 13, no. 1 (2005): 12–26.

Ross, Alistair. "Managing Cervical Spondylosis," *The Practitioner,* no. 11 (November 10, 2005): 762–769.

cervical spondylotic myelopathy (CSM)   Sometimes OSTEOPHYTE (bone spur) formation, FACET JOINT DISORDER, ARTHRITIS, SPINAL STENOSIS, or other problems can cause neck VERTEBRAE to become narrow enough to squeeze the spinal cord. In a Spine-health.com article, Dr. Thomas M. Wascher said this compression commonly occurs at the C4 to C7 vertebrae of the CERVICAL SPINE. As he described, "The end result is chronic compression of the spinal cord and nerve roots leading to impaired blood flow and . . . frank damage within the spinal cord itself."

In an article for the *Internet Journal of Neurology,* M. Hochman explained, "At the C1 level the spinal cord occupies just one half of the canal. It occupies three quarters of the canal at the C5-C7 levels, however, which helps to explain why CSM predominately occurs in the lower cervical spine." The article also pointed out, "Cervical spondylotic myelopathy (CSM) is the most common cause of spinal cord dysfunction in older patients."

Symptoms and Diagnostic Path

According to the familydoctor.org Web site, "Symptoms of CSM may develop slowly. Some symptoms of CSM may include neck stiffness, arm pain, numbness in the hands and weakness of the arms and legs. A person with CSM may have stiff legs. CSM may make it difficult for a person to use his or her hands or to walk steadily." To assist a diagnosis, the physician may recommend MAGNETIC RESONANCE IMAGING and refer the patient to a neurologist or neurosurgeon.

Treatment Options and Outlook

Surgical treatment of CSM includes ANTERIOR CERVICAL DISCECTOMY or disc decompression. If instability occurs in neck joints, ARTHRODESIS will likely be used to fuse those vertebrae. A BONE GRAFT, special hardware, BONE MORPHOGENETIC PROTEIN, or a combination of implants may be inserted to aid spinal fusion. In milder cases, TRACTION and temporary use of an ORTHOTIC device offer alternatives to surgery. In either case, advanced CSM may necessitate the use of a cane or walker.

Risk Factors and Preventive Measures

Regarding other concerns associated with CSM, Dr. William F. Young wrote, "The presence of myelopathy on neurologic examination is not unique to CSM. Therefore, it is important to exclude other diagnoses that present in a similar fashion. In one study, it was found that 14.3 percent of patients who underwent surgery for CSM were later found to have other diagnoses." For example, SYRINGOMYELIA, SPINAL TUMOR, and VITAMIN B deficiency reportedly mimic CSM.

If CSM has been confirmed and surgery needed, ELDERLY patients with OSTEOPOROSIS present a particular challenge. After researching a combination of therapies, doctors from the Israel Spine Center in Tel Aviv reported their results in the *Journal of Neurosurgery: Spine,* saying, "Our hybrid decompression fixation technique allows multilevel anterior decompression, avoids bone graft donor site morbidity, and provides a basis for stable mechanical reconstruction." These combined procedures may fail in 4 percent of the cases, but for most patients, stability in the neck can be achieved.

Ashkenazi, Ely, M.D., Yossi Smorgick, M.D., Nahshon Rand, M.D., Michael A. Millgram, M.D., Yigal Mirovsky, M.D., and Yizhar Floman, M.D. "Anterior Decompression Combined with Corpectomies and Discectomies in the Management of Multilevel Cervical Myelopathy: a Hybrid Decompression and Fixation Technique," *Journal of Neurosurgery: Spine* 3 (September 2005): 205–209.

familydoctor.org. "Cervical Spondylotic Myelopathy (CSM)," American Academy of Family Physicians. Available online. URL: http://familydoctor.org/622. xml. Downloaded December 12, 2005.

Hochman, M. and S. Tuli. "Cervical Spondylotic Myelopathy: A Review," *Internet Journal of Neurology* 4, no. 1 (2005): 24–42.

Wascher, Thomas M., M.D. "Understanding Cervical Spondylotic Myelopathy," Spine-health.com. Available online. URL: http://www.spine-health.com/topics/cd/undermy/undermy01.html. Downloaded December 12, 2005.

Young, William F., M.D. "Cervical Spondylotic Myelopathy: A Common Cause of Spinal Cord Dysfunction in Older Persons," *American Family Physician,* September 1, 2000, American Academy of Family Physicians. Available online. URL: http://www.aafp.org/afp/20000901/1064.html. Downloaded December 12, 2005.

cervicogenic headache   In describing this type of headache, Dr. Daniel J. Hurley of the Chicago Institute of Neurosurgery and Neuroresearch wrote, "Whether from chronic tension or acute whiplash injury, intervertebral disc disease or progressive facet joint arthritis, the neck can be a hidden and severely debilitating source of headaches. Such headaches are grouped under the term 'cervicogenic headache,' indicating that the primary contributing structural source of the headache is the cervical spine." Since upper neck VERTEBRAE support the weight and movement of the head, "fatigue, postural malalignment, injuries, disc problems, joint degeneration, muscular stress and even prior neck surgeries all can compound the wear and tear on this critical region of the human skeletal anatomy."

Symptoms and Diagnostic Path

While potential causes may be visible on X-RAY, COMPUTED TOMOGRAPHY SCAN, or MAGNETIC RESONANCE IMAGING, a cervicogenic headache itself can not be shown. As an alternative method of diagnosis, Mitchell Elkiss from the Department of Neurology at Wayne State University wrote, "A thorough history with particular attention to the quality of the pain, its severity . . . and particularly its localiza-tion is mandatory. Pain sensitive structures include the eyes, ears, nose, and mouth." The doctor may also ask a patient about TENSION or depression and assess biomechanical problems caused by CERVICAL SPONDYLOSIS, DEGENERATIVE DISC DISEASE, or spinal imbalances.

Treatment Options and Outlook

Depending on the cause of the headache, treatments vary from PAIN RELIEVERS to ACUPRESSURE to orthopedic correction of POSTURE. As an article in the *American Journal of Pain Management* said, "The ideal treatment approach is to address the underlying neck disorder, but this is not always possible," since cervicogenic headache "can be mistaken for other forms of . . . headache, especially . . . common migraine. . . . Therefore, the best approach is to start with conservative treatments and move to more invasive ones if necessary."

Often, a whiplash or FLEXION-EXTENSION INJURY shifts the neck vertebrae, rearranging the natural C-curve into a straight line. This can make the head feel as if it sits on a rigid pole. Assuming no FRACTURE exists, an osteopath or chiropractor may be able to ease the vertebrae back into place with SPINAL MANIPULATION done over a few weeks. Therapeutic EXERCISE commonly follows this course of treatment with STRENGTH TRAINING added after the neck has healed. Other treatment options include TRIGGER POINT THERAPY, radiofrequency treatment, SPINAL INJECTION, ACUPUNCTURE, or in extreme instances, SURGERY. In any case, the outlook may depend on whether a treatment successfully reestablishes the neck curve.

Risk Factors and Preventive Measures

A diagnostic block may prevent further recurrence of cervicogenic headaches, especially when the reasons and risks have not been clearly ascertained. In an article posted by the American Council for Headache Education, Dr. Nikolai Bogduk of Australia explained, "A diagnostic block is a procedure in which needles are used to deliver local anesthetic, under x-ray control, to any joint suspected of being the source of pain." Assuming a physician has the necessary facilities and training, "the idea is that if a joint is the source of headache, anesthetizing that joint should promptly, although temporarily, relieve the pain; much the same way that once a painful tooth is anesthetized, toothache is promptly relieved. By testing the upper cervical joints in this way a doctor can tell if one of them is responsible for headache, and if so, which one."

Bogduk, Nikolai, M.D. " 'Is It My Neck?' Cervicogenic Headache," American Council for Headache Education, ACHE. Available online. URL: http://www. achenet.org/articles/44.php. Downloaded December 9, 2005.

Elkiss, Mitchell, D.O. "Cervicogenic Headaches: Diagnosis and Treatment with Osteopathic Manipulative Therapy and Acupuncture," U.S. Doctor. Available online. URL: http://www.usdoctor.com/sym9.htm. Downloaded December 9, 2005.

Hurley, Daniel J., M.D. "Cervicogenic Headache," Chicago Institute of Neurosurgery and Neuroresearch, CINN. Available online. URL: http://www.cinn.org/news/cervicogenicheadache.html. Downloaded December 12, 2005.

Ribeiro, S., S. N. Palmer, and F. Antonaci. "Headache. Cervicogenic Headache," *American Journal of Pain Management* 15, no. 2 (April 2005): 48–58.

children, spinal concerns for   From BIRTH DEFECTS to SHAKEN INFANT SYNDROME to a vertebral FRACTURE that breaks a fall along with a growing bone, children encounter many jolts and, sometimes, give their parents a few. Most children grow at a similar rate as shown in the "2000 CDC Growth Charts: United States" posted by the National Center for Health Statistics on http://www.cdc.gov/growthcharts/. However, NUTRITION, ENVIRONMENTAL INFLUENCES, GENETIC FACTORS, and a lack of daily ACTIVITY can make boys and girls from all socio-economic levels prone to such problems as birth defects of the spine, early onset scoliosis, GROWTH HORMONE DISORDERS, JUVENILE ARTHRITIS, JUVENILE OSTEOPOROSIS, and OSTEOGENESIS IMPERFECTA.

Risks and Complications

The risk of a spinal problem begins with a potential BIRTH INJURY and proceeds to school years when BACKPACK SAFETY becomes a weighty issue. Being overweight or having an EATING DISORDER can cause problems with young bones as can wearing improperly fitted SHOES. POSTURE affects the SPINE, too, particularly if a sedentary child seems oblivious to ERGONOMIC FACTORS or slouches during prime times of growth. Although bone growth ceases after adolescence, BONE BUILDING continues for adults, including the ELDERLY. For them, childhood offers an ironically optimal time to bank bone mass and minimize the loss of bone density that typically occurs as a person ages. However, lack of SLEEP, lack of EXERCISE, inadequate water, and a poor supply of CALCIUM lower bone quality, placing the spinal health of a child at risk.

When children experience ACUTE BACK PAIN and CHRONIC BACK PAIN, the causes will likely differ from those adults encounter. For example, "Back Pain In Children," posted on the American Academy of Orthopaedic Surgeons (AAOS) Web site said, "Compared with an adult, a child with a backache is more likely to have a serious underlying disorder. This is especially true if the child is 4 years old or younger, or in a child of any age who has back pain accompanied by: Fever or weight loss; Weakness, numbness, trouble walking or pain that radiates down one or both legs; Bowel or bladder dysfunction; Pain that interferes with sleep." A back STRAIN should improve with rest, whereas weakened PARASPINAL MUSCLES may need STRENGTH TRAINING or physical therapy. According to the AAOS, "More serious causes of back pain need early identification and treatment or they may become worse. Always see a doctor if your child's back pain lasts for more than several days or progressively worsens." Besides a physical examination, X-RAY may be needed to diagnose KYPHOSIS, LORDOSIS, SPONDYLOLISTHESIS, or other postural problems that commonly require an ORTHOTIC cast or brace.

If a SPINAL INFECTION causes back pain, a pediatrician usually prescribes bed rest and an antibiotic. As the AAOS explained, "In young children, infection in a disk space (diskitis) can lead to back pain. Diskitis typically affects children aged 1–5, although older children and teenagers can also be affected."

In addition to the risk of DISCITIS, the AAOS said, "On rare occasion, tumors can be responsible for back pain. Spinal tumors usually happen in the middle or lower back. Pain is constant and progressive; it is unrelated to activity and/or happens at night." If a SPINAL TUMOR exists, a child may also limp or lean to one side.

Statistics and Studies

An article in *The Journal of Musculoskeletal Medicine* said the prevalence of LOW BACK PAIN (LBP) in children "ranges from 11% to 50%" with "distinct differences in evaluation and management of LBP in younger and older patients." Unlike for adults, "most causes of LBP in children can be identified." Although "treatment of children with LBP can be confounded by their relative lack of descriptive terminology," their back pain "can be divided into 5 general categories: developmental, inflammatory, mechanical, neoplastic, and psychosomatic." For example, spondylosis can be categorized as developmental, JUVENILE RHEUMATOID ARTHRITIS as inflammatory, a HERNIATED DISC as mechanical, and CANCER as neoplastic. For cancer, "the spine is the most common site of skeletal metastasis, accounting for 80% of all metastatic skeletal lesions." However, the article added, "Spinal tumors rarely occur in children or adolescents."

Far more likely is a playground injury. In a fact sheet on that topic, the National Center for Injury Prevention and Control posted statistics from various studies, stating, "Each year in the United States, emergency departments treat more than 200,000 children ages 14 and younger for playground-related injuries." Of these, "about 45% of playground-related injuries are severe—fractures, internal injuries, concussions, dislocations, and amputations." With girls (55 percent) sustaining more injuries than boys, "children ages 5 to 9 have higher rates of emergency department visits for playground injuries than any other age group. Most of these injuries occur at school." In addition, "a study in New York City found that playgrounds in low-income areas had more maintenance-related hazards than playgrounds in high-income areas. For example, playgrounds in low-income areas had significantly more trash, rusty play equipment, and damaged fall surfaces."

Unfortunately, some children cannot come out to play at all. According to statistics posted by ChildStats.gov, "In 2003, approximately 8 percent of children ages 5–17 were reported by parents to have activity limitations due to chronic conditions. Six percent were identified as having activity limitation solely by their participation in special education. Two percent had limitations in their ability to

walk, care for themselves, or participate in other activities."

Disease, injuries, and other factors can keep a child from walking, but disabling accidents can often be prevented. As the online article "Child Passenger Safety: Fact Sheet" by the Centers for Disease Control and Prevention (CDC) reported, "A survey of more than 17,500 children found that only 15% of children in safety seats were correctly harnessed into correctly installed seats," thus placing growing spines at unnecessary risk.

Special Aids and Adaptations

Besides the protective aid of properly fitted car seats for INFANTS and young children, a child's spinal needs may necessitate special aids such as a crawler, walker, handrail, ramp, or wheelchair to aid age-appropriate mobility.

Since children with spinal problems often require special tests or treatments, these too must be adapted to fit. For instance, most children want to know what to expect, how long it will take, and whether it will hurt. If the child is old enough to ask questions, a helpful response will usually offer simple, direct, brief, and matter-of-fact statements. Taking a quick tour of a medical facility or leafing through a picture book about a procedure may also ease fears, as can truthful but light words to explain. For example, "That machine is noisy, but it will not hurt you."

Often, children with spinal problems can be aided by various forms of COMPLEMENTARY AND ALTERNATIVE MEDICINE. Special adaptations may then include child-appropriate treatments of ACUPRESSURE, BIOFEEDBACK, HERBAL THERAPY, HOMEOPATHIC MEDICINE, or SPINAL MANIPULATION. Some specialists have been trained in MASSAGE THERAPY techniques for children, including infants, but parents may also find a good massage for themselves can help to ease chronic worries about a child.

American Academy of Orthopaedic Surgeons. "Back Pain In Children," AAOS. Available online. URL: http://orthoinfo.aaos.org/fact/thr_report.cfm?Thread_ID=329&topcategory=Spine. Downloaded December 14, 2005.

ChildStats.gov. "America's Children: Key National Indicators of Well-Being 2005, Activity Limitation," Forum on Child and Family Statistics. Available online. URL: http://childstats.gov/americaschildren/hea2.asp. Downloaded December 14, 2005.

National Center for Injury Prevention and Control. "Child Passenger Safety: Fact Sheet," Centers for Disease Control and Prevention (CDC). Available online. URL: http://www.cdc.gov/ncipc/factsheets/childpas. htm. Last reviewed February 14, 2005.

———. "Playground Injuries: Fact Sheet," Centers for Disease Control and Prevention (CDC). Available online. URL: http://www.cdc.gov/ncipc/factsheets/playgr. htm. Downloaded December 14, 2005.

Rooney, Richard C., M.D. and John G. Devine, M.D. "Evaluating and Managing Back Pain in Children and Adolescents," *The Journal of Musculoskeletal Medicine* 22, no. 6 (June 2005): 284–293.

chordoma   See SPINAL TUMOR.

chronic back pain   Unlike the abrupt arrival of ACUTE BACK PAIN, chronic pain hangs around a while, ambles off, then frequently returns. Since this unwelcome caller keeps on calling, one might wonder what a particular pain wants.

To explain some reasons for pain, a Spine-health. com article by Dr. Ralph Rashbaum said, "With acute pain, the severity of pain directly correlates to the level of tissue damage. This provides us with a protective reflex, such as the reflex to move your hand immediately if you touch a sharp object. This type of pain is a symptom of injured or diseased tissue, so that when the underlying problem is cured the pain goes away." However, "in chronic pain, the pain does not have the same meaning as with acute pain—it does not serve a protective or other biological function. Rather, the nerves continue to send pain messages to the brain even though there is no continuing tissue damage."

Symptoms and Diagnostic Path

A precise description of pain provides an important diagnostic tool. As explained on the Back.com Web site, "Neuropathic pain is caused by damage to nerve tissue. It is often felt as a burning or stabbing pain. One example of neuropathic pain is a pinched nerve." Conversely, "nociceptive pain is caused by

an injury or disease outside the nervous system. It is often an ongoing dull ache or pressure, rather than the sharper, trauma-like pain more characteristic of neuropathic pain." To find out which is which, diagnostic tests, such as MAGNETIC RESONANCE IMAGING or nerve function tests, may be needed.

Treatment Options and Outlook

If conservative treatments, such as NONSTEROIDAL ANTI-INFLAMMATORY DRUG (NSAID) THERAPY or prescription PAIN RELIEVERS, do not ease chronic back pain, Back.com suggested another approach. As the article explained, "Neurostimulation is the stimulation of the spinal cord by tiny electrical impulses. An implanted lead (a flexible insulated wire), which is powered by an implanted battery or by a receiver, is placed near your spinal cord," which then blocks "the pain messages to your brain." Reportedly, this therapy "can offer good to excellent pain relief, and improve your ability to go about daily activities."

Without successful intervention, the brain itself eventually reacts to the effects of chronic pain. To find out how much, a medical team from Northwestern University Feinberg School of Medicine in Chicago used magnetic resonance imaging in an innovative study. According to their report in *The Journal of Neuroscience,* "Our studies show that chronic back pain (CBP) (sustained for >6 months) is accompanied by abnormal brain chemistry" that resulted in "reduced cognitive abilities." Besides this decline in reasoning powers, the article reported, "the magnitude of brain gray matter atrophy caused by CBP is equivalent to 10–20 years of aging."

Undoubtedly, chronic pain stresses the brain, and makes a NERVE BLOCK or NEUROSTIMULATION viable options for PAIN MANAGEMENT. Other possibilities include ACUPRESSURE, ACUPUNCTURE, or SPINAL MANIPULATION, assuming no FRACTURE or degenerative conditions, such as OSTEOGENESIS IMPERFECTA or OSTEOARTHRITIS, exist. To repair the cause of chronic pain, SURGERY often helps, while BIOFEEDBACK can assist a person in managing pain that does not go away.

Risk Factors and Preventive Measures

Frequently, chronic pain results from an underlying medical condition, such as ARTHRITIS or OSTEOPOROSIS, with each causative factor having its own course of treatment. Nevertheless, people can sometimes avoid painful episodes or decrease the intensity by becoming aware of what triggers the pain. For instance, the American Osteopathic Association (AOA) mentioned improper LIFTING and poor POSTURE in "Prevention: The Best Treatment for Back Pain." As the AOA article said, "Prevent back pain by making a habit of sitting up straight and using correct form when lifting heavy items or completing daily tasks. Whether you work construction or spend your days typing on a computer, the way you sit, twist, bend, lift things, and even relax may either cause or prevent back pain."

Similarly, a fact sheet on "Managing Chronic Pain" posted by The American Occupational Therapy Association, Inc. (AOTA) explained that an occupational therapist (OT) can "identify specific activities or behaviors that aggravate pain and suggest alternatives." For example, an OT can "recommend and teach the client how to use adaptive equipment to decrease pain while performing tasks such as reaching, dressing, bathing, and performing household chores." Such adaptations help patients avoid the risk of encouraging unwanted pain to come and stay.

American Occupation Therapy Association, The, Inc. "Managing Chronic Pain," AOTA. Available online. URL: http://www.aota.org/featured/area6/docs/pain. pdf. Downloaded December 15, 2005.

American Osteopathic Association. "Prevention: The Best Treatment for Back Pain," AOA Health and Wellness. Available online. URL: http://www.osteopathic. org/index.cfm?PageID=you_backpain. Downloaded December 15, 2005.

Apkarian, A. Vania, Yamaya Sosa, Sreepadma Sonty, Robert M. Levy, R. Normal Harden, Todd B. Parrish, and Darren R. Gitelman. "Chronic Back Pain Is Associated with Decreased Prefrontal and Thalamic Gray Matter Density," *The Journal of Neuroscience* 24, no. 46 (November 17, 2004): 10,410–10,415.

Medtronic Sofamor Danek. "Frequently Asked Questions," Back.com. Available online. URL: http://www. back.com/faqs_chronic_pain.html. Updated July 11, 2005.

Rashbaum, Ralph, M.D. "Types of back pain," Spine-health. com. Available online. URL: http://www.spine-health.

com/topics/cd/neuropain/neuropain02.html. Downloaded December 15, 2005.

clinical trials In defining this important option, ClinicalTrials.gov said, "A clinical trial (also clinical research) is a research study in human volunteers to answer specific health questions. Carefully conducted clinical trials are the fastest and safest way to find treatments that work in people and ways to improve health." More specifically, "interventional trials determine whether experimental treatments or new ways of using known therapies are safe and effective under controlled environments. Observational trials address health issues in large groups of people or populations in natural settings."

As a service of the U.S. National Institutes of Health, information on the ClinicalTrials.gov Web site discussed what to expect: "In Phase I trials, researchers test an experimental drug or treatment in a small group of people (20–80) for the first time to evaluate its safety, determine a safe dosage range, and identify side effects. In Phase II trials, the experimental study drug or treatment is given to a larger group of people (100–300) to see if it is effective and to further evaluate its safety. In Phase III trials, the experimental study drug or treatment is given to large groups of people (1,000–3,000) to confirm its effectiveness, monitor side effects, compare it to commonly used treatments, and collect information that will allow the experimental drug or treatment to be used safely. In Phase IV trials, post marketing studies delineate additional information including the drug's risks, benefits, and optimal use."

Risks and Complications

Besides the time involved in adhering to the requirements of a clinical trial, some treatments cause adverse side effects. Also, not all participants receive the new treatment but may, instead, be given a placebo. Other patients simply become disappointed by not being accepted for a research trial.

Special Aids and Adaptations

Before participating in a clinical trial, ClinicalTrials. gov suggested asking pertinent questions, such as:

"What is the purpose of the study? . . . What kinds of tests and experimental treatments are involved? How do the possible risks, side effects, and benefits in the study compare with my current treatment? How might this trial affect my daily life? How long will the trial last? Will hospitalization be required? Who will pay for the experimental treatment? . . . What type of long-term follow up care is part of this study?" Undoubtedly, the answers will aid a person in making this potentially life-changing decision.

ClinicalTrials.gov. Home page, a service of the U.S. National Institutes of Health, developed by the National Library of Medicine. Available online. URL: http://clinicaltrials. gov/. Downloaded December 16, 2005.

Medtronic Sofamor Danek. "Could a Clinical Trial be Right for You?" Back.com. Available online. URL: http://www.back.com/articles-clinical_trial.html. Updated February 11, 2005.

coccydynia   This pain in the tailbone can occur during childbirth but more commonly results from a backward fall. Other causative factors include a SPINAL TUMOR or a SPINAL INFECTION.

Symptoms and Diagnostic Path

If a medical history gives cause to suspect CANCER, bone FRACTURE, or bone spur (OSTEOPHYTE), a physician may request X-RAYS or MAGNETIC RESONANCE IMAGING (MRI). A pelvic or a rectal examination may be necessary too. Otherwise, tests may not be needed so much as PAIN RELIEVERS and restful reclining.

Treatment Options and Outlook

According to the coccyx.org Web site, "Coccydynia can be anything from discomfort to acute pain, varying between people and varying with time in any individual. The name describes a pattern of symptoms (pain brought on or aggravated by sitting), so it is really a collection of conditions which can have different causes and need different treatments."

While inflammation lasts, at-home treatments include COLD THERAPY and NONSTEROIDAL ANTI-INFLAMMATORY DRUG (NSAID) THERAPY. If no swelling exists, HEAT THERAPY may be more comforting. Until the tailbone heals, special devices, such as a cushion with the center cut out, can avoid painful aggravation of the problem. Patients with frequent recurrences can sometimes be helped with ULTRASOUND THERAPY and, in rare instances, SURGERY.

Risk Factors and Preventive Measures

Online information from Spine-health.com said coccydynia "is fairly uncommon and probably accounts for less than 1% of cases of low back pain." Men have fewer risks, since "women have a broader pelvis, which means that sitting places pressure not only on their ischial tuberosities ('butt bone') but also on the coccyx. (Men tend to sit only on their ischial tuberosities without a lot of pressure applied to the coccyx)." A member of either sex with a tendency toward a tender tailbone would do well to avoid prolonged sitting. For some, the best position may come in being a fine citizen who remains upstanding.

coccyx.org. "What Is Coccydynia." Available online. URL: http://www.coccyx.org/whatisit/index.htm. Downloaded December 16, 2005.

Staehler, Richard, M.D. "Coccydynia—a Real Pain in the Tailbone," Spine-health.com. Available online. URL: http://www.spine-health.com/topics/cd/coccydynia/coc01.html. Downloaded December 12, 2005.

coccygeal spine   Commonly known as the tailbone, this part of the derriere consists of three to five vertebral bones designed in a triangular pattern similar to a wall sconce. Unlike the VERTEBRAE of the THORACIC SPINE and LUMBAR SPINE, the bones of the coccygeal spine have a solid center instead of a hollow opening, since they do not need to make room for the spinal cord. Instead, spinal nerves exit in the lumbar region, fanning across the hips and down the lower body.

Risks and Complications

The coccygeal spine does not articulate well with the upper SPINE and does not have much RANGE OF MOTION. As the coccyx.com Web site says, "When you walk or bend over, the coccyx does not move much in relation to the spine. But when you sit down, this pushes the flesh of your bottom out of its normal position, making the coccyx move by up to

22 degrees." In addition to this disconcerted effort, the span of coccyx bones varies among individuals with a total of one to four inches being the typical length. People with longer tailbones have a greater risk of sustaining injuries, such as COCCYDYNIA or a tailbone FRACTURE.

Statistics and Studies

Most studies agree that the odds of a bone injury lessen with BONE BUILDING efforts such as adequate NUTRITION, daily ACTIVITY, and STRENGTH TRAINING or other EXERCISE. For example, registered nurse Debra Wood recommended these sensible steps: "Eat a diet rich in calcium and vitamin D. Do weight-bearing exercises to build strong bones. Build strong muscles to prevent falls."

Special Aids and Adaptations

Whether a person has a bone fracture or a bruised tailbone, a "doughnut" cushion can relieve coccygeal pressure. ERGONOMIC FACTORS bear consideration, too, as a person can often avoid an achy tailbone by sitting correctly—or not at all.

coccyx.org. "The Normal Coccyx." Available online. URL: http://www.coccyx.org/whatisit/normal.htm. Downloaded December 16, 2005.

Wood, Debra. "Coccyx Fracture," Holy Cross Hospital, EBSCO Publishing. Available online. URL: http://healthychoice.epnet.com/GetContent.asp?siteid=holycross&docid=/dci/coccyxfracture. Downloaded December 16, 2005.

cold therapy   Sometimes known as cryotherapy, cold therapy can involve something as simple as a bag of frozen peas on a bruise. For swelling and inflammation, cold therapy provides an instinctive and effective treatment, especially after SURGERY or injuries. A cold compress also slows bleeding and, when applied to pulse points on the forehead and wrists, can help to bring down a fever.

Procedure

Whether packaged in cubes, chilled water, or state-of-the-art equipment, this therapy applies something cold to an area of heat and swelling. As a general rule, 20 minutes on and 20 minutes off the inflamed spot provides the recommended treatment for two to four days. If numbness begins at, say, ten minutes though, the session should abruptly end. For most bone-chilling needs, 15 minutes every two hours for a day or two will suffice.

Risks and Complications

Ice constricts blood flow, so anyone with circulatory problems should avoid cold therapy. Some people have an allergic response to cold, but almost everyone reacts adversely to icy treatments of the heart or chest. In an online article for the University of Michigan Health System, Dr. Pierre Rouzier cautioned, "Certain parts of the body (including the elbow, the knee, and the foot) can be injured by cold more easily because they don't have as much padding or insulation."

To avoid the risk of frostbite at any site, ice should not be applied directly to the skin for more than a minute or two. Even then, damp skin can stick and stay when an ice cube is pulled away. Besides causing an unnecessary ouch, skin damage can easily occur in INFANTS, CHILDREN, or ELDERLY patients who cannot convey their discomfort.

Assuming a person can tolerate cold, a commercial product from a reputable manufacturer provides a good option with certain precautions taken. For instance, the chemicals or dyes in some packs can seep into the body or cause skin irritation. Also, most store-bought ice packs have enough cooling power to last two hours or more but must still be used for only 10- to 20-minute intervals. However, improvised cold packs have drawbacks too. A pack of peas will defrost too quickly but not refreeze in time for the next cooling session, while crushed ice rolled into a towel can be messy or slide around the inflamed area like a car on an icy hill.

Outlook and Lifestyle Modifications

Prior to EXERCISE or a sports event, HEAT THERAPY can literally help a patient or ATHLETE to warm up. Conversely, an ice pack promptly applied to dry skin can prevent pain and swelling after intense ACTIVITY. In the Internet article mentioned above, Dr. Rouzier gave an example of a cool form of MASSAGE THERAPY, saying, "To do ice massage, first freeze water in a paper or Styrofoam cup. Then tear away the top lip of the cup and rub the ice over the injured area for 5 to 10 minutes. Ice massage works very well for overuse injuries." The doctor did not mention this, but if an injured person does not have time to freeze ice water, a sacrificial popsicle just might suffice.

Roach, Louise. "The Power of Ice," Mamashealth.com. Available online. URL: http://www.mamashealth. com/bodyparts/coldtherapy.asp. Downloaded December 19, 2005.

Rouzier, Pierre, M.D. "Ice Therapy," University of Michigan Health System, McKesson Provider Technologies. Available online. URL: http://www.med.umich. edu/1libr/sma/sma_itherapy_sma.htm. Downloaded December 19, 2005.

complementary and alternative medicine (CAM)

Traditionally, allopathic medicine strives to restore and preserve health. Complementary and alternative medicine (CAM) has the same goal, but the method can dramatically differ. For example, instead of prescribing drug therapy for a musculoskeletal complaint, CAM often takes a hands-on approach with ACUPRESSURE, ACUPUNCTURE, MASSAGE THERAPY, SPINAL MANIPULATION, or TRIGGER POINT THERAPY. Some conditions also respond to HEAT THERAPY, HYDROTHERAPY, HERBAL THERAPY, HOMEOPATHIC MEDICINE, or ULTRASOUND THERAPY. Besides treating BACKACHE or spinal pain, CAM practitioners may use BIOFEEDBACK or other methods to alter mechanisms that affect the central nervous system, produce tension, or cause problems with SLEEP.

Risks and Complications

Even a simple form of therapy has risks. For example, patients with circulatory problems must avoid COLD THERAPY, such as applying an ice pack to a bruised shin. People with SPINAL INFECTION, OSTEOPOROSIS, VERTEBRAL COMPRESSION FRACTURE, or other type of bone FRACTURE should avoid spinal manipulation, while people with food allergies must be cautious about trying herbal treatments. Complications also arise if patients refuse appropriate allopathic tests and treatments, using CAM as a soloist instead of a natural accompaniment in orchestrating their medical care. For instance, some herbs can ease the side effects of chemotherapy yet not provide the sole treatment for CANCER.

Statistics and Studies

Consumer Reports magazine surveyed 34,000 readers then announced, "Chiropractic was ranked ahead of all conventional treatments, including prescription drugs, by readers with back pain. . . . Deep tissue massage was found to be especially effective in treating osteoarthritis and fibromyalgia, a painful musculoskeletal syndrome that conventional medicine often remains at a loss to treat." Interestingly, "our new survey found that for readers who recently used alternative medicine, nearly 75 percent told their doctors about it. Most doctors approved," and "25 percent of those readers said their doctor suggested the alternative in the first place." In addition, "*Consumer Reports* subscribers, who tend to be older, wealthier, and better educated than the population at large, are enthusiastic users of alternative medicine not only to treat specific problems but also to maintain overall health. Forty-seven percent of respondents had tried an alternative remedy during the past two years, a higher percentage than that found by other large-scale surveys." Furthermore, "readers were much more likely to try alternative remedies for conditions that don't have effective conventional treatments." Although readers lauded chiropractic treatment of CERVICAL SPINE pain, the magazine did not recommend it because, "a University of California, San Francisco, study of stroke victims published in 2003 found that chiropractic manipulation of the neck significantly increased the risk of stroke by causing the lining of a neck artery to break off and block blood flow to the brain. Other studies have echoed that concern."

With a similar warning, an article in *Patient Care* said, "For any patient, neck maneuvers demand caution, particularly exercises that involve extension and rotation. . . . Overall, patients receiving manual therapy for the treatment of neck pain have a 1–2% risk of increased symptoms as a result. . . . Dizziness is most likely to worsen," but "the risk of serious complications or death from neck manipulation is estimated at about 0.0001%." Regarding the likelihood of being that one person in one-ten-thousandth of one percent, the article also said, "The prospect of injury to the cervical spine increases when the practitioner is not a physician, is not well-versed in diagnostic techniques, uses inappropriate force, or is unaware of contraindications to cervical treatment."

Mistrust, conflicting opinions, or lack of information can influence people to treat their own vertebral pain. According to an article in *USA Today,* "When adults experience back pain, they most commonly use self-help methods like resting or lying down (55%). Others try to alleviate discomfort by taking an over-the-counter medication (52%) or using a heating pad (38%). A much smaller number go to a trained medical professional to get treated, such as visiting their primary care doctor (23%), chiropractor (20%), or spine specialist (10%)."

The report "Complementary and Alternative Medicine Use Among Adults: United States, 2002" said that, "the majority of people use CAM as a complement to conventional medicine, not as an alternative." However, this choice comes with a price. As the report stated, "It has been estimated that the U.S. public spent between $36 billion and $47 billion on CAM therapies in 1997. Of this amount, between $12.2 billion and $19.6 billion was paid out-of-pocket for the services of professional CAM health care providers such as chiropractors, acupuncturists, and massage therapists. These fees are more than the U.S. public paid out-of-pocket for all hospitalizations in 1997 and about half that paid for all out-of-pocket physician services." Explanations for this growth include "marketing forces, availability of information on the Internet, the desire of patients to be actively involved with medical decision-making, and dissatisfaction with conventional . . . medicine."

More than one-third of the adults in the United States will at least investigate complementary or alternative treatments. As the National Center for Health Statistics said, these helps range from massage therapy (5 percent) to prayer for oneself or others (67 percent) with medicinal herbs (19 percent) sprinkled between like parsley.

Special Aids and Adaptations

CAM itself offers an adaptation or aid to conventional medical treatment, particularly for CHILDREN, people sensitive to pharmaceutical drugs, and those who cannot be helped by SURGERY. However, the need for CAM and traditional medical treatments can often be prevented by tending to basic necessities with greater care. Although easy to overlook, a body just naturally prescribes to the need for ample fresh water, healthful NUTRITION, regular EXERCISE, good POSTURE, and restorative sleep. Ultimately, this could make CAM mean "Caring About Myself."

Barnes, Patricia M., Eve Powell-Griner, Kim McFann, and Richard L. Nahin. "Complementary and Alternative Medicine Use Among Adults: United States, 2002," *Advance Data From Vital and Health Statistics,* National Center for Complementary and Alternative Medicine, National Institutes of Health, Centers for Disease Control and Prevention (CDC) no. 343 (May 27, 2004): p. 1–20.

Bower, Peter J., Beverly Rubik, Steven J. Weiss, and Cynthia Starr. "Manual Therapy: Hands-on Healing," *Patient Care* 31, no. 20 (December 15, 1997): 69–81.

National Center for Health Statistics. "More Than One-Third of U.S. Adults Use Complementary and Alternative Medicine, According to New Government Survey." Available online. URL: http://www.cdc.gov/nchs/pressroom/04news/adultsmedicine.htm. Last reviewed May 27, 2004.

Staff. "Sufferers Prefer Home Remedies," *USA Today Magazine* 133, no. 2,717 (February 2005): 11.

Staff. "Which Alternative Treatments Work?" Consumer Reports (August 2005): 39–41.

complex regional pain syndrome (CRPS) See REFLEX SYMPATHETIC DYSTROPHY SYNDROME.

compression fracture See VERTEBRAL COMPRESSION FRACTURE.

computed tomography (CT) or computerized axial tomography scan (CAT scan) When X-RAYS met computer technology, it was lovely at first sight. As more seriously explained by the American Academy of Orthopaedic Surgeons (AAOS) Web site, "A CT scan (computed tomography) is a modern imaging tool that combines X-rays with computer technology to produce a more detailed, cross-sectional image of your body. A CT scan lets your doctor see the size, shape and position of structures that are deep inside your body, such as organs, tissues or tumors."

The Radiology Society of North America (RSNA) added, "CT is able to depict internal bleeding and fractures in trauma victims shortly after they arrive at the hospital." Painless and noninvasive, "spinal CT scanning is a rapid procedure and offers an accurate evaluation of bone and most soft tissues. Using the latest equipment, the spine may be displayed in multiple planes, and three-dimensional imaging is an option." Also, "CT is less expensive and more cost-effective than MRI" (MAGNETIC RESONANCE IMAGING). "In addition, it is less sensitive to patient movement. Unlike MRI, CT may be carried out in patients who have an implanted device of any kind."

Procedure

For a memorable interior portrait, the patient must be as still as needed for a photo-shoot. However, this painless outpatient procedure seems less glamorous and more like being engulfed by a doughnut-shaped camera lens. As a cylindrical tube encircles the reclining person, X-rays shot from many angles appear on a computer screen. In some cases, a contrast is injected into the vein of the patient to enhance CT pictures with colorization and show a troublesome area for what it really is. For example, a CT scan may be used to detect a HERNIATED DISC, hairline FRACTURE, SPINAL TUMOR, or other abnormality in the BACK or SPINE. To get a clear picture in about one hour or less, the procedure involves a barium sulfate injection or a special dye to drink, which may seem like downing food coloring without the juicy benefits.

Risks and Complications

Some patients react to the dye with a rash or stomach upset. Although rare, the contrast medium can cause anaphylactic shock in people who take certain medications or are highly sensitive to iodine. Minimal exposure lowers radiation risks, but pregnant women should avoid a CT scan. More likely complications occur for people in small towns or rural areas where no CT scanning equipment can be found to evaluate an injury.

Outlook and Lifestyle Modifications

To assess ELDERLY patients or monitor persons with OSTEOPOROSIS, a CT scan can be used as a BONE MINERAL DENSITY TEST every two years or so. Since the pictures show soft tissue and DISCS too, a scan provides an accurate diagnostic tool for a catalog of spinal problems, each of which may suggest an appropriate change in lifestyle.

American Academy of Orthopaedic Surgeons. "Diagnostic Imaging," AAOS. Available online. URL: http://orthoinfo.aaos.org/fact/thr_report.cfm?Thread_ID=212&topcategory=General%20Information. Downloaded December 20, 2005.

Radiology Society of North America. "Computed Tomography (CT)—Spine," RSNA. Available online. URL: http://www.radiologyinfo.org/content/spinect.htm. Last reviewed August 2, 2005.

seniorhealthchannel. "CT Scan," Healthcommunities.com, Inc. Available online. URL: http://seniorhealthchannel.com/diagnostictests/CTscan.shtml. Last modified December 20, 2005.

spine inc. "CAT Scan," Extracted from Asia Medicine Net. Available online. URL: http://www.spine-inc.com/glossary/c/ct-scan.html. Downloaded December 20, 2005.

congenital anomaly of the spine   See BIRTH DEFECTS OF THE SPINE.

corpectomy   A type of ARTHRODESIS, this surgical procedure often addresses the CERVICAL SPINE but sometimes the THORACIC SPINE and LUMBAR SPINE. In any case, the operation removes one or more vertebrae and/or adjacent DISCS, usually to relieve pressure on the SPINE, spare the spinal nerves, or prevent a SPINAL CORD injury. If a bone spur has developed, that OSTEOPHYTE will also be removed.

Procedure

Similar to an ANTERIOR CERVICAL DISCECTOMY, the surgeon makes an incision in the front (anterior) portion of the neck, removes the offending bone matter, then fills the space with a BONE GRAFT. In addition, information from the All About Back & Neck Pain Web site said, "Some method of internal fixation to hold the bones and bone graft in place is normally used. The most common method is to use metal (titanium) plates and screws. The plate sits on the front of the remaining vertebrae, covering the . . . graft. Screws are placed into the vertebral bodies above and below the graft to hold the plate in place and keep the bone graft from slipping."

Risks and Complications

Every SURGERY involves risks such as bleeding or infection, but proximity to the spinal cord makes a corpectomy a delicate and potentially dangerous operation. Most patients, however, will be released from the hospital in two to four days. Some experience immediate relief, but for others, a decrease in pain may be gradual. Few complications arise, but cigarette smoking can slow bone growth, hindering the desired bone fusion.

Outlook and Lifestyle Modifications

During the recovery period, an ORTHOTIC neck brace or halo device immobilizes the neck until natural fusion has stabilized the area. If the corpectomy involves vertebrae in the BACK, a different type of orthotic may be needed to keep the person mobile. When fusion has been established, therapeutic EXERCISE can begin to strengthen the spine and PARASPINAL MUSCLES.

All About Back & Neck Pain. "Cervical Corpectomy and Strut Graft." Available online. URL: http://www.allaboutbackpain.com/html/spine_cervical/spine_cervical_corpectomy.html. Downloaded December 20, 2005.

Mellion, B. Theo, M.D. "Surgical: Cervical Corpectomy," Medtronic Sofamor Danek, Neck Surgery.com. Available online. URL: http://www.neckreference.com/treatment-surgical-corpectomy.html. Downloaded December 20, 2005.

corticosteroid injection   When other forms of PAIN MANAGEMENT no longer ease vertebral pain or swelling in the BACK and SPINE, cortisone injections come to the rescue. The tricky part can be finding the right spot to inject this synthetic version of a naturally produced hormone. If a patient can identify the source of pain, so much the better, but pain radiating from a tendon or joint can be difficult to pinpoint. If so, an ELECTROMYOGRAM may confirm the locale. Also, the doctor may request MAGNETIC RESONANCE IMAGING (MRI) or a COMPUTED TOMOGRAPHY (CT) SCAN to clarify the site of injection.

Procedure

In an article for eMedicine.com, Dr. Jerrold N. Rosenberg explained variations in the procedure: "Some physicians prefer to give one injection (the corticosteroid preparation, perhaps mixed with a local anesthetic). Their rationale is that one needle is less painful than two; however, the cortisone injection involves a thicker material and, therefore, they use a larger gauge needle." With a two-needle technique, the physician uses a smaller needle to anesthetize the area, waits three to five minutes for an optimal numbing effect, then switches to a larger needle for the actual injection.

Risks and Complications

A corticosteroid injection should not be given to a person with a SPINAL INFECTION or other fever-producing illness. In an article for Quest Diagnostics, Kerry Cooke said, "Corticosteroids should be used with caution. Although they may provide relief from pain and inflammation, corticosteroids can also slow healing and new bone formation. You may experience an increase in pain during the first 2 to 4 days after an injection." Some people also encounter side effects, such as easy bruising or edema. In addition, long-term use can thin bones and even cause OSTEOPOROSIS. However, Cooke suggested, "To prevent osteoporosis while taking long-term or high-dose corticosteroids, also take 1000 mg to 1500 mg of calcium daily, 800 IU of vitamin D daily, and a preventive medication, such as alendronate or risedronate. Weight-bearing exercise also helps reduce the risk of osteoporosis."

Outlook and Lifestyle Modifications

An article on the Spine-dr.com Web site reported the success of corticosteroid injections in treating pain in the CERVICAL SPINE. With 80 percent of the injections at the C7 to T1 level and the other 20 at C6 to C7, "The study results show marked initial relief in 63% (19/30), with relief lasting an average of eight months in 50% (15/30) of all injected patients. Seventy-six percent of injected patients who had relief initially sustained their improved state or improved further during follow up." Although the procedure does not cure a problem such as DEGENERATIVE DISC DISEASE or SPINAL STENOSIS, a corticosteroid injection may enable a patient to delay SURGERY, resume regular ACTIVITY, or begin therapeutic EXERCISE to strengthen the back and decrease vertebral pain.

Cooke, Kerry V. "Corticosteroid Injections for Spinal Stenosis," Quest Diagnostics ® Patient Health Library. Available online. URL: http://www.questdiagnostics.com/kbase/topic/detail/drug/uh1944/detail.htm. Downloaded December 20, 2005.

Rosenberg, Jerrold N., M.D. "Corticosteroid Injections of Joints and Soft Tissues," eMedicine.com. Available online. URL: http://www.emedicine.com/pmr/topic211.htm. Downloaded December 20, 2005.

Spine-dr.com. "Cervical Epidural Corticosteroid Injection In Degenerative Disease." Available online. URL: http://www.spine-dr.com/site/surgery/block_article3.html. Downloaded December 20, 2005.

costotransverse and costovertebral joint injections   In small joints where the ribs meet the SPINE, pain invites poor company. Upper back pain or pain between the ribs may signal the arrival of rib dysfunction syndromes. Since this party of problems can masquerade as other conditions, joint injections can identify the syndrome and also relieve the unwanted pain.

Procedure

For this 15- to 30-minute procedure, the patient lies facedown as a medical specialist uses FLUOROSCOPY to locate the rib joint where an injection will occur. The needle brings a quick prick, but any ACUTE PAIN or CHRONIC PAIN emanating from that joint should soon subside, and mobility should proportionately increase.

In an article for Spine-health.com, Dr. Ray Baker discussed what happens next: "Twenty to thirty minutes after the procedure, the patient will be asked to try to provoke the usual pain. Patients may or may not obtain pain relief in the first few hours after the injection, depending upon whether or not the area injected is the main source of the patient's upper back pain. On occasion, patients may feel numb or a slightly weak/odd feeling for a few hours after the injection. This may last several hours, but the patient should be able to function safely, if proper precautions are taken." For example, the person should not drive a vehicle or resume daily ACTIVITY for about 24 hours.

Risks and Complications

Patients who take blood thinners or who experience allergic reactions to medications should not have a joint injection. In general, side effects include edema and changes in weight, mood, blood pressure, or blood sugar. Discomfort may occur in the first few days after a treatment, but an ice pack or other form of COLD THERAPY will usually bring relief. Although rare, long-term use of the injections can produce ARTHRITIS.

Outlook and Lifestyle Modifications

Since a joint injection often makes a person feel better immediately, care must be taken to increase EXERCISE gradually. With the pain eased and the RANGE OF MOTION expanded, STRENGTH TRAINING can begin with greater comfort. Also, the patient may be better able to handle SPINAL MANIPULATION or other appropriate therapies.

Baker, Ray, M.D. "Costotransverse and Costovertebral Joint Injections," Spine-health.com. Available online. URL: http://www.spine-health.com/topics/conserv/joint/joint01.html. Downloaded December 21, 2005.

Silveri, Christopher P., M.D. "Costovertebral Block," International Spine Intervention Society, Patient Information, SpineUniverse.com. Available online. URL: http://www.spineuniverse.com/displayarticle.php/article656.html. Last updated November 16, 2005.

COX-2 inhibitors   See CYCLOOXYGENASE INHIBITORS.

crush fracture   See VERTEBRAL COMPRESSION FRACTURE.

crush injury syndrome   See RHABDOMYOLYSIS.

curvature of the spine   See FLAT BACK; KYPHOSIS; LORDOSIS.

cyclooxygenase (COX-2) inhibitors   This newer class of NONSTEROIDAL ANTI-INFLAMMATORY DRUG (NSAID) blocks cyclooxygenase, an enzyme commonly known as COX-2. As a MedicineNet.com article explained, "Blocking this enzyme impedes the production of the chemical messengers (prostaglandins) that cause the pain and swelling of arthritis inflammation."

Similarly, COX-1 inhibitors such as ASPIRIN, IBUPROFEN, and NAPROXEN block inflammation. However, the COX-1 enzyme has the extra jobs of protecting the stomach and helping blood to clot. Therefore, if an NSAID inhibits COX-1 production, that same medication removes the protection of this specific enzyme. Conversely, COX-2 enzymes do not safeguard the lining of the stomach, so blocking their production does not alter stomach protection.

Dosage and Potential Side Effects

The dosage of a COX-2 inhibitor depends upon the brand as well as the condition treated. For example, celecoxib (Celebrex) may be prescribed in 100 mg capsules twice a day or 200 mgs once a day to ease symptoms of pain and inflammation caused by ARTHRITIS, OSTEOARTHRITIS, or RHEUMATOID ARTHRITIS. Also, *Drug Topics* announced, "The FDA has approved a sixth indication for Pfizer's selective COX-2 inhibitor Celebrex (celecoxib). The drug can now be used for the relief of the signs and symptoms associated with ankylosing spondylitis." If all goes well with the daily dose initially recommended for about six weeks, 400 mg daily may be tried.

In general, the side effects for COX-2 inhibitors range from more common episodes of headache or queasiness to the rare but severe allergic reaction apparent in a rash. If itching, chest pain, or respiratory distress occur, the product should immediately be discontinued and medical attention sought.

Statistics and Studies

In a document updated on July 18, 2005, the U.S. Food and Drug Administration (FDA) issued a statement requiring manufacturers of both OVER-THE-COUNTER and prescription COX-2 inhibitors to change their labels. Specifically, "all sponsors of marketed prescription Non-Steroidal Anti-Inflammatory Drugs (NSAIDs), including Celebrex (celecoxib), a COX-2 selective NSAID, have been asked to revise the labeling (package insert) for their products to include a boxed warning, highlighting the potential for increased risk of cardiovascular (CV) events and the well described, serious, potential life-threatening gastrointestinal (GI) bleeding associated with their use." Besides this directive, "FDA has also requested that the package insert for all NSAIDs be revised to include a contraindication for use in patients immediately post-operative from coronary artery bypass . . . surgery."

Regarding COX-2 inhibitors previously withdrawn from the market, FDA will be unlikely to reissue approval unless benefits can be shown to outweigh those of other NSAIDs. According to an article in *Family Practice News*, the FDA requested the manufacturer to continue post-marketing studies of Celebrex. The article also said, "So far, the FDA has stopped short of asking other NSAID manufacturers to perform additional studies, but it has asked them to review all available safety data from both short- and long-term studies and look for additional safety signals."

As RESEARCH and debates continue, patients with painful inflammation not helped by SURGERY may turn to older NSAIDs or centuries-old HOMEOPATHIC MEDICINE, HERBAL THERAPY, or other forms of COMPLEMENTARY AND ALTERNATIVE MEDICINE. For most people, healthy habits of daily ACTIVITY, EXERCISE, and NUTRITION also offer gentle but reliable long-term help.

MedicineNet.com, Inc. "Cox-2 Inhibitors." Available online. URL: http://www.medicinenet.com/cox-2_inhibitors/article.htm. Last reviewed October 2, 2005.

Staff. "Celebrex Gains New Indication; Boxed Warning Added," *Drug Topics* 149, no. 16 (August 22, 2005): 10.

Sullivan, Michelle G. "COX-2 Withdrawals Complicate Pain Relief Decisions: Few Options Left for Patients with Pain," *Family Practice News* 35, no. 10 (May 1, 2005): 1–2.

U.S. Food and Drug Administration. "COX-2 Selective (includes Bextra, Celebrex, and Vioxx) and Non-Selective Non-Steroidal Anti-Inflammatory Drugs (NSAIDs)," FDA Center for Drug Evaluation and Research, Department of Health and Human Services. Available online. URL: http://www.fda.gov/cder/drug/infopage/COX2/default.htm. Last updated July 18, 2005.

degenerative disc disease A normal spine comes naturally cushioned with sturdy gel packs. Between the VERTEBRAE, each DISC acts as a shock absorber to keep one bone from rubbing another and causing painful friction. If a HERNIATED DISC ruptures, the gelatinous matter seeps from the tough outer ring, generating ACUTE PAIN. If discs in general degenerate, the news comes as a spinal shock.

Symptoms and Diagnostic Path

An article posted by the Spine Institute of New York described symptoms, saying, "The most common early symptom of degenerative disc disease is back pain that often spreads to the buttocks and upper thighs. The degenerating disc(s) can also cause 'discogenic' pain (which just means pain that originates in a damaged disc) and bulging discs."

As spinal discs bulge, so may the stomach. This occurs because the bones of the SPINE shift and settle, decreasing overall height. Subsequently, a person may feel the pudgy effects of WEIGHT even though none has been gained. For an official diagnosis, a physician will assess RANGE OF MOTION in a physical examination and inquire into a medical history. In addition, X-RAYS answer questions about vertebral changes, while MAGNETIC RESONANCE IMAGING or a DISCOGRAM can clarify the condition of each questionable disc.

Treatment Options and Outlook

DISC REPLACEMENT or other type of SURGERY may be needed to alleviate spinal nerve pressure or stabilize spinal joints. Often though, NONSTEROIDAL ANTI-INFLAMMATORY DRUG (NSAID) THERAPY or modifications in daily ACTIVITY can arrest degenerate disc behavior. Also, solving such problems as poor POSTURE or adverse ERGONOMIC FACTORS can reform a wayward spine into maintaining proper disc function.

As explained in a Spine-health.com article, "The treatment options for degenerative disc disease are either passive [done to the patient] or active [done by the patient]. Usually a combination of treatments is used to help control the symptoms. Passive treatments are rarely effective on their own—some active component is almost always required." For example, passive therapy might include a TRANSCUTANEOUS ELECTRONIC NERVE STIMULATOR (TENS) UNIT, PAIN RELIEVERS, or an EPIDURAL INJECTION, whereas active treatments may mean physical therapy and STRENGTH TRAINING. As the article summarized, "Pain from degenerative disc disease is caused by instability at the motion segment and inflammation from the degenerated discs. Both the instability and the inflammation have to be addressed for the treatment to be effective."

Risk Factors and Preventive Measures

As discs fail to cushion vertebrae in the BACK or spine, bones often shift, which, in turn, can cause VERTEBRAL SUBLUXATION or OSTEOPHYTE formation. In the latter case, bone spurs sometimes grow into the spinal column, pressing nerves or causing SPINAL STENOSIS. If neck discs degenerate, CERVICAL SPONDYLOSIS may result.

Regardless of whether problems occur in the CERVICAL SPINE, THORACIC SPINE, or LUMBAR SPINE, treatments such as therapeutic EXERCISE and SPINAL MANIPULATION can slow or lessen deterioration. So can healthful NUTRITION, ample water, and adequate SLEEP, mainly by giving the body what it needs to hydrate, nourish, and restore cells. Other preventives include low-impact dancing, swimming, rowing, and riding a stationary bicycle, preferably in front of a gorgeous view to ease the mind, please the senses, and appease boredom. Biking in front of a television set can also keep an otherwise inert body motivated into movement. This works particularly well with a program of three to four one-hour sessions regularly scheduled each week.

Spine Institute of New York. "Degenerative Disc Disease," Beth Israel Medical Center. Available online. URL: http://www.spineinstituteny.com/conditions/degenerative.html. Downloaded December 22, 2005.

Ullrich, Peter F., M.D. "Degenerative Disc Disease—Non-surgical Treatment Options," Spine-health.com. Available online. URL: http://www.spine-health.com/topics/conserv/degendisc/degendisc01.html. Downloaded December 22, 2005.

degenerative joint disease   See OSTEOARTHRITIS.

diclofenac sodium   See NONSTEROIDAL ANTI-INFLAMMATORY DRUG THERAPY.

dietary needs for spinal health   See NUTRITION.

diffuse idiopathic skeletal hyperostosis (DISH)
Also known as Forestier's Disease, this form of degenerative ARTHRITIS occurs as soft tissue hardens. What should be supple, malleable matter may become rigid, thereby binding tendons, ligaments, and joints from normal movement. As hardening continues, the condition often affects the THORACIC SPINE, but the CERVICAL SPINE and LUMBAR SPINE may lose flexibility too.

Symptoms and Diagnostic Path

Besides obvious signs of rigidity and decreased RANGE OF MOTION, the disease may be asymptomatic. Confirmation may be accidental as a doctor rules out similar conditions or detects DISH via such imaging tests as X-RAY, MRI (MAGNETIC RESONANCE IMAGING), or CT (COMPUTED TOMOGRAPHY) SCAN.

Treatment Options and Outlook

If a bone spur (OSTEOPHYTE) forms or bony overgrowth hinders a joint, SURGERY may be needed to free movement. Otherwise, DISH can usually be treated with SPINAL MANIPULATION and PAIN RELIEVERS. In addition, NONSTEROIDAL ANTI-INFLAMMATORY (NSAID) DRUG THERAPY can keep down the inflammation, subsequently reducing DISH-producing calcification.

Risk Factors and Preventive Measures

An article on the PatientPlus Web site said, "The prevalence in European men over the age of 50 years is 5.8% and in women is 1.3%." People under 40 very rarely have this problem, but, regardless of the age or sex, "thoracic vertebrae are involved in 100%, lumbar in 68–90%, and cervical in 65–78% of affected individuals."

Until causal factors have been identified, preventive measures may be hit or miss. However, an article in *Orthopaedic Nursing* gave a clue by saying, "Environmental causes question the relationship of fluoride in air and drinking water in the development of Forestiers disease." Fluoride may have a role because, "chronic fluorine exposure looks like DISH on radiographs." Also, "another area of investigation into the pathogenesis of DISH is toxic properties," such as bone changes caused by prolonged use of high doses of VITAMIN A supplements.

Besides those potential causes, one might say that being sedentary almost ensures sedimentary deposits. Therefore, regular daily ACTIVITY, stretching EXERCISES, and a healthy plate of NUTRITION may put away DISH problems.

Childs, Sharon G. "Diffuse Idiopathic Skeletal Hyperostosis," *Orthopaedic Nursing* 23, no. 6 (November/December 2004): 375–382.

Shiel, William, M.D. "Diffuse Idiopathic Skeletal Hyperostosis ('DISH' or Forestier Disease)," MedicineNet.com. Available online. URL: http://www.medicinenet.com/diffuse_idiopathic_skeletal_hyperostosis/article.htm. Last reviewed May 3, 2005.

Tidy, Colin, M.D. "Forestier's Disease," PatientPlus. Available online. URL: http://www.patient.co.uk/showdoc/40002443/. Last issued November 2, 2005.

diflunisal   See NONSTEROIDAL ANTI-INFLAMMATORY DRUG THERAPY.

disc, disk   Like bubble wrap, vertebral discs cushion bones. Instead of air though, the interior holds a gelatinous substance that aids a disc in doing its cushy job. Beginning with the second vertebra of the CERVICAL SPINE, discs go through the THORACIC SPINE and LUMBAR SPINE, then end just above the SACRAL VERTEBRAE.

An online article for ChiroGeek.com explained, "The disc is made up of three basic structures: the nucleus pulposus, the anulus fibrosus, and the vertebral end-plates. Although their composition percentage differs, the latter three structures are made of three basic components: proteoglycan (protein), collagen (cartilage), and water." Indeed, "in order for a disc to function properly, it MUST have high water content." Assuming all is well, "water is held within the disc by tiny sponge-like molecules. . . . These 'super sponges' have an amazing ability to attract and hold water molecules, and can in fact hold over 500 times their own weight in water; this gives the non-dehydrated disc the tremendous 'hydrostatic pressure' which is needed to bear the axial load of the body."

Risks and Complications

Besides absorbing the shocks of daily ACTIVITY, the button-like discs have a buttoning effect on the spine. As long as they hold up, the VERTEBRAE usually do too. However, with DEGENERATIVE DISC DISEASE and aging, spinal joints may shift, making the vertebral column feel like a wavering tower of blocks. Because of the wear and tear on weight-bearing bones in the lower back, discs in the lumbar region normally receive more pressure, but this increases even more with added WEIGHT. If the discs cannot hold up under the pressure, vertebrae may shift from alignment, subsequently decreasing spinal stability. SPINAL MANIPULATION can sometimes help to realign the spine and relieve disc pressure, but in some cases, a DISC REPLACEMENT or other type of SURGERY may be needed to stabilize the spine.

Statistics and Studies

A SpineUniverse article offered these enlightening statistics: "The average spine . . . segment undergoes approximately 100,000,000 cycles" of motion "in a lifetime, and about 6 million each year." Since "the center of rotation is mobile and not static," this puts considerable wear on discs. If they need replacing though, the article reported, "The average implant

survivorship is estimated to be 30 million cycles (5 years of clinical usage), and therefore the demands on spine . . . implants will be challenged."

Special Aids and Adaptations

Lots of fresh water, raw fruit, uncooked vegetables, and, if needed, vitamin supplements can aid disc health. However, one cannot pop a collagen pill. Instead, blue-black and red-black fruits, such as blueberries, raspberries, or black cherries, help the body produce collagen. Dark berries also help to retain the moisture that dry or worn-out discs need to bounce back after long, jolting, dehydrating hours at work.

Besides the help of NUTRITION, disc protection can come in gel-packs inserted into SHOES. Like spinal discs, synthetic gel insoles absorb vibration as a person walks or runs. Eventually, this silicone-based protection wears out too. Unlike real discs though, additional stores can usually be found at a relatively minimal cost.

Gillard, Douglas M. "Disc Anatomy," ChiroGeek.com. Available online. URL: http://www.chirogeek.com/000_Disc_Anatomy.htm. Downloaded December 23, 2005.
Janssen, Michael E. and Chi Lam. "Fusion vs. Disc Replacement for Discogenic Pain: Part 2," SpineUniverse. Available online. URL: http://www.spineuniverse.com/displayarticle.php/article165.html. Downloaded December 23, 2005.

disc disease   See DEGENERATIVE DISC DISEASE.

discectomy   A HERNIATED DISC does not always need complete removal or a DISC REPLACEMENT. Some problems resolve themselves. If not, a discectomy can provide a better surgical option by removing only a portion of the disc that presses spinal nerves and causes the pain of SCIATICA.

Procedure

The actual procedure depends on whether the patient can have MINIMALLY INVASIVE SURGERY or whether an open discectomy gives better access in stabilizing the disc. In discussing the latter, the North American Spine Society (NASS) said, "Open discectomy is the most common surgical treatment for ruptured or herniated discs of the lumbar spine. . . . During the procedure, the surgeon will make an approximate one-inch incision in the skin over the affected area of the spine. Muscle tissue is removed from the bone above and below the affected disc and retractors hold the muscle and skin away from the surgical site so the surgeon has a clear view of the vertebrae and disc. In some cases bone and ligaments may have to be removed for the surgeon to be able to visualize and then gain access to the bulging disc without damaging the nerve tissue; this is called a laminectomy or laminotomy depending on how much bone is removed."

Risks and Complications

Although most patients experience relief from the CHRONIC PAIN of a herniated disc after the discectomy has healed, some continue to have symptoms. About 5 to 10 percent of patients experience repeated disc herniation. To avoid stressing the SPINE or causing further disc damage, patients should take care in LIFTING objects correctly and pick up no more than five pounds during the first month of recovery. Driving a vehicle should be avoided during that time too.

Outlook and Lifestyle Modifications

For the first few weeks following a discectomy, PAIN MANAGEMENT may include NONSTEROIDAL ANTI-INFLAMMATORY DRUG (NSAID) THERAPY and COLD THERAPY to keep down swelling. As healing begins, daily ACTIVITY gradually resumes with the eventual addition of therapeutic EXERCISE or physical therapy. Since discs require hydration to work well, lots of fresh drinking water can be therapeutic too.

North American Spine Society. "Open Discectomy," NASS. Available online. URL: http://www.spine.org/articles/discectomy.cfm. Downloaded January 5, 2006.
Spine Institute of New York. "Discectomy," Beth Israel Medical Center. Available online. URL: http://www.spineinstituteny.com/treatments/discectomy.html. Downloaded December 23, 2005.

discitis or diskitis With this type of infection, an inflammatory lesion occurs in the DISC space between two or more VERTEBRAE. Adults can acquire this problem, for instance, as a complication after a DISCOGRAM. More commonly, discitis affects the THORACIC SPINE or LUMBAR SPINE of CHILDREN under 10.

Symptoms and Diagnostic Path

Besides a painful BACKACHE that emanates from the area of infection, ACUTE PAIN may radiate into the lower body or legs. Characteristic symptoms also include fever, fatigue, chills, and a poor appetite. As a Back.com article said, "Young children with this condition are usually irritable and uncomfortable and refuse to sit up, stand or walk."

Treatment Options and Outlook

According to the same Back.com article, "The treatment of discitis generally involves antibiotics, rest, and a brace. Surgery is rarely needed."

Risk Factors and Preventive Measures

Since discitis usually results from the invasion of a virus or bacteria into a vertebral space, preventives include such simple steps as showering thoroughly or regularly tending a wound on the BACK or nearby area. However, discitis can occur as foreign matter enters the skin through a needle. In extremely rare and curious circumstances, this could happen in a well-sanitized setting where a clean patient has a highly hygienic surgical test or well-scrubbed procedure involving sterilized instruments. A more likely culprit, however, could be drug abuse involving dirty needles.

Medtronic Sofamor Danek. "Inflammatory & Infectious Disorders: Discitis," Back.com. Available online. URL: http://www.back.com/causes-inflammatory-discitis.html. Downloaded December 23, 2005.
Young, Michael J., M.D. "Discitis: Disc Space Infection," SpineUniverse. Available online. URL: http://www.spineuniverse.com/displayarticle.php/article203.html. Downloaded December 23, 2005.

disc nucleoplasty This MINIMALLY INVASIVE SURGERY brings new voice to the surgical scene. For the procedure, a needle injects radio waves into the compact little DISC normally at play between the VERTEBRAE. If age or injury cause a disc to rupture or bulge, radio waves of nucleoplasty may be called upon to make repairs.

Procedure

In describing what happens in disc nucleoplasty, a SpineUniverse article explained, "The procedure begins with a local (or topical) anesthetic and light sedative. While the patient is awake, small amounts of radio wave energy are released into the damaged disc through a catheter-like device that is about the thickness of a dime. The energy creates a molecular reaction that causes some of the spongy tissue inside the damaged disc to dissolve. As pressure inside the disc is reduced, the herniation in the shell retracts, the irritation to the nearby nerve roots is reduced, and pain is relieved. Typically, the entire Nucleoplasty radio wave injection procedure takes 20 to 30 minutes, and the patient is ready to walk out of the clinic in about an hour."

Risks and Complications

Approved by the Food and Drug Administration and the American Medical Association, disc nucleoplasty avoids the risks of invasive SURGERY and lowers costs, financially and physically. As explained online by the Spine Institute of New York, "Recovery from this outpatient procedure is usually very quick because, like most minimally invasive surgery, it does not require the cutting of muscles or bone. With limited bed rest and a program of physical therapy, patients should resume normal activity within one to six weeks."

Disc nucleoplasty will not work well for everyone though. For a herniated disc, MICRODISCECTOMY offers the preferred treatment, whereas patients with severe DEGENERATIVE DISC DISEASE, FRACTURE, SPINAL STENOSIS, or SPINAL TUMOR may need other forms of surgery or alternatives.

Outlook and Lifestyle Modifications

Often, LOW BACK PAIN resolves itself within a few weeks. If conservative medical treatment or COMPLEMENTARY AND ALTERNATIVE MEDICINE do not help, nucleoplasty may keep disc pain from becoming an unbroken record.

DISC Nucleoplasty ™. "DISC Nucleoplasty Overview," ArthroCare Corporation. Available online. URL: http://

www.discnucleoplasty.com/dphy/dphy.aspx?s=0201. Downloaded December 23, 2005.

Maywood, Sam, M.D. "Nucleoplasty® Radio Wave Injection Offers Quick, Lasting Relief—Without Drugs," SpineUniverse. Available online. URL: http://www.spineuniverse.com/displayarticle.php/article1882.html. Last updated July 25, 2005.

Spine Institute of New York. "Intradiscal Percutaneous Procedures: Disc Nucleoplasty," Beth Israel Medical Center. Available online. URL: http://www.spineinstituteny.com/treatments/intradiscal.html. Downloaded December 23, 2005.

discogram, discography   This diagnostic test uses X-RAY to show a damaged DISC or confirm a DEGENERATIVE DISC as the source of CHRONIC LOW BACK PAIN. Since the procedure itself may be painful, most physicians try less invasive tests or treatments first, but they may turn to discography to confirm a need for SURGERY.

Procedure

To take the edge off this outpatient test, a MUSCLE RELAXANT and PAIN RELIEVER will be given. A special dye injected into the area(s) of concern will show disc bulging or scarring as white on the x-ray. If a physician suspects multiple disc involvement or needs a COMPUTED TOMOGRAPHY (CT) SCAN to get a clearer image, the procedure may take an hour instead of the usual 20 to 30 minutes. After the procedure, patients should not drive themselves home but should rest for the remainder of the day.

Risks and Complications

On the day of the test, no food can be eaten, which causes a problem for some patients. Also, the primary physician will assess any risks in taking regular medications that day. In addition, some patients experience allergic reaction to the dye used in a discogram.

According to an article posted by the North American Spine Society, "There is a risk of complications associated with discography. The most common is discitis (an infection of the disc space.) On average, this occurs in about one out of 400 patients undergoing discography. Discitis usually results in very intense pain but can be treated with antibiotics. Other complications that have been reported (but are rare) include nerve root injury, urticaria (a vascular reaction on the skin), injection of dye into the dural sac (surrounding the spinal cord), bleeding . . . , nausea, headache and increased pain."

Outlook and Lifestyle Modifications

Information from the International Spinal Intervention Society said that a discogram can recreate "painful symptoms if the disc/discs is abnormal," and provide, "confirmation of a diagnosis and/or determination of which disc/discs is the source of pain."

An Orthospine.com article further explained, "In some cases it may be difficult to clearly identify a source of pain in the lower back. In other instances surgery may be planned and yet it is uncertain at which level to end a fusion." With the results of a discogram, however, the doctor or surgical team can determine the best course of treatment for each individual.

Farcy, Jean-Pierre C., M.D. and Frank J. Schwab, M.D. "Medical Tests, Discography," Orthospine.com. Available online. URL: http://www.orthospine.com/?frameSrc=/medical_tests/medical_tests.html. Downloaded December 23, 2005.

International Spinal Intervention Society. "Discogram: What Is It?" ISIS. Available online. URL: http://www.spinalinjection.com/a/pes/disco.htm. Downloaded December 23, 2005.

North American Spine Society. "Discography," NASS. Available online. URL: http://www.spine.org/articles/discography.cfm. Downloaded December 23, 2005.

disc replacement   On October 26, 2004, the *FDA Talk Paper* announced, "The Food and Drug Administration (FDA) has approved an artificial spinal disc for use in treating pain associated with degenerative disc disease (DDD). The device is intended to replace a diseased or damaged intervertebral disc." Specifically, the announcement said, "The device—the first of its kind—is the Charité artificial disc manufactured by DePuy Spine, Inc., of Raynham, Mass. It was approved for use in patients who have DDD at one level in the lumbar spine (from L4-S1) and who have had no relief from low back pain after at least six months of non-surgical treatment."

Procedure

Describing a DISC replacement, an article on the Web site of the Chicago Institute of Neurosurgery and Neuroresearch said, "The goal of the procedure is to restore the intervertebral disc height . . . while restoring physiologic motion. The surgery is approached from the front, with a small incision in the abdomen below the belly button. Organs are gently moved to the side so that the surgeon can visualize the spine while protecting important anatomic structures. The collapsed degenerated disc is removed and the Charité prosthesis is implanted. . . . The artificial disc stays in place by the spinal ligaments and remaining part of the . . . disc, as well as the compressive force of the spine. Bending X-rays of patients after the surgery show that the motion of the artificial disc (flexion, side bending and rotation) can closely approximate the normal motion of a healthy disc."

Risks and Complications

Writing for SpineUniverse, Dr. Thomas G. Lowe said, "At this relatively early stage of disc replacement development, we do not know all of the problems that may be encountered following these procedures. Because the surgical approach is through the abdomen . . . (around/through the stomach), there are some predictable complications," such as vein inflammation, blood clot, or nerve root injuries.

Some patients, however, should not risk a disc replacement at all. According to the North American Spine Society (NASS), "There are several conditions that may prevent you from receiving a disc replacement. These include spondylolisthesis (the slipping of one vertebral body across a lower one), osteoporosis, vertebral body fracture, allergy to the materials in the device, spinal tumor, spinal infection, morbid obesity, significant changes of the facet joints (joints in the back portion of the spine), pregnancy, chronic steroid use or autoimmune problems. Also, total disc replacements are designed to be implanted from an anterior approach (through the abdomen). You may be excluded from receiving an artificial disc if you previously had abdominal surgery or if the condition of the blood vessels in front of your spine increases the risk of significant injury during this type of spinal surgery."

Outlook and Lifestyle Modifications

For patients who do have a disc replacement, recovery will usually be much faster than occurs after ARTHRODESIS since a disc replacement involves neither a BONE GRAFT nor spinal fusion. To compare the two procedures, the NASS said, "With fusion there also is a possibility that the fusion of one part of the spine forces the discs and vertebra above and/or below to carry more load and motion. This may result in more wear and tear than normal. The artificial disc may significantly reduce this risk."

In the announcement mentioned earlier, the FDA also compared disc replacement with fusion and noted that the study "showed that two years after surgery, patients treated with the artificial disc did no worse than patients treated with intervertebral body fusion. The rates of adverse events from use of the artificial disc were similar to those from treatment with fusion." In accordance with the FDA requirements, post-approval studies continue "to assess the product's long-term safety and effectiveness, including its impact on other discs and on the bony structures on the back of the spine."

Chicago Institute of Neurosurgery and Neuroresearch. "Beyond Spinal Fusion: CINN Tests The New Artificial Disc," CINN. Available online. URL: http://www.cinn.org/isc/artificialdiskoutcomes.html. Downloaded December 23, 2005.

FDA Talk Paper. "FDA Approves Artificial Disc; Another Alternative to Treat Low Back Pain," U.S. Food and Drug Administration, Department of Health and Human Services. Available online. URL: http://www.fda.gov/bbs/topics/ANSWERS/2004/ANS01320.html. Downloaded December 23, 2005.

Lowe, Thomas G., M.D. "Back Pain and Degenerative Disc Disease: Are Artificial Discs the Solution?" SpineUniverse. Available online. URL: http://www.spineuniverse.com/displayarticle.php/article2652.html. Last updated May 2, 2005.

North American Spine Society. "Artificial Discs: What Is an Artificial Disc?" NASS. Available online. URL: http://www.spine.org/fsp/prob_action-new-artifdisc.cfm. Last updated April 17, 2005.

disease modifying anti-rheumatic drug (DMARD)

This type of drug alters the progress of a rheu-matic condition, such as RHEUMATOID ARTHRITIS (RA), JUVENILE RHEUMATOID ARTHRITIS, or ANKYLOSING SPONDYLITIS, thus avoiding the permanent joint damage that commonly occurs with chronic inflammation. However, a DMARD takes time to take effect. Since CHRONIC PAIN and inflammation seldom go away, these slow-acting anti-rheumatic drugs do not replace the need for fast-acting NONSTEROIDAL ANTI-INFLAMMATORY DRUG (NSAID) THERAPY, such as ASPIRIN.

Dosage and Potential Side Effects

Most doctors prescribe a DMARD within three months of diagnosing RA or other rheumatic illness. Taken as a tablet or capsule, the dosage may be twice a day or once a week, while the liquid form requires a weekly injection. For example, the fastest-acting DMARD, methotrexate, may be given to CHILDREN with the juvenile form of RA either as a weekly injection or as tablets taken each week.

Since each DMARD may be a different drug with a different kind of action, the dosage varies as does the speed of treatment. For example, daily tablets of azathioprine may take effect in two to three months. Other daily options include hydroxychloroquine/chloroquine and sulfasalazine in one to two tablets with benefits usually arriving in three to six months. Slower-working gold salts may take a year to be effective. However, the Arthritis Society said, "The essence of DMARDS, clearly, isn't speed; rather, it's the medication's ability to control your symptoms, and your ability to tolerate the medication over the long haul. The goal is to have you taking the least amount of medication necessary to keep your inflammatory arthritis under control. As your symptoms slowly fade away, your rheumatologist may start gradually cutting back on the medications one at a time."

To clarify the options, an article from DrugDigest.org explained, "Some of the drugs are cytotoxic agents, which means they kill rapidly dividing cells as are seen in inflammatory conditions like RA or in cancer. Methotrexate, for example, interferes with DNA synthesis, which prevents cell replication, and suppresses the immune reaction in the body." As other choices, "gold compounds (auranofin, aurothioglucose, and gold sodium thiomalate) appear to stop the immune system from producing proteins and antibodies, which are the primary elements that cause joint damage. Penicillamine seems to interfere with the production of immune system proteins called immunoglobulin," whereas "sulfasalazine may interfere with a variety of inflammatory processes in the body. Hydroxychloroquine, which is usually used to treat malaria, is also used as a DMARD because it appears to suppress the effects of arthritis. Azathioprine is an immunosuppressant that also reduces inflammation."

With additional options available, a rheumatologist or other physician monitors the effectiveness of a DMARD and adjusts the prescription, depending on the side effects encountered. Often, symptoms of general dryness, pain, and numbness come from the rheumatic disease itself rather than the DMARD. However, some patients experience flu-like symptoms, such as stomach upset or nausea, that may be alleviated by changing the medication or the dosage. During powerful infections, such as bacterial pneumonia, a DMARD that suppresses the immune system may be temporarily suspended. DMARD treatments usually continue, though, in the presence of a less severe infection or virus.

Statistics and Studies

According to an article in *Consultant,* "New knowledge about the . . . progression of joint damage in RA has had a major impact on therapy for this disease. The onset of . . . joint damage varies among patients with RA, but it is now known that erosive disease develops in more than 50% within the first 2 years. Once erosive disease develops, it is irreversible with currently available treatment. Thus, DMARD therapy is now being initiated earlier in the disease course to prevent joint damage." Furthermore, "a growing body of evidence indicates that 2- and 3-drug combinations of DMARDs are superior to DMARD monotherapy for improving outcomes in RA. With better understanding of the progression of RA and the availability of more effective drugs, the goals of therapy have been broadened from simply reducing the signs and symptoms of RA to include preventing joint damage. It is hoped that timely and intensive DMARD therapy will improve quality of life, reduce disability, and prolong survival—as well as reduce the economic burden associated with the disease."

Arthritis Society, The. "Disease-Modifying Anti-Rheumatic Drugs (DMARDs)." Available online. URL: http://www.arthritis.ca/tips%20for%20living/understanding%20medications/disease%20modifying/default.asp?s=1. Downloaded December 26, 2005.

DrugDigest.org. "Disease Modifying Antirheumatic Drugs." Available online. URL: http://www.drugdigest.org/DD/Comparison/NewComparison/0,10621,32-4,00.html. Downloaded December 26, 2005.

Savage, Christine, William St. Clair, and John S. Sundy. "Emerging Treatments for Rheumatoid Arthritis: Update," *Consultant* (August 1, 2005): 984.

dislocated vertebra The sudden impact of an injury or the ongoing pressure of inflammation on a swollen joint can shift bones in the SPINE, causing VERTEBRAL SUBLUXATION. If, however, a rib, neck, or back bone dislodges completely from its joint, a dislocated vertebra results. That particular joint will cease to function, but the damage can also affect surrounding tendons, ligaments, and PARASPINAL MUSCLES. Far more seriously, a dislocated vertebra can injure the SPINAL CORD and even cause paralysis. In any case, medical attention should be sought, not only to avoid permanent damage but to get an orthopedic physician, osteopath, or chiropractor to pop the joint carefully back into place.

Symptoms and Diagnostic Path

ACUTE PAIN, slow swelling, and, sometimes, skin discoloration mark the spot of dislocation. X-RAYS or other imaging tests may be needed to rule out a FRACTURE.

Treatment Options and Outlook

Whether a RIB INJURY or an underlying medical condition such as RHEUMATOID ARTHRITIS causes a dislocated joint, a trained physician must relocate the vertebra. The joint should function again immediately or within a day or two. Meanwhile, the RICE METHOD of rest, ice, compression, and, if appropriate, elevation, comes commonly recommended. Since inflammation usually occurs, a NONSTEROIDAL

ANTI-INFLAMMATORY DRUG (NSAID) can keep down pain and swelling.

Risk Factors and Preventive Measures

Care should be taken in moving an injured patient, especially if dislocation has occurred in the CERVICAL SPINE. If a joint has been weakened by a previous injury or a BIRTH DEFECT OF THE SPINE, temporary use of an ORTHOTIC device such as a neck or back brace may prevent future dislocation. For most people, ample water, NUTRITION, and EXERCISE will strengthen the BACK and keep spinal joints from getting out of line.

MamasHealth.com. "Joint Dislocation." Available online. URL: http://www.mamashealth.com/bodyparts/jointdis. asp. Downloaded December 26, 2005.

Powell, Don R., *Health At Home*, ©1999, American Institute for Preventive Medicine. "Neck/Spine Injuries, Chapter 23. Emergency Conditions," Saints Self-Care Medical Library. Available online. URL: http://www.saintsok.com/pages/medicallibrary/DISLOCAT.HTM. Downloaded December 26, 2005.

dowager's hump   See KYPHOSIS.

dual photon absorptiometry (DPA)   See ABSORPTIOMETRY.

dual x-ray absorptiometry (DEXA or DXA)   See ABSORPTIOMETRY.

dwarfism   This bone growth disorder frequently results from GENETIC FACTORS, but about 80 percent of the CHILDREN with dwarfism have parents of average size. The most common form of dwarfism, achondroplasia, may be immediately apparent through head and body proportions unlike those of most newborn INFANTS. In many growth disorders, body proportions look similar to the general public, but characteristically, achondroplasia produces shortened limbs and a large head. Because of the latter, prenatal testing can prepare parents to expect a Caesarian section to avoid damage to the mother.

Risks and Complications

In 10 percent or less of infants with dwarfism, SPINAL CORD compression increases the risk of death. Potentially life-threatening conditions can also occur at any age if vertebrae in the CERVICAL SPINE become unstable. Often, SURGERY, such as ARTHRODESIS with a BONE GRAFT, can stabilize the SPINE and alleviate pressure on the spinal cord.

Sometimes dwarfism involves BIRTH DEFECTS OF THE SPINE, but SPINAL STENOSIS and POSTURE problems such as KYPHOSIS or LORDOSIS may develop as the child grows. To keep bones from damaging internal organs, surgery may help, but this adds the minimal risk of bleeding, infection, or other complications. In addition, the Little People of American (LPA) stated, "As a general statement of philosophy, most members of the dwarf community believe that no child should undergo surgery unless it is for a treatable medical condition that will improve her or his health. Limb-lengthening surgery, by contrast, does not address any medical condition, although certainly there are dwarfs who have undergone the procedure and are quite happy with the results."

When a bone growth condition exhibits proportions similar to those of people without dwarfism, GROWTH HORMONE THERAPY may increase overall stature at maturity. However, hormonal therapy carries other risks, such as bone overgrowth or OSTEOPHYTES, and may worsen conditions such as SCOLIOSIS.

Since height seldom exceeds 4-foot 10 inches, a primary complication occurs in the psychological or emotional damage caused by small-minded people who make unkind remarks, including name-calling. Most dwarfs prefer to be called dwarfs or little people, but far more desirable would be the sound of his or her name.

Statistics and Studies

According to the Little People of America (LPA), "Achondroplasia is caused by a gene mutation that is the same in 98% of the cases. The mutation, affecting growth, especially in the long bones, occurs early in fetal development in one out of every twenty thousand births. Since the achondroplasia gene discovery, genes for many other forms of dwarfism have been located and identified."

Special Aids and Adaptations

Ironically, the most challenging adaptation has occurred with medical breakthroughs in genetic testing. As LPA explained, "On one hand, the breakthrough may be used to help achondroplastic couples to identify a fetus with . . . a fatal condition that occurs in 25% of births to those couples." However, "it is also possible that the tests for genes causing short stature will become part of the increasingly routine and controversial genetic screening given to all expectant mothers." Since screening may cause some parents to abort a pregnancy, LPA continues to educate people and overcome fears or myths. For example, in expressing the general consensus of its members, LPA said, "We as short statured individuals are productive members of society who must inform the world that, though we face challenges, most of them are environmental (as with people with other disabilities), and we value the opportunity to contribute a unique perspective to the diversity of our society." To aid and encourage those contributions, such considerations as lowered countertops and appropriately sized furniture can lower the risk of accidents and allow little people to perform daily ACTIVITY with greater ease.

Francomano, Clair A., M.D. "Achondroplasia," GeneReviews. Available online. URL: http://www.geneclinics. org/profiles/achondroplasia/details.html. Downloaded December 29, 2005.

Little People of America. "Dwarfism Resources: Frequently Asked Questions," LPA Online. Available online. URL: http://www.lpaonline.org/resources_faq. html. Last updated November 20, 2005.

Roye, Benjamin D., M.D. "Achondroplasia," MedlinePlus, U.S. National Library of Medicine and the National Institutes of Health. Available online. URL: http://www.nlm.nih.gov/medlineplus/ency/article/001577. htm. Last updated December 13, 2005.

early onset scoliosis See IDIOPATHIC SCOLIOSIS.

eating disorders, bone loss caused by A strong connection between health and healthy food often becomes apparent as people learn about NUTRITION or focus on such topics as CALCIUM intake, MINERAL BALANCE, and an alphabet of VITAMINS from A to E. However, someone with an eating disorder may not be able to see beyond a distorted view found in a mirror. On that flat surface, dissatisfaction may appear in an emotionally rendered portrait, outlined with self-loathing or self-talk of being fat. A more accurate picture, though, might reveal someone of either sex and almost any age who has binged into a series of bulges or who may be slowly starving to death. Because the skeletal bones also lack the nutrients they require, bone loss and other serious health problems eventually occur.

Symptoms and Diagnostic Path

The National Eating Disorders Association (NEDA) identified three types of eating disorders as anorexia nervosa, bulimia nervosa, and binge-eating. The last does not usually result in bone loss but may add stressful WEIGHT to the backbone and spinal joints. Regarding bulimia, the NEDA said, "The recurrent binge-and-purge cycles of bulimia can affect the entire digestive system and can lead to electrolyte and chemical imbalances in the body that affect the heart and other major organ functions. . . . Electrolyte imbalance is caused by dehydration and loss of potassium, sodium, and chloride from the body as a result of purging behaviors." That imbalance affects bone health with initial signs seen in tooth stains and decay caused by regularly induced vomiting. Other symptoms include esophagus problems caused by bingeing then purging food. For bulimia

patients who abuse laxatives with the same goal of ridding the body of calories, symptoms include ulcerations or other disorders of the digestive tract.

With anorexia, however, patients simply do not eat. As the NEDA explained, "In anorexia nervosa's cycle of self-starvation, the body is denied the essential nutrients it needs to function normally. Thus, the body is forced to slow down all of its processes to conserve energy, resulting in serious medical consequences." Those consequences include dehydration, loss of concentration, loss of coordination, loss of energy, dry or yellowed skin, hair loss, and loss of bone density that eventually results in dry, brittle bones, OSTEOPENIA, or OSTEOPOROSIS. Also, muscle loss affects the PARASPINAL MUSCLES and, more seriously, the heart muscle, so that "the risk for heart failure rises as the heart rate and blood pressure levels sink lower and lower."

In addition to heart irregularities, female anorexia patients typically experience irregular menstrual cycles or conditions similar to menopause. A fact sheet posted by the National Institutes of Health (NIH) explained, "Both nutritional and endocrine factors set the stage for bone loss in anorectics. One of the most significant factors is estrogen deprivation. Low body weight causes the body to stop producing estrogen. This disruption in the menstrual cycle, known as amenorrhea, is associated with estrogen levels similar to those found in postmenopausal women. Significant losses in bone density typically occur."

According to an article in *The Mount Sinai Journal of Medicine,* "Considerable evidence is mounting that patients with either anorexia or bulimia have elevated serotonin metabolites," or chemicals that constrict blood flow, which "seems to correlate directly with the severity of symptoms" such as dizziness and heart palpitations. To obtain a timely diagnosis, a BONE MINERAL DENSITY TEST, laboratory tests, medical history, and low-key questioning can help.

Treatment Options and Outlook

Without medical intervention and professional counseling, people with anorexia nervosa and bulimia nervosa have a similar outlook of poor health, low energy, and, too often, an untimely death. In most cases, bulimia may be easier to admit and, therefore, treat. Also, the moments of bingeing provide some nutrients the body may retain, whereas anorexic patients have few or no nutrients with which to sustain themselves.

The National Alliance on Mental Illness (NAMI) summarized a common course of treatment: "Some form of psychotherapy is needed to deal with underlying emotional issues. Cognitive-behavioral therapy is sometimes used to change abnormal thoughts and behaviors. Group therapy is often advised so people can share their experiences with others. Family therapy is important particularly if the individual is living at home and is a young adolescent. A physician or advanced-practice nurse is needed to prescribe medications that may be useful in treating the disorder. Finally, a nutritionist may be necessary to advise the patient about proper diet and eating regimens."

To help a patient, literally, hold on to food for dear life, easy-to-digest meals and small portions provide the first course of dietary treatment. Some patients may need to be hospitalized so that vital signs can be monitored and intravenous feedings begun. At home or in the hospital, caregivers must take care not to overload patients with heavy foods and calories in an attempt to fatten them up. Too much weight too soon taxes the digestive tract and heart. Optimally, a slow gain of one to two pounds per week offers the best outlook for recovery as patients establish and maintain a healthy body weight.

Risk Factors and Preventive Measures

The NIH provided these statistics: "According to the American Anorexia Bulimia Association, approximately ten percent of eating disorder sufferers are male. While men are much less commonly affected by anorexia than women, research suggests that male victims also experience significant bone loss."

The greatest risks to bone health occur in ADOLESCENT boys and girls. As the NIH said, "Key studies have found significant decreases in bone density in anorectic adolescents. For example, affected teens have been shown to have spinal density 25% below that of healthy controls." Not only does this place a teenager at risk, but "studies suggest that half of peak bone density is achieved in adolescence. Anorexia typically develops between mid to late adolescence, a critical period for bone accretion. Affected teens experience decreases in bone density at a time when bone formation should be occurring." As a result, eating disorders developed in CHILDHOOD or teen years put a person at risk for BACK and SPINE problems throughout life.

Unfortunately, eating disorders often go unnoticed. Regarding anorexia nervosa (AN), an article in *Pediatrics* stated, "AN represents the third most common chronic illness among adolescent girls, and the true prevalence may be even higher because it goes undiagnosed in up to 50% of cases." Left untreated, "AN is associated with the mortality rate of 5.6% per decade in adults, the highest among all psychiatric illnesses." However, very thin persons of any age who are obsessed by weight and physical appearance rarely recognize the dire dietary risks they take each day. Therefore, the intervention of family and friends may be needed to prevent irreversible problems, such as early bone loss or, worse, the premature loss of that child, that spouse, or that friend.

Misra, Madhusmita, Avichal Aggarwal, Karen K. Miller, Cecilia Almazan, Megan Worley, Leslie A. Soyka, David B. Herzog, and Anne Kilbanski. "Effects of Anorexia Nervosa on Clinical, Hematologic, Biochemical, and Bone Density Parameters in Community-Dwelling Adolescent Girls," *Pediatrics* 114, no. 6 (December 2004): 1,574–1,583.

National Alliance on Mental Illness. "What Is Anorexia Nervosa?" NAMI. Available online. URL: http://www.nami.org/Template.cfm?Section=By_Illness&template=/ContentManagement/ContentDisplay.cfm&ContentID=7409. Downloaded December 29, 2005.

National Eating Disorders Association. "General Eating Disorders Information," NEDA. Available online. URL: http://www.nationaleatingdisorders.org/p.asp?WebPage_ID=291. Downloaded December 29, 2005.

National Institutes of Health (NIH) Osteoporosis and Related Bone Diseases, National Resource Center. "Skeletal Effects of Anorexia," National Institute of Arthritis and Musculoskeletal and Skin Diseases. Available online. URL: http://www.osteo.org/newfile. asp?doc=r709i&doctitle=Skeletal+Effects+of+Anorexia&doctype=HTML+Fact+Sheet. Downloaded December 29, 2005.

Seidenfield, Marjorie E., M.D., Elyse Sosin, and Vaughn I. Rickert. "Nutrition and Eating Disorders in Adolescents," *The Mount Sinai Journal of Medicine* 71, no. 3 (May 2004): 155–161.

elderly, spinal concerns of As Baby Boomers and others reach retirement age, weight-bearing joints age and boom. Disco gives way to DEGENERATIVE DISC DISEASE and HERNIATED DISCS. Bones wear. Backs ache, and spines decline. Undesirable companionships form with ARTHRITIS, OSTEOARTHRITIS, OSTEOPOROSIS, SPINAL STENOSIS, and an overall loss of bone density. People live longer, but at a height of an inch or so less than in younger days. If perpetual problems with POSTURE begin to affect balance, just one false step and a spinal FRACTURE can lead to the fall of independence and mobility.

Despite the CHRONIC PAIN and worries that often accompany advanced age, the good news is that most older people have the time and focus to alter their gloomy prospects. For instance, instead of hopping on an elevator, a retired person might take the time to take the stairs. Instead of passing up daily ACTIVITY in a neighborhood or religious center, a retired person might participate more fully and actually have fun. Instead of backing four wheels out of a driveway, a two-wheeler may do. If knee pain or BACK problems cause a nosedive in EXERCISE, swimming can move the body without undue wear and tear on the joints. For upper body strength, rowing a fishing boat may reel in a tighter tummy and tighten PARASPINAL MUSCLES too.

Risks and Complications

A general lack of energy may indicate the need to treat an underlying medical condition, dehydration, SLEEP problem, or inadequate NUTRITION. According to the U.S. Department of Agriculture (USDA), "Older people may not know that their nutrient requirements can change from their younger years." Furthermore, "the process of aging can introduce other factors—chronic disease, physical disabilities, poor economic status, social isolation, prescription medications, and altered mental status—that may cause poor eating habits that do not meet an older person's current nutrient needs." Therefore, "the elderly face the challenge of choosing a nutrient dense diet, one that provides an adequate intake of nutrients at a time when their activity levels and energy needs decline." For instance, dairy foods high in CALCIUM, whole grains high in fiber, and fruits high in VITAMIN C and other vitamins may be particularly significant.

Besides dietary concerns, the National Institute of Arthritis and Musculoskeletal Skin Diseases (NIAMS) pointed out that "among Americans age 65 and older, fall-related injuries are the leading cause of accidental death." Often, this occurs because "aging slows a person's reaction time and makes it harder to regain one's balance following a sudden movement or shift of body weight." Changes in vision also contribute to missteps, as do loose rugs, poor lighting, and obstacles in a walkway.

Statistics and Studies

According to the American Academy of Orthopaedic Surgeons (AAOS), "Many of the changes in our musculoskeletal system result more from disuse than from simple aging. Fewer than 10 percent of Americans participate in regular exercise, and the most sedentary group is over age 50."

The National Center for Injury Prevention and Control offered these statistics: "Older adults are hospitalized for fall-related injuries five times more often than they are for injuries from other causes. Of those who fall, 20% to 30% suffer moderate to severe injuries that reduce mobility and independence, and increase the risk of premature death." With hip fractures presenting the biggest problem, "the most common fall-related injuries are osteoporotic fractures . . . of the hip, spine, or forearm."

A hip or spine-damaging fall that lands a person in the hospital may also pave the way to a nursing home. As an article in *BMC Geriatrics* pointed out, "Many older adults develop functional decline and impaired walking while in the hospital. Preventing and treating hospital-related deconditioning is, therefore, of great importance." Unfortunately, "few studies . . . examine the role of exercise in the hospital."

An article in *The Journal of the American Osteopathic Association* said, "People are living longer but are dying with more disabilities. The fastest growing segment of the population is those older than 85 years. Frailty and disability increase with age. Many patients will require assistance with activities of daily living (ADL) which may necessitate institutionalization if adequate resources are not available. . . . Of those who enter nursing homes, it is estimated that one third will die within 12 months of admission."

Special Aids and Adaptations

As suggested by the *BMC Geriatrics* article, resistance exercises for elderly patients can be adapted to "(1) allow the subject to exercise from bed . . . , (2) provide enough resistance so that muscle fatigue occurs before 10 repetitions, (3) strengthen the major muscle groups of the lower extremities, (4) utilize safe, effective procedures and postures, and (5) standardize and describe the exercise program so that it can be precisely reproduced."

For patients who have not been confined to a bed, NIAMS suggested practicing balancing exercises every day. "While holding the back of a chair, sink, or countertop, practice standing on one leg at a time for a minute. Gradually increase the time. Try balancing with your eyes closed. Try balancing without holding on."

As the AAOS reminded, "An exercise program doesn't have to be strenuous to be effective. Walking, square dancing, swimming and bicycling are all recommended activities for maintaining fitness into old age. The 30 minutes of moderate activity can be broken up into shorter periods; you might spend 15 minutes working in the garden in the morning and 15 minutes walking in the afternoon. It all adds up."

To aid ease of movement, well-fitted walking SHOES with gel insoles help to cushion aging bones and discs. However, not just any exercise will do. Each individual has individual needs and circumstances. Therefore, a medical evaluation not only assesses potential risks involved in exercise but helps a specialist to design a sensible program. An article in *The Journal of Musculoskeletal Medicine* explained, "Mobility testing and determination of which positions induce pain and which relieve it can help devise an exercise program and identify the nature of the underlying pathology." For example, RANGE OF MOTION testing may show less restriction with one movement than another, thus clarifying the type of exercise that can be performed for optimal effect. Regardless of personal limitations, "Older patients who present with spinal complaints do not need to accept the aches and pains as a consequence of aging. Many of the spinal problems associated with aging can be mollified greatly by finding and maintaining the right balance of physical activity and healthful living habits. Judicious use of exercise, proper body mechanics, medications, and surgery can result in improvement of function and quality of life."

For new retirees and the very elderly, ENVIRONMENTAL INFLUENCES and ERGONOMIC FACTORS can affect the quality of life either positively or negatively. Beneficial changes can come, however, as a person acknowledges his or her physical limitations and sensibly adapts movements in LIFTING objects, bending, and finding a manageable pace. For many people, the quality of life and overall outlook also improve through regular interaction with nature. This may mean meandering on a scenic trail, training a pet, tending garden plants, or cultivating the ageless company of particularly pleasant people, including, of course, oneself.

American Academy of Orthopaedic Surgeons. "Effects of Aging," AAOS. Available online. URL: http://orthoinfo. aaos.org/fact/thr_report.cfm?Thread_ID=224&topcategory=General%20Information. Downloaded December 29, 2005.

Insight 14. "A Focus on Nutrition for the Elderly: It's Time to Take a Closer Look," *Nutrition Insights,* two-page brochure, July 1999, a Publication of the USDA Center for Nutrition Policy and Promotion, U.S. Department of Agriculture.

Mallery, Laurie H., Elizabeth A. MacDonald, Cheryl I. Hubley-Kozey, Marie E. Earl, Kenneth Rockwood, and Chris MacKnight. "The Feasibility of Performing Resistance Exercise with Acutely Ill Hospitalized Older Adults," *BMC Geriatrics* 3, no. 3 (October 7, 2003).

Marx, Tracy L. "Partnering With Hospice to Improve Pain Management in the Nursing Home Setting," *JAOA, The Journal of the American Osteopathic Association* 105, no. 3 (March 2005): 22–26.

National Center for Injury Prevention and Control. "A Tool Kit to Prevent Senior Falls: The Costs of Fall Injuries Among Older Adults," Centers for Disease Control and Prevention. Available online. URL: http://www.cdc.gov/ncipc/factsheets/fallcost.htm. Last updated July 26, 2004.

National Institute of Arthritis and Musculoskeletal and Skin Diseases (NIAMS). "Preventing Falls and Related Fractures," National Institutes of Health (NIH), Department of Health and Human Services. Available online. URL: http://www.niams.nih.gov/bone/hi/prevent_falls.htm. Downloaded December 29, 2005.

Zucherman, James, M.D. and Judy Silverman, M.D. "Managing Spinal Conditions in Older Persons," *The Journal of Musculoskeletal Medicine* 22, no. 5 (May 2005): 214–222.

electrical stimulation See NEUROSTIMULATION.

electromyogram (EMG) Similar to a NERVE CONDUCTION STUDY, this type of nerve function test examines the condition of spinal nerves by studying the electrical impulses they send into the muscles to which they are attached. As explained by the American Academy of Orthopaedic Surgeons, "Injuries or diseases that affect nerves and muscles can slow or halt the movement of these electrical signals. If you have pain, weakness or numbness in your back, neck or hands, measuring the speed and degree of electrical activity in your muscles and nerves can help your doctor make a proper diagnosis."

Procedure

In less than an hour, an electromyogram (EMG) can assess one muscle or many. First, a tiny electrode goes into each muscle being tested. The muscle then remains at rest or actively contracts. Either way, an EMG records the information onto a monitor for the doctor to evaluate and report.

Risks and Complications

Metal objects and lotions can mar test results. Otherwise, an EMG is generally accurate and safe, although bruising and soreness may occur where an electrode has been injected into a muscle. Patients on a daily regimen of ASPIRIN or another blood thinner need to ask their doctors about the risk of bleeding.

Outlook and Lifestyle Modifications

If an EMG shows improper functioning of a muscle, this may indicate spinal nerve compression caused, for example, by SPINAL STENOSIS or a HERNIATED DISC. Therefore, the outlook may depend on the results of other tests, such as an X-RAY or MAGNETIC RESONANCE IMAGING (MRI). Once the source of a problem has been identified, appropriate treatments or other modifications can begin.

American Academy of Orthopaedic Surgeons. "Electrodiagnostic Testing," AAOS. Available online. URL: http://orthoinfo.aaos.org/fact/thr_report.cfm?Thread_ID=356&topcategory=General%20Information. Downloaded December 29, 2005.

Spine Institute of New York. "EMG (Electromyogram)," Beth Israel Medical Center. Available online. URL: http://www.spineinstituteny.com/conditions/EMG.html. Downloaded December 29, 2005.

endoscopic surgery See MINIMALLY INVASIVE SURGERY.

environmental influences on spine health Can RHEUMATISM forecast the weather? Does barometric pressure weigh heavily on the BACK? Can rain drop spinal pain? Maybe, but after a study of hundreds of patients over the course of a few years, the report in *Rheumatology* stated, "Among individuals with arthritis, in spite of increasingly sophisticated . . . methods, the purported association between weather and pain largely remains an enigma."

Everybody talks about the weather connection to joint and back pain. However, a throng of environmental irritants may damage spinal health. In random disorder, these include harsh chemicals, microbiological or infectious agents, radiation, toxic vapors, allergens, fungicides, herbicides, pesticides, mold, dust, dyes, and artificial additives to foods.

Most commonly, irritants in the air, water, and soil affect the skin and other filtering organs, such as the nose, lungs, kidneys, and liver, but toxins influence vertebral health too. For example, eating unwashed raw vegetables can introduce a pesticide that harms the kidneys, which can mar CALCIUM absorption, thus leading to loss of bone density. Other environmental influences may affect the BACK or SPINE directly by producing CANCER cells or SPINAL TUMOR. Usually, risks increase with long-term exposure or high doses of toxins that can adversely affect anyone, especially INFANTS and ELDERLY patients. Also, different locales and lifestyles bring differing degrees of environmental risks.

Risks and Complications

A fact sheet on aluminum from the Agency for Toxic Substances and Disease Registry (ATSDR) warned, "Children with kidney problems who were given aluminum in their medical treatments developed bone diseases. . . . It is not known whether aluminum affects children differently than adults, or what the long-term effects might be in adults exposed as children. Large amounts of aluminum have been shown to be harmful to unborn and developing animals because it can cause delays in skeletal and neurological development." To reduce risks, the ATSDR said, "The most important way families can lower exposure to aluminum is to know about the sources of aluminum and lessen exposure to these sources. Since aluminum is so common and widespread in the environment, families cannot avoid exposure to aluminum. Exposure to the low levels of aluminum that are naturally present in food and water and the forms of aluminum present in dirt and aluminum cookware is generally not harmful." Regardless, "The best way to reduce exposure to aluminum is to avoid taking large quantities of soluble forms of aluminum such as aluminum-containing antacids and buffered aspirin. Make sure these products have child-proof caps so children will not accidentally eat them." Food additives and antiperspirants often contain aluminum too, but as a special concern, the ATSDR said, "Some soy-based formulas may contain high levels of aluminum, so parents may want to consult with their physician when choosing an infant formula," or, perhaps, read product labels carefully.

Communal concerns commonly arise about adding fluoride to drinking water and toothpaste. In a fact sheet on the subject, the ATSDR said, "Small amounts of fluoride help prevent tooth cavities, but high levels can harm your health. In adults, exposure to high levels of fluoride can result in denser bones. However, if exposure is high enough, these bones may be more fragile and brittle and there may be a greater risk of breaking the bone." To lessen the risk of getting too much fluoride, the ATSDR advised parents that "in the home, children may be exposed to high levels of fluorides if they swallow dental products containing fluoridated toothpaste, gels, or rinses. Parents should supervise brushing and place at most, a small pea size dab of toothpaste on the brush and teach children not to swallow dental products. People who live in areas with high levels of naturally-occurring fluoride in the water should use alternative sources of drinking water, such as bottled water."

Statistics and Studies

Sometimes environmental influences and lifestyle choices have more effect on bone health than GENETIC FACTORS do. For example, *Spine* presented the results of a Danish study conducted "to determine the relative contribution of genetic and environmental factors to back pain in old age." As the article reported, "A current or previous diagnosis of osteoporosis, degenerative joint disease, or lumbar disc prolapse was found to significantly affect the risk of back pain. Additive genetic effects explained approximately one fourth of the liability to report back pain in men and none of the occurrence in women. Individual environmental effects were found to explain roughly 75% of the occurrence of back pain in men and 100% in women."

Environmental influences cover a wide range of possibilities, which, unlike genetic factors, usually offer a choice of some kind. For example, *Genetic Epidemiology* reported on a study that allowed researchers to evaluate "the contribution of genetic and life-style factors (exercise, smoking, and alcohol consumption) and the interactions between non-genetic factors in determining bone mineral density (BMD) of the hip and spine" with adjustments made for age, weight, and height. According to the report, "Exercise had significant beneficial effects for male spine BMD and female hip BMD. Alcohol consumption experienced in our sample had significant beneficial effects on hip BMD in both sexes. Although the main effect of smoking was not significant, there were significant interaction effects between smoking and other important factors (e.g., exercise, weight, alcohol consumption). For example, for female spine BMD, exercise had significant beneficial effects in smokers; however, its effect in non-smokers was non-significant. This result indicates that exercise may reduce deleterious effects of smoking (if any) on BMD, but may have minor effects in increasing BMD in non-smokers."

Special Aids and Adaptations

With so many environmental influences and so many factors interacting in a unique way, study may well begin at home. For example, reading product labels, asking pertinent questions, and investigating questionable practices help consumers to become informed about hazards to their spinal health. Each person can also be aware of such symptoms as a rash, stomach upset, and breathing problems that occur after touching, ingesting, or inhaling something questionable. If any evidence exists, say, of a toxic metal in the body, a blood test or urinalysis can show the level. To lessen the likelihood of ingesting chemicals in fresh produce and meat, natural foods can be washed with water and, often, with vinegar water to reduce contaminants. One part vinegar to four parts water provides a natural way to disinfect countertops and other surfaces too.

Drinking lots of filtered water, distilled water, or natural apple juice may also help to cleanse the body of toxins that accumulate from adverse environmental influences. In addition, well-balanced NUTRITION with daily supplies of VITAMINS A, C, and E help to build up the immune system as does EXERCISE. Seen or unseen factors continuously affect bone quality in varying degrees, but at best, environmental influences offer fresh water, fresh air, and fresh produce from unpolluted soil.

Agency for Toxic Substances and Disease Registry. "Tox-FAQs ™ for Aluminum," ATSDR Information Center. Available online. URL: http://www.atsdr.cdc.gov/tfacts22.html. Downloaded December 30, 2005.

Agency for Toxic Substances and Disease Registry. "Tox-FAQs ™ for Fluorine, Hydrogen Fluoride, and Fluorides," ATSDR Information Center. Available online. URL: http://www.atsdr.cdc.gov/tfacts11.html. Downloaded December 31, 2005.

Deng, Hong-Wen, Wel-Min Chen, Theresa Conway, Yan Zhou, K. Michael Davies, Mary Ruth Stegman, Hongyi Deng, and Robert R. Recker. "Determination of Bone Mineral Density of the Hip and Spine in Human Pedigrees by Genetic and Life-Style Factors," *Genetic Epidemiology* 19 (2000): 160–177.

Hartvigsen, Jan, Kaare Christensen, M.D., Henrik Frederiksen, M.D., and Hans Christian. "Genetic and Environmental Contributions to Back Pain in Old Age: A Study of 2,108 Danish Twins Aged 70 and Older," *Spine* 29, no. 8 (April 15, 2004): 897–901.

Wilder, F. V., B. J. Hall and J. P. Barrett. "Osteoarthritis Pain and Weather," *Rheumatology* 42, no. 8 (2003): 955–958.

epidural abscess   See SPINAL INFECTION.

epidural injection   This nonsurgical outpatient procedure treats SCIATICA pain or CERVICAL RADICULOPATHY with the injection of a synthetic steroid similar to one produced naturally in the body. An epidural injection can also be used as a diagnostic tool to locate a source of CHRONIC PAIN.

As explained by the Spine Institute of New York, "The benefits to epidural steroid injections are threefold. 1. Injecting steroids into the epidural space helps reduce the inflammation of the nerves, nerve roots, or nerve coverings, which are the source of leg pain. 2. The steroids serve as a temporary form of pain relief so the body can begin its natural healing process. 3. An epidural steroid injection is a good diagnostic tool because its blockage of the nerve pinpoints the source of your pain."

An article in the *BMJ (British Medical Journal)* said, "Mechanical back pain may often be associated with some nerve root irritation, or present as an exacerbation of chronic symptoms." Therefore, "corticosteroid delivered into the epidural space is able to attain high local concentrations. Reports on thousands of patients indicate that epidural corticosteroid injections are relatively straightforward and safe," but "a need exists for well designed trials of adequate size to determine the effectiveness of epidural injection in back pain." Also, "the evidence for and against epidural steroid injection should be clearly explained to allow patients to make an informed choice regarding their treatment."

Procedure

Prior to the procedure, a medical technician swabs the site and injects a local anesthetic. According to the Chicago Institute of Neurosurgery and Neuro-research (CINN), "After the area is numb, the anesthesiologist will insert a needle through the skin into the epidural space that surrounds the spinal cord and spinal nerves, and inject the steroid. You will feel pressure, but no pain, while the anesthesiologist injects the steroid. The nurse will then place a small adhesive bandage on the injection site and check your blood pressure and pulse." Sometimes, anxiety causes vital signs to become irregular. "If so, the nurse will continue to monitor you for approximately 30 minutes while you sit or lie down. This short period of rest will help your blood pressure and pulse return to normal. The epidural steroid injection procedure takes approximately 15 to 30 minutes to complete."

Risks and Complications

About a week before an epidural injection, the use of ASPIRIN and other blood thinners must be avoided, which presents a problem for some patients. Regarding risks in general, the CINN said, "The epidural steroid injection has a long history of safe use. There is only a 1 percent chance that you will suffer from a brief headache after receiving an epidural steroid injection. Also, whenever skin is punctured, there is a slight chance it may become infected, resulting in redness, swelling, tenderness, or warmth at the injection site."

Rare complications include SPINAL INFECTION in the spinal canal. Also, some patients may experience adverse reactions to the medication or nerve damage from needle slippage. Epidural injections should not be used for back care during PREGNANCY nor for patients with CANCER, spinal infection, or SPINAL TUMOR.

Outlook and Lifestyle Modifications

An ice pack applied for about 15 minutes every hour or so may relieve swelling and soreness until the injection itself begins to ease the pain and inflam-mation. Although the desired effect may take up to 10 days, many patients experience long-term relief. If not, a second injection can be given in about two weeks. Should this fail to alleviate pain, other types of treatment can be considered, depending on the condition. For instance, pain caused by a HERNIATED DISC, sciatica, or SPINAL STENOSIS may require SURGERY, whereas pain caused by VERTEBRAL SUBLUXATION may respond to SPINAL MANIPULATION and spine-strengthening EXERCISE. Also, effective PAIN MANAGEMENT may occur with ACUPUNCTURE or other form of COMPLEMENTARY AND ALTERNATIVE MEDICINE (CAM).

Chicago Institute of Neurosurgery and Neuroresearch. "Epidural Steroid Injection," CINN. Available online. URL: http://www.cinn.org/workinjury/services/epidural. html. Downloaded December 31, 2005.

Samanta, Ash and Jo Samanta. "Is Epidural Injection of Steroids Effective for Low Back Pain?" *BMJ (British Medical Journal)* 328, no. 26 (June 2004): 1,509–1,510.

Spine Institute of New York. "Epidural Steroid Injection," Beth Israel Medical Center. Available online. URL: http://www.spineinstituteny.com/treatments/epidural. html. Downloaded December 31, 2005.

ergonomic factors   Researchers, writers, and readers of encyclopedias may be inclined to think that ergonomics means having a stressless chair to assist POSTURE and avoid a BACKACHE while sitting at a desk, but the Occupational Safety & Health Administration (OSHA) used broader terms. According to the agency, musculoskeletal disorders affecting the BACK and SPINE encompass "Awkward Postures, which might include: prolonged work with hands above the head or with the elbows above the shoulders; prolonged work with the neck bent; squatting, kneeling, or lifting; handling objects with back bent or twisted; repeated or sustained bending or twisting of wrists, knees, hips or shoulders; forceful and repeated gripping or pinching." In addition, OSHA mentioned "Forceful Lifting, Pushing Or Pulling, which might include: handling heavy objects; moving bulky or slippery objects; assuming awkward postures while moving objects." Besides concerns about proper LIFTING and LOAD TOLERANCE, workers need to be aware of "Prolonged Repetitive Motion, which might include: keying; using tools or knives; packaging, handling, or manipulating objects," and "Contact Stress, which might include: repeated contact with hard or sharp objects, like desk or table edges." OSHA further mentioned "Vibration, which might include: overuse of power hand tools." With such broad guidelines, OSHA most likely covered almost every back.

Risks and Complications

Aging equipment used by an aging workforce can increase the risk of back and spine problems. So can a poor ergonomic design that looks good on a drafting table but proves impractical in real life. Workers can work with employers by reporting their concerns about design flaws or job safety, but implementing such changes can be costly and time-consuming. In any case, ergonomic factors aim to fit the job to the worker, not the other way around. If this does not happen, PARASPINAL MUSCLES or VERTEBRAE in the CERVICAL SPINE, THORACIC SPINE, and LUMBAR SPINE attempt to adapt to the task at hand or foot or back. Ultimately, something has to give.

Statistics and Studies

According to the Bureau of Labor Statistics, 324,935 men and 194,910 women missed work in 2001 because of musculoskeletal problems. Ergonomic injuries included teenaged workers and those over 55, but the large majority of problems occurred among young adult to middle-aged laborers. Although one might expect new employees to have the most discomfort, people who had been in their jobs for over a year actually took more days off from work. Of those recorded events, repetitive motion disorders accounted for over 60,000 cases, while another 219,665 resulted from exertion during lifting.

Special Aids and Adaptations

To aid workers and employees in preventing musculoskeletal problems, the National Institute for Occupational Safety and Health (NIOSH) offers a hotline, 1-800-35-NIOSH (1-800-356-4674). The NIOSH also suggested seven steps toward safety, beginning with, "One: Looking for signs of a potential musculoskeletal problem in the workplace, such as frequent worker reports of aches and pains,

or job tasks that require repetitive, forceful exertions." Other adaptations include "encouraging worker involvement in problem-solving activities" and training workers to evaluate musculoskeletal concerns. In addition, "gathering data to identify jobs or work conditions that are most problematic" can occur by "using sources such as injury and illness logs, medical records, and job analyses." Then follow-up will aid in "identifying effective controls for tasks that pose a risk of musculoskeletal injury and evaluating these approaches once they have been instituted to see if they have reduced or eliminated the problem." NIOSH suggested "establishing health care management to emphasize the importance of early detection and treatment of musculoskeletal disorders for preventing impairment and disability." As NIOSH also pointed out, it "is less costly to build good design into the workplace than to redesign or retrofit later."

For the retrofit of a desirable office chair, an article on Spine-health advised, "Seat height should be easily adjustable. A pneumatic adjustment lever is the easiest way to do this. A seat height that ranges from about 16 to 21 inches off the floor should work for most people. This allows the user to have his or her feet flat on the floor, with thighs horizontal and arms even with the height of the desk." An appropriately sized seat with padding and "fabric that breathes is preferable to a harder surface." Adjustable armrests "should allow the user's arms to rest comfortably and shoulders to be relaxed" with elbows but not forearms supported. Also, "an ergonomic chair should have a lumbar adjustment (both height and depth) so each user can get the proper fit to support the inward curve of the lower back." Should none of the above prove workable, recent designs in inflatable ball chairs provide a bouncy option.

American Academy of Orthopaedic Surgeons. "How to Sit at a Computer," AAOS. Available online. URL: http://orthoinfo.aaos.org/fact/thr_report.cfm?Thread_ID=323&topcategory=General%20Information. Downloaded December 31, 2005.

Bureau of Labor Statistics. "Table 11: Number of Nonfatal Occupational Injuries and Illnesses with Days Away from Work Involving Musculoskeletal Disorders by Selected Workers and Case Characteristics, 2001."

U.S. Department of Labor. Available online. URL: http://www.bls.gov/iif/oshwc/osh/case/ostb1154.pdf. Downloaded December 31, 2005.

Lefler, Rodney K., "Choosing the Right Ergonomic Office Chair," Spine-health.com. Available online. URL: http://www.spine-health.com/topics/conserv/chair/chair01.html. Posted July 2, 2004.

National Institute for Occupational Safety and Health. "Elements of Ergonomics Programs," NIOSH. Available online. URL: http://www.cdc.gov/niosh/ephome2.html. Downloaded December 31, 2005.

Occupational Safety & Health Administration. "Ergonomics: Contributing Conditions," OSHA, U.S. Department of Labor. Available online. URL: http://www.osha.gov/SLTC/ergonomics/job_analysis.html. Last revised March 6, 2003.

estrogen   See HORMONE REPLACEMENT THERAPY and PHYTOESTROGENS.

etidronate   According to the "etidronate Center" at MedicineNet.com, "Etidronate belongs to a class of medications which strengthen bone. Bone is in a constant state of remodeling in which old bone is removed by cells called osteoclasts, and new bone is laid down by cells called osteoblasts. Etidronate inhibits bone removal by the osteoclasts."

Dosage and Potential Side Effects

Used to treat conditions of bone loss, such as OSTEOPOROSIS or OSTEOGENESIS IMPERFECTA (Paget's Disease), a typical dosage is 200 to 400 mg taken orally. In a hospital setting, etidronate may be administered through an injection. In either case, this BISPHOSPHONATE may interact adversely with PARATHYROID HORMONE (PTH), OVER-THE-COUNTER PRODUCTS such as antacids, and CALCIUM or other mineral supplements. Alcohol and caffeine also interfere with this medication at any time, but etidronate must not be taken with anything but water anyway.

Information from the DrugDigest.org Web site said, "It is very important to take etidronate with a full glass of plain water (6–8 ounces). Do not take with orange juice, coffee, or other fluids as these may decrease the absorption of etidronate. Do not take etidronate with food. Wait at least 30 minutes or longer after taking etidronate before you eat, drink or take other medicines." Equally important, the patient must not sit, bend, or recline for at least a half-hour after taking this medication to avoid throat irritation. Otherwise, "serious side effects from etidronate are rare." However, "patients using etidronate for more than 6 months at a time are at an increased risk of developing bone fractures." If tar-like stools, skin rash, or bone pain occur, patients should seek immediate medical attention.

Statistics and Studies

An article of expert opinions posted by MedicineNet.com compared studies of etidronate with those for the newer drug alendronate. Reportedly, "evidence from studies demonstrates the safety and effectiveness of alendronate in the prevention of vertebral fractures . . . as well as hip and wrist fractures in postmenopausal women with low bone density. Similar evidence does not exist to support the effectiveness of etidronate in fracture prevention, although etidronate treatment is associated with an increase in lumbar spine bone mineral density. Based on these studies, alendronate should be the current bisphosphonate of choice, whereas etidronate should be reserved for patients with a contraindication to alendronate or who are intolerant of alendronate therapy."

DrugDigest.org. "Etidronate Disodium," Clinical Pharmacology©. Available online. URL: http://www.drugdigest.org/DD/DVH/Uses/0,3915,6108|Etidronate%2BDisodium%2B,00.html. Last updated September 16, 2005.

MedicineNet.com. "Ask The Experts! Question Regarding: Alendronate vs. Etidronate for Osteoporosis." Available online. URL: http://www.medicinenet.com/script/main/ques.asp?qakey=2699. Downloaded January 3, 2006.

———. "etidronate Center." Available online. URL: http://www.medicinenet.com/etidronate/article.htm. Downloaded December 31, 2005.

etodolac   See NONSTEROIDAL ANTI-INFLAMMATORY DRUG THERAPY.

Ewing's sarcoma   See SPINAL TUMOR.

exercise   As a form of heightened ACTIVITY, exercise often has a specific theme, purpose, or goal. Movements may aim to regain flexibility, maintain mobility, or address spinal concerns of the ELDERLY. Exercise can also strengthen the BACK of an ATHLETE, engage CHILDREN in play, and coax ADOLESCENTS outdoors. For those concerned about adverse effects of WEIGHT on the SPINE, exercise can trim pounds and tighten tummies. Whether active or passive, aerobic or anaerobic, low impact or high impact, regular exercise firms muscles, including the heart, and increases circulation in all parts of the body. General themes of STRENGTH TRAINING and RESISTANCE TRAINING can meet their respective goals. Before beginning any exercise program though, older or sedentary people and patients with a medical condition should walk the idea by a primary care physician. When medical approval has been obtained, the patient begins each round of exercise by warming up and ends by cooling down.

The American Academy of Orthopaedic Surgeons (AAOS) defined warm-ups as "slow, rhythmic exercises" that can be accomplished simply by walking around a bit. With instructions to "inhale deeply before each repetition of an exercise and exhale when performing each repetition," the AAOS described exercises such as wall slides to strengthen the PARASPINAL MUSCLES: "Stand with your back against a wall and feet shoulder-width apart. Slide down into a crouch with knees bent to about 90 degrees. Count to five and slide back up the wall. Repeat 5 times."

That exercise requires at least enough energy to get out of bed, but a couple of the AAOS exercises work well on awakening: "Lie on your back with your arms at your sides. Lift one leg" and hold "for a count of 10" As that leg eases back onto the mattress, "Do the same with the other leg. Repeat five times with each leg. If that is too difficult, keep one knee bent and the foot flat . . . while raising the leg." This exercise strengthens the hips, aids mobility, and tightens the stomach, while loosening stress on the lower back. To ease a BACKACHE even more, "Lie on your back with your knees bent and feet flat on your bed or floor. Raise your knees toward your chest. Place both hands under your knees and gently pull your knees as close to your chest as possible. Do not raise your head. Do not straighten your legs as you lower them. Start with five repetitions, several times a day."

Risks and Complications

People with a SPINAL INFECTION, FRACTURE, or fever should avoid exercise as should anyone requiring bedrest. For almost everyone else, the primary risk of exercise lies in not doing any. As a Back.com article stated, "Strengthening the abdominal and trunk muscles, and the core of your body, is one of the first steps towards improving your upright posture and alleviating low back pain. Poor posture is common for those who lead a sedentary lifestyle, and this places a tremendous strain on the lower back and discs. By training your abdominal muscles to encourage a proper upright posture, back pain can be reduced to a significant degree." Initially, exercise can make a person sore. However, Back.com assured readers, "If you have not been exercising regularly, then it is common to feel more pain immediately after exercising and especially the next day. This is the beginning of a long-term process. Conditioning takes time and it is very natural to experience more pain at the beginning of an exercise program."

Overdoing can complicate matters, particularly if people sprint out of a recliner. To run away from muscle STRAIN or SPRAIN, a "Basic Training" article in *Runner's World* recommended "the 10% rule. Ensure that your weekly distance does not increase by more than 10% compared to the preceding week. Going too far too fast will soon bring on tiredness, soreness, injury and a premature end to all your good intentions. If you have had to shelve your training for a while, perhaps due to illness, injury or vacation, make sure that you start back at a much lower level and build up again."

Besides mentioning the importance of correct technique and correctly fitted SHOES, the article suggested "the hard-easy rule," which basically means, "ensure that every hard workout is alternated by either a day of rest, an alternative form of exercise or by a slower, less intense, easy walk. This allows your muscles to recover and recuperate from the previous day's hard training." According to the article, a hard workout means anything that involves "walking faster, harder or longer than what is normal for you." However, "listen to your body. When your body tells you it needs a rest, listen to it. Taking heed of your body's warning signals can mean the difference between getting injured or ill, and walking pain-free and staying healthy. . . . If something aches or hurts for more than two or three days, consult a sports practitioner." Also, "monitor your waking pulse rate. If it is five to ten beats higher than normal, take a rest day."

Statistics and Studies

People concerned about falls or balance may want to dance away the plight. As a *Men's Health* article reported, "Swedish researchers found that 12 weeks of dance training improved skiers' joint mobility, range of hip motion, and spinal flexibility. The subjects also experienced 67 percent less back pain after the training. According to the study, any type of dance that forces you to balance can help. The skiers in the study performed modern or jazz dance or ballet."

An article published in *Physical Therapy* considered classic trunk exercises versus general exercise in treating patients with LOW BACK PAIN: "Classic trunk exercises performed in physical therapy activate the abdominal and paraspinal muscles as a whole and at a relatively high contraction level." Unless a patient had spinal instability, "a general exercise program reduced disability in the short term to a greater extent than a stabilization-enhanced exercise approach in patients with recurrent nonspecific low back pain."

Special Aids and Adaptations

To protect the spine and paraspinal muscles from injury during exercise, warm-ups or gentle stretches work especially well. Generally speaking, stretching also aids RANGE OF MOTION. As an article posted by the University of Michigan Health System explained, "With static stretching, your muscle is slowly lengthened to the point where you feel a mild stretch. You then hold the position for 15 to 30 seconds and then slowly release the stretch. The most important rule to follow for any stretching exercise is that it must not be painful. If you stretch to the point of pain, the muscle will not relax and might even become tighter!" Done correctly, light stretches not only aid relaxation, flexibility, agility, and balance but give most people an overall sense of well-being.

While muscle flexibility aids one goal of exercise, bone strengthening adapts another important theme for back care. As an article on the National Osteoporosis Foundation (NOF) Web site explained, "Just as a muscle gets stronger and bigger the more you use it, a bone becomes stronger and denser when you place demands on it." BONE BUILDING may not be obvious to the eye, but "if you x-ray the arms of a tennis player, you would see that the bones in the playing arm are bigger and denser than the bones in the other arm." In addition, "two types of exercises are important for building and maintaining bone mass and density: weight-bearing and resistance exercises. Weight-bearing exercises are those in which your bones and muscles work against gravity. This is any exercise in which your feet and legs are bearing your weight. Jogging, walking, stair climbing, dancing and soccer are examples of weight-bearing exercise with different degrees of impact. Swimming and bicycling are not weight-bearing. . . . The second type of exercises are resistance exercises or activities that use muscular strength to improve muscle mass and strengthen bone. These activities include weight lifting, such as using free weights and weight machines found at gyms and health clubs."

With a go-ahead from a doctor, almost anyone without a broken bone or illness can gradually adapt to sensible activity. However, an exercise program must also adapt well to each person with a particular purpose or personal theme ready to be exercised.

American Academy of Orthopaedic Surgeons. "Back Pain Exercises," AAOS. Available online. URL: http://orthoinfo.aaos.org/fact/thr_report.cfm?Thread_ID=17&topcategory=Spine. Downloaded January 3, 2006.

Clapis, Phyllis. "Stretching," University of Michigan Health System. Available online. URL: http://www.med.umich.edu/1libr/sma/sma_stretch_sma.htm.

Koumantakis, George A., Paul J. Watson, and Jacqueline A. Oldham. "Trunk Muscle Stabilization Training Plus General Exercise Versus General Exercise Only: Randomized Controlled Trial of Patients with Recurrent Low Back Pain," *Physical Therapy* 85, no. 3 (March 2005): 209–225.

Mackintosh, Terry. "Basic Training," *Runner's World*. Available online. URL: http://www.runnersworld.com/article/0,5033,s6-51-183-0-1917,00.html. Downloaded January 3, 2006.

Medtronic Sofamor Danek. "Spine Exercise Frequently Asked Questions," Back.com. Available online. URL: http://www.back.com/articles-spine.html. Updated February 17, 2005.

National Osteoporosis Foundation. "Bone Is Living Tissue That Responds to Exercise by Becoming Stronger,"

Prevention, Exercise for Healthy Bone, NOF. Available online. URL: http://www.nof.org/prevention/exercise.htm. Downloaded January 4, 2006.

Quill, Scott. "Muscle News Briefs: Back Relief," *Men's Health* 20, no. 1 (January/February 2005): 42.

facet joint disorder Also known as facet joint syndrome, this disorder involves small joints between and behind each VERTEBRA. These joints occur as vertebral bones connect, with the exception of the SACRAL VERTEBRAE and the first neck bone in the CERVICAL SPINE. Working correctly, facet joints stabilize the spinal column while allowing the SPINE to twist, turn, and bend backward, forward, or sideways in a normal RANGE OF MOTION.

If the facet joints themselves get bent out of shape, a multitude of spinal problems may begin. Under degenerative conditions, for example, inflamed joints can indicate OSTEOARTHRITIS or produce muscle spasm in the PARASPINAL MUSCLES. Problems with POSTURE may also arise, while bone overgrowth can cause formation of OSTEOPHYTES. As those bone spurs form, their growth can produce SPINAL STENOSIS or other painful BACK conditions that press the spinal nerves. Conversely, nerves can be damaged if loosened facet joints allow excessive movement in the spine.

Symptoms and Diagnostic Path

ACUTE PAIN emanating from inflamed facet joints may resemble other conditions, such as a HERNIATED DISC, FRACTURE, or SPINAL INFECTION. On the other hand, an underlying condition, such as ARTHRITIS, may seem to be a facet joint disorder. To differentiate, X-RAY or COMPUTED TOMOGRAPHY SCAN can reveal abnormalities or changes in a joint. If tests and a physical examination remain inconclusive, a SPINAL INJECTION may be needed to locate and treat the source of pain.

Treatment Options and Outlook

To treat this disorder, Dr. Charles Dean Ray suggested therapeutic EXERCISE and posture training. For example, "A very useful posture when standing or sitting is the pelvic tilt—where one pinches together the buttocks and rotates forward the lower pelvis—and holding that position for several seconds, done several times per day." Other treatments include COLD THERAPY, HEAT THERAPY, SPINAL MANIPULATION, and NONSTEROIDAL ANTI-INFLAMMATORY DRUG (NSAID) THERAPY. If PAIN MANAGEMENT does not prove successful with conservative medical treatment or COMPLEMENTARY AND ALTERNATIVE MEDICINE, a BONE GRAFT or other type of SURGERY may be needed. As another option, a FACET RHIZOTOMY INJECTION may help by destroying the inflamed nerve, thereby removing that source of CHRONIC PAIN.

Risk Factors and Preventive Measures

To clarify risks and preventive measures, an article posted by Neck and Back Pain Info.com said, "These small joints are prone to injury, deterioration, and inflammation. Facet joint syndrome can occur anywhere in the spine including the low back. Pain arising from the facet joints is usually at the level of the affected facet joint(s), and is made worse by activities that put pressure on these joints, i.e. leaning backwards and 'extending' the lower back or twisting at the waist." In addition, "poor body mechanics or how we use our body can also cause problems with the facet joints." Therefore, proper posture, proper LIFTING, and problem-solving ERGONOMIC FACTORS may prevent recurrence, so that "most individuals with facet joint syndrome will recover and return to normal activities."

Neck and Back Pain Info.com. "Facet Joint Syndrome," Joint Pain Info.com. Available online. URL: http://jointpaininfo.com/back/backFacetJointSyndrome.html. Downloaded January 4, 2006.

Ray, Charles Dean, M.D. "Facet Joint Disorders and Back Pain," Spine-health.com. Available online. URL:

http://www.spine-health.com/topics/cd/facetjoint/
facetjoint01.html. Downloaded January 4, 2006.

facet joint injection   See FACET JOINT DISORDER;
SPINAL INJECTION.

facet neurotomy or facet rhizotomy injection

Sometimes used to treat FACET JOINT DISORDER, this
procedure, in essence, disconnects a hot-wired
nerve. Although a neurotomy seldom provides the
first course of treatment, the procedure may be used
if a SPINAL INJECTION, COLD THERAPY, PAIN RELIEVERS,
or other forms of PAIN MANAGEMENT fail to help.

Procedure

After anesthesia has taken effect in the patient, a
medical specialist uses the guidance of a fluoroscope
to apply heat from a needlelike probe. As a SpineUniverse article explained, "Once the needle is injected,
a mild electrical current is used to stimulate the nerve
and confirm its exact location. You may feel slight
pressure or tingling during this part of the procedure.
Then the electrode is heated to deaden the sensory
nerves. When the procedure is completed, the needle
is removed and the injection site is bandaged."

A Spine-health article said, "Theoretically, by
deadening the sensory nerve to the facet joint, a
facet rhizotomy effectively prevents the pain signals from getting to the brain." Since more than
one facet may be addressed, the time needed for
this outpatient procedure varies from ten minutes
to an hour or so.

Risks and Complications

Any soreness resulting from the injection can usually be eased with an ice pack applied for about 15
minutes every hour or two. Regarding the facet
pain for which the treatment was intended, about
50 to 60 percent of the patients experience pain
relief within a few days. This means, however, that
a neurotomy provides little or no pain relief about
40 percent of the time. Besides the risk of failure,
an injection can destabilize a facet joint, although
that complication seldom occurs. A more likely risk
arises as growing nerve fibers later replicate the
original problem.

Outlook and Lifestyle Modifications

If the procedure offers little or no relief, patients
may need to consider such other options as BIO-
FEEDBACK to manage pain. With a successful outcome, the injection can give patients pain-free time
in which to begin therapeutic EXERCISE, increase
their daily ACTIVITY, or tackle STRENGTH TRAINING.

Richeimer, Steven, M.D., and Mary Claire Walsh. "Facet
    Rhizotomy: Procedure Preparation and Aftercare,"
    SpineUniverse. Available online. URL: http://www.
    spineuniverse.com/displayarticle.php/article221.
    html. Last updated November 21, 2005.
Spine-health.com. "Injections: Facet Rhizotomy Injec-
    tion." Available online. URL: http://www.spine-health.
    com/topics/conserv/overview/inj/inj04.html. Down-
    loaded January 4, 2006.

failed back surgery syndrome (FBSS)   Not really a
syndrome, but the result of failed SURGERY, this condition may cause disability as a person encounters
CHRONIC PAIN. In the overview, "Failed Back Surgery
Syndrome: What It Is and How to Avoid It," Dr. Peter
Ullrich Jr. explained, "Spine surgery is only basically
able to accomplish two things: 1) Decompressing a
nerve root that is pinched, or 2) Stabilizing a painful joint." In some cases, the area thought to be the
source of pain is not, but "some types of back surgery are far more predictable in terms of alleviating
a patient's symptoms than others." For example, "a
spine fusion for spinal instability (e.g. spondylolisthesis) is a relatively predictable operation. However, a
spine fusion for multi-level lumbar degenerative disc
disease is far less likely to be successful in reducing a
patient's pain."

The site of the BACK problem can be a factor too.
According to Dr. Ullrich, "A discectomy (or microdiscectomy) for a lumbar disc herniation that is causing
leg pain is a very predictable operation. However, a
discectomy for a lumbar disc herniation that is causing lower back pain is far less likely to be successful." Even if the surgery goes well, pain may return
as scar tissue forms. For example, "the one time that
scar tissue . . . may be symptomatic is for a patient
who initially does well . . . only to have recurrent
pain come on slowly between 6 to 12 weeks after
surgery. This is the time period that scar tissue takes

to form." Conversely, "pain that starts years after surgery, or pain that continues after surgery and is never relieved, is not from scar tissue."

Symptoms and Diagnostic Path

An article posted by Back.com said, "Symptoms may include diffuse, dull, and achy pain located primarily in the back and/or legs" or "sharp, pricking, and stabbing pain that radiates from the legs." In either case, "A joint may become irritated because surgery altered the person's posture and way of moving." Symptoms may also include depression and lack of SLEEP.

To rule out such painful possibilities as a HER-NIATED DISC, a diagnostic X-RAY or MAGNETIC RES-ONANCE IMAGING may be needed. In addition, an ELECTROMYOGRAM can assess potential damage involving the spinal nerves.

Treatment Options and Outlook

Options include ACUPUNCTURE, EXERCISE, NEURO-STIMULATION, SPINAL MANIPULATION, and, in some instances, additional surgery. For example, if a BONE GRAFT has failed to complete spinal fusion, ARTHRODESIS may help. For some patients, a SPINAL INJECTION or FACET NEUROTOMY may relieve pain, at least temporarily.

Risk Factors and Preventive Measures

Sometimes failed back surgery occurs because the patient resumes daily ACTIVITY too soon, disrupting the spinal fusion meant to take place over the natural course of recovery. At other times, inadequate NUTRITION and lack of EXERCISE cause further weakening in the BACK or VERTEBRAE. For instance, a person may not get enough dietary CALCIUM to aid BONE BUILDING. Or a patient may not be able to perform stretching exercises that keep scar tissue to a manageable minimum. During the first few weeks after surgery, stretching and LIFTING should be avoided as should other stresses on the surgical site.

Medtronic Sofamor Danek. "Mechanical Disorders: Failed Back Syndrome (FBS)," Back.com. Available online. URL: http://www.back.com/causes-mechanical-failed. html. Last updated March 11, 2005.

Ullrich, Peter F., Jr., M.D. "Failed Back Surgery Syndrome: What It Is and How to Avoid It," Spine-health. com. Available online. URL: http://www.spine-health. com/topics/surg/failed_back/failed_back01.html. Last updated June 1, 2004.

female athlete triad   The coining of this phrase in 1992 publicized a syndrome among female ATH-LETES that involves three main symptoms, but more may exist. Primarily, symptoms include loss of bone density, loss of menses (amenorrhea), and loss of weight with the latter sometimes caused by an EAT-ING DISORDER, such as anorexia nervosa or bulimia nervosa. Typically, loss of energy also occurs.

Symptoms and Diagnostic Path

As explained in *The Lancet,* "Energy restriction is common in sports, and for many athletes it is necessary to achieve the sport-specific bodyweight and composition that result in optimum performance. Because of the importance of fat loss, female athletes in many sports consume 30% less energy per unit of bodyweight than male athletes. The prevalence of disordered eating, involving dietary restriction and purgative behaviours such as vomiting and misuse of laxatives, ranges from 1% to 62% dependent on the sport, and is highest in sports in which low bodyweight conveys a competitive advantage." However, this short-term advantage pales beside such disadvantages as hormonal changes that disrupt the menstrual cycle and bone formation, which "can lead to irreversible bone loss in adults and can impair the accretion of bone mass in adolescents."

To confirm a diagnosis, a medical history, physical examination, evaluation of symptoms, and BONE MINERAL DENSITY TEST will usually be needed. In addition, a blood test to determine any mineral imbalance may help to diagnose the syndrome and individualize the course of treatment.

Treatment Options and Outlook

According to an online article first published in the *American Family Physician,* "Preservation of bone mineral density is one of the many reasons to screen female athletes and diagnose the female athlete triad early in its course. Postmenopausal women lose most of their bone mass and density in the first four to six years after menopause. If this is also true of amenorrheic athletes, intervention is needed before bone mass is irreversibly lost." To re-establish the menstrual cycle, HORMONE REPLACE-MENT THERAPY may be prescribed. "While hormonal therapy will treat the amenorrhea, the ultimate goal is the return of regular menses through proper nutrition, revised training regimens and maintenance of reasonable body weight." To do this, the article further suggested, "Optimal treatment of the female athlete triad includes instruction from a dietician to educate and monitor the patient for adequate nutrition and to help the patient attain and maintain a goal weight. The patient, dietician and physician should agree on a goal weight, with consideration for the weight requirements for participation in the patient's chosen sport. A weight gain of 0.23 to 0.45 kg (0.5 to 1 lb) per week until the goal weight is achieved is a reasonable expectation. Helping the patient focus on optimal health and performance instead of weight is important. The patient need not stop exercising completely. Exercise activity should be decreased by 10 to 20 percent, and weight should be monitored closely for two to three months."

Risk Factors and Preventive Measures

An article in the *Journal of Strength and Conditioning Research* reported that female gymnasts have a lower risk of bone loss than do cross-country runners. Therefore, the latter group might "include more high-impact activities in their training regimen to optimize their bone health."

BONE BUILDING efforts, such as increased CALCIUM intake, can lower the risk of OSTEOPOROSIS and VERTEBRAL COMPRESSION FRACTURE. Also, a BISPHOSPHONATE drug may help, but studies have not adequately focused on its effects in treating female athlete triad. For most patients, psychological counseling, hydration, and a sensible course of NUTRITION will prevent life-threatening damage and restore the athlete to health. To encourage her success in reaching that goal, her coach, family members, and friends must quickly become her biggest fans.

Bemben, Debra A., Torey D. Buchanan, Michael G. Bemben, and Allen W. Knehans. "Influence of Type of Mechanical Loading, Menstrual Status, and Training Season on Bone Density in Young Women Athletes," *Journal of Strength and Conditioning Research* 18, no. 2 (May 2004): 220–226.

Hobart, Julie A., M.D. and Douglas R. Smucker, M.D. "The Female Athlete Triad," *American Family Physician* 61, no. 11 (June 1, 2000): Available online. URL: http://www.aafp.org/afp/20000601/3357.html. Downloaded January 4, 2006.

Loucks, Anne B. and Aurelia Nattiv. "The Female Athlete Triad," *The Lancet* 366, no. 9503 (December 17, 2005): 49–50.

fenoprofen   See NONSTEROIDAL ANTI-INFLAMMATORY DRUG THERAPY.

fibromyalgia   Once unkindly proclaimed as being all in the head, this complex syndrome exhibits tender points almost everywhere but the skull. Characteristically, the dull but widespread pain occurs in fibrous tissue of muscles, ligaments, and tendons. Unlike ARTHRITIS and other rheumatic or degenerative conditions, however, fibromyalgia does not inflame or damage vertebral joints and bone. Therefore, by ruling out the conditions that cause those symptoms, a rheumatologist or primary care physician may come to a diagnostic conclusion.

Symptoms and Diagnostic Path

Since no evidence of this chronic disorder will be found in blood work, X-RAYS, or any other tests, the doctor relies on a medical history and symptoms, which include fatigue, depression, difficulty focusing, and sensitivity to noise or climatic change. Stomach upset often occurs too. Interestingly, each of these symptoms commonly relates to a chronic lack of SLEEP, which fibromyalgia patients typically encounter.

The most telling symptoms occur in pain located at tender points in precise locations. According to the National Fibromyalgia Association (NFA), diagnostic criteria include "tenderness or pain in at least 11 of the 18 specified tender points when pressure is applied." From the front, these points appear on either side of the throat, at a midpoint below each collarbone, on the inner fold of each elbow, and the inside edge of each knee. From the back, tender points reside on either side of the VERTEBRAE at the base of the skull, along the top edge of each shoulder, around the dimpled area on each cheek of the hip, and on each outer thigh just below the buttock. The NFA also specified another diagnostic determinant as "widespread pain in all four quadrants of the body for a minimum duration of three months."

Treatment Options and Outlook

PAIN RELIEVERS, MASSAGE THERAPY, SPINAL MANIPULATION, ACUPRESSURE, and other forms of COMPLEMENTARY AND ALTERNATIVE MEDICINE offer some measure of relief. For example, HERBAL THERAPY might include ginkgo biloba capsules to stimulate circulation in the morning and a cup of passionflower tea to relax muscles at night. Besides taste and visual appeal, culinary herbs sometimes have medicinal value too. For instance, a dash of cayenne pepper or a crushed clove of garlic can boost the immune system while enhancing the flavor of tomato sauce. A little turmeric rubbed into fish or ginger sprinkled onto carrots and chicken may provide a pain-killer of a gourmet meal.

The National Pain Foundation (NPF) suggested a variety of treatment options, which, with the approval of a doctor, includes gradually working up to a half hour of aerobic EXERCISE four or five times a week. According to the NPF, "Flexibility is the other form of exercise that is necessary to reduce the symptoms of pain for people with fibromyalgia. . . . The old statement, 'if you don't use it, you lose it,' is true when it comes to muscles, tendons, and ligaments. They stiffen up and tight muscles are uncomfortable muscles. You can actually decrease pain by increasing flexibility. Stretches should be done daily, but remember to go about all of these exercises slowly, gently, and yet progressively." Besides strengthening the body, exercise improves mental outlook too.

Risk Factors and Preventive Measures

Preventing a condition usually depends on addressing the causal factors, but an article on the Web site of the American College of Rheumatology said, "No one knows what causes fibromyalgia. However, we do know that people with fibromyalgia may have abnormal levels of Substance P, a chemical that helps transmit and amplify pain signals to and from the brain. For the person with fibromyalgia, it is as though the 'volume control' is turned up too high in the brain's pain processing areas. Current studies are underway to examine how the brain and spinal cord (the central nervous system) process pain and the role Substance P plays."

GENETIC FACTORS and ENVIRONMENTAL INFLUENCES also warrant study. Meanwhile, young to middle-aged women have seven times the risk men have of developing fibromyalgia.

Clauw, Daniel J., M.D. and Denise Taylor-Moon. "Fibromyalgia," American College of Rheumatology, ACR. Available online. URL: http://www.rheumatology.org/public/factsheets/fibromya_new.asp. Downloaded January 5, 2006.

Holistic online.com. "Treatment of Fibromyalgia." Available online. URL: http://holistic-online.com/Remedies/cfs/fib_herbal.htm. Downloaded January 4, 2006.

National Fibromyalgia Association. "About Fibromyalgia," NFA. Available online. URL: http://fmaware.org/fminfo/brochure.htm. Downloaded January 4, 2006.

National Pain Foundation, The. "Fibromyalgia Treatment Options," My Pain. Available online. URL: http://www.nationalpainfoundation.org/MyTreatment/TreatmentOptionsContinuum_Fibromyalgia.asp. Last updated August 19, 2005.

fibrous dysplasia This skeletal disorder causes abnormal growth in one bone or many, with the ribs a more likely location than the VERTEBRAE. Brittleness and deformity can occur at a single site, at random sites, or on one side of the body, including the face.

Symptoms and Diagnostic Path

A fact sheet from the National Institutes of Health (NIH) listed bone pain, bone deformity, and FRACTURE as common symptoms of this uncommon disorder. Characteristically, "bone pain may occur due to the expanding fibrous tissue in the bone. The onset of pain may signal an impending fracture in a bone that has been weakened by this gradual expansion. A fracture may cause a sudden increase in severe pain. It is also possible, although less common, for abnormal bone to produce pain by pressing on an adjacent nerve. In patients with considerable deformity of the weight-bearing long bones (thighs and shins), arthritis can develop in the hips and knees." Besides ARTHRITIS, some individuals develop hormonal problems, such as early puberty or high blood calcium from PARATHYROID HORMONE (PTH). Although rare, patients may also encounter the skeletal deformities of RICKETS. In any case, X-RAYS confirm the diagnosis.

Treatment Options and Outlook

Regarding treatments, the NIH recommended various specialists, such as "orthopedic surgeons, since most symptomatic patients have bone pain and/or skeletal deformity; Craniofacial or plastic surgeons who are needed for correction of facial deformities; Neurosurgeons who are needed for treatment of brain or spinal complications; and Endocrinologists who are best for treating patients who develop hormonal problems."

For most patients, appropriate EXERCISE assists skeletal health and joint mobility. An improved outlook also comes through ongoing RESEARCH of GENETIC FACTORS. As the NIH reported, "Recent studies indicate that fibrous dysplasia may be caused by a chemical abnormality in a protein in the bone that leads to an overgrowth of bone cells that produce fibrous tissue. The chemical abnormality occurs because of a mutation or change in the structure of the gene that produces the protein. Fibrous dysplasia is thought to be a congenital disorder, meaning that individuals who have it probably had it when they were born. There is no evidence, however, that the disorder can be inherited."

Risk Factors and Preventive Measures

For a potential preventive of bone malformation and pain, the American Academy of Orthopaedic Surgeons (AAOS) said, "Bisphosphonates are medications that decrease the activity of cells that dissolve bone. . . . These medications have not been used extensively in the treatment of fibrous dysplasia, but early studies have demonstrated effective relief of the pain associated with fibrous dysplasia." With or without BISPHOSPHONATES, some patients may need SURGERY to prevent spinal deformity. If so, the AAOS said, "stabilization of the bone with metal implants such as rods or plates and screws can be useful to fix a fracture or deformity, or pre-

vent bone breakage." Also, "braces may occasionally be used to prevent fracture, but they have not been effective in preventing deformity."

In assessing the risks of this chronic disorder, the NIH reported, "Young patients who have fibrous dysplasia in many bones may have more problems." However, "patients with one or only a few lesions may have mild or no symptoms. Related hormonal abnormalities are usually successfully treated once a problem is recognized."

American Academy of Orthopaedic Surgeons. "Fibrous Dysplasia," AAOS. Available online. URL: http://orthoinfo. aaos.org/fact/thr_report.cfm?Thread_ID=485&topcategory=Tumors. Downloaded January 4, 2006.

National Institutes of Health Osteoporosis and Related Bone Diseases, The. "Information for Patients about Fibrous Dysplasia," NIH, National Resource Center. Available online. URL: http://www.osteo.org/newfile.asp?doc=p111i&doctitle=Fibrous+Dysplasia&doctype=HTML+Fact+Sheet. Downloaded January 5, 2006.

flat back or flatback   Normally, the BACK has a forward curve (KYPHOSIS) and a backward curve (LORDOSIS.) These natural curves enable the SPINE to maintain POSTURE, flexibility, and balance in standing, walking, or carrying a load. With a flat back, however, the VERTEBRAE form a straight line, causing a forward-motion look even if the person is standing still. Since that rigid posture throws the body off balance, a cane or walker may be needed to retain mobility.

Sometimes, flat back results from a BIRTH DEFECT OF THE SPINE, but the problem can occur later. For instance, the doctor who performs a spinal fusion must take the natural curve of the back into account, or flat configuration will occur.

Symptoms and Diagnostic Path

The appearance of rigidity and presence of CHRONIC PAIN make this disorder readily apparent. Nevertheless, a diagnosis will likely include X-RAYS, a physical examination, and a medical history.

Treatment Options and Outlook

Prompt treatment of SCOLIOSIS or other contributing factors, such as a VERTEBRAL COMPRESSION

FRACTURE and DEGENERATIVE DISC DISEASE, can prevent flat back from occurring. Mild cases may be helped with SPINAL MANIPULATION and more severe ones with a BONE GRAFT, osteotomy, or other type of SURGERY. However, ORTHOTIC devices may not provide an optimal form of treatment. In an article for eSpine.com, Dr. Robert S. Pashman explained, "Since symptoms are produced through abnormal mechanics of the spine, pelvis and upper legs, a brace intended to support a decompensated spine would have to cross each of these structures. Such braces are not usually effective. Similarly, trunk braces, which also capture the leg are not well tolerated by most individuals. In general, bracing is not an option for symptomatic flat back. When conservative methods fail and the patient is symptomatic to the point of being dysfunctional due to the pain, surgery is indicated."

Risk Factors and Preventive Measures

According to iScoliosis.com, "Patients can develop a painful flat back deformity as the result of degenerative arthritis of the spine, or as a consequence of a previous spinal fusion operation. . . . Today, surgeons are often able to correct scoliosis while still preserving as much of the normal alignment of the spine as possible. This is largely the result of advances in the techniques and types of instruments that are used to correct scoliosis."

Medtronic Sofamor Danek. "Flat Back Syndrome," iScoliosis.com. Available online. URL: http://www.iscoliosis.com/symptoms-flat.html. Downloaded January 5, 2006.

Pashman, Robert S., M.D. "Back to Basics: Flatback," eSpine.com. Available online. URL: http://www.espine.com/flatback.html. Downloaded January 5, 2006.

flexion-extension injury A flexion-extension injury can occur in any joint as a person exceeds his or her grasp. For instance, a tennis player might overextend a racquet to score a tennis elbow, or a surfer might catch a wave of hip pain. In the BACK, VERTEBRAE, and CERVICAL SPINE, however, a flexion-extension injury most often results from what is commonly known as a whiplash.

Symptoms and Diagnostic Path

Similar to a STRAIN or SPRAIN, a flexion-extension injury usually occurs after a precipitous event, such as a sports accident or car crash. Although the latter may involve other areas of the SPINE, an information page from the National Institute of Neurological Disorders and Stroke (NINDS) addressed the neck, saying, "Symptoms such as neck pain may be present directly after the injury or may be delayed for several days. In addition to neck pain, other symptoms may include neck stiffness, injuries to the muscles and ligaments (myofascial injuries), headache, dizziness, abnormal sensations such as burning or prickling (paresthesias), or shoulder or back pain. In addition, some people experience . . . conditions such as memory loss, concentration impairment, nervousness/irritability, sleep disturbances, fatigue, or depression." If a flexion-extension injury involves the cervical spine, CERVICOGENIC HEADACHES may be present too.

Treatment Options and Outlook

A MUSCLE RELAXANT, NONSTEROIDAL ANTI-INFLAMMATORY DRUG THERAPY, SPINAL MANIPULATION, and ORTHOTIC device, such as a cervical collar or brace, usually begin the conservative treatment. Initially, COLD THERAPY may be needed to reduce inflammation, but after swelling subsides, HEAT THERAPY can relieve the muscle TENSION. According to the NINDS, "Most patients recover within 3 months after the injury, however, some may continue to have residual neck pain and headaches." Sometimes this lasts up to two years.

If CHRONIC PAIN extends beyond a normal recovery time, X-RAYS or MAGNETIC RESONANCE IMAGING may reveal FACET JOINT DISORDER, a HERNIATED DISC, or SACROILIAC JOINT PAIN SYNDROME, each of which involves various treatments. In any case, the best outlook comes by identifying and treating damage to a joint, bone, muscle, or soft tissue. To ease inflammation in spinal nerves or locate a damaged nerve, a SPINAL INJECTION may help. If, however, an injured DISC or vertebra causes spinal nerve pressure, SURGERY may be needed.

The North American Spine Society (NASS) offered this insight into chronic pain after a flexion-extension injury: "Muscle strain of the neck and upper back can cause acute pain. However, there is no evidence that neck muscles are a primary cause of chronic neck pain, although muscles can hurt if they are working too hard to protect injured discs, joints, or the nerves of the neck or there is something else wrong that sustains the muscle pain, such as poor posture and work habits."

In addition to improving POSTURE, the NASS suggested, "Strength training is necessary to develop sufficient muscle strength to be able to hold the head and neck in positions of good posture at rest and during activity. Strengthening the muscles will also improve their range of motion."

Risk Factors and Preventive Measures

Automobile safety measures, such as proper seat belt usage, airbag installation, and impact-resistant designs, offer the best preventives for whiplash, while sturdy equipment can ease spinal worries for ATHLETES. Therapies typically begun after a flexion-extension injury can act as preventives too. For instance, STRENGTH TRAINING builds PARASPINAL MUSCLES and neck muscles, enabling them to endure greater levels of stress while increasing flexibility and RANGE OF MOTION.

National Institute of Neurological Disorders and Stroke. "NINDS Whiplash Information Page," NINDS, National Institutes of Health. Available online. URL: http://www.ninds.nih.gov/disorders/whiplash/whiplash.htm. Last updated November 23, 2005.

North American Spine Society. "Whiplash and Whiplash Associated Disorders," NASS. Available online. URL: http://www.spine.org/articles/whiplash.cfm. Downloaded January 5, 2006.

fluoride   See ENVIRONMENTAL INFLUENCES ON SPINE HEALTH.

fluoroscopy   Instead of an X-rated movie, fluoroscopy offers an X-RAY movie. As explained on the University of Maryland Medical Center (UMMC) Web site, "A continuous x-ray beam is passed through the body part being examined, and is transmitted to a TV-like monitor so that the body part and its motion can be seen in detail. . . . Fluoroscopy is used in many types of examinations and procedures, such as barium x-rays, cardiac catheterization, and placement of intravenous (IV) catheters (hollow tubes inserted into veins or arteries)."

In treating or testing SPINE problems, fluoroscopy may be used for a biopsy, MYELOGRAM, or SPINAL INJECTION, such as a LUMBAR PUNCTURE or facet joint injection. While fluoroscopy provides a picture of the VERTEBRAE and other BACK bones, the Baptist Memorial Health Care Web site said, "It reveals less detail than a standard still X-ray. It exposes the person to somewhat more radiation than a standard X-ray. Therefore, doctors use it only when they need to see internal movement."

Procedure

Depending on the reason for the test, fluoroscopic procedures can be performed in either an outpatient clinic or a hospital setting. As an article from OhioHealth.com explained, "Although the specifics vary depending on the type of fluoroscopic test you undergo, in general you will be asked to lie or stand between the X-ray machine and a fluorescent screen after putting on a hospital gown. An intravenous line may be started in your arm or a catheter may be inserted. An X-ray scanner produces fluoroscopic images of the body part being examined. The procedure itself is generally painless."

Risks and Complications

Pregnant women should generally avoid fluoroscopy because of the radiation exposure. Most patients, however, encounter only the minimal risks usually associated with low-dose radiation. Some patients react to barium, but with a lot of water, this quickly washes from the digestive system.

Outlook and Lifestyle Modifications

Often, fluoroscopy provides only a small role in the overall picture. Satisfactorily solving a mystery determines whether this medical scene ends on an upbeat scene.

Baptist Memorial Health Care. "Fluoroscopy." Available online. URL: http://www.baptistonline.org/health/library/test3236.asp. Downloaded January 5, 2006.

OhioHealth.com. "Fluoroscopy," American Radiology Services, Inc., Radiological Society of North America. Available online. URL: http://www.ohiohealth.

com/facilities/outpatient_facilities/imaging/details/ fluoroscopy.htm. Downloaded January 5, 2006.

University of Maryland Medical Center. "Radiology: Fluoroscopy," UMMC. Available online. URL: http://www. umm.edu/radiology/fluroscopy.html. Downloaded January 5, 2006.

flurbiprofen   See NONSTEROIDAL ANTI-INFLAMMATORY DRUG THERAPY.

folate or folic acid (B9)   As a member of the VITAMIN B-COMPLEX family, this nutrient has been singled out for its fine contribution to the SPINE of a healthy baby. Most notably, folate or folic acid can prevent neural tube defects, such as SPINA BIFIDA. To be effective though, this vitamin must be in the system before a woman becomes pregnant. As the Centers for Disease Control and Prevention (CDC) explained, "Birth defects of a baby's brain or spine happen in the first few weeks of pregnancy, often *before* a woman knows that she is pregnant."

Dosage and Potential Side Effects

According to the Office of Dietary Supplements, National Institutes of Health (NIH), "Folate is a water-soluble B vitamin that occurs naturally in food," whereas "folic acid is the synthetic form of folate that is found in supplements and added to fortified foods."

Most multi-vitamin supplements for INFANTS, CHILDREN, and adults include the daily minimum requirement of folic acid as do fortified breakfast cereals and bread products. As a good source of NUTRITION in general, fresh foods also contain the natural form of folate. Named from the Latin word, folium, for leaf, folate leafs out in spinach, turnip greens, and asparagus but can also be found in citrus fruits and dried peas or beans.

Since vitamin B9 is water soluble, an excessive dose washes out of the system. In adults, however, the NIH said, "Intake of supplemental folic acid should not exceed 1,000 micrograms (mcg) per day to prevent folic acid from triggering symptoms of vitamin B12 deficiency." For children and ADOLESCENTS, the maximum daily dosage lowers to 300 micrograms for one- to three-year-olds; 400 mcg for children four to eight; 600 mcg for ages nine to 13; 800 mcg for 14- to 18-year old teens; and 1,000 mcg for anyone older.

Concerns about B12 deficiency can be resolved by taking more of that vitamin. Regarding a B9 deficiency, the NIH said, "In infants and children, folate deficiency can slow overall growth rate." For most age groups, "other signs of folate deficiency are often subtle. Digestive disorders such as diarrhea, loss of appetite, and weight loss can occur, as can weakness, sore tongue, headaches, heart palpitations, irritability, forgetfulness, and behavioral disorders."

Statistics and Studies

According to the CDC, "Scientists don't know how folic acid works to prevent birth defects. But they do know that folic acid is needed to make healthy new cells, like the ones that make up a baby's brain and spine. Taking folic acid every day, starting before and during pregnancy, can reduce the risk for these serious birth defects by 50% to 70%."

Despite the ongoing efforts of the CDC, March of Dimes, and other groups who try to educate the public about B9, only about 30 percent of the people in the United States have an adequate amount in their diets. An update in *Nutraceuticals World* said, "A team of researchers . . . reported that folic acid fortification accounted for a 36% decline in neural tube defects (NTDs) in the Hispanic population and a 34% drop among the white, non-Hispanic population between 1995 and 2002." However, "the prevalence of NTDs in the black, non-Hispanic population did not decrease significantly." As awareness rises in all races, the race may be on to protect the spinal health of every unborn child.

Centers for Disease Control and Prevention. "Folic Acid Topic: Home," CDC, Department of Health and Human Services. Available online. URL: http://www.cdc.gov/ncbddd/folicacid/index.htm. Downloaded January 5, 2006.

Kurtzweil, Paula. "How Folate Can Help Prevent Birth Defects," U.S. Food and Drug Administration, *FDA Consumer* July 1996, revised February 1999. Available online. URL: http://vm.cfsan.fda.gov/~dms/fdafolic. html. Downloaded January 6, 2006.

Office of Dietary Supplements. "Dietary Supplement Fact Sheet: Folate," National Institutes of Health. Available online. URL: http://ods.od.nih.gov/factsheets/folate. asp. Downloaded January 6, 2006.

Staff. "More Folic Acid Consumption Emphasized," *Nutraceuticals World* 8, no. 9 (October 2005): 14–15.

footwear See SHOE CHOICE, SPINAL EFFECTS OF.

foraminotomy In a pinch, this surgical procedure takes the pressure off spinal nerves, specifically those exiting through holes in the side of the spine known as the foramina. For example, a HERNIATED DISC or OSTEOPHYTE around the VERTEBRAE may press or pinch a nerve, causing pain, tingling, or numbness in the corresponding limbs. If SPINAL STENOSIS occurs in the LUMBAR SPINE, weakness may be felt in the legs and feet, whereas an obstruction in the CERVICAL SPINE often radiates pain or numbness into the arms and hands.

Procedure

X-RAYS or other imaging tests show the problem area then guide the surgeon in making an incision. In an article for NeckSurgery.com, Dr. B. Theo Mellion explained, "Bone from the . . . spine and joint over the nerve are removed using special cutting instruments and/or a drill. Thickened ligament, bone spurs and/or bulging discs are removed to decompress the exiting nerve, which is checked with a probe to insure adequate space around the nerve root. . . . Depending on many factors such as the location of the compressed nerve or severity of the patient's symptoms, a foraminotomy may be combined with other procedures such as a laminotomy or laminectomy." If a LAMINECTOMY is needed, additional steps may be involved. Otherwise, "when the spine surgeon is satisfied that ample space has been created around the nerve root, the muscles and interior tissues are closed in layers using absorbable sutures."

Risks and Complications

In assessing potential problems, a SpineUniverse article stated, "All surgical procedures carry some risk. The risks from a foraminotomy include the risks inherent to every operation (i.e. a small risk of infection, bleeding etc.)." Although rare, "there is a small risk of injury to the nerve or spinal cord and this should be discussed specifically with the surgeon."

Outlook and Lifestyle Modifications

Pain can be expected at the surgical site, but most patients notice immediate improvement. Others may find symptoms disappearing gradually. To ease discomfort during recovery, PAIN MANAGEMENT usually includes NONSTEROIDAL ANTI-INFLAMMATORY DRUG (NSAID) THERAPY and COLD THERAPY. After recovery, gradual increase in daily ACTIVITY and EXERCISE can aid flexibility and build strength. Physical therapy may also help to increase the RANGE OF MOTION and prevent spinal nerves from getting in a future pinch.

Mellion, B. Theo, M.D. "Surgical: Foraminotomy," NeckSurgery.com. Available online. URL: http://www. necksurgery.com/treatment-surgical-foraminotomy. html. Updated April 20, 2005.

Sekhon, Lali, M.D. and Susan Spinasanta. "Foraminotomy: Taking Pressure off Spinal Nerves," SpineUniverse. Available online. URL: http://www.spineuniverse. com/displayarticle.php/article554.html. Downloaded January 5, 2006.

Forestier's disease See DIFFUSE IDIOPATHIC SKELETAL HYPEROSTOSIS (DISH).

fractures Broken bones can occur anytime any place for any age group, but an undue number of fractures fall onto ATHLETES, CHILDREN, or ELDERLY persons. As stated in the article "Fractures" on the American Academy of Orthopaedic Surgeons (AAOS) Web site, "Fractures can happen in a variety of ways, but there are three common causes: Trauma accounts for most fractures. For example, a fall, a motor vehicle accident or a tackle during a football game can all result in a fracture." Secondly, "osteoporosis also can contribute to fractures. Osteoporosis is a bone disease that results in the 'thinning' of the bone. The bones become fragile and easily broken." Finally, "overuse sometimes results in stress fractures. These are common among athletes." Most of the time, an external device, such as a cast or splint, will assist a bone in mending properly. However, a bone-crushing blow may require corrective SURGERY to affix the bone with metal screws, plates, or pins.

In considering spinal fractures in need of surgical repair, a SpineUniverse article said, "When describing and diagnosing spinal fractures, spine surgeons divide the spinal column into 3 sections: 1. Anterior column," which includes the front portion of the VERTEBRAE, along with the related ligaments and discs. "2. Middle column—made up of the posterior one-half of the vertebral body, disc, and . . . the posterior . . . ligament. 3. Posterior column—made up of the facet joints . . . and the interconnecting ligaments." Besides the location and bone matter, the stability of a fracture must be assessed. As the article explained, "Generally, a fracture is considered stable if only the anterior column is involved, as in the case of most wedge fractures. When the anterior and middle columns are involved, the fracture may be considered more unstable. When all three columns are involved, the fracture is by definition considered unstable, because of the loss of the integrity of the posterior stabilizing ligaments."

Risks and Complications

The AAOS article "Fracture of the Thoracic and Lumbar Spine" said, "Fracture of one or more parts of the spinal column (vertebrae) of the middle (thoracic) or lower (lumbar) back is a serious injury usually caused by high-energy trauma like a car crash, fall, sports accident or act of violence (i.e., gunshot wound). Males experience the injury four times more often than females do." If the fracture occurs in the LUMBAR SPINE or CERVICAL SPINE, moving the person can cause a spinal cord injury that results in permanent paralysis, disability, or death.

In discussing the complication of burst fractures, Dr. Thomas A. Zdeblick said this "is a descriptive term for an injury to the spine in which the vertebral body is severely compressed." In a severe trauma, "a great deal of force vertically onto the spine" can crush a vertebra. While a compression fracture has a wedge shape, a burst fracture goes in all directions. Therefore, "this is a much more severe injury than a compression fracture for two reasons. With the bony margins spreading out in all directions the spinal cord is liable to be injured. The bony fragment that is spread out toward the spinal cord can bruise the spinal cord causing paralysis or partial neurologic injury." If this happens in vertebrae between the THORACIC SPINE and lumbar spine, "paralysis of the legs and loss of control of the bowel and bladder may result." To avoid this risk, Dr. Zdeblick said, "At the scene of the accident, patients complaining of severe back pain should not be placed into a seated or flexed position. They should be kept lying flat and transported in the flat position. A patient who stands or sits with a burst fracture may increase their neurologic injury." This may or may not be true of every fracture, but with a burst fracture, "however, often the amount of pain that is present is severe enough that patients know it is a good idea not to walk."

Amazingly, a burst fracture does not necessarily require surgery. Treatment may require only a molded turtle shell brace or body cast for eight to twelve weeks. If surgery is later needed, Dr. Zdeblick said, "The degree of recovery may depend on the timing of surgery, the degree of spinal canal compromise and the stability of the spine. The most important factor in how much neurologic recovery occurs is how severe the original injury was."

Statistics and Studies

To prevent a fracture from happening spontaneously, medical specialists often focus on BONE MINERAL DENSITY TEST results, particularly in older women. However, an article in *Geriatrics* summarized concerns about the reliability of those predictors. As the article reported, "A large number of women sustained osteoporotic fractures within 1 year after . . . bone mineral density (BMD) testing, although they had T-scores greater than -2.5. . . . Approximately 82% of the women suffered fractures of the wrist, forearm, hip, rib, or spine. Nevertheless, just 18% of these women would have been recommended for treatment if the intervention threshold was set at -2.5 or less." In other words, "the study showed that if you use -2.5 as a treatment threshold, which we believe many physicians do, you would have missed 82% of the women who actually fractured."

Special Aids and Adaptations

In bone-compromising conditions, such as OSTEOPOROSIS, OSTEOPENIA, FIBROUS DYSPLASIA, CANCER, or OSTEOGENESIS IMPERFECTA, a patient can sustain a VERTEBRAL COMPRESSION FRACTURE simply by getting out of bed. For people with fair to normal bone structure, complications from a fracture mainly occur by exerting too much pressure on the bone too soon. Often, a broken bone means adapting to crutches or an ORTHOTIC device until the bone has healed, but those aids rarely include a walking cast. As the AAOS article "Fractures" explained, "Pain usually stops long before the fracture is solid enough to handle the stresses of normal activity. Even after your cast or brace is removed, you may need to continue limiting your activity until the bone is solid enough to use in normal activity." Another complication arises with muscle weakness or tight ligaments caused by lack of use. However, the gradual increase of EXERCISE and daily ACTIVITY can restore muscle tissue and ultimately aid bone strength.

American Academy of Orthopaedic Surgeons. "Fracture of the Thoracic and Lumbar Spine," AAOS. Available online. URL: http://orthoinfo.aaos.org/fact/thr_report.cfm?Thread_ID=299&topcategory=Spine. Downloaded January 5, 2006.

———. "Fractures," AAOS. Available online. URL:http://orthoinfo.aaos.org/fact/thr_report.cfm?Thread_ID=125&topcategory=General%20Information. Downloaded January 6, 2006.

Holwerda, Teri and Mary Claire Walsh. "Spinal Fractures: The Three-Column Concept," SpineUniverse. Available online. URL: http://www.spineuniverse.com/displayarticle.php/article2718.html. Last updated April 1, 2005.

Staff. "Fracture Risk Intervention Relies on More than T-scores," *Geriatrics* 59, no. 7 (July 2004): 16–17.

Zdeblick, Thomas A., M.D. "Burst Fractures: Defined and Diagnosed," SpineUniverse. Available online. URL: http://www.spineuniverse.com/displayarticle.php/article1434.html. Last updated December 28, 2005.

gene therapy   See RESEARCH.

genetic factors, genomics   When a person has amber eyes, black curls, creamy skin, or long fingers, those genetic factors can be summed up at a glance. A closer look into that attractive cover may show an inherited tendency toward art, mathematics, mechanics, music, or sports. Whether at birth or over time, genetic factors can also be seen in bone quality, musculoskeletal development, or a tendency toward conditions that affect the BACK and SPINE. For example, parents may have spinal concerns for INFANTS born into a family history of ANKYLOSING SPONDYLITIS, GROWTH HORMONE DISORDERS, OSTEOGENESIS IMPERFECTA, OSTEOPOROSIS, or SCOLIOSIS. They may not know, however, of genetic influences such as iron metabolism dysfunction that often occurs in patients with RHEUMATOID ARTHRITIS or other inflammatory disorders. With more information, though, people find more pertinent questions to ask.

An article posted by the Office of Genomics at the Centers for Disease Control and Prevention (CDC) defined genetics as "the study of inheritance, or the way traits are passed down from one generation to another." As the CDC explained, "Genes carry the instructions for making proteins, which in turn direct the activities of cells and functions of the body that influence traits such as hair and eye color. Genomics is a newer term that describes the study of all the genes in a person, as well as interactions of those genes with each other and with that person's environment."

In "Genomics Lingo," Elizabeth Mahanna explained that "genetics usually refers to the study of single genes, while genomics refers to the study of all the genes in a person or organism. The human genome is a person's complete set of DNA." Regarding DNA, she explained, "The chemical DNA (deoxyribonucleic acid) is in all the cells of our body. . . . Genes are pieces of DNA that contain instructions for making cells or for what cells do. Each gene contains instructions for building one or more proteins, but a gene can contain millions of bases, so deciphering how it works or what a mutation is can be very difficult." Basically, "a mutation is a change in the order of the bases in a gene." Interestingly though, "scientists have found that, of the 3 billion or so bases in the human genome, 99.9% are exactly the same from person to person. About 3 million (or 0.1%) are different, and that's what makes us unique. Three million may seem like a big number, but it's not much compared to 3 billion." Also, "scientists now think that there are more genetic differences between people of the same race than between people of different races."

Risks and Complications
Many problems affect the back and spine because of genetic factors. To assess the likelihood of such occurrences, the Office of Genomics and Disease Prevention of CDC said, "The key features of a family history that may increase risk are: Diseases that occur at an earlier age than expected . . . ; Disease in more than one close relative . . . ; Certain combinations of diseases within a family. . . . If your family has one or more of these features, your family history may hold important clues about your risk for disease." Therefore, "people with a family history of disease may have the most to gain from lifestyle changes and screening tests. . . . You can't change your genes, but you can change unhealthy behaviors, such as smoking, inactivity, and poor eating habits. In many cases, adopting a healthier lifestyle can reduce your risk for diseases that run in your family."

Statistics and Studies

According to the CDC, "Geneticists have long recognized the value of family history for diagnosing disorders due to mutations in single genes, including certain forms of common diseases. Although typically associated with a very high individual risk of disease, single-gene mutations account for a small proportion of cases. Most common diseases result from the interactions of multiple genes with multiple environmental factors in complex patterns that, despite progress in sequencing the human genome, are unlikely to be understood fully in the near future. In the meantime, family medical history represents a 'genomic tool' that can capture the interactions of genetic susceptibility, shared environment, and common behaviours in relation to disease risk."

Special Aids and Adaptations

No one wants to experience a disabling deformity, CHRONIC PAIN, or shortened life span, but parents in particular just want their children to be happy and healthy. When genetic factors decrease the likelihood of physical, mental, social, or financial health, a family may have difficulty accepting a condition or seeing a child for the individual she or he is. High genetic factors trigger high emotions, but these can often be calmed as a genetic counselor or medical specialist answers questions and overcomes fears with facts. If someone already faces a spinal disorder, that person may find the aid of organizations who assist with that condition. Clinical RESEARCH provides an option for adaptation, too, by giving individuals active means of participating in their own health and aiding others in finding effective treatments.

Online information from the March of Dimes said, "Identifying disease-causing genes can be a first step toward developing specific treatments, such as new drugs or gene therapy, in which a healthy gene is used to replace one that is missing or faulty." Furthermore, "knowing more about our genetic makeup also should lead to a more individualized approach to preventive medicine." For example, "you may be able to be tested to learn whether you are specially susceptible to certain diseases, so that you can take steps to prevent them."

While genetic factors affect everyone in one way or another, most people have at least some measure of control through their choices. For example, ENVIRONMENTAL INFLUENCES that affect the back or spine may necessitate a move to a place deemed healthier for that person. More often, restorative aids of daily ACTIVITY, EXERCISE, ample fresh water, NUTRITION, and SLEEP can help people overcome a tendency toward a particular condition and better adapt to the unique life they have been given.

Mahanna, Elizabeth. "Genomics Lingo," Office of Genomics & Disease Prevention, Centers for Disease Control and Prevention (CDC), Department of Health and Human Services. Available online. URL: http://www.cdc.gov/genomics/activities/ogdp/2003/2003_lingo.htm. Last updated December 30, 2005.

March of Dimes Birth Defects Foundation. "Genetic Science on the Move," March of Dimes. Available online. URL: http://www.marchofdimes.com/pnhec/4439_4134.asp. Downloaded January 7, 2006.

Office of Genomics & Disease Prevention, Centers for Disease Control and Prevention. "Frequently Asked Questions," CDC, Department of Health and Human Services. Available online. URL: http://www.cdc.gov/genomics/faq.htm. Last updated December 30, 2005.

———. "General Public: Family History," CDC. Available online. URL: http://www.cdc.gov/genomics/fHix.htm. Last updated December 30, 2005.

geriatrics   See ELDERLY, SPINAL CONCERNS OF THE.

gigantism   See GROWTH HORMONE DISORDERS.

glucosamine   Found naturally in the body, glucosamine is a type of amino sugar thought to aid formation of healthy cartilage. Another naturally occurring substance, chondroitin sulfate is part of a protein believed to help cartilage elasticity. Together or separately, synthetic versions of these substances may be used to treat OSTEOARTHRITIS (OA).

As a Spine-health article explained, "Perhaps the most important aspect of glucosamine and chondroitin sulfate supplements is that they are thought to help slow or prevent the degeneration of joint cartilage, the underlying cause of osteoarthritis pain. Glucosamine and chondroitin sulfate dietary supplements may also help alleviate existing joint pain."

Dosage and Potential Side Effects

In an article for the *Cleveland Clinic Journal of Medicine,* Dr. Michele Hooper wrote, "Although no study has addressed the correct dose of glucosamine or the actual time to onset of pain relief, the human clinic trials seem to suggest that a 12-week course of treatment is required at a dosage of 500 mg three times a day." People who are allergic to shellfish may not be able to take glucosamine since it is derived from crustaceans, but for most people, "glucosamine is less toxic than nonsteroidal anti-inflammatory drugs."

Glucosamine can be extracted from a number of sources, such as crab, lobster, or shrimp, so people may react to a product by one manufacturer and not another. According to the Arthritis Foundation, "In most cases, however, allergies are caused by proteins in shellfish, not chitin, a carbohydrate from which glucosamine is extracted. . . . Because glucosamine is an amino sugar, people with diabetes should check their blood sugar levels more frequently when taking this supplement."

Adding chondroitin may add other concerns. For example, "if you are taking chondroitin sulfate in addition to a blood-thinning medication or daily aspirin therapy, have your blood clotting time checked more often. This supplement is similar in structure to the blood-thinning drug heparin, and the combination may cause bleeding in some people." Otherwise, the Arthritis Foundation said, "The most common side effects are increased intestinal gas and softened stools. If you experience these problems, you might want to try another supplement brand before you stop using them altogether." However, "if you don't experience any difference in your symptoms within a few months, you probably will not get any relief from using the supplements."

Patients who cannot tolerate glucosamine sulfate might try supplementing with glucosamine hydrochloride. As a Spine-health article reported, "Glucosamine hydrochloride, another form of glu-

cosamine, is considered to be equally effective as the sulfate form. . . . It is absorbed more easily by the body and can be taken in lower dosages with the same effectiveness as glucosamine sulfate."

Statistics and Studies

With new studies underway, the Arthritis Foundation said, "Past studies show that some people with mild to moderate osteoarthritis (OA) taking either glucosamine or chondroitin sulfate reported pain relief at a level similar to that of nonsteroidal anti-inflammatory drugs (NSAIDs) such as aspirin and ibuprofen. Some research indicates that the supplements might also slow cartilage damage in people with OA."

Arthritis Foundation. "Glucosamine and Chondroitin Sulfate." Available online. URL: http://www.arthritis.org/conditions/alttherapies/Glucosamine.asp. Downloaded January 7, 2006.

Hooper, Michele, M.D. "Is Glucosamine an Effective Treatment for Osteoarthritic Pain?" *Cleveland Clinic Journal of Medicine* 68, no. 6 (June 2001): 494–495.

Hyde, Thomas E. "Effectiveness of Glucosamine and Chondroitin Sulfate for Osteoarthritis," Spine-health.com. Available online. URL: http://www.spine-health.com/topics/conserv/gluco/gluco01.html. Posted April 19, 2005.

gold salt treatment Gold salt may offer a dash of help, especially when such treatments as NONSTEROIDAL ANTI-INFLAMMATORY DRUG (NSAID) THERAPY or STEROID THERAPY have not eased RHEUMATOID ARTHRITIS. Considered a second-line drug, gold salts can be administered in a capsule or as an injection to reduce inflammation, relieve joint pain, and lower the likelihood of bone or joint damage. Either form, however, may take two to six months to become effective.

Dosage and Potential Side Effects

As a therapy for JUVENILE RHEUMATOID ARTHRITIS (JRA), gold salt treatments often start with weekly injections that taper to bi-weekly then once-a-month. However, an article for BCHealthGuide reported, "Gold salts treatment is often discontinued because the shots are painful, testing is necessary with every treatment, and reactions to the medication are common." If the treatment causes soft tissue to inflame, this side effect may first become apparent in a rash or other inflammation of the skin.

A MedicineNet article cautioned that, "Side effects of gold salts can occur any time during treatment or months after treatment has been discontinued," but the treatment "should be avoided by patients with a history of serious reaction to any gold medication. . . . It should also be avoided in patients with blood, liver or kidney diseases, recent radiation treatment, or uncontrolled diabetes."

According to information from the University of Washington (UW) Web site, "When injected, gold is given as gold sodium thiomalate (brand name: Myochrysine) or as aurothioglucose (brand name: Solganal). Injections must be given by your doctor or nurse. First, you'll be given a small dose, to make sure you do not have a severe reaction to the medicine. Then, you'll gradually be given larger doses until the full dose is reached. The full dose is given every week for four to five months. The dose is then adjusted, depending on how your arthritis improves and whether you have any side effects. When things are going well, the periods between injections will be increased, usually up to four weeks. Since everyone reacts differently to gold, some people will require more frequent injections than other people." In capsule form, "gold is given as auranofin (brand name: Ridaura). It is usually given as two capsules every day. Some doctors prefer to start treatment with a single capsule for the first several weeks. You may be given slightly higher or lower doses from time to time, depending on the side effects and how well your arthritis responds."

Statistics and Studies

To date, studies have not shown the means by which gold salts work for any age group, but for CHILDREN under six, neither safety nor effectiveness has been established. For other ARTHRITIS or RA patients, the UW reported, "Two or three of every 10 people do not benefit from gold," but "arthritis usually improves in about one-half of all people treated early in the course of the disease. Many 'late starters' may also benefit from gold."

Cooke, Kerry V. and Richard P. Terra. "Gold Salts for Juvenile Rheumatoid Arthritis," BCHealthGuide.org, British Columbia Ministry of Health. Available online. URL: http://www.bchealthguide.org/kbase/topic/detail/drug/hw102829/detail.htm. Last updated October 8, 2004.

MedicineNet.com. "Aurothioglucose Center." Available online. URL: http://www.medicinenet.com/aurothioglucose/article.htm. Downloaded January 7, 2006.

UW Medicine, Orthopaedics and Sports Medicine. "Gold Treatment." University of Washington, Seattle. Available online. URL: http://www.orthop.washington.edu/uw/medications/tabID__3376/ItemID__76/Articles/Defau lt.aspx. Last updated December 30, 2004.

graft   See BONE GRAFT.

growth hormone (GH) disorders   During childhood, the pituitary gland produces a growth hormone that stimulates development of the musculoskeletal system. Too much of this good thing causes gigantism in CHILDREN or ADOLESCENTS, and too little GH causes a type of DWARFISM. Unlike the more common form of dwarfism known as achondroplasia, the type related to growth hormones may not be apparent in newborns since the proportions of head, body, and limbs look like those of most INFANTS.

Risks and Complications

Usually, parents must decide whether a child with GH disorder will undergo injections on a weekly basis or continue as a little person at maturity. Similarly, parents of children with gigantism may be the ones who elect treatments that slow growth. Either choice can bring physical and emotional complications felt throughout the family.

If GH production occurs in a normal manner until the teen years then becomes excessive in adult years, a condition known as acromegaly may result. With acromegaly, the increased production of GH becomes apparent as hands, feet, and skin thicken, grow, and eventually, become misshapen. Also, bony overgrowth in the SPINE can press spinal nerves, causing CHRONIC PAIN or numbness in the limbs. Sometimes this adult form of gigantism occurs from GH stimulation due to a tumor, which, often, can be surgically removed. If not, treatments to normalize GH may cause side effects or begin too late to be effective. Untreated, gigantism and acromegaly often result in early death.

A GH deficiency that has been noticed and treated during childhood may cause complications in adults when treatments end. Also, GH affects muscle mass and bone composition throughout life, so an adult could be more prone to develop such conditions as OSTEOPOROSIS or experience adverse affects of WEIGHT. To prevent these complications, follow-up testing will be needed with GH therapy often resumed during the adult years.

Statistics and Studies

In considering a maintenance dose for GH deficiency during the transition from adolescent to adult years, Dr. Madhusmita Misra said, "This is an important question, which has not yet been fully addressed. Based on higher GH concentrations in children and adolescents compared with adults, the replacement dose in children is higher" than for adults. "The optimal dose during the transition from adolescent to adult replacement is likely somewhere in between, given that GH concentrations gradually decrease after puberty to adult levels." Besides the best dosage, timing may be a factor. Discontinuation of therapy for a period of one to three months is advisable prior to re-testing, but "Current data suggest that the duration of discontinuation of GH therapy should not last longer than two years pending further data."

GH levels bear watching in patients with an excess of growth hormones too. To offer some statistics, an eMedicine.com article said, "Gigantism is extremely rare, with approximately 100 reported cases to date. Acromegaly is found more frequently, with an incidence of 3–4 cases per million people per year and a prevalence of 40–70 cases per million population." With acromegaly, the mortality rate may be up to three times higher than a national average. However, normalization of GH levels usually brings an average life expectancy.

Special Aids and Adaptations

An adult who has previously had no excess of GH may encounter overproduction because of a tumor, or a person can acquire GH deficiency. As Dr. Steven Grinspoon explained, "Acquired growth hormone (GH) deficiency results from the destruction of normal pituitary and/or hypothalamic tissue, usually from a tumor or secondary to surgical and/or radiation therapy." Whether a patient has too much growth hormone or too little, an endocrinologist or other specialist can adapt an appropriate course of treatment for that individual, regardless of the age.

Grinspoon, Steven, M.D. "Advances in Recombinant Human Growth Hormone Replacement Therapy in Adults," The Neuroendocrine Clinical Center, Massachusetts General Hospital, Harvard Medical School. Available online. URL: http://pituitary.mgh.harvard.edu/e-f-944.htm. Downloaded January 9, 2006.

Misra, Madhusmita, M.D. "Growth Hormone Treatment: Transitioning Care from Adolescence to Adulthood," The Neuroendocrine Clinical Center, Massachusetts General Hospital, Harvard Medical School. Available online. URL: http://pituitary.mgh.harvard.edu/NCBV11I2.htm#GH. Downloaded January 9, 2006.

Shim, Melanie, M.D. and Pinchas Cohen, M.D. "Gigantism and Acromegaly," eMedicine.com. Available online. URL: http://www.emedicine.com/ped/topic2634.htm. Last updated July 29, 2004.

heart, effects of the spine on the Does the SPINE affect the cardiovascular system? Can SPINAL MANIPULATION ease chest pain or regulate a heartbeat? Can cardio-static on the line of a misaligned spine clear up by adjusting the vertebral joint that connects the neck to the upper BACK? Answers to such questions may stir controversy, yet the heart does not live alone. With the aid of imaging tools, an inside glimpse into the cardiovascular system reveals a complex arrangement of blood, spinal nerves, and soft tissue connecting this vital muscle to a variety of protective ribs and VERTEBRAE. Also, less obvious connections between the heart and spine can be found.

Chapter 10 of *Somatovisceral Aspects of Chiropractic: An Evidence-Based Approach* discussed the relationship between the heart and various pathways involving spinal nerves. For example, the vagus nerve with its cardiac branches extends into and beyond the THORACIC SPINE, which consists of the vertebrae numbered T1–T12. Because of this mid-point connection with the spine, stimulating the vagus nerve will lessen heart muscle contractions and slow the heartbeat, and "very strong stimulation of the vagi can cause cardiac arrest for up to 10 seconds." Furthermore, spinal misalignment or VERTEBRAL SUBLUXATION "may affect the rate, rhythm, and power of heart contraction through . . . pathways originating from T1–T5." In addition, "cervical subluxation at any level could also affect . . . pathways to the heart." For example, if the vertebrae in the CERVICAL SPINE shift or lose alignment, "the heart could be disturbed by upper cervical subluxation, primarily because of the passage of the vagus nerve through the jugular foramen."

Risks and Complications

A simple comparison of spinal misalignment might equate a cardiac problem to a washing machine with an out-of-balance load. That figurative example may or may not hold water, but another metaphorical glimpse comes in considering the hose. For example, a clogging agent, such as the formation of a blood clot at the site of a spinal injection, could produce cardiovascular complications that risk shutting the heart down.

Other cardiac imbalances may occur from something akin to electric impulses, or the lack thereof, affecting the natural pacemaker or sinus rhythm of the heart. An article in the *Canadian Journal of Anesthesia* discussed the risks of a spinal injection inducing a dangerously low heart rate and causing bradycardia then warned, "Given that bradycardia can occur at times after subarachnoid injection, immediate availability of atropine is a wise precaution." Regardless of the procedure that requires anesthesia injected into the spine, "deviations from normal sinus rhythm can be insignificant or have effects that range from discomfort for the awake patient to serious morbidity requiring resuscitative intervention." Therefore, "the importance of an arrhythmia lies in its impact on the patient's cardiovascular status." However, "this may be difficult to separate from the physiological effects of the spinal anesthetic itself or the interventions employed to manage side effects."

Statistics and Studies

After gathering evidence of studies spanning many decades, Masarsky and Cremata summarized the findings. In 1922, for example, "Henry K. Winsor, a medical anatomist at the University of Pennsylvania, reported autopsy results correlating regions of spinal curvature to 20 cases of heart . . . pathology. Spinal curvature was found in the T1–T5 region," of the thoracic spine, "in 18 cases, and at C7," of the cervical spine through, "T1 in 2 cases." In 1939, researcher A. D. Becker reported on manipulative osteopathy in cardiac therapy with particular emphasis on the upper cervical spine and T1 to T6 vertebrae in the thoracic region. Similarly, in 1961, Richard Koch presented a review of 150 cases of heart disease. Reporting highlights from that study, Masarsky and Cremata said, "In 93% of the functional group and 100% of the organic group, . . . evidence of vertebral dysfunction was noted in the T2–T6 region, with findings clustering at T4–6. In summarizing the histories of these patients, Koch found that they all experienced upper thoracic symptoms. Furthermore, the majority of these patients reported that they developed upper thoracic spine symptoms months or years before the onset of their cardiac symptoms." More recently, M. E. Jarmel considered the possible role of spinal joint dysfunction in the genesis of sudden cardiac death in a 1989 issue of the *Journal of Manipulative and Physiological Therapeutics*. Masarsky and Cremata also mentioned a 1995 study by Jarmel and associates that used a monitoring system to record improvements of cardiac arrhythmias after manipulation had corrected vertebral shifts in the cervical or upper thoracic regions of the spine.

Special Aids and Adaptations

To prove and replicate treatments and, thus, aid health in the cardio-spinal connection, medical science requires well-documented evidence. Masarsky and Cremata, who are themselves members of the chiropractic community, mentioned a "treatment package" consisting of spinal manipulation, EXERCISE, and NUTRITION, but they found scanty documentation to report the effectiveness of that package. As they said, "Unfortunately, the levels of chiropractic adjustment were not noted and the dietary and exercise programs were not described." This loss may be lamentable, not only for individuals seeking treatment, but also for those who may not know to treat the spine as a bodyguard intended to protect a healthy heart.

Masarsky, Charles S. and Edward E. Cremata. "Chiropractic Care and the Cardiovascular System," *Chapter 10, Somatoviscral Aspects of Chiropractic: An Evidence-Based Approach*, © 2001, Churchill Livingstone, UK, pages 143–154. Available online. URL: http://www.intl.elsevierhealth.com/e-books/pdf/184.pdf. Downloaded January 10, 2006.

Youngs, Paul J. and Judith Littleford, M.D. "Arrhythmias during Spinal Anesthesia/ L'arythmie pendant la rachianesthésie," *Canadian Journal of Anesthesia* 47, no. 5 (2000): 385–387.

heat therapy   A nice hot bath comes with the connotation of soothing relaxation that helps to lessen pain. Although COLD THERAPY brings down inflammation and swelling, heat works well in loosening stiff joints, muscle spasms, and soreness in PARASPINAL MUSCLES. To obtain this therapeutic value, some wet and dry options include the use of comfortably warm water, electric heating pads, steam baths, hot tubs, heated cloths, and hot packs with air-activated discs that retain their warmth for several hours. For most people, though, that would be too long to roast.

Procedure

Regardless of the heat source, the basic procedure applies warmth wherever something hurts. Exceptions include inflammation, bruising, and bleeding, since heat accelerates swelling and blood flow. Pending the approval of a doctor, some patients may need to warm an area for hours, but usually 15 to 20 minutes every couple of hours will suffice.

Risks and Complications

Patients with problems of vein fragility or high blood pressure should avoid heat therapy since the treatment can increase their symptoms or cause an adverse event. Anyone with nerve damage or a cognitive impairment may risk burning the skin. Also, heat can parch soft tissue, irritate sensitive skin, and aggravate dermatological eruptions.

Outlook and Lifestyle Modifications

In an online article, Dr. Pierre Rouzier said, "Moist heat is more effective than dry heat because it penetrates more deeply, which increases the effect on muscles, joints, and soft tissue. . . . Heat can be used to help loosen tight muscles and joints during a warm-up period before exercise."

In an article for Spine-health, Dr. Vert Mooney discussed the relief heat therapy brings to LOW

BACK PAIN. For instance, "heat therapy dilates the blood vessels of the muscles surrounding the lumbar spine. This process increases the flow of oxygen and nutrients to the muscles, helping to heal the damaged tissue." Also, "heat application facilitates stretching the soft tissues around the spine, including muscles, connective tissue, and adhesions. Consequently, with heat therapy, there will be a decrease in stiffness as well as injury, with an increase in flexibility and overall feeling of comfort. Flexibility is very important for a healthy back."

Mooney, Vert, M.D. "Benefits of Heat Therapy for Lower Back Pain," Spine-health. Available online. URL: http://www.spine-health.com/topics/conserv/heat_therapy/heat_therapy01.html. Downloaded January 10, 2006.

Rouzier, Pierre, M.D., for McKesson Provider Technologies. "Heat Therapy," University of Michigan Health System (UMHS). Available online. URL: http://www.med.umich.edu/1libr/sma/sma_htherapy_sma.htm. Last reviewed July 22, 2002.

herbal therapy With the variety produced by nature, herbal therapy comes in varied forms. Depending on the intended usage, herbs may be mashed into a paste or into a pasta sauce. They can be ground into powder, pressed into a pill, or sprinkled over a baked potato. Leaves can be steeped for hot tea, soaked in cold water, or fermented with sugar and made into wine. With the addition of honey, herbs can be cooked down into a syrup for pancakes or for a rib-wrenching cough. Soaking them in olive or grapeseed oil for a week or so produces an herb-enhanced lubricant to rub into a wound or mix with vinegar and tastefully toss onto a salad. Added to petroleum jelly, herbs produce a salve or ointment. When wetted and liberally applied, an herb poultice can ease a BACKACHE or sore muscles and leave a soggy mess of leaves.

Often, herbal treatments come with fair warning: the FDA may not approve. Since the *F* in FDA stands for foods including herbs, the U.S. Food and Drug Administration (FDA) has issued warnings to manufacturers of herbal products, taking them to task for making unsubstantiated claims. As the November 10, 2005, "FDA News" explained,

"under the federal Food, Drug, and Cosmetic Act (FDCA), a product is considered to be a drug if it claims to diagnose, cure, mitigate, treat or prevent disease or, for products other than foods and dietary supplements, if it claims to affect the structure or function of the body. The Warning Letters further state that FDA considers these products to be 'new drugs' that require FDA approval before marketing." While some patients may resent governmental interference with herb use, others see the FDA stance as standing up for better testing, safety, and standardization of herbal products.

Risks and Complications

Versatile though herbs may be, people with skin sensitivities or food allergies know that natural does not always mean safe. For example, black walnut offers herbal therapy that can either detox the body or poison it. Anyone who reacts strongly to any food allergen risks anaphylactic shock just by tasting an herb with properties similar to the offending food. To avoid this risk, a physician can prescribe medication to keep on hand for an antidote. However, the shelf-life of such medications may not be very long, so sensitive patients should stock OVER-THE-COUNTER antihistamines as well as chewable VITAMIN C to help the body produce its own antihistamine. In a squeeze, sucking a lemon may keep skin from breaking out in hives or lips from swelling. If, however, those lips pucker with lipstick from an herb shop, a rash of events may follow, especially since some natural cosmetics contain that nut-allergy nightmare, black walnut.

Another nightmare can arrive with adverse interactions between an herb and a pharmaceutical drug. As a general guideline, no herb should be taken for the same condition being treated with a prescription or an over-the-counter medication such as an NSAID (NONSTEROIDAL ANTI-INFLAMMATORY DRUG). To treat pain, for example, ASPIRIN should not be used in conjunction with the white willow bark from which it is derived, nor should it be used with any herb, such as garlic, that shares its ability to thin the blood. Natural foods boost any medicinal effects they share with a drug, but herbs and vegetables can also interfere with medications that have the opposite effect. For instance, the VITAMIN K in broccoli and eggplant interrupts the action of drugs meant to slow blood clotting. Such herb-food-drug combinations can cause serious complications, especially for sensitive people, CHILDREN, ELDERLY patients, and anyone who takes medication for an ongoing condition. In addition, some herbs may be combined in a single capsule or tonic, which makes label reading even more important.

An article on the interactions between medicines and herbs posted by Holistic-online.com said that goldenseal may be used to treat ARTHRITIS but warned "the plant's active ingredient will raise blood pressure, complicating treatment for those taking antihypertensive medications, especially beta-blockers. For patients taking medication to control diabetes or kidney disease, this herb can cause dangerous electrolyte imbalance. High amount of consumption can lead to gastrointestinal distress and possible nervous system effects." Furthermore, goldenseal is "not recommended for pregnant or lactating women." Similarly, turmeric "should be avoided by persons with symptoms from gallstones."

Statistics and Studies

Historically, turmeric has been used to lessen joint pain and ease an aversion to the taste of catfish, but recent studies took a closer look at this herb, which has no known side effects and can be found in the spice section of most grocery stores. In an article for *Better Nutrition,* Amber D. Ackerson wrote, "Numerous medical studies indicate that turmeric has significant anti-inflammatory action, primarily due to its active constituent, curcumin. Curcumin has been shown to prevent platelet aggregation (clumping) associated with the development of atherosclerosis. Preliminary studies indicate curcumin may have benefits in preventing numerous cancers and cancer metastasis (spread), and it may be used to enhance the effectiveness of chemotherapy and radiation." While this medicinal herb can be used for culinary purposes, therapeutic amounts beyond a kitchen dash include "standardized extract containing 90–95 percent curcumin: 250–500 mg three times daily," "tincture (1:5 concentration): 3–3.5 mL three times daily," or "fluid extract (1:1 concentration): 0.5–1.5 mL three times daily." In most herbal instances, a tincture or extract will be stronger than a fresh or dried kitchen herb.

An article by Sara Altshul discussed the use of devil's claw, which is an herb not found on a spice rack but frequently found by patients racked with OSTEOARTHRITIS and other sources of LOW BACK PAIN. According to the 2005 article in *Prevention,* "Last fall, researchers from the universities of Toronto, Freiburg (Germany), Sydney, and Maryland published a thorough review and analysis of 12 devil's claw studies that involved a total of 1,105 participants. . . . The researchers concluded that there is good evidence for using devil's claw at certain dosages as a treatment for chronic lower-back pain and osteoarthritis." Specifically, "a daily dose of 60 mg of the devil's claw compound, called harpagoside, relieved back pain as effectively as did a standard dose of rofecoxib (Vioxx)."

With future studies needed for most herbal therapies, the National Center for Complementary and Alternative Medicine (NCCAM) warned, "The active ingredient(s) in many herbs and herbal supplements are not known. There may be dozens, even hundreds, of such compounds in an herbal supplement." Therefore, "scientists are currently working to identify these ingredients and analyze products, using sophisticated technology. Identifying the active ingredients in herbs and understanding how herbs affect the body are important research areas."

Special Aids and Adaptations

Besides the ongoing aid of NCCAM and the FDA in regulating and standardizing herbal therapies, some patients may prefer their own garden plants. A good place to start would be culinary herbs traditionally used to ease pain and inflammation. Home-grown herbs not only provide the freshest source of herb therapy but may aid in reducing the side effects that often come when only part of a plant is used.

An article in the *Western Journal of Medicine* explained, "Practitioners of herbal medicine generally use unpurified plant extracts containing several different constituents. Typically, they claim that these can work together synergistically so that the effect of the whole herb is greater than the sum total of the effects of its components. They also claim that toxicity is reduced when whole herbs are used instead of isolated active ingredients ('buffering')." In other words, unidentified constituents in a natural herb may be inadvertently removed during processing yet be the very ingredients needed to prevent the side effects found in a pharmaceutical version.

While this alleged advantage of fresh herbs bears scientific scrutiny, most people agree that fresh herbs just naturally taste better, smell better, and look better as an aid to NUTRITION. For most gardeners, spine-strengthening benefits also come naturally with the daily ACTIVITY of tending plants intended, in turn, to tend them.

Ackerson, Amber D. "Turmeric (Curcuma longa)," *Better Nutrition* 67, no. 3 (March 2005): 12.

Altshul, Sara. "Low-Back Pain Relief," *Prevention* 57, no. 4 (April 2005): 90.

Holistic-online.com. "Medicine—Herb/Food Interactions." Available online. URL: http://holistic-online.com/Herbal-Med/hol_herb_med_reac.htm. Downloaded January 10, 2006.

National Center for Complementary and Alternative Medicine. "Herbal Supplements: Consider Safety, Too," NCCAM, National Institutes of Health. Available online. URL: http://nccam.nih.gov/health/supplement-safety/. Last modified October 19, 2005.

U.S. Food and Drug Administration. "FDA News, FDA Issues Warning Letters to Marketers of Unapproved 'Alternative Hormone Therapies' Items Promoted for Treatment or Prevention of Cancer, Heart Disease, and Osteoporosis," FDA, Department of Health and Human Services. Available online. URL: http://www.fda.gov/bbs/topics/news/2005/NEW01260.html. Originally issued November 10, 2005.

Vickers, Andrew, Catherine Zollman, and Roberta Lee. "Herbal Medicine," *Western Journal of Medicine* (WJM) 175, no. 2 (August 2001): 125–128.

heredity   See GENETIC FACTORS.

herniated disc   Whether ruptured, prolapsed, slipped, or herniated, a misshapen disc causes ACUTE PAIN. Usually, the discomfort begins when the bulging area of a vertebral disc presses against spinal nerves.

Symptoms and Diagnostic Path

Although sharp, shooting pain characteristically occurs, some people experience tingling or numb-ness as the first sign of a herniated disc. If herniation happens in the CERVICAL SPINE, symptoms often include neck pain that radiates into the arms or causes numbness in the arms and hands. In the THORACIC SPINE, chest pains may be felt, whereas a herniated disc in the LUMBAR SPINE presents the intense pain, weakness, or numbness of SCIATICA. If a patient loses mobility or control of bowel and bladder function, those symptoms may signify CAUDA EQUINA SYNDROME or other medical emergency that, most likely, will require SURGERY.

UCLA Neurosurgery offered an online chart showing various levels of disc herniation and resultant symptoms. For instance, spinal root compression emanating from the C5 neck vertebra may be felt as shoulder weakness. A herniation at C6–C7 produces sensory loss in the middle finger, while a herniated disc between C7 and the first vertebra in the thoracic spine, T-1, causes numbness in the ring and little fingers.

To locate the specific area of herniation, X-RAYS may help, but MAGNETIC RESONANCE IMAGING or a COMPUTED TOMOGRAPHY SCAN provide clearer details. Also, a MYELOGRAM may highlight any spinal nerve involvement.

Besides tests and a medical history, a diagnosis includes a physical examination such as Dr. James C. Farmer described for patients with LOW BACK PAIN: "The physical examination of a patient suspected to have a lumbar disk herniation should include a thorough motor and sensory as well as reflex examination." For example, straightening and raising each leg may help to identify patients with lumbar disk herniations, since "the maximal tension within the sciatic nerve itself occurs between 35° and 70° of elevation of the leg . . . In the higher-level disk herniations involving the L2, L3, and L4 nerve roots, testing is performed using a . . . stretch test or a reverse straight leg raise."

Treatment Options and Outlook

Regardless of the location of a herniated disc, TRACTION may relieve painful pressure caused by disc compression. Usually though, conservative treatment begins with bed rest alternated with EXERCISE or physical therapy a doctor has prescribed. For general pain, NONSTEROIDAL ANTI-INFLAMMATORY DRUG THERAPY helps most patients, about 80 to 90 percent of whom eventually improve without surgery. If a DISCECTOMY or MICRODISCECTOMY is needed, patients often return to normal daily ACTIVITY within a few weeks.

In discussing various types of surgery to treat herniated discs, the American Association of Neurological Surgeons (AANS) listed several options on their Web site. For example, a discectomy involves "surgical removal or partial removal of an intervertebral disc," whereas a LAMINECTOMY means, "surgical removal of most of the bony arch, or lamina of a vertebra." Laminotomy requires "an opening made in a lamina, to relieve pressure on the nerve roots," while spinal fusion is "a procedure in which bone is grafted onto the spine, creating a solid union between two or more vertebrae; and in which instrumentation such as screws and rods may be used to provide additional spinal support." The AANS also said, "Fortunately, the majority of herniated discs do not require surgery. However, a very small percentage of people with herniated, degenerated discs may experience symptomatic or severe and incapacitating low back pain which significantly affects their daily life."

Information from the North American Spine Society reported, "Most patients respond well to discectomy; however, as with any surgery, there are some risks involved. These include bleeding, infection and injury to the nerves or spinal cord. It is also possible that pain will not improve following surgery or that symptoms may return. In about 3–5% of patients, the disc will rupture again and cause symptoms at a later time."

Risk Factors and Preventive Measures

People whose jobs involve LIFTING or other manual tasks that exceed their LOAD TOLERANCE may be particularly at risk for a disc herniation. People with poor POSTURE and those adversely affected by WEIGHT or ERGONOMIC FACTORS encounter more risks too. So do ELDERLY patients prone to a fall and CHILDREN or ADOLESCENTS who disregard BACKPACK SAFETY. For almost everyone though, general dehydration makes vertebral discs less flexible. Therefore, most people do well to drink lots of water. Regular exercise also aids overall flexibility and strength, whereas a good mattress can aid the repairs a body needs during restful SLEEP.

Dawson, Edgar G., M.D. "Herniated Discs," SpineUniverse. Available online. URL: http://www.spineuniverse.com/displayarticle.php/article1431.html. Last updated July 7, 2005.

Farmer, James C., M.D. "Lumbar Disk Herniation," AAOS Clinical Topic, American Academy of Orthopaedic Surgeons. Available online. URL: http://www3.aaos.org/memdir/academic/eletter/2004/topics/Lumbar%20Disk%20Herniations.htm. Downloaded January 10, 2006.

NeurosurgeryToday.org. "Herniated Disc," American Association of Neurological Surgeons (AANS.) Available online. URL: http://www.neurosurgerytoday.org/what/patient_e/herniated.asp. Downloaded January 10, 2006.

North American Spine Society. "Herniated Cervical Disc, Herniated Lumbar Disc," NASS. Available online. URL: http://www.spine.org/fsp/prob_action-degen-hern.cfm. Downloaded January 10, 2006.

Scholten, Amy. "Herniated Disc (Ruptured Disk, Prolapsed Disk, Slipped Disk)," Holy Cross Hospital. Available online. URL: http://healthychoice.epnet.com/GetContent.asp?siteid=holycross&docid=/dci/herniatedisk. Downloaded January 10, 2006.

University of California. "What Is Cervical Disc Disease," UCLA. Available online. URL: http://neurosurgery.ucla.edu/Diagnoses/Spinal/SpinalDis_1.html. Downloaded December 5, 2005.

University of Michigan Health Center. "Herniated Disk," UMHC, McKesson Provider Technologies. Available online. URL: http://www.med.umich.edu/1libr/sma/sma_herndisk_crs.htm. Downloaded January 10, 2006.

homeopathic medicine   Similar to many pharmaceutical drugs and OVER-THE-COUNTER PRODUCTS, homeopathic remedies stem from natural sources that can usually be obtained directly from HERBAL THERAPY or regular NUTRITION. Unlike other therapies, however, homeopathic medicine treats like with like, which means the remedy produces the same symptoms as those of the condition being treated.

The concept originated in the late 18th century when German doctor and chemist Samuel Hahnemann apparently tired of bloodletting and other treatments in common use at the time. After carefully observing and recording the natural responses of the body in an attempt to heal itself, Dr. Hahnemann derived the principle of like curing like. For instance, as a response to chest congestion, a person typically coughs. Therefore, a homeopathic remedy would not suppress a cough but provoke one, thus relieving the congestion. Figuratively speaking, the concept seems like fighting fire with fire.

Dosage and Potential Side Effects

Because of substantial dilutions, most homeopathic remedies are considered safe. As with any new medicine, herb, or food, however, a person should proceed with caution, trying only one ingredient at a time. If a remedy comes as a combination product, a minimal amount should be taken only once on the first day. If the person has no side effects, the amount can be gradually increased each day until reaching the recommended dosage.

For BACKACHE, FIBROMYALGIA, OSTEOARTHRITIS, or RHEUMATOID ARTHRITIS, homeopathic remedies often include arnica, which reportedly relieves CHRONIC PAIN. For OSTEOPOROSIS, a product may contain silica, phosphorus, calcarea carbonica, calcarea fluorica, or other significant names.

An article posted by the National Center for Complementary and Alternative Medicine (NCCAM) discussed another unique aspect of homeopathy. Instead of relying on potency, a homeopathic medicine will be diluted numerous times. As the NCCAM explained, "A concept that became 'potentization,' which holds that systematically diluting a substance, with vigorous shaking at each step of dilution, makes the remedy more, not less, effective by extracting the vital essence of the substance. If dilution continues to a point where the substance's molecules are gone, homeopathy holds that the 'memory' of them—that is, the effects they exerted on the surrounding water molecules—may still be therapeutic." In traditional allopathic medicine, for example, a correlation might be made with some types of inoculation, which, in essence, place the memory of a previous illness into the body in order to prevent that particular ailment.

To describe the dilution process further, information from the National Center for Homeopathy said, "A plant substance, for example, is mixed in alcohol to obtain a tincture. One drop of the tincture is mixed with 99 drops of alcohol (to achieve a ratio of 1:100) and the mixture is strongly shaken.

This shaking process is known as succussion. The final bottle is labeled as '1C.' One drop of this 1C is then mixed with 100 drops of alcohol and the process is repeated to make a 2C. By the time the 3C is reached, the dilution is 1 part in 1 million! Small globules made from sugar are then saturated with the liquid dilution. These globules constitute the homeopathic medicine."

The online article, "Understanding Homeopathic Potency," explained, "Homeopathic potencies are designated by the combination of a number and a letter (for example, 6X or 30C). The number refers to the number of dilutions the tincture has undergone within a series to prepare that remedy. The letter refers to the proportions used in each dilution of the series (the Roman numeral X means 10, and the Roman numeral C means 100), as well as the number of succussions the vial of solution undergoes in each successive stage."

Statistics and Studies

Today, the research begun by Dr. Hahnemann continues, often with mixed reviews. As the NCCAM article reported, "Research studies on homeopathy have been contradictory in their findings. Some analyses have concluded that there is no strong evidence supporting homeopathy as effective for any clinical condition. However, others have found positive effects from homeopathy. The positive effects are not readily explained in scientific terms."

That assessment is not surprising in light of the individualization of the treatment. As the NCCAM described the concept, "treatment should be selected based upon a total picture of an individual and his symptoms, not solely upon symptoms of a disease. Homeopaths evaluate not only a person's physical symptoms but her emotions, mental states, lifestyle, nutrition, and other aspects. In homeopathy, different people with the same symptoms may receive different homeopathic remedies." Although some may view this very old medicinal approach as a hoax, others see the value of different treatments coaxing cures for different folks. For example, patients with sensitivities to medicines may prefer the idea that, with homeopathy, less is usually more.

Homeopathy. "Understanding Homeopathic Potency," VitaminShoppe and HealthNotes Online. Available online.

URL: http://www.homeopathyhome.com/services/rshop/vshoppe/remguide/potency.shtml#HN. Downloaded January 11, 2006.

National Center for Complementary and Alternative Medicine. "Questions and Answers About Homeopathy," NCCAM, National Institutes of Health. Available online. URL: http://nccam.nih.gov/health/homeopathy/. Last modified August 24, 2004.

National Center for Homeopathy. "What Are the Medicines?" Available online. URL: http://www.homeopathic.org/meds.htm. Downloaded January 11, 2006.

hormone replacement therapy (HRT)   This treatment option may combine estrogen with progestin to lessen the risk of a VERTEBRAL COMPRESSION FRACTURE in postmenopausal women and younger women prone to OSTEOPOROSIS or other bone-thinning conditions that affect the BACK and SPINE. However, hormone replacement therapy (HRT) may not present the best choice for every woman.

The American Medical Association (AMA) cautioned readers that "the 2004 Surgeon General's report stated that any decision to use HT must take into consideration its impact on overall health outcomes, including not only its potential to reduce the risk of fractures, but also its potential to increase the risk of other health problems. The FDA has advised that postmenopausal women who use or are considering using estrogen or estrogen with progestin discuss its benefits (e.g., relief from moderate to severe hot flashes . . .) and risks with their physicians. Although HT is effective for the prevention of postmenopausal osteoporosis, it should only be considered for women at significant risk of osteoporosis who cannot take non-estrogen medications." HERBAL THERAPY and HOMEOPATHIC MEDICINE also offer options but without the proven benefits of HRT.

Dosage and Potential Side Effects

Available in pill, patch, or gel forms, hormone therapy often provides daily continuous treatment. However, MedicineNet advised, "Because the risks outweigh the benefits of long-term hormone therapy (HT) for most women, women who are at risk of, or who have been diagnosed with, osteoporosis should talk to their doctors about non-estrogen

medications . . . in preventing and treating osteoporosis." Those choices might include ALENDRONATE (Fosamax), CALCITONIN (Miacalcin) RISEDRONATE (Actonel), raloxifene (Evista), teriparatide (Forteo), and other BISPHOSPHONATES, SELECTIVE ESTROGEN RECEPTOR MODULATORS (SERMS), or ANTIRESORPTIVE DRUGS.

Statistics and Studies

In considering BONE MINERAL DENSITY (BMD), the AMA discussed trials by the Women's Health Initiative (WHI), a prevention study begun in 1991 to address the most common causes of death, disability, and impaired quality of life in postmenopausal women, that "confirmed for the first time the effects of combined continuous hormone therapy on osteoporotic fracture reduction at several sites, including the hip. Hip and vertebral fractures decreased by at least one-third in both of the trials and total fractures decreased by 24%–30%." However, "the clear fracture benefits of postmenopausal hormone therapy (HT) are offset by the adverse effects (e.g., increased risk of stroke, cognitive impairment . . .) encountered in the women taking HT. The WHI trials also found that HT provided no cardioprotective benefit, and increased the risk of breast cancer."

Karin H. Humphries and Sabrina Gill spoke of the importance of individualized choices to consider the personal risks and benefits. In considering the back and spine, the authors said, "HRT has been shown to increase bone mineral density, but data supporting reduction of vertebral and nonvertebral osteoporotic fractures with HRT are inconsistent. Consequently, the U.S. Food and Drug Administration indicates HRT for the prevention, not the treatment, of osteoporosis. Similarly, the Scientific Advisory Council of the Osteoporosis Society of Canada recommends HRT as first-line preventative therapy in postmenopausal women who have low bone density but as second-line treatment in postmenopausal women who have osteoporosis. Alternatively, there are considerable data demonstrating vertebral and nonvertebral fracture reduction with bisphosphonates, and vertebral fracture reduction with selective estrogen-receptor modulators and calcitonin."

While estrogen and other hormonal treatments have been shown to slow bone loss in women, similar studies of testosterone for men seem to be lacking. As quoted in an article for *Geriatrics,* Dr. E. Darracott Vaughan Jr. of Weill Medical College at Cornell University in New York said, "I was surprised at the weakness of the literature. We looked at over 400 articles and there were fewer than 50 with any evidence-based research." As testosterone levels decline with age, so do muscle mass and bone strength. Yet men frequently request this form of hormone replacement therapy, not to strengthen bones but to enhance sexual function. Since 1999, the number of doctors who prescribed testosterone increased 170 percent. Seeing the trend as "patient driven," Dr. Vaughan pointed out that available studies indicate escalation in prostate cancer too, so he suggested that physicians test for present testosterone levels before prescribing more.

American Medical Association. "Antiresorptive Therapy: Hormone Therapy," AMA. Available online. URL: http://www.ama-cmeonline.com/osteo_mgmt/module05/04anti/index.htm. Downloaded January 10, 2006.

Humphries, Karen H. and Sabrina Gill. "Risks and Benefits of Hormone Replacement Therapy: the Evidence Speaks," *Canadian Medical Association Journal* (CMAJ) 168, no. 8 (April 15, 2003): 1,001–1,010.

Mathur, Ruchi, M.D. "Hormone Therapy (Estrogen Therapy, Estrogen/Progestin Therapy)," MedicineNet, Inc. Available online. URL: http://www.medicinenet.com/hormone_therapy/article.htm. Downloaded January 10, 2006.

MedicineNet.com. "Estrogen/Progestins—Oral," First DataBank, Inc. Available online. URL: http://www.medicinenet.com/estrogenprogestins-oral/article.htm. Last reviewed March 2, 2005.

Staff. "Testosterone Prescriptions Jump 170% since 1999, yet Uses Remain Unproven," *Geriatrics* 59, no. 1 (January 2004): 15.

humpback or hunched back   See KYPHOSIS.

hydrotherapy   From therapeutic baths in ancient Greece and Rome to the natural hot springs found in the United States, hydrotherapy usually joins HEAT THERAPY in easing an aching BACK or SPINE.

At home treatments include whirlpool baths or hot tubs, while professional spas offer soothing hot towels wrapped up with MASSAGE THERAPY.

Procedure

Each type of hydrotherapy follows its own method, but basically, hydrotherapy involves relaxing in water. Being in a pool also offers a way to EXERCISE without adding pressure to joints affected by ARTHRITIS, OSTEOARTHRITIS, or DEGENERATIVE DISC DISEASE. To encourage 45-minute to one-hour exercises two to three times a week, the Arthritis Foundation developed the Aquatics Program for exercising in a swimming pool. Simply walking in knee-high water can strengthen muscles and bones too, while swimming improves flexibility and tones PARASPINAL MUSCLES.

Risks and Complications

Holistic-online.com warned, "Saunas should not be taken by persons with acute rheumatoid arthritis, acute infection, active tuberculosis, sexually transmitted diseases, acute mental disorder, inflammation of an inner organ or blood vessels, significant vascular changes in the brain or heart, circulatory problems or acute cancer." Patients with high blood pressure, RHEUMATOID ARTHRITIS, and SPINAL INFECTIONS should avoid heated forms of hydrotherapy. Although CHILDREN and ELDERLY patients often respond well to a sauna, care should be taken to avoid dehydration and damage to sensitive skin. "For overall tension reduction, use a neutral bath (temperature between 92 to 94 degree F) that is close to the skin temperature." While higher temperature may work better for easing stress and encouraging restful SLEEP, temperatures over 105 degrees can induce a fever. As a precaution, Holistic-online advised, "Do not spend more than 15 to 20 minutes at a time in a sauna. Wipe your face frequently with a cold cloth to avoid overheating."

Water therapy does not have to tap into heat, however. In comparing hot and cold therapies, a SpineUniverse article said, "Warmer water induces vasodilation: drawing blood into the target tissues. Increased blood flow delivers needed oxygen and nutrients, and removes cell wastes. The warmth decreases muscle spasm, relaxes tense muscles, relieves pain, and can increase range of motion."

Conversely, "cold-water therapy produces vasoconstriction, which slows circulation reducing inflammation, muscle spasm, and pain."

Outlook and Lifestyle Modifications

To keep from becoming dehydrated from hydrotherapy or other heated treatments, people should drink plenty of water throughout the day. Fresh fruit and raw vegetables also bring moisture and add good NUTRITION too.

Davis, Dana L. and Susan Spinasanta. "Hydrotherapy and Aquatic Therapy," SpineUniverse. Available online. URL: http://www.spineuniverse.com/displayarticle.php/article1489.html. Last updated July 6, 2004.

Holistic-online.com. "Hydrotherapy." Available online. URL: http://www.holistic-online.com/hydrotherapy.htm. Downloaded January 11, 2006.

Tilden, Helen M. "Water Exercise," Arthritis Foundation. Available online. URL: http://www.arthritis.org/conditions/Exercise/water_exercise.asp. Downloaded January 11, 2006.

hyperparathyroidism   See PARATHYROID HORMONE.

hyperpituitarism   See GROWTH HORMONE DISORDERS.

hypoparathyroidism   See PARATHYROID HORMONE.

hypophosphatasia   GENETIC FACTORS cause this metabolic disorder that produces skeletal problems similar to OSTEOGENESIS IMPERFECTA or RICKETS. The age of onset determines whether the person has the infantile, childhood, or adult type of hypophosphatasia, but INFANTS have the most severe symptoms and shortest life span.

Symptoms and Diagnostic Path

A fact sheet from the National Institutes of Health (NIH) reported, "The severity of hypophosphatasia is remarkably variable from patient to patient. The most severely affected fail to form a skeleton in the womb and are stillborn." To diagnose patients of all ages, a routine blood test will show low levels of an enzyme called alkaline phosphatase (ALP) but, as NIH pointed out, "it is important that the doctors use appropriate age ranges for normal ALP levels when interpreting the blood test."

According to the online report "Hypophosphatasia, Infantile" posted by Johns Hopkins University, "three more or less distinct types can be identified: (1) type 1 with onset in utero or in early postnatal life, . . . severe skeletal abnormalities . . . and death in the first year or so of life; (2) type 2 with later, more gradual development of symptoms, moderately severe . . . skeletal changes and premature loss of teeth; (3) type 3 with no symptoms, the condition being determined on routine studies."

For any age group, X-RAYS help to assess the severity of the disease and the presence of skeletal deformity. With severe chest distortion, for example, frequent episodes of pneumonia may occur. Patients may also experience recurrent FRACTURES.

Treatment Options and Outlook

According to the NIH, "severe forms of hypophosphatasia occur in approximately one per 100,000 live births. The more mild childhood and adult forms are probably somewhat more common. About one out of every 300 individuals in the United States is thought to be a carrier for hypophosphatasia." Regarding the overall outlook, the NIH stated, "Cases detected in the womb or with severe deformities at birth almost invariably result in death within days or weeks."

The report "Hypophosphatasia, Adult Type" from Johns Hopkins University said, "The dominant disorder may be one of osteoblasts, whereas the recessive form is a defect of alkaline phosphatase." Differentiating between the two can be crucial since treatments vary. For instance, VITAMIN D therapy may help the form of hypophosphatasia similar to rickets, but that same treatment can cause kidney damage in patients with other types of the disease.

Risk Factors and Preventive Measures

If instances of hypophosphatasia have been diagnosed within a family, potential parents may want to seek genetic counseling. As yet, no established medical treatments have been determined nor preventives found.

McKusick, Victor A., M.D. et al. "Hypophosphatasia, Adult Type," OMIM™, Online Mendelian Inheritance in Man™, Johns Hopkins University. Available online. URL: http://www.ncbi.nlm.nih.gov/entrez/dispomim.cgi?id=146300. Downloaded January 9, 2006.

———. "Hypophosphatasia, Infantile," OMIM™, Online Mendelian Inheritance in Man™, Johns Hopkins University. Available online. URL: http://www.ncbi.nlm.nih.gov/entrez/dispomim.cgi?id=241500. Downloaded January 9, 2006.

Whyte, Michael, M.D. "Hypophosphatasia," The National Institutes of Health (NIH) Osteoporosis and Related Bone Diseases, National Resource Center. Available online. URL: http://www.osteo.org/newfile.asp?doc=i102i&doctitle=Hypophosphatasia&doctype=HTML+Fact+Sheet. Downloaded January 9, 2006.

ibandronate This treatment for OSTEOPOROSIS became the third BISPHOSPHONATE approved by the U.S. Food and Drug Administration. Then advertising fame quickly came with the brand Boniva, approved as the first bisphosphonate tablet for once-a-month use.

Dosage and Potential Side Effects

Other bisphosphonates, such as ALENDRONATE, can be injected every three months or even annually, but ibandronate can be taken monthly by mouth in a dosage of 150 mg. For daily dosage, ibandronate is also available in tablets of 2.5 mg. Either way, the tablet must be taken with a full glass of water at least one hour before ingesting any other beverage or food.

As Dr. Jay W. Marks explained in an article for MedicineNet, "Absorption of ibandronate from the intestine is poor, and any potential further decrease in absorption by food or medications needs to be avoided." Equally important, "ibandronate tablets also should be swallowed whole with six to eight ounces of plain water while in an upright position, in order to be certain that the tablets enter the stomach." If the medication sticks along the way, severe irritation of the mouth, throat, or esophagus will almost inevitably occur. Therefore, neither ibandronate nor any other bisphosphonate should be given to patients who can not remain upright for an hour or who can not delay eating.

Other than side effects that result from not following instructions, ibandronate is considered safe for anyone who does not have a blood calcium problem. Pregnant women should discuss other options with their doctor since the effects on an unborn child have not been adequately studied. Although patients in general may experience back pain or stomach upset, allergic reactions rarely occur. If, however, a patient erupts in hives or has difficulty breathing, emergency medical attention should be sought immediately.

Statistics and Studies

Highlights from the 2005 National Osteoporosis Foundation meeting addressed interim findings of the two-year MOBILE (Monthly Oral Ibandronate in Ladies) study. With the participation of nearly 1,600 postmenopausal women, the trial studied the effects of four different dosages of ibandronate: 2.5 mg daily, 50 mg on two consecutive days (50/50), once-a-month doses of 100 mg, and once-a-month doses of 150 mg. According to the summary reported in *Contemporary OB/GYN,* "all of the monthly regimens were at least as effective as daily administration, but the 150-mg dosage produced the best response." Specifically, "lumbar spine bone mineral density (BMD) increased 4.9% in that group, compared to 4.3%, 4.1%, and 3.9% in the 50/50, 100-mg, and daily groups, respectively." Those who received the highest dose of ibandronate had the most flu-like symptoms, yet none of the women experienced gastrointestinal problems, including those who previously had that medical history.

Drug.com™. "Boniva," Drug Information Online. Available online. URL: http://www.drugs.com/boniva.html. Last revised March 30, 2005.

Marks, Jay W., M.D. "Ibandronate," MedicineNet. Available online. URL: http://www.medicinenet.com/ibandronate/article.htm.

National Osteoporosis Foundation: Meeting Highlights. "Monthly Ibandronate Effective for Osteoporosis," *Contemporary OB/GYN* 50, no. 6 (June 2005): 17.

ibuprofen Like other NONSTEROIDAL ANTI-INFLAMMATORY (NSAID) DRUGS, ibuprofen relieves pain and inflammation. Patients with painful inflammatory conditions of the BACK and SPINE, such as OSTEOARTHRITIS or RHEUMATOID ARTHRITIS, may find ibuprofen especially helpful in easing symptoms and slowing the deterioration that often comes with CHRONIC PAIN and swelling. Ibuprofen also dulls ACUTE PAIN, loosens PARASPINAL MUSCLES, eases BACKACHE, and reduces the joint pain of ARTHRITIS.

Dosage and Potential Side Effects

Available in various strengths, ibuprofen comes in a variety of generic forms and brand names, such as Motrin, Nuprin, and Advil. Whether in a tablet or a liquid, this popular NSAID is often combined with other ingredients in products used to ease fevers, coughs, or muscle cramps. However, ibuprofen should not be combined with diuretics or blood-thinners, nor should it be taken with HERBAL THERAPY containing feverfew, ginger, garlic, or ginkgo biloba. By itself, side effects may include mild stomach upset, headache, or drowsiness. Anything more should be reported to a doctor.

Statistics and Studies

If preferred, patients who take a daily maintenance dose of 81 mg ASPIRIN can use ibuprofen later that day for pain. As a MayoClinic.com article reported, "Studies indicate that aspirin is still effective if taken two hours before a single daily dose of ibuprofen. But taking multiple doses of ibuprofen daily or taking ibuprofen before aspirin can impair the protective effect of aspirin." Also, "a recent study showed that occasional use of ibuprofen—less than 60 days a year—doesn't seem to impair aspirin's ability to reduce the risk of heart attack."

Some people prefer one over the other, but both ibuprofen and aspirin have anti-clotting effects similar to a blood thinner. Because of this, doctors often recommend that patients refrain from using an NSAID up to a week before scheduled SURGERY. To find out if that were necessary though, a group of doctors tested 11 healthy adults not in need of surgery. For one week, volunteers took 600 mg of ibuprofen, orally, every eight hours. At the end of that time, researchers tested blood platelet formation in each participant at intervals of 40 minutes, eight hours, and 24 hours. Less than one hour after the last dose of ibuprofen,

seven of the 11 showed abnormal platelet function. In 24 hours, none did, as their blood had returned to normal clotting time. Whether such results will be replicated with aspirin or other NSAIDs has yet to be studied.

DrugDigest.com. "Ibuprofen." Available online. URL: http://www.drugdigest.org/DD/DVH/Uses/0,3915,335%7CIbuprofen,00.html. Last updated May 18, 2005.

Goldenberg, N. A., L. Jacobson, and M. J. Manco-Johnson. "Brief Communication: Duration of Platelet Dysfunction after a 7-Day Course of Ibuprofen," *Annals of Internal Medicine* 142, no. 7 (April 5, 2005): 506–509. http://www.annals.org/cgi/content/full/142/7/I-54.

MayoClinic.com. "Ibuprofen: Does It Counteract the Benefits of Aspirin?" Mayo Foundation for Medical Education and Research. Available online: http://www.mayoclinic.com/health/ibuprofen/AN00803. Last updated October 7, 2005.

MedlinePlus. "Ibuprofen," U.S. National Library of Medicines and the National Institutes of Health. Available online. URL: http://www.nlm.nih.gov/medlineplus/druginfo/medmaster/a682159.html. Last updated January 10, 2006.

idiopathic juvenile osteoporosis See JUVENILE OSTEOPOROSIS.

idiopathic scoliosis Lack of a clear cause defines this type of SCOLIOSIS that presents side-to-side curvature of the SPINE and affects POSTURE in INFANTS, CHILDREN, or ADOLESCENTS. Babies diagnosed before age three are classified as having early onset or infantile idiopathic scoliosis, while juvenile idiopathic scoliosis may first be detected in children three to 10. Adolescent idiopathic scoliosis occurs after the 10th birthday but prior to adulthood.

Symptoms and Diagnostic Path

Spinal curvatures in babies or young children can usually be seen with the eye, particularly during bath time or when readying a child for bed. With fast-growing adolescents though, parents may not notice a worsening curvature in the BACK unless a misshapen shirt provides a clue. Since teenagers often avoid the medical checkups they once had regularly as children, a school nurse may be the first to spot a problem.

In an article for Spine-health, Dr. Peter F. Ullrich described a typical examination: "Most students are given the Adam's forward bend test routinely in school to determine whether or not they may have scoliosis. The test involves the student bending forward with arms stretched downward toward the floor and knees straight, while being observed by a healthcare professional. This angle most clearly shows any asymmetry in the spine and/or trunk of the adolescent's body."

Should abnormal spinal development be suspected, a pediatrician or other physician will exam the child and order X-RAYS to assess the degree of curvature. An MRI (MAGNETIC RESONANCE IMAGING) will not usually be needed unless the child has other symptoms, such as pain, that might suggest spinal nerve involvement or an underlying medical condition.

According to Dr. Ullrich, "curves that are less than 10 degrees are not considered to even represent scoliosis but rather spinal asymmetry. These types of curves are extremely unlikely to progress and generally do not need any treatment." If the curve ranges between 20 and 30 degrees, follow-up examinations will be needed about every four months during periods of growth. As Dr. Ullrich recommended, "If the curve progresses more than 5 degrees, then the curve will need treatment." However, "the only curves that tend to continue to progress after skeletal maturity are those that are greater than 50 degrees in angulation, so the treatment objective is to try to get the child into adulthood with less than a 50 degree curvature."

Treatment Options and Outlook

To arrest the development of spinal curvature, a back brace can be molded to fit a growing child. This type of brace can be taken off as needed but is usually worn throughout the day. Unfortunately, other children may notice and comment on the ORTHOTIC, which can be socially and emotionally upsetting to young patients. In some instances, this problem can be resolved with the use of a bending back brace that works against the curve while the child sleeps at night. However, neither type of orthotic device works well for a mature spine.

Although idiopathic scoliosis has no commonly accepted cause, this is not true for all types of scoliosis. An article in GP explained, "In non-structural curves, the spine is structurally normal but is curved due to an underlying condition such as differing leg length, muscle spasms or even appendicitis." Regarding treatment, "non-structural scoliosis resolves if the underlying cause is dealt with." For example, "a non-structural (postural) scoliosis reduces on forward bending. It is usually a mild lumbar curve compensating for a short leg. It is not progressive and should correct with a heel raise."

Patients with excessive spinal curvatures may require spinal fusion to redirect the curve and avoid a poor outlook during adult years. For example, a severe 90-degree curve can compromise the function of the heart or lungs. However, in lieu of SURGERY, another treatment option may be forthcoming. In 2004, a Pediatric Health News Release announced, "Scientists at Cincinnati Children's Hospital Medical Center have developed a 'spine staple' that could eliminate the need for thousands of invasive spine surgeries in children each year. . . . The spine staple would be implanted in a minimally invasive procedure in children who are at high risk of needing surgery in adolescence. The staple would slow progression of the curvature or actually decrease the curvature as the child grows."

Risk Factors and Preventive Measures

Growing children between the ages of 10 and 18 account for about 80 percent of the cases of idiopathic scoliosis diagnosed in this country and, therefore, encounter the greatest risks of developing this condition. Nevertheless, a 2005 report from the U.S. Preventive Services Task Force (USPSTF) stated, "The USPSTF did not find good evidence that screening asymptomatic adolescents detects idiopathic scoliosis at an earlier stage than detection without screening." With "variable" results cited from the forward bending test typically used in schools, "the USPSTF found fair evidence that treatment of idiopathic scoliosis during adolescence leads to health benefits (decreased pain and disability) in only a small proportion of persons. Most cases detected through screening will not progress to a clinically significant form of scoliosis. . . . Scoliosis needing aggressive treatment, such as surgery, is likely to be detected without screening."

Other governmental agencies, such as the U.S. Department of Health and Human Services or the U.S. Public Health Service, have the option of following the USPSTF recommendation or not. In any case, parents who keep a watchful eye on a growing child of any age will be most likely to obtain the most timely treatment.

Calonge, Ned, M.D., Chair, U.S. Preventative Services Task Force. "Screening for Idiopathic Scoliosis in Adolescents: Recommendation Statement," *American Family Physician* 71, no. 10 (May 15, 2005): 1,975–1,976.

Cincinnati Hospital Children's Medical Center. "August 10, 2004—Cincinnati Children's Scientists Develop New Spine Staples," 2004 Pediatric Health News Release. Available online. URL: http://www.cincinnatichildrens.org/about/news/release/2004/8-spine-staples.htm. Downloaded December 29, 2005.

McAfee, Paul C., M.D. "Bracing Treatment for Idiopathic Scoliosis," Spine-health.com. Available online. URL: http://www.spine-health.com/topics/conserv/brace/feature/bracescolio.html. Downloaded December 29, 2005.

National Institute of Arthritis and Musculoskeletal and Skin Diseases. "Questions and Answers about Scoliosis in Children and Adolescents," NIAMS, National Institutes of Health (NIH), Department of Health and Human Services. Available online. URL: http://www.niams.nih.gov/hi/topics/scoliosis/scochild.htm. Downloaded December 29, 2005.

Staff. "GP Clinical: The Basics—Recognising and Identifying a Scoliosis," *GP* (October 28, 2005): 56.

Ullrich, Peter F., M.D. "Understanding Idiopathic Scoliosis," Spine-health.com. Available online. URL: http://www.spine-health.com/topics/cd/scoliosis/scoliosis01.html. Last updated March 30, 2004.

image-guided surgery This computer-assisted SURGERY provides clear imagery and guides a surgeon in reconstructing VERTEBRAE or stabilizing the SPINE.

Procedure

Prior to image-guided surgery, a COMPUTED TOMOGRAPHY (CT) SCAN or MAGNETIC RESONANCE IMAGING (MRI) provide preliminary information. Those tests also reduce the need for X-RAYS during the actual procedure, thereby eliminating additional exposure to radiation.

In describing image-guided surgery in an article for SpineUniverse, Dr. Mark R. McLaughlin wrote, "An optical camera is stationed in the operating room to receive signals from special digitized instruments equipped with light emitting diodes (LEDs). During surgery the camera receives and sends the signals to a high-speed computer. The signals are received from both the instrument (its position) and the patient (anatomy)." Using a geometric form of triangulation, the optical camera establishes "the distance between two points (instrument position and patient anatomy). The computer integrates the 'triangulated signals' onto the patient's CAT or MRI scan images. An image is then generated projecting the instrument's exact location in relation to the patient's anatomy. The surgeon views the image on a nearby screen (e.g. computer monitor) to see the exact location of his instrument."

Risks and Complications

Precise imaging may be difficult to obtain in patients with spinal abnormalities, such as those caused by SCOLIOSIS. Too much movement can complicate the visuals too. If needed, FLUOROSCOPY can be added to the procedure.

Outlook and Lifestyle Modifications

Based on the Global Positioning System the military uses to track vehicles by satellite, an image-guided procedure offers a high-tech form of MINIMALLY INVASIVE SURGERY. An article posted by the University of Maryland Medical Center explained, "Because the image-guided technology is so precise and accurate, surgeons can decide how best to get to a targeted area and avoid healthy tissue before an incision is ever made. . . . All of this precision shortens operating times and allows for smaller incisions, which translates into speedier recoveries and better results for patients. It also means that patients with conditions considered 'inoperable' in the past now have an option."

McLaughlin, Mark R., M.D. "Image-Guided Spinal Surgery," SpineUniverse. Available online. URL: http://

www.spineuniverse.com/displayarticle.php/article774.
html. Last updated October 22, 2005.

University of Maryland Medical Center. "Image-Guided
Surgery," UMMC. Available online. URL: http://www.
umm.edu/neurosciences/image_guided.html. Downloaded January 12, 2006.

indocid   See NONSTEROIDAL ANTI-INFLAMMATORY
DRUG THERAPY.

indomethacin   See NONSTEROIDAL ANTI-INFLAMMA-
TORY DRUG THERAPY.

infantile scoliosis   See IDIOPATHIC SCOLIOSIS.

infant massage therapy   Unlike vigorous types of
MASSAGE THERAPY for adults, infant massage treats
PARASPINAL MUSCLES with light pressure and loving
care. Not only does this form of tender touch provide comfort and relaxation, the baby also receives
healthy stimulation.

Assuming that no fever or infection exists, infant
massage can aid the tiniest newborn, but this was
not always allowed. As an article by Christopher
Vaughan reported, "In the early 1960s, doctors
treating premature babies feared infection above
all else. So they isolated the infants completely in
sterile boxes; no one could touch them directly. . . .
In the late '60s, psychiatrist Herbert Liederman
became concerned about the effect of isolation
on the parent-child relationship. When parents
finally brought their babies home after weeks of
fretting, they often felt alienated and unsure how
to care for them." Therefore, clinical settings, such
as Stanford's Lucile Packard Children's Hospital,
encouraged parents to wash their hands and handle their babies. "This research sparked the term
'bonding' and the idea that physical contact is an
important part of the parent-infant relationship."
In subsequent studies, "researchers at other universities later established that holding and caress-
ing premature infants also helps them develop
physically and emotionally."

Procedure

To develop a procedure for preterm infants, the
Touch Research Institute at the University of Miami
School of Medicine began conducting studies in the
mid 1980s. As Tiffany Field reported, "The massage
sessions were comprised of 3 five-minute phases.
During the first and third phases, tactile stimulation
was given. The newborn was placed in a prone position and given moderate pressure stroking of the
head and face region, neck and shoulders, back, legs
and arms for five one-minute segments." Studies
eventually showed "The massaged infants gained
47 percent more weight, even though the groups
did not differ in calorie intake; The massaged infants
were awake and active a greater percentage of the
observation time (much to our surprise, since we had
expected that the massage would stimulate a sopo-
rific state and greater sleep time, leading to weight
gain via lesser energy expenditure and calories);
The massaged infants showed better performance
on the Brazelton Scale on habituation, orientation,
motor activity and regulation of state behavior; The
massaged infants were hospitalized, on average, six
fewer days than the control infants."

Once home, parents might begin by lightly coat-
ing their hands with a natural, perfume-free oil to
avoid chafing the baby's sensitive skin. The massage then involves gentle strokes with light pressure, but not too light or the infant will perceive
this as unpleasant tickling. In general, the caretaker should remain aware of each response the
baby gives. If an infant becomes cranky, startled, or
tense, the massage should cease immediately but be
tried another time.

Risks and Complications

Rough treatment and careless handling present the most obvious risks. Whether perceived as
pleasant or unpleasant, most babies quickly react
to stimuli, but an abused infant loses that natural
ability and withdraws into fear. To overcome an
acquired revulsion to touch, massage sessions can
initially be confined to a minute or less then gradually increased over a few weeks, depending on the
readiness of the child.

Outlook and Lifestyle Modifications

For all babies, a good massage should provide a
safe time that aids mental, physical, and emotional

development, not only for the infant, but also for the parent. As information from the International Loving Touch Foundation Web site explained, infant massage "helps the parent to feel more confident and competent in caring for their children." For example, massaging a baby "helps parents understand their infants' cues and states of awareness" and also "promotes bonding and attachment." If an infant has been ill, massage can help parents to "feel a greater part of the healing process." If the mother herself has been ill or depressed, infant massage will be likely to aid her healing too.

Field, Tiffany. "Infant Massage," Touch Research Institute, University of Miami School of Medicine, edited from the *Zero to Three Journal,* October/November 1993. Available online. URL: http://www.zerotothree.org/massage.html. Downloaded January 13, 2006.

International Loving Touch Foundation. "Benefits for Parents and Primary Caregivers." Available online. URL: http://www.lovingtouch.com/2/mfi-benefitsp.php. Downloaded January 13, 2006.

Vaughan, Christopher. "Holding On," *Stanford Magazine.* Available online. URL: http://www.stanfordalumni.org/news/magazine/2002/sepoct/features/neonatal.html. Downloaded January 13, 2006.

infants, spinal concerns for   Concern for the SPINE of an infant begins before the arrival of a baby but also before the arrival of a fetus. As explained by MayoClinic.com, "the fourth week marks the beginning of the embryonic period, when the baby's brain, spinal cord, heart and other organs begin to form. Your baby is now $^1/_{25}$ of an inch long." During that embryonic state, "the embryo is now made of three layers. The top layer—the ectoderm—will give rise to a groove along the midline of your baby's body. This will become the neural tube, where your baby's brain, spinal cord, spinal nerves and backbone will develop." By the seventh week of pregnancy, the baby "weighs less than an aspirin tablet." With the umbilical cord now taking shape, "the cavities and passages needed to circulate spinal fluid in your baby's brain have formed, but your baby's skull is still transparent." By week nine, "the embryonic tail at the bottom of your baby's spinal cord is shrinking, helping him or her look less like a tadpole and more like a developing person." As neurons multiply in week 10, "the bones of your baby's skeleton begin to form." In week 13, ribs may take shape, and by week 15, bone marrow develops. About a month later, the mother may feel the child begin to move. Shortly thereafter, bone marrow awakens to its job of making blood cells. At week 29, fully developed bones begin to store minerals, such as IRON and CALCIUM, yet bones remain pliable to ease into the world sometime around week 40.

Risks and Complications

At any time prior to birth, alcohol consumption, inadequate NUTRITION, smoke, or other ENVIRONMENTAL INFLUENCES can disrupt skeletal development. GENETIC FACTORS also contribute to BIRTH DEFECTS OF THE SPINE, whereas accidents and womb-crowding complicate the formation of healthy VERTEBRAE. After prenatal development has ceased, the minimal risk of a BIRTH INJURY TO THE SPINE arises during the actual delivery. Afterward, spinal damage most often comes during transportation, for example, if someone drops a baby or a vehicular accident occurs.

In addressing car safety, the American Academy of Orthopaedic Surgeons (AAOS) said, "Most car crashes happen within 25 miles of home. That's why it is important to put your child in a safety seat every time you drive. Adults often think that holding a child on their lap is as safe as using a safety seat. It is not. Experts refer to the 'on-lap' position as the 'child-crusher' position. In a crash at 30 miles per hour, a 10 pound child could be thrown from the adult's lap into the dashboard or windshield with a force of 200 pounds."

Only a certified, age-appropriate seat should be purchased for a child, but if the parent does not find it manageable, even the priciest equipment does no good. As an article posted by SafetyBeltSafe USA said, "The 'best' seat is the one that fits your child, fits your car, and fits your family's needs in terms of comfort and convenience, so that you'll use it on every single ride." Also, "babies should ride rear facing as long as possible to protect the spine. They must ride rear facing until they are at least one year old to prevent possible death or lifelong disability. Babies have heavy heads and weak necks with soft bones and stretchy ligaments. In a frontal collision, which is the type most likely to cause death or severe injury, a forward-facing baby's neck may stretch up to two inches, but the spinal cord ruptures if it stretches more than one-fourth of an inch."

Statistics and Studies

Car safety affects spinal health throughout a person's life, but in the earliest moments, deformities of the BACK or spine cause more fatalities. Among black families, National Vital Statistics listed premature birth or low birth weight as the primary cause of infant death with the second cause being "congenital malformations, deformations and chromosomal abnormalities." Among Native American, Caucasian, Hispanic, and Asian families, spinal abnormalities presented the first cause of infant death.

Special Aids and Adaptations

Prospective parents concerned about a family history of severe spinal problems might seek the aid of a pediatrician or other physician who specializes in orthopedic concerns. Regarding safety in transportation, the AAOS reported, "Research on child safety seats has found that they can reduce fatal injuries by 71 percent for infants who are less than 1 year old." Also, anyone who carries a child should be physically and mentally able to hold that valuable cargo with care. As one hand cradles a diapered bottom, the other lightly supports the CERVICAL SPINE and upper THORACIC SPINE until the infant develops enough neck strength to hold the head upright. During the crawling and toddling stages, stair gates and other protective aids provide limits yet encourage young children to explore the safe surroundings personally adapted to and for them.

American Academy of Orthopaedic Surgeons. "Car Seat Safety," AAOS. Available online. URL: http://orthoinfo.aaos.org/fact/thr_report.cfm?thread_id=61&topcategory=Injury%20Prevention. Downloaded January 12, 2006.

MayoClinic.com. "Fetal Development," Mayo Foundation for Medical Education and Research. Available online. URL: http://www.mayoclinic.com/health/prenatal-care/PR00112. Last updated October 7, 2005.

National Vital Statistics. "Table 7. Infant Deaths and Mortality Rates for the Five Leading Causes of Infant Death by Race and Hispanic Origin of Mother: United States," National Vital Statistics Report 50, no. 12 (August 28, 2002): 21.

SafetyBeltSafe USA. "Which Safety Seat Is 'the Best' for My Child?" Available online. URL: http://www.carseat.org/Resources/624_bestseat.pdf. Downloaded January 12, 2006.

infection of the spine   See SPINAL INFECTION.

injection   See SPINAL INJECTION.

injury   See SPINAL INJURY.

intradiscal electrothermal therapy (IDET)   If the nonsurgical methods of PAIN MANAGEMENT fail, intradiscal electrothermal therapy (IDET) may offer a pain-relieving option. IDET can be used to treat patients with SCIATICA, less severe cases of DEGENERATIVE DISC DISEASE, and other disc-related conditions that affect the BACK and SPINE.

Procedure

In an article for SpineUniverse, Dr. Steven Richeimer wrote, "This procedure involves the insertion of a needle into the affected disc with the guidance of an x-ray machine. A wire is then threaded down through the needle and into the disc until it lies along the inner wall of the annulus," which is the ring-like portion of the intervertebral disc body. "The wire is then heated which destroys the small nerve fibers that have grown into the cracks and have invaded the degenerating disc. The heat also partially melts the annulus, which triggers the body to generate new reinforcing proteins in the fibers of the annulus."

Risks and Complications

IDET takes only about an hour, but discomfort may actually increase for the first few days after the procedure. As happens with any type of SURGERY, IDET offers no guarantee of pain relief, but pain lessens for most patients within a few weeks. Some, however, may encounter additional DISC problems in the future.

According to the American Academy of Orthopaedic Surgeons (AAOS), IDET is not recommended for patients with SPINAL STENOSIS, spinal instability, or spinal nerve compression. Long-term results remain unknown. Therefore, the AAOS cautioned, "Because this is a relatively new procedure, you should make sure that the practitioner you see is adequately trained in using the equipment."

Outlook and Lifestyle Modifications
Online information from The Virginia Spine Institute said, "During the disc healing process, from 8 to 16 weeks following the procedure, it is very important to treat your discs with care. Your physician may prescribe temporary lumbar support as well as activity and physical rehabilitation guidelines." However, "in a small study of 700 patients, nearly 80% enjoyed reduced pain and greater mobility. Half of those patients taking narcotic pain-killers ended up drug-free."

Sensible care during recovery may include lifestyle changes to aid disc health. Also, ample drinking water, well-balanced NUTRITION, and doctor-approved EXERCISE will improve the long-term outlook for almost any disc.

American Academy of Orthopaedic Surgeons. "IDET (Intradiscal Electrothermal Annuloplasty)," AAOS. Available online. URL: http://orthoinfo.aaos.org/fact/thr_report.cfm?Thread_ID=339&topcategory=Spine. Downloaded January 12, 2006.

Richeimer, Steven, M.D. "New Technologies for Treating Sciatica and Back Pain," SpineUniverse. Available online. URL: http://www.spineuniverse.com/displayarticle.php/article1485.html. Last updated November 8, 2005.

Virginia Spine Institute, The. "IntraDiscal ElectroThermal Therapy." Available online. URL: http://www.spinemd.com/idet.htm. Downloaded January 12, 2006.

intrathecal spinal pump If nonsurgical methods of PAIN MANAGEMENT no longer help, INTRADISCAL ELECTROTHERMAL THERAPY (IDET) offers a pain-

relieving option. If various types of SURGERY fail to ease CHRONIC PAIN, an intrathecal spinal pump can deliver pain relief directly to the site.

Procedure
To explain the reasoning behind this procedure, Dr. Steven Richeimer wrote, "Medicines taken orally get diffused throughout the entire body which means that a great deal of medication must be ingested in order to get the appropriate quantities to the place it is needed most to ease pain: the spinal cord." However, "by surgically implanting a pump under the skin of a person's abdomen, and running a catheter to the precise location in the spine where the pain is, we can pump medication directly into the spinal fluid, allowing for a much more potent effect on the spinal cord. This drastically cuts down the dose of medication that is needed, and the medication often provides even better pain relief with much fewer side effects."

Risks and Complications
The use of a spinal pump carries a minimal risk of infection. Also, strong narcotics, such as morphine, will be used, which can be costly as well as potentially addictive.

Outlook and Lifestyle Modifications
As Dr. Ralph F. Rashbaum explained in a Spine-health article, "medication in the pump is added periodically (e.g. monthly) by injecting medication through the skin into the pump reservoir." Presumably, this means regular follow-ups with a physician.

To find out whether an intrathecal spinal pump will work well, a trial phase allows the patient to try the treatment on a short-term basis. If needed though, the actual implant can also be removed.

Rashbaum, Ralph F., M.D. "Spinal Cord Stimulators and Pain Pumps—Implantable Systems for Neuropathy," Spine-health. Available online. URL:http://www.spine-health.com/topics/conserv/neuropaintr/neuropaintr04.html. Downloaded January 13, 2006.

Richeimer, Steven, M.D. "Spinal Pumps and Stimulators," SpineUniverse. Available online. URL: http://www.spineuniverse.com/displayarticle.php/article1612.html. Last updated October 22, 2005.

iron   In healthy red-blooded people, this mineral aids red cell production. Those cells then carry oxygenated blood throughout the body, enabling a person to perform daily ACTIVITY or EXERCISE with vitality. Such vigorous efforts aid BONE BUILDING and strengthen PARASPINAL MUSCLES too.

All iron, however, is not created equal. According to the National Institutes of Health (NIH) Office of Dietary Supplements, "there are two forms of dietary iron: heme and nonheme. Heme iron is derived from hemoglobin, the protein in red blood cells that delivers oxygen to cells. Heme iron is found in animal foods that originally contained hemoglobin, such as red meats, fish, and poultry. Iron in plant foods such as lentils and beans is arranged in a chemical structure called nonheme iron. This is the form of iron added to iron-enriched and iron-fortified foods. . . . Heme iron is absorbed better than nonheme iron, but most dietary iron is nonheme iron."

Dosage and Potential Side Effects

The Weightlossforall.com Web site from England listed "Foods Rich With Iron," which included 20 mg of heme iron found in a traditional British dish known as blood pudding. As another blood source from which most high-heme springs, liver offers 9 mg of iron, but even a can of shrimp contains 5 mg of heme iron, while lean beef has about 2.5 mg. To avoid blood sources and cholesterol, nonheme iron can be found in many culinary herbs, with the understanding, of course, that the heaping amounts required to meet the Recommended Daily Allowance (RDA) would ruin a meal. Nevertheless, dietary sources of nonheme iron include thyme, curry, cinnamon, rosemary, and paprika but with more substantial amounts found in cashews, almonds, and other nuts. Despite the numerous natural sources for iron-rich NUTRITION, people with dietary restrictions may not get enough. Since each age group has unique requirements for iron, supplements should be taken according to the RDA shown on a product label or as recommended by a doctor.

Statistics and Studies

At almost any age or place, signs of iron deficiency can be seen. As the NIH reported, "The World Health Organization considers iron deficiency the number one nutritional disorder in the world. As many as 80% of the world's population may be iron deficient, while 30% may have iron deficiency anemia." Besides blood loss and low dietary intake, iron deficiency commonly occurs because of adverse interactions with medications or interference from other foods.

The NIH Office of Dietary Supplements further advised, "Some researchers have raised concerns about interactions between iron, zinc, and calcium. When iron and zinc supplements are given together in a water solution and without food, greater doses of iron may decrease zinc absorption. However, the effect of supplemental iron on zinc absorption does not appear to be significant when supplements are consumed with food. There is evidence that calcium from supplements and dairy foods may inhibit iron absorption, but it has been very difficult to distinguish between the effects of calcium on iron absorption versus other inhibitory factors such as phytate." According to other studies cited by the NIH, "tannins (found in tea), calcium, polyphenols, and phytates (found in legumes and whole grains) can decrease absorption of nonheme iron. Some proteins found in soybeans also inhibit nonheme iron absorption."

While CALCIUM hinders iron absorption, and vice versa, VITAMIN A and VITAMIN C help the body better absorb iron, similar to the way VITAMIN D boosts calcium uptake. Too much boosting, however, is seriously inadvisable. As the NIH warned, "In children, death has occurred from ingesting 200 mg of iron."

Since iron deficiency anemia seldom occurs in men or in postmenopausal women, they, too, must take care not to overload. As the NIH said, "As far back as the 1980s, some researchers suggested that the regular menstrual loss of iron, rather than a protective effect from estrogen, could better explain the lower incidence of heart disease seen in premenopausal women. After menopause, a woman's risk of developing coronary heart disease increases along with her iron stores." Whether the culprit is too much iron or too much cholesterol, vigorous exercise makes use of both. Conversely, the NIH warned, "the need for iron may be 30% greater in those who engage in regular intense exercise."

Office of Dietary Supplements. "Dietary Supplement Fact Sheet: Iron," National Institutes of Health. Available online. URL: http://ods.od.nih.gov/factsheets/iron.asp. Downloaded January 12, 2006.

Weightlossforall.com. "Foods Rich in Iron." Available online. URL: http://www.weightlossforall.com/iron-rich-food.htm. Downloaded January 13, 2006.

juvenile arthritis "Arthro" refers to joints and "itis" to the inflammation that characterizes this rheumatic condition. Unfortunately, juvenile arthritis (JA) often goes undetected. People usually think of ARTHRITIS as occurring in the ELDERLY, but JA begins sometime during childhood, usually before age 15.

According to the article "Arthritis in Children" posted by the Arthritis Foundation (AF), "about 285,000 children in the United States have a form of juvenile arthritis. The most common form of arthritis in children is juvenile rheumatoid arthritis (JRA.)" Besides JUVENILE RHEUMATOID ARTHRITIS, "Children also are affected by arthritis as a feature of more than 100 other diseases including diseases that affect the spine, connective tissue diseases, and non-inflammatory disorders such as fibromyalgia." However, "the cause of most forms of juvenile arthritis remains unknown. Juvenile arthritis is not contagious and there is no evidence that foods, toxins, allergies or vitamin deficiencies play a role. Current research indicates that there may be a genetic predisposition to juvenile arthritis. Most of the symptoms are due to inflammation as a result of the immune system. Nonetheless, there are many effective treatments available to help you and your child manage juvenile arthritis."

Symptoms and Diagnostic Path

Joint pain, BACK pain, fatigue, and stiffness in the SPINE sometimes occur during normal growth spurts in CHILDREN and ADOLESCENTS, but those growing pains can also be symptoms of JA. In general, CHRONIC PAIN indicates the presence of some type of disorder. To investigate the possibilities, a rheumatologist may request a blood test. Although this test may not identify JA, it may rule out similar conditions, such as JUVENILE SPONDYLOARTHRI-

TIS or ANKYLOSING SPONDYLITIS. A medical history, physical examination, and an eye examination can also assist the diagnosis. If joint inflammation has affected RANGE OF MOTION, a rheumatologist, pediatrician, or other doctor may use X-RAYS to evaluate the condition of those joints.

Although the AF mentioned a lack of evidence implicating ENVIRONMENTAL INFLUENCES, such factors might be considered on an individual basis, with diagnostic clues often found at home. For instance, if symptoms begin in more than one person after a family has moved into an old house, the lead on a painted surface or in the well-water might be the cause. More often, JA symptoms arise because of undetected food allergies. To begin that detective work, meals and snacks must be restricted to bland food for about 10 days. Then one potential allergen, such as wheat, tomatoes, shellfish, or chocolate, can be returned to the diet each week. If a skin rash or stomach upset occurs, the food should be removed to see if this eliminates the symptoms. If so, at least one food allergen has been identified, which may indicate the presence of others. If no problem arises, that food can be returned to the regular diet and the next potential allergen tested.

Treatment Options and Outlook

Traditionally, PAIN MANAGEMENT of JA includes NONSTEROIDAL ANTI-INFLAMMATORY DRUG (NSAID) THERAPY or prescription medication. Depending on the presence of other symptoms, such as inflammation around the eyes or a skin rash on the body, regular eye examinations and visits to a dermatologist may be needed.

Various types of COMPLEMENTARY AND ALTERNATIVE MEDICINE, such as HOMEOPATHIC MEDICINE or HERBAL THERAPY, may help some JA patients. In general, appropriate EXERCISE, adequate liquids, and well-balanced NUTRITION offer everyday benefits. For example, cold water fish, such as cod or salmon, aid the body in lubricating joints inflamed by dryness, while cayenne pepper or ginger sprinkled over foods may reduce pain. The bromelain enzyme found in fresh pineapple may ease inflammation, whereas products containing processed sugar may increase the symptoms.

If needed, counseling and antidepressant drugs can improve the mental outlook, relieve the anxiety common to JA patients, and increase an overall sense of well-being. Counseling may also ensure timely treatment of pain.

Risk Factors and Preventive Measures

Online information from the National Institute of Arthritis and Musculoskeletal and Skin Diseases said, "Juvenile arthritis is one of the most prevalent chronic diseases in children in the United States. While arthritis pain has been the focus of much research in adults, there is an increasing awareness of the need to focus on pain in children. Children with juvenile arthritis may have pain that can be intense and disabling, and comprehensive treatment optimizes their ability to fully participate in school and social activities."

Unfortunately, children may not let parents know about discomfort. As explained in the article "Childhood Pain" posted by the AF, "children are sometimes reluctant to complain of pain, and may deny or under report pain because they: fear it will result in additional unpleasant procedures or treatments; do not understand the pain can be treated; wish to protect their parents from the reality of their disease; desire to please others."

With ongoing pain, a risk comes in avoiding exercise and social contact. If a child receives treatment though, pain may subside long enough to allow enjoyable daily ACTIVITY. Also, as inflammation eases, joint damage may be less likely to occur.

Arthritis Foundation. "Arthritis in Children," AF. Available online. URL: http://www.arthritis.org/AFStore/StartRead.asp?idProduct=3369. Downloaded January 14, 2006.

———. "Childhood Pain," AF. Available online. URL: http://www.arthritis.org/communities/juvenile_arthritis/

Taking_Control/Childhood_Pain.asp. Downloaded January 14, 2006.

National Institute of Arthritis and Musculoskeletal and Skin Diseases. "Pain of Juvenile Arthritis May Reduce School and Social Activity," NIAMS, National Institutes of Health. Available online. URL: http://www.niams.nih.gov/ne/highlights/spotlight/2003/pain-juvenile.htm. Downloaded January 14, 2006.

juvenile osteoporosis   Although primary juvenile osteoporosis (JO) has no known cause, treatments for such conditions as JUVENILE RHEUMATOID ARTHRITIS can produce a secondary form of OSTEOPOROSIS in CHILDREN and ADOLESCENTS. Disorders that affect bone mass, such as OSTEOGENESIS IMPERFECTA, can also produce the porous bones that mark JO.

Symptoms and Diagnostic Path

Most common in children between eight and 14, symptoms include ACUTE or CHRONIC PAIN in the BACK, compression of the VERTEBRAE, and, sometimes, FRACTURE of long bones in the legs or small bones in the SPINE. Often, young patients experience difficulties in walking or just going about their daily ACTIVITY. KYPHOSIS or other problems with POSTURE may develop too.

In addition to a medical history and physical examination, X-RAYS may be needed for a diagnosis. To assess bone strength, a BONE MINERAL DENSITY (BMD) TEST, such as ABSORPTIOMETRY, establishes a baseline for annual follow-up testing to assess new bone growth. To get an accurate reading though, a BMD test must use pediatric software for comparative analysis with the appropriate age group.

Treatment Options and Outlook

According to The Pediatric Orthopaedic Society of North America, "the outlook for spontaneous recovery is good, usually in 2–4 years or at skeletal maturity, but protracted disability has been reported in a small number of adults."

Besides various forms of PAIN MANAGEMENT, treatment may include ANTIRESORPTIVE DRUGS. An article in the 2005 annual *Pediatric Drugs* explained, "Bone mass increases progressively during childhood, but mainly during adolescence when approximately 40% of total bone mass is accumulated." However, "many disorders, by various mechanisms, may affect the acquisition of bone mass." This not only affects present bone strength in children and teenagers but determines their future bone mass as adults and ELDERLY patients. Therefore, "the use of bisphosphonates in children and adolescents with osteoporosis is increasing and their positive effect in improving bone mineral density is encouraging."

Recent studies focused on treating childhood osteoporosis with alendronate (Fosamax). To explain the rationale for using this particular BISPHOSPHO-NATE, ClinicalTrial.gov said, "Bones grow and stay strong through a continuous process of formation (building) and resorption (break down). When more bone is formed than resorbed, the density (level of calcium) in bone increases and the bones become stronger. However, if more bone is resorbed than formed, the density of bone decreases and the bones become weak." Since "alendronate (Fosamax) is a drug that works by stopping bone resorption (break down)," ClinicalTrial.gov said, "Researchers believe that children treated with alendronate will improve bone strength and decrease the amount of fractures caused by osteoporosis."

Risk Factors and Preventive Measures

Some medications, such as prednisone, used to treat juvenile rheumatoid arthritis, can decrease bone density, thus causing secondary juvenile osteoporosis or OSTEOPENIA. Also, if children and teenagers have almost any ongoing illness or disorder, they become less likely to have the EXERCISE needed to aid spinal health and BONE BUILDING. Although WEIGHT-BEARING EXERCISE would place porous bones at greater risk during periods of growth, other types of daily activity can be tailored to the child.

NUTRITION provides another natural preventive, but dietary whims increase the risks. For example, soft drinks contain PHOSPHORUS that can affect MINERAL BALANCE, especially if sodas replace bone-building dairy products. To ensure adequate CALCIUM intake, individual tastes can be assessed. For example, a child who dislikes milk may have a lactose intolerance not triggered by yogurt. If the texture of yogurt seems too unappetizing, the frozen version offers the same amount of calcium and, for many people, tastes better than ice cream. Most dairy products also add VITAMIN D to increase cal-

cium absorption, but playing in the sun for a few minutes without sunscreen will provide the daily vitamin D needed and add spine-strengthening exercise too.

Baroncelli, Giampiero Igli, Silvano Bertelloni, Federica Sodini, and Giuseppe Saggese. "Osteoporosis in Children and Adolescents: Etiology and Management," *Pediatric Drugs* annual issue 7, no. 5 (2005): 295–323.

ClinicalTrials.gov. "Treatment of Childhood Osteoporosis with Alendronate (Fosamax)," U.S. National Institutes of Health. Available online. URL: http://www.clinicaltrials.gov/ct/show/NCT00001720. Downloaded January 12, 2006.

National Institute of Arthritis and Musculoskeletal and Skin Diseases. "Juvenile Osteoporosis," NIAMS, National Institutes of Health. Available online. URL: http://www.niams.nih.gov/bone/hi/osteoporosis_juv.htm. Downloaded January 12, 2006.

Pediatric Orthopaedic Society of North America, The. "Juvenile Osteoporosis," POSNA. Available online. URL: http://www.posna.org/index?service=page/core Curriculum&article=juvenileOsteoporosis.html. Downloaded January 12, 2006.

juvenile rheumatoid arthritis   As the most common form of JUVENILE ARTHRITIS, juvenile rheumatoid arthritis (JRA) can occur in CHILDREN or ADOLESCENTS of any age but rarely in INFANTS under six months. A family history of ARTHRITIS or RHEUMATOID ARTHRITIS may imply involvement of GENETIC FACTORS in this chronic inflammatory disease.

Symptoms and Diagnostic Path

According to the Arthritis Foundation, symptoms vary with each child, and sometimes with each day, but "the most common features of JRA are: joint inflammation, joint contracture (stiff, bent joint), joint damage and/or alteration or change in growth. Other symptoms include joint stiffness following rest or decreased activity level (also referred to as morning stiffness or gelling), and weakness in muscles and other soft tissues around involved joints. However, because JRA affects each child differently, your child may not experience all of these changes. Children also vary in the degree to which they are affected by any particular symptom."

In an online article posted by the American College of Rheumatology, Dr. Leslie Abramson said, "Systemic onset JRA affects about 10 percent of children with arthritis. It begins with a recurrent fever that can be 103°F or higher, often accompanied by a pink rash that comes and goes. Systemic onset JRA may cause inflammation of the internal organs as well as the joints. Swelling of the joints may not be present at onset and may appear months or even years after the onset of fevers." While various types of JRA can affect various areas of the body, "all cause joint inflammation and begin before the age of 16, but otherwise are often associated with distinct symptoms and complications and may require different approaches to treatment."

Besides taking a medical history and performing a physical examination, a rheumatologist or other specialist will request a blood test to see if a child tests positive for the rheumatoid factor. If so, this may indicate the need for more aggressive treatment.

Treatment Options and Outlook

Incorporating varied approaches to treatment may provide the best outlook. For example, a medical team commonly includes a pediatrician, rheumatologist, occupational therapist, physical therapist, and mental health counselor. If symptoms present a concern about eye health, an ophthalmologist will be needed, whereas an orthopedic surgeon may become involved if joints show severe structural damage.

As Dr. Abramson recommended, "The overall goal of treatment of JRA is to control symptoms, prevent joint damage and maintain function." This typically begins with NONSTEROIDAL ANTI-INFLAMMATORY DRUG (NSAID) THERAPY, which, to avoid stomach upset in children, should be taken with food. If JRA remains active, a DISEASE MODIFYING ANTI-RHEUMATIC DRUG (DMARD) may be added.

Risk Factors and Preventive Measures

Pain or inflammation may make a child want to withdraw from school or social activities, but the National Institute of Arthritis and Musculoskeletal and Skin Diseases (NIAMS) recommended otherwise: "Although pain sometimes limits physical activity, exercise is important to reduce the symptoms of JRA and maintain function and range of motion of the joints. Most children with JRA can take part fully in physical activities and sports when their symptoms are under control. During a disease flare-up, however, the doctor may advise limiting certain activities depending on the joints involved. Once the flare-up is over, a child can start regular activities again."

Abramson, Leslie S., M.D. "Arthritis in Children," American College of Rheumatology. Available online. URL: http://www.rheumatology.org/public/factsheets/arth_in_children.asp?aud=pat. Downloaded January 14, 2006.

Arthritis Foundation. "Juvenile Rheumatoid Arthritis," AF. Available online. URL: http://www.arthritis.org/conditions/DiseaseCenter/jra.asp. Downloaded January 12, 2006.

National Institute of Arthritis and Musculoskeletal and Skin Diseases. "Questions and Answers about Juvenile Rheumatoid Arthritis," NIAMS, National Institutes of Health. Available online. URL: http://www.niams.nih.gov/hi/topics/juvenile_arthritis/juvarthr.htm. Downloaded January 12, 2006.

juvenile scoliosis   See IDIOPATHIC SCOLIOSIS.

juvenile spondyloarthritis   Like other types of ARTHRITIS, juvenile spondyloarthritis (JSpA) inflames the joints and often affects the VERTEBRAE. Although various forms exist, the most common is juvenile ANKYLOSING SPONDYLITIS. The term indicates a bent SPINE, which describes what occurs unless treatment intervenes.

Online information from the Spondylitis Association of America (SAA) said, "Juvenile-onset spondyloarthritis (JSpA), also known as Juvenile Spondyloarthropathy, is the medical term for a group of childhood rheumatic diseases, which cause arthritis before the age of 16 and may span through adult life. The juvenile spondyloarthropathies include undifferentiated spondyloarthropathy, juvenile ankylosing spondylitis, psoriatic arthritis, reactive arthritis and spondylitis of inflammatory bowel diseases."

Symptoms and Diagnostic Path

According to the SAA, "JSpA typically causes pain and inflammation in the joints in the lower part of the body, for example, the pelvis, hips, knees and ankles. Other areas of the body can also be affected, such as the spine, eyes, skin and bowels. Fatigue and lethargy can also occur."

An article on the Cincinnati Children's Hospital Medical Center Web site said, "In SpA, the inflammation often occurs where tendons attach our muscles to bones, or where ligaments attach to bones." Comparing the symptoms of JSpA with JUVENILE RHEUMATOID ARTHRITIS (JRA), the article continued, "In general, SpA tends to occur in older boys and involve a small number of large joints (i.e. hips, knees and ankles). Back pain or stiffness is more frequent in pediatric SpAs than JRA."

Information from the New York-Presbyterian Hospital reported, "Juvenile spondyloarthropathies usually affect the spine and the sites where the muscles, tendons, and ligaments are attached to bone. The disease causes inflammation of the spine and large joints, resulting in stiffness and pain. When severe, the disease may result in erosion at the joint between the spine and the hip bone (the sacroiliac joint), and the formation of bony bridges between vertebrae in the spine, fusing those bones." X-RAYS and blood tests may help to confirm the condition.

Treatment Options and Outlook

Treatment often begins with PAIN MANAGEMENT that includes NONSTEROIDAL ANTI-INFLAMMATORY DRUG (NSAID) THERAPY. Should this fail to relieve pain, DISEASE-MODIFYING ANTI-RHEUMATIC DRUGS (DMARDs) may be added.

Some children may need POSTURE training or other forms of physical therapy to aid flexibility in the SACRAL VERTEBRAE and LUMBAR SPINE. Although WEIGHT-BEARING EXERCISE can damage inflamed joints, other types of EXERCISE, such as swimming or stretching exercises, will usually be recommended. Also, programs of daily ACTIVITY and NUTRITION can be designed to fit the child and his or her specific needs and interests. To encourage an active outlook, ORTHOTIC devices or cushioned insoles for SHOES usually make walking more comfortable.

Risk Factors and Preventive Measures

Although juvenile spondyloarthritis may be more severe than similar conditions arising in adults, early treatment reduces the risk of CHRONIC PAIN and lessens the likelihood of permanent disability. No cure exists, but JSpA may go into remission, providing the child with an opportunity to build strength. Should flare-ups return, prompt treatment can prevent the condition from getting out of hand and also encourage the child to continue participating in activities important to childhood.

Cincinnati Children's Hospital Medical Center. "Juvenile Spondyloarthritis." Available online. URL: http://www. cincinnatichildrens.org/health/info/rheumatology/ diagnose/spondyloarthritis.htm. Downloaded January 12, 2006.

New York-Presbyterian. "Juvenile Spondyloarthritis," The University Hospitals of Columbia and Cornell. Available online. URL: http://wo-pub2.med.cornell.edu/ cgi-bin/WebObjects/PublicPediatrics.woa/2/wa/ viewContent?contentID=1721&wosid=A7T1Ockk9t 1wbr1mXsjQP0. Downloaded January 12, 2006.

Spondylitis Association of America. "Juvenile Spondyloarthritis (JSpA)," SAA. Available online. URL: http:// www.spondylitis.org/about/juvenile.aspx. Downloaded January 12, 2006.

ketoprofen See NONSTEROIDAL ANTI-INFLAMMA-TORY DRUG THERAPY.

kyphoplasty This MINIMALLY INVASIVE SURGERY uses X-RAY guidance to stabilize the SPINE after a VERTEBRAL COMPRESSION FRACTURE. Although not appropriate for young patients or people with SPINAL STENOSIS, kyphoplasty provides a new and encouraging surgical option for many ELDERLY patients, OSTEOPOROSIS patients, and CANCER patients. Since the procedure can be used to treat one or more compression fractures, it can restore height and prevent severe POSTURE problems, such as KYPHOSIS, from progressing.

Procedure

Dr. Arya Nick Shamie of the UCLA Spine Center explained, "Kyphoplasty is performed with a probe placed into the fractured vertebral body through two small skin incisions. A deflated balloon is then inserted and expanded to bring the compressed bone back to its desired height. Bone cement is injected to hold the fracture in place. The cement acts as an internal cast to hold the bone in place until it heals. About 80 to 90 percent of patients have immediate pain relief after the procedure." Usually, each quarter-inch slit can then be closed with a single stitch.

Risks and Complications

An article in *Neurosurgical Focus* compared kyphoplasty with VERTEBROPLASTY, stating, "Complications are rare, but they can be serious, and their exact incidence is unknown." For example, bone cement can leak outside the vertebrae or damage the spinal cord. Although "complications have been reported for both procedures, ... a review of Food and Drug Administration safety data revealed 58 reported complications from 1999 through 2003 of approximately 200,000 procedures performed."

Outlook and Lifestyle Modifications

The American Academy of Orthopaedic Surgeons advised, "For the best results, kyphoplasty should be performed as soon as possible after spinal bone collapse or fracture. The results are less predictable in older fractures but in certain circumstances may still be beneficial." Although pain may persist in some patients, "Most patients have excellent pain relief and straighter backs. This may result in added height. More than 95 percent of patients rate their treatment as successful and report that they are able to return to all their pre-fracture activities." Other than continuing the pre-operative treatment for an underlying medical condition, "most patients do not need physical therapy or any other form of rehabilitation."

American Academy of Orthopaedic Surgeons. "Spinal Surgery for Fractured Vertebrae," AAOS. Available online. URL: http://orthoinfo.aaos.org/fact/thr_report.cfm?Thread_ID=464&topcategory=Spine. Downloaded January 12, 2006.

Burton, Allen W., M.D. Laurence D. Rhines, M.D. and Ehud Mendel, M.D. "Vertebroplasty and Kyphoplasty: a Comprehensive Review," *Neurosurgical Focus* 18, no. 3 (March 2005).

UCLA Healthcare. "New Spine Surgeries Allow Quicker, Less Painful Recovery," UCLA Health Sciences. Available online. URL: http://www.healthcare.ucla.edu/vital-signs/article-display?article_id=315. Downloaded January 21, 2006.

kyphosis In this type of POSTURE problem, the upper BACK acquires a rounded look, but kyphosis can also develop in the lower back or LUMBAR SPINE. Often, spinal problems become apparent during teen years, but congenital kyphosis occurs in INFANTS whose bones did not form correctly prior to birth. One type of the disorder known as Scheuermann's kyphosis begins in an older child or young adult and typically presents a smooth curve in the THORACIC SPINE. Also, ELDERLY patients can develop secondary kyphosis if bones have been weakened by OSTEOPOROSIS or if bone CANCER produces VERTEBRAL COMPRESSION FRACTURES.

Regarding kyphosis among CHILDREN, the Spine Center of the Colorado Springs Orthopaedic Group said, "The cause of Scheuermann's kyphosis has not been discovered, but there are many possible theories about its development. Scheuermann, the Danish radiologist for whom the disease is named, was the first to notice the problem. He proposed that the problem was a result of a process of 'avascular necrosis' of the cartilage ring of the vertebral body. This means the cartilage of the spinal bone's ring died because it lacked the necessary blood supply. Scheuermann believed that this interrupted bone growth during development, leading to wedge-shaped vertebrae." Indeed, "most researchers think that some sort of damage to the growth area of the vertebrae starts the process. The abnormal growth that follows is what causes the excessive kyphosis."

Symptoms and Diagnostic Path

While kyphosis can usually be seen with the eye, a physical examination and X-RAYS reveal the extent of curvature. Over 50 degrees is considered abnormal, but SURGERY will seldom be needed unless the curve exceeds 75 degrees.

Treatment Options and Outlook

To treat postural kyphosis, the American Academy of Orthopaedic Surgeons (AAOS) said, "Exercises to strengthen the abdomen and stretch the hamstrings may help take away associated discomfort. But exercises probably won't result in significant correction of the postural kyphosis." If needed, NONSTEROIDAL ANTI-INFLAMMATORY DRUG (NSAID) THERAPY can be used to treat pain, but the AAOS said, "This condition does not lead to problems in adult life."

For Scheuermann's kyphosis, the AAOS advised, "An initial program of conservative treatment is also recommended for patients with Scheuermann's kyphosis. This includes exercises and anti-inflammatory medications. If the child is still growing, the doctor may prescribe a brace. The child wears the brace until skeletal maturity is reached."

Back.com further explained, "Other forms of treatment, including bracing and surgery, are considered when there is a rapid increase in the size of the curve; worsening of the vertebral body wedging, back pain that will not improve with conservative measures, and difficulties with pulmonary function that are related to the kyphotic deformity. The decision about when and how to brace the spine of a patient with Scheuermann's disease, or to perform surgery, is made on an individual basis."

For elderly patients who develop kyphosis because of vertebral compression fracture, treatment may include MINIMALLY INVASIVE SURGERY, such as KYPHOPLASTY or VERTEBROPLASTY. Young infants may need other types of corrective surgery to straighten the SPINE and avoid respiratory problems.

Risk Factors and Preventive Measures

In growing children and ADOLESCENTS, an ORTHOTIC brace will commonly be prescribed to prevent further development of the curvature and avoid spinal deformity. Also, well-designed EXERCISE can lessen pain, improve posture, and strengthen the spine. Although slouching can exaggerate curvature, kyphosis may cease to progress after the child or teenager reaches full growth.

American Academy of Orthopaedic Surgeons. "Kyphosis (Curvature of the Spine)," AAOS. Available online. URL: http://orthoinfo.aaos.org/fact/thr_report.cfm?Thread_ID=247&topcategory=Spine. Downloaded January 12, 2006.

Medtronic Sofamor Danek. "Developmental Disorders: Scheuermann's Kyphosis," Back.com. Available online. URL: http://www.back.com/causes-developmental-scheuermann.html. Last updated March 11, 2005.

SpineUniversity. "Introduction," Spine Center, Colorado Springs Orthopaedic Group. Available online. URL: http://www.spineuniversity.com/public/spinesub.asp?id=52. Downloaded January 12, 2006.

laminaplasty See CERVICAL LAMINAPLASTY.

laminectomy, laminotomy Often referred to as spinal decompression, this type of SURGERY removes all or part of the bony lamina covering the spinal canal at a particular point of pressure. Commonly, the procedure involves the lower back, but spinal decompression can reduce pressure on spinal nerves in the CERVICAL SPINE or the THORACIC SPINE as well as the LUMBAR SPINE. A laminectomy can be done alone, but the surgery may be an aspect of LUMBAR SPINAL FUSION or other type of ARTHRODESIS used to fuse VERTEBRAE and stabilize or strengthen the SPINE.

Procedure

According to the North American Spine Society (NASS), "after an incision is made in the midline of the neck or back, the muscle is moved away to expose the lamina, which are the bony shingles. . . . The lamina can be removed in whole or in part to expose a single nerve . . . or more . . . as needed." Partial removal of lamina in a laminotomy may suffice, but "In the case of spinal stenosis, a more extensive laminectomy is performed, and may require removal of an entire lamina, on both sides of the midline, and including the spinous process," the column of bony ridges that can be felt on the BACK, "where the lamina from both sides meet. This permits the surgeon to uncover the canal containing the nerves and to extend the decompression laminectomy to the area of the facet joints, where bony spurs can be removed. In some cases, it is necessary to remove the entire lamina and a portion of the facet joint (through the same exposure). If the surgeon is concerned that instability will occur, a fusion may be performed in addition."

Besides removing some portion of the lamina, the surgeon eliminates bone spurs (OSTEOPHYTES), scar tissue, or ruptured areas of a DISC. Typically, the procedure takes about two hours and includes insertion of a small drainage tube to keep blood from collecting in the surgical site. The next day, the drain will be removed and the dressing changed, but an intravenous (IV) pump may remain for two or three days to administer antibiotics or pain medication. An IV may also be inserted to ensure adequate intake of food and liquids.

As an alternative to laminectomy, a new MINIMALLY INVASIVE SURGERY uses the recently approved X STOP implant to allow room for exiting nerves. Like a laminectomy, this procedure relieves pressure on the spinal nerves, but the X STOP decreases recovery time. As the Center for Devices and Radiological Health said, "The X STOP® is a titanium implant that fits between the spinous processes of the lower (lumbar) spine. It is made from titanium alloy and consists of two components: a spacer assembly and a wing assembly." Implanted at one or two lumbar levels, "The X STOP® is designed to limit extension of the spine in the affected area, which may relieve the symptoms of lumbar spinal stenosis."

Risks and Complications

In patients who undergo spinal decompression surgery, depression and fatigue typically set in by the second or third day. A number of sources mention the importance of an optimistic attitude during recovery, presumably to prevent discouragement when pain continues. However, the stress of surgery, the proximity of the spinal cord in a laminectomy, and the residual effects of anesthesia complicate attempts at cheeriness. Most patients need rest, time to heal, and gradual restoration of activities before a full recovery occurs.

Patients also risk CHRONIC PAIN of FAILED BACK SURGERY SYNDROME and the dangerous complication of CAUDA EQUINA SYNDROME (CES), particularly if spinal decompression involves extensive removal of lamina in a laminectomy. In an article for *Neurosurgical Focus,* Dr. John P. Kostuik said, "The generally accepted frequency of CES is between 2 and 6% of all laminectomies performed for lumbar disc herniation. . . . One of the most common errors that arises following discharge from the hospital includes the failure of the physician or other medical personnel to ask appropriate questions over the telephone or in an office setting. This situation is particularly unfortunate if the patient has experienced changes in any symptoms including increased back pain and/or radicular pain and perhaps difficulty in urination. Bladder function inquiries are crucial." The potential of CES arising after surgery increases if a patient experiences ACUTE PAIN in the back, limited leg raising, or sensory motor loss. In the same issue of *Neurosurgical Focus,* Dr. Randy L. Jensen also addressed the potential complication of CES, adding, "Factors that might precipitate postoperative CES include inadequate decompression, nerve root swelling, hematoma," or blood clot, and "retained disc fragments."

Outlook and Lifestyle Modifications

Spine Inc. described what commonly occurs after a laminectomy: "Initially, you are permitted to get out of bed following surgery with assistance from a nurse. Thereafter, you should be up walking as much as tolerated. The goal is to do more walking each day. Start with short trips and set a graduated pace so that each day more activity is accomplished." For those who have difficulty getting up, "the easiest way for you to get out of bed is to raise the head of the bed as far as it will go, balance yourself in a sitting position, then stand with weight distributed on the skeletal frame, to avoid straining of back muscles. Avoid prolonged sitting. Initially, you should only sit for meals."

At home, ERGONOMIC FACTORS should be addressed with upright furniture to encourage proper POSTURE and correctly support the spine. Not only does this design provide the best positioning for the lower back but for the upper back and neck too.

Regarding other modifications, Spine Inc. said, "Follow-up to remove staples will be scheduled for ten to fourteen days following surgery. Another follow-up to see progress will be scheduled four to six weeks following surgery. Other follow-ups, which may continue for as long as a year after surgery, will be scheduled depending on progress."

To aid that progress, the patient should completely refrain from bending over for several weeks. Except for light-weight objects under two pounds, LIFTING should be totally avoided in the first weeks, but daily ACTIVITY, physical therapy, and doctor-recommended EXERCISE should gradually increase. An abundance of fresh water and fresh fruit or other natural forms of NUTRITION also assist recovery.

If a sensation of pressure continues after an incision has healed, COLD THERAPY may relieve the swelling that commonly causes that pressure. Some patients find relief in alternating HEAT THERAPY with cold. For example, after a hot shower, an ice pack can be applied for five minutes. Otherwise, either hot or cold treatments may help, depending on which feels best to the patient. For general pain, prescription medication or NONSTEROIDAL ANTI-INFLAMMATORY DRUG (NSAID) THERAPY can be used as needed during the recovery, which may take a few months.

CDRH Consumer Information. "New Device Approval X STOP® Interspinous Process Decompression System (XSTOP) - P040001," Center for Devices and Radiological Health, U.S. Food and Drug Administration, Department of Health and Human Services. URL: http://www.fda.gov/cdrh/mda/docs/p040001.html. Last updated January 4, 2006.

Jensen, Randy L. "Cauda Equina Syndrome as a Postoperative Complication of Lumbar Spine Surgery," *Neurosurgical Focus* 16, no. 6 (June 2004): 34–38.

Kostuik, John P., M.D. "Medicolegal Consequences of Cauda Equina Syndrome: an Overview," *Neurosurgical Focus* 16, no. 6 (June 2004): 39–41.

North American Spine Society. "Laminectomy or Laminotomy," NASS. Available online. URL: http://www.spine.org/fsp/prob_action-surgical-laminectomy.cfm. Last updated March 3, 2005.

Spine Inc. "Laminectomy." Available online. URL: http://www.spine-inc.com/glossary/l/laminectomy.html. Downloaded January 16, 2006.

lifting   After almost any type of SURGERY, patients should avoid lifting more than a pound or two during the recovery period. At any time, however, CHILDREN, ADOLESCENTS, younger adults, and ELDERLY adults need to be aware of the LOAD TOLERANCE of the BACK and SPINE, especially as relates to their particular age or condition. By taking care not to overload spinal DISCS and VERTEBRAE, such back conditions as a HERNIATED DISC or SPINAL INJURY can often be prevented.

To provide tips on safe means of lifting, the Occupational Safety & Health Administration (OSHA) of the U.S. Department of Labor said, "Lift loads close to the body." Also, "limit the number of allowed lifts per worker per day. Avoid heavy lifting especially with spine rotated." To avoid the back injuries that often occur among hospital personnel and home caretakers, OSHA further advised, "Never transfer patients/residents when off balance. Never lift alone, particularly fallen patients/residents." Instead, "use team lifts or use mechanical assistance."

Risks and Complications

Homes and small medical facilities may not have mechanical patient lift systems or other equipment needed to assist caretakers in lifting patients. For other types of lifting, complications commonly arise if the person happens to twist slightly at the moment of lift-off. Additional risks occur if a person has weak PARASPINAL MUSCLES or bone loss due to OSTEOPENIA, OSTEOPOROSIS, and other conditions. People with DEGENERATIVE DISC DISEASE should also avoid lifting heavy objects because of the pressure this exerts on the spinal discs.

Statistics and Studies

An abstract of "Prevention of Disabling Back Injuries in Nurses by the Use of Mechanical Patient Lift Systems" stated, "According to the National Institute for Occupational Safety and Health (NIOSH), occupational back injury is the second leading occupational injury in the United States. Among health care personnel, nurses have the highest rate of back pain, with an annual prevalence of 40–50% and a lifetime prevalence of 35–80%." Studies consistently show, however, that assistive equipment can enable caretakers to handle patients safely, thereby reducing risk of musculoskeletal disorders and injuries, not only in themselves but also in their patients.

Similarly, an article in *Spine* addressed the effects of wearing a back belt. Although studies offer conflicting evidence about belt usage, this study of 28 workers determined that belts helped to reduce torso motions and remind workers to lift slowly. Furthermore, back belts caused workers to rely on squat-lift techniques that distributed weight evenly around the body, thus lessening the spinal load.

Special Aids and Adaptations

An article posted by Back.com defined the two most common mistakes in lifting as using back muscles instead of muscles in the legs and buttock and lifting an object too far from the body. As the article said, "Just to illustrate, if you lift a 10-pound weight at arms length, it will put 150 pounds of pressure on your back. Lifting an object that weighs 86 pounds puts over 700 pounds of force on the discs in the lower back. An object that weighs over 86 pounds should not be lifted more than a distance of 12 to 13 inches and should not be lifted more than once every five minutes if possible. The heavier the object, the shorter distance it should be lifted." Besides the extra lift of a stepping stool or ladder, motions should be adapted "to limit twisting when lifting." Likewise, the person must take care not to twist the neck or head in order to prevent injuries in the CERVICAL SPINE and THORACIC SPINE.

Edlich, Richard E. "Prevention of Disabling Back Injuries in Nurses by the Use of Mechanical Patient Lift Systems," *Journal of Long-Term Effects of Medical Implants* 14, no. 6 (2004): 521–533.

Giorcelli, Rebecca J., Richard E. Hughes, James T. Wassell, Hongwei Hsiao. "The Effect of Wearing a Back Belt on Spine Kinematics during Asymmetric Lifting of Large and Small Boxes," *Spine* 26, no. 16 (August 15, 2001): 1,794–1,798.

Medtronic Sofamor Danek. "Lifting Techniques," Back.com. Available online. URL: http://www.back.com/articles-lifting.html. Updated April 15, 2005.

Occupational Safety & Health Administration. "Health-Care Wide Hazards Module—Ergonomics," OSHA, U.S. Department of Labor. Available online. URL: http://www.osha.gov/SLTC/etools/hospital/hazards/ergo/ergo.html. Downloaded January 9, 2006.

liniment See TOPICAL ANALGESIC.

load tolerance How much weight can one SPINE carry? Does a back belt keep a BACK from buckling? Should parents of CHILDREN and ADOLESCENTS peer into schoolbags to help each child bear BACKPACK SAFETY? Will poor LIFTING techniques bring a load of load intolerance no matter how little something weighs?

With cautions about POSTURE also arising, load tolerance takes into account the age, biomechanics, and condition of the spine, joints, and vertebral DISCS of each individual. Therefore, load tolerance varies from one person to the next. For example, the spinal concerns of ELDERLY persons or OSTEOPOROSIS patients differ greatly from those of a young adult using STRENGTH TRAINING and other forms of EXERCISE to pump up PARASPINAL MUSCLES.

In a report on load tolerance, Robin Burgess-Limerick stated, "Injuries occur when loads on anatomical structures are, either instantly or over time, greater than the structures can withstand. Anatomical complexity, individual variability in tissue tolerances, and the interactions between biomechanical, environmental, and psychosocial risk factors make the determination of valid threshold limit values for exposure to biomechanical risk factors exceptionally difficult." Yet "more attention has been paid to determining threshold limits for preventing back injury than any other region." However, "these approaches predominately focus on the compressive forces applied to the lumbar spine, comparing estimates of spinal compression based on biomechanical models of varying complexity. . . . The general problems with this approach are: a) tissue tolerances vary with age and sex, and load history; b) compression is only one contributing factor; c) accurate estimates of tissue load require complex measurement techniques; and d) exposure to whole body vibration interacts with other risk factors."

Risks and Complications

A large risk factor comes not necessarily with limitations but with lack of awareness of those limits. For example, children and teenagers may not realize the undue pressure exerted on growing bones as they lug around a backpack weighing more than 10 percent of their own body weight. Stepping on scales could sidestep that problem, but parents may need to intervene by weighing a backpack or helping a child sort out necessary items from those best left in a bedroom or school locker.

People of all ages risk load intolerance each time they lift items over their heads, twist their bodies while lifting, or bend their backs and necks instead of their knees. Equally important, all weights are not created equal. For example, lifting ten pounds away from the body places not ten but 150 pounds of pressure on the back. Besides the risk of improper lifting, load intolerance increases with each repetition of weight until fatigue presents a final straw in overloading the spine.

Statistics and Studies

An article in *Occupational Ergonomics* reported on a study comparing the effects of continuous and discontinuous loads. Using ELECTROMYOGRAM (EMG) to measure and analyze data "showed that constant load caused higher muscular fatigue than intermittent loads despite the lower value of the external force and lower muscle activation." Furthermore, "the results of the study support the thesis that all biomechanical factors which influence upper limb load and fatigue (upper limb posture, external force and time sequences) should be considered when work stands and work processes are designed. They also indicate that constant load should be especially avoided."

Regarding the influence of posture on spinal overload, a *Spine* article reported on a study of "Muscle Activation Strategies and Symmetry of Spinal Loading in the Lumbar Spine with Scoliosis." For this study, "spinal loading was estimated in a lumbar spine model with increasing degrees of scoliosis. External loading was each of three pure moments or forces acting at T12" in the THORACIC SPINE, "with magnitudes of either 50% or 75% of maximum effort." Focusing on SCOLIOSIS patients, the researchers concluded, "We speculate that individuals with scoliosis can adopt different muscle activation strategies and that these strategies may determine whether or not the spinal loading causes scoliosis progression during growth." In other words, different movements produce different effects. Therefore, patients can be shown how to move in ways most helpful to their spine health, especially if they still have growing bones.

Another study considered the "Structural Injury Tolerance of the Spine: Stability and Lumbar Lordosis in Lifting." According to those conclusions presented to the North American Congress on Biomechanics, "These results confirm our hypotheses that 1) the stability of the lumbar spine during lifting exertions is influenced by the lordotic shape," or the inward curve in the lower back, "of the spine, and 2) the curvature of the spine necessary to maintain stability changes," particularly as the person bends forward. As author K. P. Granata concluded, "Hence, injuries may occur due to instability" of the spinal column, "despite spinal loads well within recommended safety levels."

In an article for *Ergonomics*, Granata and Marras discussed the "relation between spinal load factors and the high-risk probability of occupational low-back disorder." Studies often apply external or mechanical forces to compress the spine, since "spinal compression is traditionally assumed the principal biomechanical mechanism associated with occupationally related low-back disorder (LBD). One of the criteria that the NIOSH lifting guide uses to discriminate between safe and hazardous tasks is based . . . on estimates of compressive loads on the spine. . . . Consequently, research examining the risk of low-back pain often focuses on axial" or mid-body "compression loads associated with occupational tasks." However, "studies indicate that other factors, including repetitive twisting or lateral," sideways, "bending and lifting, even with relatively light loads, are significant risk factor for LBD." With tissue strain also a factor, the article stated, "No single biomechanical factor completely describes the probability of high-risk classification. . . . Thus, estimates of spinal compression alone cannot fully predict the risk of LBD, because the injury mechanism is influenced by multidimensional loading patterns" that affect many areas. Interestingly, a pattern of job satisfaction may also affect workers. As researchers noted, "employees with low approval ratings and who 'hardly ever' enjoyed their jobs were at high risk of subsequently filing a back injury claim."

Special Aids and Adaptations

Apparently, job satisfaction lifts the load tolerance. Although disgruntled workers might prefer to reassign their spines to job training for a new position, the present task may put the person in the position of straining under a load. If so, an ORTHOTIC device or back belt seldom does more than remind a person to lift with the legs and not twist or overdo. A more productive aid comes in strengthening paraspinal muscles and lessening the load.

Burgess-Limerick, Robin, UniQuest Pty Ltd. "Issues Associated with Force and Weight Limits and Associated Threshold Limit Values in the Physical Handling Work Environment," Issues Paper 2: Commissioned by NOHSC for the Review of the National Standard and Code of Practices on Manual Handling and Associated Documents, February 2003, pages 4 and 7. Available online. URL: http://ergonomics.uq.edu.au/download/tlv.pdf. Downloaded January 16, 2006.

Gielo-Perczak, Krystyna. "Differences in Muscular Activation and Fatigue for Intermittent and Constant Load," *Occupational Ergonomics* 5, no. 1 (2005): 43–56.

Granata, K. P. "Structural Injury Tolerance of the Spine: Stability and Lumbar Lordosis in Lifting," North American Congress on Biomechanics. Available online. URL: http://asb-biomech.org/onlineabs/NACOB98/188/. Downloaded January 16, 2006.

Granata, Kevin P. and William S. Marras. "Relation between Spinal Load Factors and the High-risk Probability of Occupational Low-back Disorder," *Ergonomics* 42, no. 9 (1999): 1,187–1,199.

Stokes, Ian A. F. and Mack Gardner-Morse. "Muscle Activation Strategies and Symmetry of Spinal Loading in the Lumbar Spine With Scoliosis," *Spine* 29, no. 19 (October 1, 2004): 2,103–2,107.

lordosis   Also known as swayback, lordosis creates a vertebral curvature opposite that of KYPHOSIS. While the latter usually presents an outward bow-curve in the THORACIC SPINE, lordosis curves the LUMBAR SPINE inward, just above the hips. Whether mild or severe, both of those POSTURE problems exaggerate the natural curvature of the SPINE. Conversely, SCOLIOSIS presents a side to side abnormality in the spinal column with the VERTEBRAE forming an *S* or *C*.

Symptoms and Diagnostic Path

Severe instances of lordosis in a newborn may indicate a BIRTH DEFECT OF THE SPINE, especially if the normal flexibility of the spinal column seems rigid or fixed. More commonly, parents may notice a curve when holding the baby. To check this at home, the infant can be placed, face up, on a flat surface. If a gap exists between that surface and the lower back of the baby, treatment may be needed.

If lordosis later occurs in CHILDREN or growing ADOLESCENTS, a medical history and physical examination can clarify an underlying cause, such as DISCITIS, SPONDYLOLISTHESIS, or a previously undetected case of DWARFISM. To investigate those conditions or rule out other possibilities, X-RAYS may be needed.

An article posted online by the University of Utah Health Science Center said, "Each child may experience symptoms differently. The major clinical feature of lordosis is a prominence of the buttocks. Symptoms will vary depending if lordosis occurs with other defects," such as MUSCULAR DYSTROPHY, bone abnormalities, or disorders caused by spinal nerves. Back pain, while not characteristic of lordosis, can occur, but more commonly, that symptom indicates the presence of another problem.

Treatment Options and Outlook

As long as the spine remains flexible rather than fixed, most infants need no treatment. If an older child develops a lordotic curve, the cause must be medically investigated to ensure appropriate therapy. For postural problems with no underlying medical cause, treatment may include an ORTHOTIC device, such as a back brace, to stop progression of the curvature.

Risk Factors and Preventive Measures

Early detection and treatment lessen the risk of spinal deformity, especially if regular physical examinations assess the direction of new bone growth. Usually, lordosis patients improve with EXERCISE to strengthen PARASPINAL MUSCLES. Physical therapy, posture training, good NUTRITION, and other forms of BONE BUILDING often prevent the condition from worsening.

Chen, Andrew L., M.D. "Lordosis," MedlinePlus, A.D.A.M. Available online. URL: http://www.nlm.nih.gov/medlineplus/ency/article/003278.htm. Last updated December 13, 2005.

University of Utah Health Science Center. "Lordosis," University Health Care. Available online. URL: http://uuhsc.utah.edu/healthinfo/pediatric/orthopaedics/lordosis.htm. Downloaded January 16, 2006.

low back pain Sometimes called lumbago or, more commonly, a bad BACKACHE, nagging back pains eventually nag most people. According to an online report from the American Association of Neurological Surgeons (AANS), "more than 65 million Americans suffer from low back pain every year. Back aches are the most common reason for doctor visits, after cold and flu symptoms," and, like those pesky health bugs, backaches often come again. As the AANS reported, "Fifty percent of all patients who suffer from an episode of low back pain will have another occurrence within one year." While the severity may differ with each episode, the AANS said, "In the vast majority of cases back pain is caused by the irritation of a nerve root near the spine, not by problems with the muscles, ligament or bone." For example, pain in the lower LUMBAR SPINE may arise from spinal nerve inflammation produced by DEGENERATIVE DISC DISEASE, HERNIATED DISC, SCIATICA, SPONDYLOLISTHESIS, or SPINAL STENOSIS.

Despite a multitude of potential causes, medical professionals generally agree that most low back pain resolves itself within a few weeks. However, patients with symptoms of CAUDA EQUINA SYNDROME, SPINAL INFECTION, SPINAL TUMOR, or bone FRACTURE need immediate treatment. So do those who suffer a trauma or encounter such symptoms as a fever, rash, bladder problem, or muscle weakness.

An article in *American Family Physician* advised, "Imaging studies are generally not recommended in the first month of acute low back pain." Although a BONE SCAN, COMPUTED TOMOGRAPHY SCAN, MAGNETIC RESONANCE IMAGING, or other imaging device will seldom be needed, "patients who do not improve within one month should obtain magnetic resonance imaging if a herniated disc is suspected. Computed tomographic scanning is useful in demonstrating osseous structures" of bone and their relations to spinal nerves "and for assessment of fracture." Also, "bone scans can be used to determine the extent of . . . disease throughout the skeletal system." In general, "all imaging results should be correlated with the patient's signs and symptoms because of the high rate of positive imaging findings in asymptomatic persons." Therefore, patients with no symptoms but a backache could have something going on, such as an undetected kidney problem that causes low back pain.

Risks and Complications

ELDERLY persons and patients with OSTEOPOROSIS or other bone-weakening condition, such as CANCER, may encounter unprovoked episodes of ACUTE PAIN in the lower back, which could suggest a spontaneous VERTEBRAL COMPRESSION FRACTURE. Low back pain that begins after a fall may indicate a fracture in the BACK, SPINE, or ribs.

In discussing "Low Back Pain," The Merck Manuals Online Medical Library said, "One of the most common causes is muscle and ligament strains and sprains. Strains and sprains may result from lifting, exercising, or moving in an unexpected way (such as when falling or when in a car accident)."

Adult workers especially risk back pain that arises from improperly LIFTING or exceeding LOAD TOLERANCE, but CHILDREN and ADOLESCENTS carry this risk too. For example, young people may not adhere to BACKPACK SAFETY, or they might heap heavy items on a high shelf or participate in contact sports without using safety equipment. Also, skeletal conditions or POSTURE problems can cause low back pain.

As explained by the National Institute of Neurological Disorders and Stroke (NINDS), "Skeletal irregularities produce strain on the vertebrae and supporting muscles, tendons, ligaments, and tissues supported by the spinal column." Similarly, strain on the lumbar spine increases a need for back care during PREGNANCY. Also, heavy men, women, and young people risk the adverse effects WEIGHT can have on the lower back.

Statistics and Studies

An article in *Health* reported, "Northwestern University researchers found that people who experienced lower-back pain for more than a year had up to 11 percent less brain matter in areas responsible for learning, higher thought, and reasoning than those without chronic pain. Our brains do shrink as we grow older, but only by about ½ percent per year." However, "the loss seen in folks with persistent pain is equivalent to what occurs in up to 20 years of normal aging."

To lessen the discomfort and potential damage that pain can cause, the National Institute of Neurological Disorders and Stroke (NINDS) said, "Scientists are examining the use of different drugs to effectively treat back pain, in particular daily pain that has lasted at least 6 months. Other studies are comparing different health care approaches to the management of acute low back pain (standard care versus chiropractic, acupuncture, or massage therapy). These studies are measuring symptom relief, restoration of function, and patient satisfaction. Other research is comparing standard surgical treatments to the most commonly used standard nonsurgical treatments to measure changes in health-related quality of life among patients suffering from spinal stenosis."

Measuring pain levels and developing diagnostic guidelines continue to provide themes for RESEARCH of low back pain. For example, an article in the *Southern Medical Journal* said, "The goal of clinical practice guidelines is to provide busy clinicians with . . . 'best practice' alternatives . . . based on careful evaluation of the evidence. Ideally, clinical practice guidelines focus on common problems with significant morbidity or mortality. Back pain fits this ideal. It is very common, accounting for 200,000 (1.8%) office visits in the United States per year, and since only one fourth of patients with physical symptoms seek medical attention, those presenting for care represent only the tip of the iceberg." While most patients return to their regular daily ACTIVITY in a month, "others incur serious disability and consume substantial health care resources." For example, "20% of claimants having back pain for more than 4 months account for 60% of the back pain health care costs." Unfortunately, however, the article reported that the governmental Agency for Health Research and Quality "guidelines for the management of acute low back pain had a modest impact on physician behavior, increasing the use of acetaminophen and nonsteroidals and decreasing the use of muscle relaxants and physical therapy referrals."

While physicians have reportedly decreased referrals to physical therapists, that group of medical professions has continued to research ways to assist clinicians in decision-making. As explained in "Relationship of Physical Examination Findings and Self-Reported Symptom Severity and Physical Function in Patients with Degenerative Lumbar Conditions" in *Physical Therapy,* "physical therapists use physical examination (PE) procedures routinely when making clinical decisions. Yet, limited data are available to guide the clinical decision-making process." Therefore, "clinicians rely on inductive reasoning, intuition, and evidence to formulate clinical decisions." However, "by identifying subgroups with similar PE findings, clinical researchers can determine which patients are likely to benefit most from a particular intervention."

Similarly, an article in the *Canadian Medical Association Journal* reported, "So-called red flags to identify pain that is specific (i.e., pain in the back originating from tumours, fractures, infections, cauda equina syndrome, visceral pain and systemic disease) account for about 3% of all cases of back pain." However, "the overwhelming majority of back-pain problems are nonspecific. One important feature of nonspecific back pain among workers is that a small proportion of cases (<10%) accounts for most of the costs (>70%). This fact has led investigators to focus on the early identification of patients who are at higher risk of disability, so that specialized interventions can be provided earlier, whereas other patients can be expected to recover with conservative care." Usually though, "potential predictors are often limited to administrative or clinical data, whereas it is clear that back pain is a multidimensional health problem."

Special Aids and Adaptations

Considering the complexity of low back pain, a timely diagnosis and appropriate treatment can be hard to find. To complicate the matter, the best form of therapy depends on the individual person and individual set of circumstances surrounding a particular condition. Although SURGERY provides the primary course of treatment for such emergency conditions as CAUDA EQUINA SYNDROME, spinal tumors, and severe bone fractures, most low back pain can be relieved through NONSTEROIDAL ANTI-INFLAMMATORY DRUG (NSAID) THERAPY, doctor-prescribed EXERCISE, and prescription PAIN RELIEVERS. Other conservative

treatments involve COLD THERAPY, HEAT THERAPY, HYDROTHERAPY, SPINAL MANIPULATION, TRIGGER POINT THERAPY, MASSAGE THERAPY, and BIOFEEDBACK. While not clinically proven to help, time-tested COMPLEMENTARY AND ALTERNATIVE MEDICINE approaches to low back pain, such as ACUPRESSURE, ACUPUNCTURE, HERBAL THERAPY, and HOMEOPATHIC MEDICINE, go back hundreds, sometimes thousands, of years.

To aid healing and protect the back from future problems, the International Association of Fire Fighters adapted these rules: "Stand smart—Maintain a neutral pelvic position. If you must stand for long periods of time, alternate placing your feet on a low footstool to take some of the load off your lower back." Also, "Sit smart—Choose a seat with good lower back support or place a pillow or rolled towel in the small of your back to maintain its normal curve. Keep your knees and hips level." Besides those aids to the joints, "Lift smart—Let your legs do the work. Move straight up and down. Keep your back straight and bend only at the knees. Hold the load close to your body. Avoid lifting and twisting simultaneously." Finally, "Sleep smart—Lie on a firm mattress. Use pillows for support, but don't use a pillow that forces your neck up at a severe angle."

Regarding SLEEP, the article, "Bed Rest or Normal Activity for Patients with Acute Low Back Pain," in *Spine* reported, "For patients with acute low back pain, normal activity is at least equivalent to bed rest. The findings of this study indicate that prescriptions for bed rest, and thus for sick leaves, should be limited when the physical demands of the job are similar to those for daily life activities."

For those who want to stay home or change occupations, an occupational therapist (OT) may help. No, an OT is not in the job-placement business, but the therapist will be apt to notice TENSION held in the lower back because of job dissatisfaction. Also, an OT will investigate ERGONOMIC FACTORS at work then show the patient how to support the spine, keep joints in a neutral position, and utilize time, equipment, and talent well. As information from The American Occupational Therapy Association Web site explained, "Occupational therapists are trained in recognizing both psychological and physical issues that may influence the treatment of back pain. By looking at all factors that could contribute to low back pain, occupational therapists can provide the tools to help people accomplish their daily tasks at work and at leisure activities."

American Association of Neurological Surgeons. "Low Back Pain," AANS. Available online. URL: http://www.neurosurgerytoday.org/what/patient_e/low.asp. Downloaded January 12, 2006.

American Occupational Therapy Association, The. "Tackling Low Back Pain," AOTA. Available online. URL: http://www.aota.org/featured/area6/links/link02bc.asp. Downloaded January 12, 2006.

Dionne, Clermont E., Renee Bourbonnais, Pierre Fremont, Michel Rossignol, Susan R. Stock, Isabelle Larocque. "A Clinical Return-to-work Rule for Patients with Back Pain," *Canadian Medical Association Journal, CMAJ* 172, no. 12 (June 7, 2005): 1,559–1,567.

Humphreys, S. C., J. C. Eck, and S. D. Hodges. "Neuroimaging in Low Back Pain," *American Family Physician* 65, no. 11 (June 2002): 299–306.

International Association of Fire Fighters. "Back Injuries and the Fire Fighter," IAFF. Available online. URL: http://www.iaff.org/safe/content/BackPain/BackPain.htm. Downloaded January 12, 2006.

Jackson, Jeffrey L., M.D. and Robert Browning, M.D. "Impact of National Low *Back Pain* Guidelines on Clinical Practice," *Southern Medical Journal* 98, no. 2 (February 2005): 139–143.

Lyle, Mark A., Sarah Manes, Michael McGuinness, Sarah Ziaei, and Maura D. Iversen. "Relationship of Physical Examination Findings and Self-Reported Symptom Severity and Physical Function in Patients with Degenerative Lumbar Conditions," *Physical Therapy* 85, no. 2 (February 2005): 120–133.

Merck.com. "Low Back Pain," The Merck Manuals Online Medical Library. Available online. URL: http://www.merck.com/mmhe/sec06/ch094/ch094a.html. Downloaded January 12, 2006.

National Institute of Neurological Disorders and Stroke. "Low Back Pain Fact Sheet," National Institutes of Health. Available online. URL: http://www.ninds.nih.gov/disorders/backpain/detail_backpain.htm. Last updated November 23, 2005.

Patel, Atul T., M.D. and Abna A. Ogle, M.D. "Diagnosis and Management of Acute Low Back Pain," *American Family Physician* (March 15, 2000). Available online. URL: http://www.aafp.org/afp/20000315/1779.html. Downloaded January 12, 2006.

Rozenberg, Sylvie, M.D., Cecile Delval, M.D., Yvonne Rezvani, M.D., Nicole Olivieri-Apicella, M.D., Jean-Louis Kuntz, M.D., Eric Legrand, M.D., Jean-Pierre Valat, M.D., Francis Blotman, M.D., Jean Meadeb, Denis Rolland, M.D., Stephanie Hary, M.D., Bernard Duplan, M.D., Jean-Louis Feldmann, M.D., Pierre Bourgeois, M.D. "Bed Rest or Normal Activity for Patients with Acute Low Back Pain: A Randomized Controlled Trial," *Spine* 27, no. 14 (July 15, 2002): 1,487–1,493.

Woodbury, M. A. "Beware the Aching Back," *Health* 19, no. 4 (May 2005): 142.

lumbago　See LOW BACK PAIN.

lumbar disc replacement　See DISC REPLACEMENT.

lumbar epidural steroid injection　See EPIDURAL INJECTION.

lumbar laminectomy　See LAMINECTOMY.

lumbar microdiscectomy　See MICRODISCECTOMY.

lumbar puncture　Commonly known as a spinal tap, a lumbar puncture (LP) provides a diagnostic tool to assess various neurological conditions, such as spinal meningitis or MENINGOCOCCAL DISEASE, that affect the SPINE.

Procedure

An article in *RN* referred to this procedure as a means of, "injecting contrast agents or administering spinal anesthesia. . . . An LP is usually done at the bedside, and involves inserting a needle into the subarachnoid space of the spinal column." Since that space occurs beneath the delicate arachnoid membrane that covers the spinal cord, vital signs must be "monitored continuously for 24 hours," which necessitates a hospital stay.

Risks and Complications

Because a lumbar puncture invades the sensitive arachnoid membrane, patients encounter a very small but, nevertheless, dangerous risk of developing ARACHNOIDITIS. A more likely development after an LP is a headache, which an article in *European Neurology* called "trivial and usually self-limited. However, there are other less common but serious complications that physicians should bear in mind whenever they perform this procedure." For instance, the article mentioned potential leakage of spinal fluids and also a risk of blood clots, the latter of which "should not be considered a benign condition, since up to 44% of them may become complicated with progressive deterioration of consciousness and life-threatening symptoms," requiring surgical removal. Regarding the LP itself, the article concluded, "Although it is not usually a dangerous procedure, clinicians should keep in mind that it should be performed only when necessary."

Outlook and Lifestyle Modifications

An article from MedicineNet.com said, "Headaches occur less frequently when the patient remains lying flat 1–3 hours after the procedure." More importantly, "LP can provide lifesaving information." For example, "spinal fluid obtained from the lumbar puncture can be used to diagnose many important diseases such as bleeding around the brain; increased pressure from hydrocephalus; inflammation of the brain, spinal cord, or adjacent tissues (encephalitis, meningitis); tumors of brain or spinal cord, etc. Sometimes spinal fluid can indicate diseases of the immune system, such as multiple sclerosis."

Beanie Dulak, Sally. "Lumbar Puncture," *RN* 68, no. 6 (June 2005): 36–39.

Martin-Millan, M., J. L. Hernandez, P. Matorras, A. Oterino, and J. Gonzalez-Macias. "Multiple Subdural Haematomas following Lumbar Puncture," *European Neurology* 53, no. 3 (2005): 159–160.

MedicineNet.com. "Lumbar Puncture (LP)." Available online. URL: http://www.medicinenet.com/lumbar_puncture/article.htm. Downloaded January 18, 2006.

lumbar radiculopathy   This type of LOW BACK PAIN radiates with SCIATICA and often causes numbness or weakness in the lower part of the body.

Symptoms and Diagnostic Path

To assess RANGE OF MOTION and strength, a physical examination focuses on the LUMBAR SPINE and legs. As an article for SpineUniverse said, "You may be asked to stand, walk or lie down on the exam table during the physical examination. In a lying position, your physician will raise each of your legs to demonstrate flexibility and strength in your low back and legs." The specific symptoms and location of pain also aid a diagnosis. For example, nerve involvement of the second VERTEBRA in the lumbar region (L2) may lessen the strength in the hip. Spinal nerve involvement at L3 may lessen reflexes in the knee, whereas L4 will be more likely to cause a sensory loss in the foot. L5 may have that effect, too, but that level can also affect the large toe with pain felt down the side of the leg. Conversely, the S1 SACRAL VERTEBRA may affect the little toe with "pain down the back of the leg into the bottom or side of the foot."

Besides a medical history, the doctor may request X-RAYS to evaluate the condition of the vertebrae and MAGNETIC RESONANCE IMAGING to assess the DISCS and other soft tissue.

Treatment Options and Outlook

An article posted by the Spine Center of the University of Rochester Medical Center said, "In most cases, surgery is offered after physical therapy, rest, and medications have failed to adequately relieve the symptoms of pain, numbness and weakness over a period of time." More commonly, treatment requires "bed rest for 48 hours, occasionally up to 7 days." Other conservative treatments include physical therapy and NONSTEROIDAL ANTI-INFLAMMATORY DRUG (NSAID) THERAPY. Occasionally, steroids, an EPIDURAL INJECTION or SPINAL INJECTION may be used to relieve inflammation or pain. Depending on the causal factor, an ORTHOTIC back brace or lumbar support may be prescribed, but only for temporary support.

Risk Factors and Preventive Measures

Again, the underlying condition must be addressed to assess both the risks and the means of prevention. For most patients, doctor-recommended EXERCISE will help. Whether those exercises provide RESISTANCE TRAINING, STRENGTH TRAINING, or a means of improving flexibility depends on the cause and severity of the condition.

Skelton, Alta. "Lumbar Radiculopathy," SpineUniverse. Available online. URL: http://www.spineuniverse.com/displayarticle.php/article1469.html. Last updated June 20, 2005.

Strong Health. "Lumbar Radiculopathy," Orthopaedics, Spine Center, University of Rochester Medical Center. Available online. URL: http://www.stronghealth.com/services/orthopaedics/spinecenter/backcare/lumbar.cfm. Downloaded January 10, 2006.

lumbar spinal fusion A type of ARTHRODESIS, lumbar fusion surgery may be needed if conventional medicine and COMPLEMENTARY AND ALTERNATIVE MEDICINE fail to alleviate LOW BACK PAIN or weakness and numbness in the lower limbs. SCIATICA may be the most common reason for spinal fusion, but the procedure can also be used to treat SPONDYLOLISTHESIS, DEGENERATIVE DISC DISEASE, and less frequently, ARTHRITIS. A lumbar spinal fusion can also address FAILED BACK SURGERY SYNDROME and other causes of instability in the LUMBAR SPINE. With the use of an autologous BONE GRAFT from the patient's own body and BONE MORPHOGENETIC PROTEIN (BMP) to encourage new bone growth, spinal fusion eventually stops movement in painful segments of VERTEBRAE, thus making the spine more stable but less flexible.

An online article posted by the North American Spine Society (NASS) explained, "The ultimate goal of fusion is to obtain a solid union between two or more vertebrae. Fusion may or may not involve use of supplemental hardware (instrumentation) such as plates, screws and cages. Instrumentation is sometimes used to correct a deformity, but usually is just used as an internal splint to hold the vertebrae together while the bone grafts heal."

After referring to autologous bone grafts as the "gold-standard material for achieving successful spinal fusions," an international group of researchers reported in the *Journal of Neurosurgery: Spine,* "Nevertheless, attempts at arthrodesis of the lumbar spine, even when performed using an autologous bone graft, result in a failure of fusion . . . in 5 to 35% of patients." Also, the use of devices that

aid "spinal fusion by applying rigid internal fixation thus far has failed to eradicate the incidence of nonunion." Since the whole point of the procedure is to get the vertebrae to unite, fuse, and hold, BMP helps to enhance the process by speeding up formation of new bone tissue.

Procedure

In writing for Spine-health, Dr. Peter F. Ullrich Jr. described four types of lumbar spinal fusion, each of which involves a slightly different method or approach. For example, one "surgical approach to the spine is from the back through a midline incision that is approximately three inches to six inches long. . . . This type of spinal fusion, which involves placing bone graft in . . . a region just outside the spine . . . , has a long history and is considered by many surgeons to be the 'tried and true' method of spinal fusion." However, "the principal risk of this type of low back surgery is that a solid fusion will not be obtained (nonunion) and further surgery to re-fuse the spine may be necessary. Nonunion rates of between 10% and 40% have been quoted in the medical literature."

Another option involves a similar incision in the back but "achieves spinal fusion in the low back by inserting a bone graft and/or spinal implant (e.g. cage) directly into the disc space." This procedure involves a LAMINECTOMY, but "not as much of the disc space can be removed with a posterior approach (from the back.)" In a frontal or anterior approach to lumbar fusion, the procedure "is similar to the posterior lumbar interbody fusion . . . , except that . . . the disc space is fused by approaching the spine through the abdomen instead of through the lower back." With a three- to five-inch incision made on the left side of the abdomen, the nearness of large blood vessels in the legs adds to the surgical risks. Therefore, some procedures add endoscopy for MINIMALLY INVASIVE SURGERY that reduces the size of surgical incision. However, Dr. Ullrich cautioned, "The endoscopic approach has more limited visualization, and it usually leads to larger surgical times and carries with it a much higher technical learning curve for the surgeon." Despite the increased risks, an advantage is that "both the back muscles and nerves remain undisturbed. Another advantage is that placing the bone graft in the front of the spine places it in compression, and bone in compression tends to fuse better."

Finally, lumbar fusion can combine front and back approaches. As Dr. Ullrich explained, "This anterior/posterior lumbar fusion procedure is usually done for patients with a high degree of spinal instability (e.g. fractures), or in revision surgery (if the initial fusion did not set up), although some spine surgeons do prefer the anterior/posterior fusion surgery as a primary spinal fusion technique." Fusing the front and the back of the vertebrae produces the greatest stability with about a 95 percent success rate. However, "a drawback of the procedure is that both an anterior incision in the abdomen and a posterior incision in the low back need to be done."

Risks and Complications

In an article for SpineUniverse, Dr. Todd Albert said, "As with any operation, there are risks involved with spine fusion surgery. Some patients may develop a distended abdomen and may not be able to eat. If this happens, a special tube may be inserted to relieve the distension." Although rare, some patients may not respond well to an antibiotic given to avoid infection, while others may develop urinary tract problems or a potentially dangerous blood clot. Also, "some patients may continue to have pain at the bone graft donor site. If the fusion does not heal, (a condition known as pseudoarthrosis) the instrumentation, such as rods, screws, hooks, may break, and further surgery may be required. People who smoke are at a higher risk for pseudoarthrosis complications."

The risk of a failed fusion increases for patients who previously had SURGERY in the same area. As Dr. Albert explained, "Revision surgery often involves correcting a deformity caused by a previously failed back surgery, breakage of instrumentation or pseudoarthrosis. The type of revision depends on the problem. The procedure may include operating on both the front and back of the spine. The incidence of complications from revision lumbar spine fusion surgery is higher than in first-time procedures. It is also more difficult to relieve pain and restore nerve function in revision surgery. Patients should be aware that the chance of having long-term spinal pain is increased."

Outlook and Lifestyle Modifications

After surgery, deep-breathing exercises will be encouraged, but smoking assuredly will not. Since motion must remain limited for three months, patients will be instructed on ways to move without straining the lower back. Short walks in the hospital hallway begin regular ACTIVITY that can gradually increase each day. For about a month though, patients should not drive a car nor lift heavy objects. During the postoperative visit four to six weeks after lumbar fusion, the doctor may recommend EXERCISE and physical therapy to strengthen PARASPINAL MUSCLES and keep the spine flexible.

As the NASS cautioned, "Recovery following fusion surgery is generally longer than for other types of spinal surgery. . . . It also takes longer to return to a normal active lifestyle after spinal fusion than many other types of surgery. This is because you must wait until your surgeon sees evidence of bone healing. The fusion process varies in each patient as the body heals and incorporates the bone graft to solidly fuse the vertebrae together. The healing process after fusion surgery is very similar to that after a bone fracture. In general, the earliest evidence of bone healing is not apparent on X-ray until at least six weeks following surgery. During this time, the patient's activity is generally restricted. Substantial bone healing does not usually take place until three or four months after surgery. At that time activities may be increased, although continued evidence of bone healing and remodeling may continue for up to a year after surgery." Since lumbar fusion decreases the RANGE OF MOTION, this "can put added strain on the vertebrae above and below the fusion. Fortunately, once a fusion has healed it rarely, if ever, breaks down."

Albert, Todd, M.D. "Understanding Lumbar Fusion Surgery," SpineUniverse. Available online. URL: http://www.spineuniverse.com/displayarticle.php/article1562.html. Last updated December 12, 2005.

Hasharoni, Amir, M.D., Yoram Zilberman, M.D., Gadi Turgeman, M.D., Gregory A. Helm, M.D., Meir Liebergall, M.D., and Dan Gazit, M.D. "Murine Spinal Fusion Induced by Engineered Mesenchymal Stem Cells that Conditionally Express Bone Morphogenetic Protein-2," *Journal of Neurosurgery: Spine* 3, no. 1 (July 2005): 47–52.

North American Spine Society. "Spinal Fusion Surgery," NASS. Available online. URL: http://www.spine.org/articles/spinalfusion.cfm. Downloaded January 18, 2006.

Ullrich, Peter F. Jr., M.D. "Lumbar Spinal Fusion Surgery," Spine-health.com. Available online. URL: http://www.spine-health.com/topics/surg/overview/lumbar/lumb05.html. Updated January 20, 2004.

lumbar spinal stenosis   See SPINAL STENOSIS.

lumbar spine   Better known as the lower back, the lumbar spine offers a familiar site for BACKACHE and LOW BACK PAIN. Anatomically speaking, this portion of the spinal column consists of five VERTEBRAE numbered L1 through L5. Some individuals may have a sixth lumbar bone labeled L6, which may actually be part of the SACRAL VERTEBRAE. Regardless of the number, vertebrae come well-padded with DISCS. In addition to that cushy effect, strengthening occurs through knobby aspects that protrude on either side of each vertebra then connect to create facet joints.

In describing the lumbar spine, Dr. Stewart G. Eidelson said, "The vertebrae and discs are held together by groups of ligaments. Ligaments connect bone to bone, whereas tendons connect muscle to bone. In the spine, tendons connect muscles to the vertebrae. The ligaments and tendons help to stabilize the spine and guard against excessive movement in any one direction." That stability not only keeps a person upright and mobile, but protects the spinal cord that runs through vertebrae in the spinal column. Whether the vertebrae are located in the CERVICAL SPINE, THORACIC SPINE, or lumbar, "small nerve roots branch off from the spinal cord through spaces between each vertebra and extend out into the entire body. The spinal cord and the nerves are part of the central nervous system that includes the brain. The nerves are the body's neural message system."

As a Back.com article explained, "The true spinal cord ends at approximately the L1 level, where it divides into many different nerve roots that travel to the lower body and legs. This collection of nerve roots is called the 'cauda equina,' which means horse's tail and describes the continuation of the nerve roots at the end of the spinal cord."

Besides providing this avenue for CAUDA EQUINA SYNDROME, Back.com said, "The lumbar vertebrae, L1–L5, are most frequently involved in back pain because these vertebrae carry the most amount of body weight and are subject to the largest forces and stresses along the spine."

Risks and Complications

In discussing the anatomy of the lumbar spine, The Mount Sinai Medical Center reviewed these risks: "Low back pain is a very common complaint for a simple reason. Since the lumbar spine is connected to your pelvis, this is where most of your weight bearing and body movement takes place. Typically, this is where people tend to place too much pressure, such as: lifting up a heavy box, twisting to move a heavy load, or carrying a heavy object. Such repetitive injuries can lead to damage to the parts of the lumbar spine." This damage may include HERNIATED DISC, FACET JOINT DISORDER, and even a FRACTURE.

Complications in the lumbar spine begin prior to birth with GENETIC FACTORS, such as DWARFISM, that can affect the lower back. At delivery, INFANTS may exhibit BIRTH DEFECTS OF THE SPINE, such as LORDOSIS or SCOLIOSIS. Although problems with POSTURE usually arise later, newborns may have frail or weakened bones, such as occurs with OSTEOGENESIS IMPERFECTA. If the mother had insufficient FOLIC ACID prior to pregnancy, a newborn may have SPINA BIFIDA. Later, other factors related to NUTRITION, such as CALCIUM intake or VITAMIN D, can increasingly affect bone strength.

Even with healthy vertebrae, injuries cause spinal concerns for ATHLETES, CHILDREN, and ADOLESCENTS. During periods of growth, young spines can be particularly vulnerable in exceeding LOAD TOLERANCE or forgetting BACKPACK SAFETY. Teenaged and adult workers untrained in proper methods of LIFTING may be especially prone to injury. In addition, ELDERLY persons or OSTEOPOROSIS patients can sustain VERTEBRAL COMPRESSION FRACTURES simply by bearing the weight of their own bodies.

Statistics and Studies

RESEARCH often tests the outer limits of load tolerance by loading the lumbar spine with mechanical devices or external force. As an article in the *Journal of Rehabilitation Research & Development* said, "For a full understanding of the mechanical response of the spine . . . , measuring the forces and the movements produced simultaneously is essential." Also, medical staff may measure the movements or rotation in the hips to indicate spinal stiffness, but "in future studies, researchers may employ the present method to study various factors that may affect the bending stiffness of the spine—for instance, breathing and muscular contraction."

Special Aids and Adaptations

To aid the lumbar spine, adequate nutrition, adequate daily ACTIVITY, adequate fresh water intake, adequate EXERCISE, and adequate SLEEP are needed. Throughout life, though, the lower back must constantly adapt to changing conditions, inside the body and out. For most people, ongoing aid comes by adapting a lifestyle to a simple adage: be kind to the spine.

Eidelson, Stewart G., M.D. "Lumbar Spine," SpineUniverse. Available online. URL: http://www.spineuniverse.com/displayarticle.php/article1394.html. Last updated June 30, 2005.

Lee, Raymond Y. W., Bonnie Y. S. Tsung, Pin Tong, and John Evans. "Bending Stiffness of the Lumbar Spine Subjected to Posteroanterior Manipulative Force," *Journal of Rehabilitation Research & Development* 42, no. 2 (March/April 2005): 167–174.

Medtronic Sofamor Danek. "Lumbar Spine," Back.com. Available online. URL: http://www.back.com/anatomy-lumbar.html. Last updated March 17, 2005.

Mount Sinai Medical Center, The. "Anatomy: The Parts of Your Spine and How They Work," Orthopaedic Spine Surgery at Mount Sinai. Available online. URL: http://www.mountsinai.org/msh/msh_frame.jsp?url=clinical_services/orthospine_lbp.htm#Anatomy. Downloaded January 12, 2006.

magnesium   Craving chocolate may signal a need for magnesium. Of course, it can also mean a person really likes chocolate. Either way, people in the United States seldom have a magnesium deficiency. Low levels of this essential nutrient, the fourth highest ranking mineral in the body, can be detrimental to the BACK, SPINE, and health in general.

According to the Office of Dietary Supplements at the National Institutes of Health (NIH), "Magnesium is needed for more than 300 biochemical reactions in the body. It helps maintain normal muscle and nerve function, keeps heart rhythm steady, supports a healthy immune system, and keeps bones strong. Magnesium also helps regulate blood sugar levels, promotes normal blood pressure, and is known to be involved in energy metabolism and protein synthesis."

Half of the magnesium in the body can be found in the bones with about 49 percent in organ and tissue cells. The remaining 1 percent sails through the bloodstream as the whole body strives to maintain MINERAL BALANCE. Alcohol consumption tips that scale as can some medications and supplements, such as ZINC and VITAMIN D.

If something interferes with magnesium absorption, low levels of the mineral can cause high levels of TENSION. In addition, the NIH said, "Early signs of magnesium deficiency include loss of appetite, nausea, vomiting, fatigue, and weakness. As magnesium deficiency worsens, numbness, tingling, muscle contractions and cramps, seizures, personality changes, abnormal heart rhythms, and coronary spasms can occur." Furthermore, "severe magnesium deficiency can result in low levels of calcium in the blood (hypocalcemia). Magnesium deficiency is also associated with low levels of potassium in the blood." Eventually, a mineral imbalance can affect the strength and quality of VERTEBRAE and

other bones, but a diet balanced well with CALCIUM, VITAMIN E, and VITAMIN B-COMPLEX aids magnesium uptake and, thus, helps to avoid mineral imbalances and deficiencies.

Dosage and Potential Side Effects

Dark chocolate may taste best, but other dietary sources provide more magnesium and more NUTRITION too. For example, shellfish, bananas, apricots, watermelon, uncooked English peas, almonds, and other types of nuts offer a tasty variety of magnesium-rich foods. Dark green vegetables, such as kale, mustard greens, or collards, also provide an excellent source, mainly because magnesium is to chlorophyll what IRON is to the blood. Straight from the tap, hard water delivers more magnesium than soft water, but bottled water may have none. Some types of filtering and softening systems completely remove this vital mineral, whereas Epsom salts add too much.

A case report in the *Southern Medical Journal (SMJ)* discussed a fatal incident in which a seven-year-old boy had been given an Epsom salt enema. Since "Epsom salt is essentially 100% magnesium sulfate," the article warned, "this is a considerable amount, considering that the recommended daily allowance for an adult is only 300 to 400 mg per day." Therefore, "because of the possibility of toxicity, the use of Epsom salt enemas should be discouraged. Rectal absorption of magnesium can be significant and difficult to predict, leading to toxic levels, even in patients with normal renal function."

To avoid toxicity, natural foods high in magnesium and other vital nutrients provide the safest sources unless, of course, a person has food allergies. For those who take supplements, the Recommended Daily Allowance (RDA) for CHILDREN one to three is 80 mg, while four- to eight-year-olds need

130 mg each day. For nine- to 13-year-old ADOLESCENTS, the RDA is 240 mg. Males from 14 through the ELDERLY adult years need about 400 mg daily. Although women usually require less magnesium than men, their RDA of around 300 mg increases during pregnancy and lactation.

Statistics and Studies

Reporting on a study presented by the *Journal of the American Geriatrics Society,* a News-Medical.net article said, "Over 2,000 black and white men and women ages 70–79 years old were asked to complete a questionnaire to determine how much magnesium they were receiving from food and various supplements." After incorporating BONE MINERAL DENSITY TESTS into the RESEARCH, "the study revealed that those who ingested more magnesium had significantly higher bone density than those who got the least amount of magnesium. For every 100 milligram per day increase in magnesium intake, data showed a 1% increase in bone density. . . . However, this link was only true for the older white men and women. Previous research has demonstrated that black men and women may process vitamin D and other calcium regulating hormones differently than whites, thus possibly explaining the lack of association between magnesium and bone density among them in this study."

News-Medical.net. "Magnesium for Stronger Bones," Medical Research News. Available online. URL: http://www.news-medical.net/?id=15170. Posted January 5, 2006.

Office of Dietary Supplements, National Institutes of Health. "Magnesium," NIH Clinical Center. Available online. URL: http://ods.od.nih.gov/factsheets/magnesium.asp. Downloaded January 27, 2006.

Tofil, Nancy M., M.D., Kim W. Benner, and Margaret K. Winkler, M. D. "Fatal Hypermagnesemia Caused by an Epsom Salt Enema: a Case Illustration," *Southern Medical Journal* 98, no. 2 (February 2005): 253–256.

magnetic resonance imaging (MRI)   This newer type of imaging test takes longer and can be more expensive than an X-RAY, but magnetic resonance imaging exposes neither hard nor soft tissue to radiation. Like X-rays, an MRI pictures bones in the BACK and SPINE. Unlike X-rays though, an MRI shows soft tissue too.

Information from the Spine Institute of New York Web site said, "One of the most advanced diagnostic imaging methods available, the MRI provides detailed information about the body and is often used to evaluate the spine." For example, an MRI helps to diagnose DEGENERATIVE DISC DISEASE, a HERNIATED DISC, KYPHOSIS, SCIATICA, SCOLIOSIS, SPINAL TUMOR, SPINAL INFECTION, or other conditions "in which the anatomy of the spine and its soft tissues need to be seen clearly." For a VERTEBRAL COMPRESSION FRACTURE, though, COMPUTED TOMOGRAPHY (CT or CAT) SCAN may be used, whereas the condition of the SPINAL CORD may best be seen with a CT scan following MYELOGRAPHY. Unlike a myelogram, an MRI is not invasive. As with most MEDICAL TESTS for the spine, patients must not move during an MRI but often feel as if they have been inserted into a giant thermos bottle.

Procedure

In describing an MRI for the University of Michigan Health System Web site, Dr. Pierre Rouzier said, "You lie down on a cushioned bed that moves into a tunnel-shaped magnet that is open on both ends. If you get nervous when you are in small closed spaces you should talk to your health care provider about this before you have your MRI. He or she may be able to give you a medicine that will help you feel less nervous." During this confining but painless procedure, "you will hear loud knocking and a whirring sound while the pictures are being taken. You will wear earplugs or music will be provided so that the noise doesn't sound so loud." Usually, an MRI takes less than an hour, during which time the person must remain still.

According to the Radiological Society of North America (RSNA), "a typical MRI exam includes two to six imaging sequences, which produce sectional views or 'slices' of the spine in different planes: left to right, front to back, upper to lower. The sections are often about a quarter-inch apart, providing a detailed look at the tissues making up the spinal column. The images may be stored in a computer and subsequently viewed on screen, or they may be printed on film much like a conventional x-ray. Depending on the location of symptoms, you probably will have only part of your spine imaged: the cervical (neck) portion, the thoracic (chest) spine or the lumbar (lower) spine."

Risks and Complications

Since an MRI utilizes magnetic fields to provide images, patients with a cardiac pacemaker and women in the first trimester of pregnancy should avoid this test. Also, any metal items or metallic fragments in and around the body can cause problems. Some patients experience a panic attack inside the tube, but they must remain still since movement blurs the images. If the imagery needs enhancement to provide sharper detail, the patient may be given gadolinium, which can trigger an allergic reaction, although this rarely occurs.

Outlook and Lifestyle Modifications

An MRI can help a physician or orthopedic team to identify spinal conditions and determine future treatments. As an example, the RSNA said, "MRI is able to detect subtle changes in the vertebral column that may be an early stage of infection or tumor. The procedure may be better than CT scanning for evaluating tumors, abscesses and other masses near the spinal cord." Since an MRI also helps to monitor diseases and disorders already diagnosed in the back or spine, the first test can provide a baseline with follow-up tests to show the progression or, preferably, successful treatment of that condition.

RadiologyInfo™. "Magnetic Resonance Imaging (MRI)— Spine," Radiological Society of North America, Inc. (RSNA). Available online. URL: http://www.radiology info.org/content/spinemr.htm. Last reviewed August 2, 2005.

Rouzier, Pierre, M.D., for McKesson Provider Technologies. "Magnetic Resonance Imaging (MRI)," University of Michigan Health System. Available online. URL: http:// www.med.umich.edu/1libr/sma/sma_mriimage_sma. htm. Last modified April 11, 2005.

Spine Institute of New York. "Magnetic Resonance Imaging (MRI)," Beth Israel Medical Center. Available online. URL: http://www.spineinstituteny.com/conditions/mri. html. Downloaded January 27, 2006.

magnetic therapy   The pull of a magnet directs a compass and commonly keeps a calendar or crayon drawing from falling off a refrigerator. In centuries past though, people used this present form of COMPLEMENTARY AND ALTERNATIVE MEDICINE to pull PAIN from the body or an iron nail from the foot. This typically involved a magnetic object with a static field of energy. Once electricity had been harnessed, however, inert objects could be charged and electromagnets produced.

Currently, magnets draw big businesses with big claims investigated by the U.S. Food and Drug Administration (FDA). For example, information from the FDA Center for Devices and Radiological Health said, "Magnets marketed with medical claims are considered to be medical devices because they are promoted to treat a medical condition or to affect the structure or function of the body. The law requires that manufacturers of medical devices, including magnets intended for medical use, obtain marketing clearance for their products from the Food and Drug Administration (FDA) before they may offer them for sale. This helps protect the public health by ensuring that new medical devices are shown to be either safe and effective or substantially equivalent to other devices already legally marketed in this country." However, "to date, the FDA has not cleared for marketing any magnets promoted for medical uses. Because these devices do not have marketing clearance, they are in violation of the law, and are subject to regulatory action. Action is taken on a case by case basis depending on the significance of the medical claims being made." For example, some companies laud magnets as a way to treat CHRONIC PAIN in such conditions as ARTHRITIS or RHEUMATISM. Others rely on magnets to stimulate the nerves.

While magnet therapies may be poles apart, all magnets draw iron in some form or another. Presumably, this can be IRON in blood and body cells or iron in the fragment of a weapon lodged in the BACK. Regarding the various types and power of magnets used for treatments, the National Center for Complementary and Alternative Medicine (NCCAM) said, "Magnets come in different strengths, most often measured in units called gauss (G). For comparison purposes, the Earth has a magnetic field of about 0.5 G; refrigerator magnets range from 35 to 200 G; magnets marketed for the treatment of pain are usually 300 to 5,000 G; and MRI (magnetic resonance imaging) machines widely used to diagnose medical conditions noninvasively produce up to 200,000 G."

Procedure

With the notable exception of MAGNETIC RESONANCE IMAGING (MRI), used to diagnose and monitor conditions of the SPINE, most magnets have been designed for home use. Often, these treatments merely require a person to put on an object or lie down since some manufacturers insert static magnet disks into SHOE inserts or mattress pads. Another type of magnet therapy draws arthritis patients to the jewelry store where they fasten on a bracelet to unclasp the pain. While the effectiveness of that ancient practice remains dubious, the NCCAM said, "There are some uses of electromagnets within conventional medicine. For example, scientists have found that electromagnets can be used to speed the healing of bone fractures that are not healing well. Even more commonly, electromagnets are used to map areas of the brain. However, most uses of magnets by consumers in attempts to treat pain are considered CAM, because they have not been scientifically proven and are not part of the practice of conventional medicine."

With further studies needed, static magnets and electromagnets have both been used to treat a variety of conditions, such as NECK PAIN, LOW BACK PAIN, SLEEP problems, pain of POST-POLIO SYNDROME, and the pain of FLEXION-EXTENSION INJURIES. Sometimes results sound promising, but they usually come with mixed reviews.

Risks and Complications

Pregnant women, people with pacemakers or metallic inserts of any kind, and patients who receive medication through a skin patch should avoid magnetic therapies. Anyone with a bad SPRAIN, open wound, SPINAL INFECTION, or other type of inflammation should exercise caution too. In most cases, magnets cause no complications except for the money spent on a treatment that may not work. Also, anyone who "feels weird" after magnetic therapy should resist the pull of this treatment.

Outlook and Lifestyle Modifications

To experiment with magnets, patients might investigate the criteria for participating in a CLINICAL TRIAL. Meanwhile, the NCCAM offered this advice: "In the studies that did find benefits from magnetic therapy, many have shown those benefits very quickly. This suggests that if a magnet does work, it should not take very long for the user to start noticing the effect. Therefore, people may wish to purchase magnets with a 30-day return policy and return the product if they do not get satisfactory results within 1 to 2 weeks."

Center for Devices and Radiological Health. "Magnets," CDRH Consumer Information, U.S. Food and Drug Administration. Available online. URL: http://www.fda.gov/cdrh/consumer/magnets.html. Last updated March 1, 2000.

National Center for Complementary and Alternative Medicine. "Questions and Answers About Using Magnets To Treat Pain," NCCAM, National Institutes of Health. Available online. URL: http://nccam.nih.gov/health/magnet/magnet.htm. Last modified January 31, 2006.

marble bone disease See OSTEOPETROSIS.

Marfan syndrome Some people think Abraham Lincoln exhibited symptoms of this connective tissue disorder. Regardless, GENETIC FACTORS undoubtedly caused the loose, lanky appearance characteristic of Marfan syndrome.

Symptoms and Diagnostic Path

Wobbly joints, exceptionally long limbs, and a slim build commonly mark this disorder. As online information from Holy Cross Hospital explained, "Connective tissues hold other body tissues together and provide support for many structures in the body."

Marfan syndrome often affects the eyes, lungs, and heart, but its effects on the BACK include curvature of the SPINE, weakened PARASPINAL MUSCLES, and LOW BACK PAIN. Reportedly, one in 5,000 to 10,000 people in the United States have the disorder, but a diagnosis can be difficult to obtain. With no laboratory test to confirm Marfan syndrome, a physician relies on a physical examination, eye examination, medical history, and tests using ultrasound.

Treatment Options and Outlook

According to The National Marfan Foundation (NMF), "Aspects of the skeleton that are unique in individuals with the Marfan syndrome are differences in the growth of bone and decreased ligamentous support. There is great variability among people who are affected with the disorder in the severity of these manifestations. In only about one-third of people with the Marfan syndrome do these orthopedic concerns become severe enough to see an orthopedic doctor." Besides KYPHOSIS, SCOLIOSIS, or other problems with POSTURE, "Some people with the Marfan syndrome have aches and pains in the back, arms, legs or feet. These can be partially prevented by keeping in good physical condition with regular exercise (four or five times per week) that does not stress the aorta, applying ice or heat, stretching or taking a mild analgesic (such as Tylenol®) in accordance with a doctor's recommendation."

Risk Factors and Preventive Measures

The National Center for Biotechnical Information said, "Beta blockers have been used to control some of the cardiovascular symptoms of Marfan syndrome; however, they are not effective against the skeletal and ocular problems, which can also be serious."

In discussing those skeletal concerns, the NMF said, "Treatment is sometimes recommended because scoliosis can cause many problems, including back pain, decreased lung function, and posture and shape disturbances. A child with scoliosis should have his or her back checked one or two times per year. An adult with scoliosis should have it examined every one to three years. If the curve is increasing and is more than 20°, some treatment, such as a back brace, "is usually recommended in growing children and adolescents because exercise alone will not prevent a curve from progressing." For all ages of Marfan patients, special SHOES and other ORTHOTICS may help. In general, therapeutic EXERCISE can be strengthening.

Alan, Rick. "Marfan Syndrome," Holy Cross Hospital. Available online. URL: http://healthychoice.epnet.com/GetContent.asp?siteid=holycross&docid=/dci/marfan. Downloaded January 27, 2006.

Genes and Disease. "Marfan Syndrome," National Center for Biotechnical Information (NCBI), U.S. National Library of Medicine. Available online. URL: http://www.ncbi.nlm.nih.gov/books/bv.fcgi?call=bv.View.ShowSection&rid=gnd.section.247. Downloaded January 27, 2006.

National Marfan Foundation, The. "Orthopedic Concerns," NMF. Available online. URL: http://www.marfan.org/nmf/GetSubContentRequestHandler.do?sub_menu_item_content_id=8&menu_item_id=42. Downloaded January 27, 2006.

Marie-Strumpell disease   See ANKYLOSING SPONDYLITIS.

massage therapy   Long before Hippocrates avowed, "First, do no harm," medical texts in China referred to the therapeutic value of massage. Doctors and nurses in the United States treated patients with massages, too, until that practice ended in the early 20th century. Today, SPINAL MANIPULATION rates the highest among people who try various forms of COMPLEMENTARY AND ALTERNATIVE MEDICINE (CAM) treatments, but most CAM patients, including INFANTS, welcome a good massage.

Reporting the results of a survey on massage therapy, an online article in *BMC Complementary and Alternative Medicine* said, "Visits to massage therapists were for a limited number of conditions. About 60% of visits were for musculoskeletal symptoms, particularly back, neck, and shoulder symptoms. Visits for 'wellness' (i.e., relaxation) accounted for another 20% of visits and mental health concerns, largely anxiety and depression, for another 6 to 9% of visits. Virtually all other visits were for general body symptoms (mostly generalized pain) or 'nervous system' symptoms (most commonly headache)." With massage typically sought for CHRONIC PAIN in the BACK or CERVICAL SPINE, "virtually all visits included a massage that emphasized at least two techniques. The most commonly emphasized techniques were Swedish massage, deep tissue, and trigger point/pressure point techniques."

Procedure

Since newborns and older babies require unique considerations, a separate entry addresses INFANT

MASSAGE THERAPY, which pertains to young CHIL-DREN too. For ADOLESCENTS through ELDERLY adults, massage may also begin at home.

The *Consumer Reports on Health* article, "Handy Techniques You Can Learn," focused on five basic but "relatively gentle" techniques used in Swedish massage. With mineral oil or other skin lubricant to reduce the friction, a massage begins and ends with a technique known as effleurage. As the article instructed, "Using the palms and fingers, glide slowly and rhythmically across the skin, applying light to moderate pressure. Push toward the heart when working on arms and legs." For friction massage, the fingertips are used to "apply deep, circular movements near joints and on either side of the spine. Manipulate one spot at a time, focusing on the underlying muscles or tendons, without sliding over the skin." With the petrissage technique, the motion resembles kneading bread dough, whereas tapotement taps like a drum with the palms or edges of the hands striking "firmly but not hard enough to cause any discomfort." Finally, a vibration technique applies "firm, trembling pressure with the fingertips, palms, or both."

Risks and Complications

The *Consumer Reports On Health* article cautioned, "The more vigorous the massage, the greater the potential for harm, especially for people with weak bones or skin problems. And hot oils containing wintergreen or capsaicin, which are used by some massage therapists, can cause blistering and possible infection." Since perfumes frequently bother sensitive people, the safest choice of lubricants may be grapeseed oil, olive oil, or other liquid vegetable oil the person normally uses for cooking.

The *BMC Complementary and Alternative Medicine* reported, "In the US alone an estimated 113 million visits were made to massage therapists in 1997, suggesting that serious adverse experiences due to massage are extremely rare." After reviewing case reports to ascertain general safety, the researchers said, "Only 3 reports (including 7 cases) described adverse effects that were probably attributable to treatments by massage therapists practicing Western forms of massage." For example, deep tissue massage produced a blood clot, whereas neck massage affected hearing with "three additional reports

of adverse events associated with shiatsu" on the neck. Yet, "despite these scattered reports of adverse experiences, common forms of massage (e.g., Swedish, deep tissue, and neuromuscular) are considered very low risk, especially when massage is tailored appropriately to the individual (e.g., possible pressure or anatomic site restrictions), as massage therapists are commonly trained to do." However, patients "with deep vein thrombosis should not receive massage to the lower extremities."

Burn victims and anyone with skin problems or wounds should avoid massage therapy altogether. Massage can also be risky for patients with a bone FRACTURE or bones weakened by such conditions as OSTEOPOROSIS and OSTEOGENESIS IMPERFECTA. Mild complications, such as dryness or queasiness, may arise from dehydration after a massage, but lots of water or a glass of pineapple juice can ease that concern and assist the natural detoxification process that typically occurs in the body. Also, all patients risk bruising at the untrained hands of a careless masseuse, but usually, bruises develop simply because the person refrained from saying, "Ouch!"

Outlook and Lifestyle Modifications

The article "Massage Treatment for Back Pain" in the *British Medical Journal (BMJ)* addressed the outcome and outlook to expect. As the article explained, "The mechanical action of the hands on cutaneous and subcutaneous structures" on and beneath the skin "is believed to enhance circulation of blood and lymph resulting in increased supply of oxygen and removal of waste products or mediators of pain. Certain massage techniques have been shown to increase the threshold for pain and reduce muscular tone. Most importantly perhaps, a massage can relax the mind and reduce anxiety, which may affect the perception of pain positively."

An article in *Holistic Nursing Practice* reported the results of a study on "Massage Therapy Versus Traditional Therapy for Low Back Pain Relief." The report stated, "Although traditional therapy showed slightly greater pain relief, the decline in pain using massage therapy was significant." While a massage may bring "slightly less relief than traditional therapy, this noninvasive treatment offers several potential benefits." For example, "Massage therapy for relief of low back pain allows patients an alternative to traditional medical therapy. For patients wanting to control their healthcare choices, an alternative option is a plus." Also, "massage therapy affords patients relief without overriding their desire not to use drugs." Besides the naturalness of this treatment, "massage therapy can be self-referred, allowing patients to choose this intervention without gatekeepers." Most importantly, "massage therapy rarely has adverse effects. Because massage can be taught to laypersons, the potential to use laypersons trained in massage as part of the caregiving team may appeal to certain patients desiring involvement of significant others or family members. Likewise, massage may appeal to caregivers who wish hands-on involvement in caring for their loved ones."

Ernst, E. "Massage Treatment for Back Pain," Editorial, *British Medical Journal (BMJ)* 326 (March 15, 2003): 562–563.

Melancon, Bryan and Lucy H. Miller. "Massage Therapy versus Traditional Therapy for Low Back Pain Relief," *Holistic Nursing Practice* 19, no. 3 (May/June 2005): 116–121.

Sherman, Karen, J., Daniel C. Cherkin, Janet Kahn, Janet Erro, Andrea Hrbek, Richard A. Deyo, and David M. Eisenberg. "A Survey of Training and Pactice Patterns of Massage Therapists in Two US States," *BMC Complementary and Alternative Medicine*. Available online. URL: http://www.biomedcentral.com/1472-6882/5/13. Downloaded January 27, 2006.

Staff. "Handy Techniques You Can Learn," *Consumer Reports on Health* 17, no. 7 (July 2005): 9.

McArdle syndrome   See METABOLIC DISEASES OF MUSCLE.

medical alternatives   See COMPLEMENTARY AND ALTERNATIVE MEDICINE.

medical tests for conditions affecting the back and spine   Since many conditions affect the BACK and SPINE, numerous tests reflect that diversity. Usually, the simplest tests can be performed during a physi-cal examination, for instance, as a doctor tests the RANGE OF MOTION in the vertebral joints. If needed, X-RAYS may provide a first portrait of the ribs or bones in the CERVICAL SPINE, THORACIC SPINE, or LUMBAR SPINE. For detailed imagery of bone density, SPINAL TUMORS, or a VERTEBRAL COMPRESSION FRACTURE, a COMPUTED TOMOGRAPHY (CT) SCAN offers a good option. However, CT scans and X-rays both require radiation, whereas MAGNETIC RESONANCE IMAGING (MRI) does not. An MRI costs more, but it examines both hard and soft matter from bones of the VERTEBRAE to soft tissue in the PARASPINAL MUSCLES as well as supportive tendons and ligaments.

For assessment of bone strength, a BONE MINERAL DENSITY TEST may be ordered, whereas a BONE SCAN may help to diagnose the primary cause of bone PAIN. If a damaged DISC produces CHRONIC PAIN, a DISCOGRAM can assess the need for SURGERY. To evaluate any spinal nerve involvement, an ELECTROMYOGRAM or a NERVE CONDUCTION velocity test may be needed. To show internal movement, a FLUOROSCOPY may be used alone or in conjunction with a LUMBAR PUNCTURE. Fluoroscopy may be included during a MYELOGRAM, too, to direct the insertion of a needle and evaluate the SPINAL CORD. To detect CANCER in soft or hard tissue of the back, a bone biopsy or a muscle biopsy will usually be required.

Besides assessing various structures of the back, tests can evaluate specific factors. For example, a TB test may rule out SPINAL TUBERCULOSIS, while a bacterial culture may determine the source of a SPINAL INFECTION. If symptoms and circumstances suggest heavy metal absorption or other adverse ENVIRONMENTAL INFLUENCE, a strand of hair may be analyzed. Similarly, a urinalysis or blood test can detect a lack of MINERAL BALANCE or the presence of a GENETIC FACTOR, such as occurs in RHEUMATOID ARTHRITIS and GROWTH HORMONE DISORDERS.

Blood tests also show abnormal levels of hormones, vitamins, minerals, and other substances affecting the condition of bones. For example, abnormal levels of creatinine may reveal a kidney problem that endangers health and causes LOW BACK PAIN. As a Healthwise article explained, "Creatinine is a waste product formed by the breakdown of a substance (creatine) important for converting food into energy (metabolism). The creatinine is filtered out of the blood by the kidneys and then passed out of the body in urine. . . . If the kidneys are damaged and cannot function normally, the amount of creatinine in the urine decreases while the amount of creatinine in the blood increases." Besides causing various degrees of BACKACHE, this condition eventually affects bone quality too.

Risks and Complications

Noninvasive tests seldom cause a problem. Although some tests involve radiation, the low level poses minimal threat of exposure, except, perhaps, in patients who have already had too much. More often, the risks associated with a test increase in proportion to the degree of penetration involved in an invasive procedure. For example, a small bruise may occur at a tiny puncture site where blood has been drawn, whereas a biopsy that extends into spinal nerves may be quite painful. If the test itself produces pain, either a local or general anesthesia will be given to lower discomfort, but then that anesthesia can produce side effects or an allergic reaction. Also, some tests introduce a contrast dye into the system, causing an allergic response in sensitive patients.

Statistics and Studies

With the ultimate test being an autopsy, the governmental Agency for Healthcare Research and Quality (AHRQ) posted an *Evidence Report/Technology Assessment* that included such statistics as, "The chance that an autopsy will reveal a misdiagnosis that may have affected outcome . . . was 10.2%," and "the base probability of the autopsy detecting a major error in a given case was 25.6%." The report further stated, "Clearly, nothing can be done to help the individual. However, there are benefits for the system, the public, and the clinicians." For example, an autopsy may document more fully the progression of a spinal condition or disease, thus aiding RESEARCH or future studies.

Special Aids and Adaptations

Medical tests aid spinal health by supplying the information needed for proper treatment. Depending on the symptoms and medical history, tests can diagnose a disorder or disease and also monitor its progression. For example, a bone mineral density test not only can detect osteoporosis but, a year

or two later, can be used to update information, thereby enabling a physician to change or continue medication and other treatments.

To help patients get the most out of a test, the AHRQ Web site provided tips on relevant questions to ask healthcare professionals, such as "What kind of information will the test provide?" and "Is this test the only way to find out that information?" If not, a patient might ask, "What are the benefits and risks of having this test?" Questions should also address the accuracy of the results, the doctor's preference for a particular laboratory, and the type of follow-up typically needed. Most importantly, patients should receive clear instructions to prepare for each test and be advised about what to expect during and after a procedure. Regarding the outcome, the AHRQ advised, "Do not assume that no news is good news. If you do not hear from your doctor, call to get your test results."

Agency for Healthcare Research and Quality. "Quick Tips—When Getting Medical Tests," AHRQ Publication No. 01-0040b. Available online. URL: http://www.ahrq.gov/consumer/quicktips/tiptests.htm. Downloaded January 30, 2006.

American Academy of Orthopaedic Surgeons. "Glossary of Orthopaedic Diagnostic Tests," AAOS. Available online. URL: http://orthoinfo.aaos.org/fact/thr_report.cfm?Thread_ID=372&topcategory=General%20Information. Downloaded January 30, 2006.

Cooke, Kerry V. and Amy Fackler. "Creatinine," Yale New Haven Health, Healthwise, Inc. Available online. URL: http://yalenewhavenhealth.org/library/healthguide/en-us/support/topic.asp?hwid=stc123819. Last updated May 27, 2005.

Washington, A. Eugene, M.D. and Kathyrn M. McDonald, University of California at San Francisco (UCSF)—Stanford University Evidence-based Practice Center. "The Autopsy as an Outcome and Performance Measure," *Evidence Report/Technology Assessment* 58, pages 14 and 146, Agency for Healthcare Research and Quality (AHRQ). Available online. URL: http://www.ahrq.gov/downloads/pub/evidence/pdf/autopsy/autopsy.pdf. Downloaded January 30, 2006.

meningitis, meningococcal disease In this type of SPINAL INFECTION, a virus or bacteria infect the meninges tissue covering the brain and the spinal cord. When caused by bacteria, contagious infection can invade fluids in the spinal cord and brain, causing brain damage, paralysis, or death unless treatment begins within 24 hours of onset. Even without treatment, meningococcal disease caused by a virus usually runs a milder course.

Symptoms and Diagnostic Path

Besides producing symptoms similar to flu, bacteria-induced meningitis characteristically produces stiffness in the CERVICAL SPINE. That stiff neck along with a high fever and, sometimes, a skin rash indicate the need for immediate medical attention. To find out which type of bacteria has caused the illness, a LUMBAR PUNCTURE (spinal tap) will likely be required.

Information from the Centers for Disease Control and Prevention (CDC) explained, "Knowing whether meningitis is caused by a virus or bacterium is important because the severity of illness and the treatment differ. Viral meningitis is generally less severe and resolves without specific treatment, while bacterial meningitis can be quite severe and may result in brain damage, hearing loss, or learning disability. For bacterial meningitis, it is also important to know which type of bacteria is causing the meningitis because antibiotics can prevent some types from spreading and infecting other people." According to the CDC, "Today, *Streptococcus pneumoniae* and *Neisseria meningitidis* are the leading causes of bacterial meningitis."

Treatment Options and Outlook

For the most promising outlook, the CDC said, "Bacterial meningitis can be treated with a number of effective antibiotics. It is important, however, that treatment be started early in the course of the disease. Appropriate antibiotic treatment of most common types of bacterial meningitis should reduce the risk of dying from meningitis to below 15%, although the risk is higher among the elderly."

Risk Factors and Preventive Measures

An overview on the Web site of the American College of Health Association (ACHA) stated, "It is estimated that 100 to 125 cases of meningococcal disease occur annually on college campuses and 5 to 15 students die as a result." Regarding the risk

of contagion, the ACHA said, "Meningococcal disease can affect people at any age. Certain groups are at increased risk for contracting the disease including those in close contact with a known case, upper respiratory infections with compromised immune systems, and persons traveling to endemic areas of the world. Since 1991, cases of meningococcal disease among 15–24 year olds have more than doubled." Vaccination lowers the risk of getting a bacteria-induced infection, and instead of spreading the disease, spreading information can prevent it. As the ACHA said, "Meningococcal bacteria are transmitted through the air via droplets of respiratory secretions and direct contact with persons infected with the disease. Oral contact with shared items such as cigarettes or drinking glasses or through intimate contact such as kissing could put a person at risk for acquiring the infection. People identified as close contacts of a patient with meningococcal disease should receive antibiotics to prevent the disease."

For people planning a trip abroad, the CDC offered this travel advisory: "Although large epidemics of meningococcal meningitis do not occur in the United States, some countries experience large, periodic epidemics. Overseas travelers should check to see if meningococcal vaccine is recommended for their destination. Travelers should receive the vaccine at least 1 week before departure, if possible. Information on areas for which meningococcal vaccine is recommended can be obtained by calling the Centers for Disease Control and Prevention at (404)-332-4565."

American College of Health Association. "Overview of Meningococcal Disease," ACHA. Available online. URL: http://www.acha.org/projects_programs/overview.cfm. Downloaded January 30, 2006.

Centers for Disease Control and Prevention. "Meningococcal Disease," CDC, National Center for Infectious Diseases/Division of Bacterial and Mycotic Diseases, Department of Health and Human Services. Available online. URL: http://www.cdc.gov/ncidod/dbmd/diseaseinfo/meningococcal_g.htm. Posted October 12, 2005.

metabolic bone disease (MBD) This group of diseases affects the bones in the BACK and SPINE, producing such conditions as OSTEOPENIA, OSTEO-POROSIS, OSTEITIS DEFORMANS (Paget's disease), and RICKETS. GENETIC FACTORS contribute to the development of many metabolic bone diseases (MBD), but some types can be acquired through ENVIRON-MENTAL INFLUENCES. Failing conditions elsewhere in the body can cause MBD too, for instance as hormones or kidney functions decline.

In discussing normal bone processes, Dr. Robert C. Mellors explained, "Mature bone consists of: an organic matrix (osteoid) composed mainly of type 1 collagen formed by osteoblasts; a mineral phase which contains the bulk of the body's reserve of calcium and phosphorus in crystalline form . . . deposited in close relation to the collagen fibers; bone cells; and a blood supply with sufficient levels of calcium and phosphate to mineralize the osteoid matrix," the basic substance from which bone forms. This process of bone turnover and bone remodeling continues throughout life. However, "the metabolic bone diseases may reflect disturbances in the organic matrix, the mineral phase, the cellular processes of remodeling, and the . . . nutritional, and other factors which regulate skeletal and mineral homeostasis." In any case, the body either does not have adequate nutrients or does not utilize them well.

Symptoms and Diagnostic Path

From CHRONIC PAIN to spontaneous VERTEBRAL COM-PRESSION FRACTURE, symptoms vary widely. Therefore, a medical history, not only of the patient but also of the family provides a diagnostic clue. With detailed information and the results of a physical examination, a physician may request X-RAYS, a BONE MINERAL DENSITY TEST, blood test, and, sometimes, a bone biopsy.

Treatment Options and Outlook

In an article for MedlinePlus, Dr. Laurence Finberg said, "Most patients are responsive to a combination of managing the underlying cause when possible and either vitamin D or calcitriol therapy." The latter is a form of vitamin D the body can produce itself if briefly exposed to sunshine.

Identifying and treating the causal factors offers the best outlook for each individual. For example, one patient may need a well-balanced diet and a few minutes of daily sunshine without sunscreen, while another may need GROWTH HORMONE therapy or surgical removal of a tumor. Treatments also include HORMONE REPLACEMENT THERAPY, CALCITO-NIN, BISPHOSPHONATES, SELECTIVE ESTROGEN RECEP-TOR MODULATORS (SERMs), or other individualized approach.

Characteristic symptoms can be monitored to detect progression of the disorder. For example, hearing loss may occur as MBD damages tiny bones in the ear. If decreased kidney function produces MBD, a urinalysis will determine the calcium to creatinine ratio. With early testing to establish a baseline, a patient can be monitored regularly, promptly benefiting from adjustments that need to be made in the ongoing treatment.

Risk Factors and Preventive Measures

Genetic factors place a person at risk for developing a bone disorder, but people with deficiencies in NUTRITION remain at high risk too. For example, lack of vitamin D, CALCIUM, or proper MINERAL BALANCE can produce MBD symptoms. Conversely, adequate intake and uptake or absorption of nutrients may prevent MBD. Also, bone-strengthening potential can naturally be found in fresh air, sunshine, daily ACTIVITY, and therapeutic EXERCISE.

Finberg, Laurence, M.D. "Metabolic Bone Disease," eMedi-cine.net. Available online. URL: http://www.emedicine.com/ped/topic2854.htm. Downloaded January 31, 2006.

Mellors, Robert C., M.D. "Bone," Weill Medical College of Cornell University. Available online. URL: http://edcenter.med.cornell.edu/CUMC_PathNotes/Skeletal/Bone_04.html. Downloaded January 31, 2006.

metabolic diseases of muscle If the human body arrived with a maintenance manual, it might mention the basic need everyone has for food. With metabolic diseases of muscle, however, patients cannot get the NUTRITION they need. Even if a person has a healthy intake of vitamins and minerals, a small genetic flaw keeps the body from using those nutrients to produce adequate energy.

In an online article, Dr. Y. Harati explained, "Metabolic muscle disorders are related to defects in the enzymes that regulate carbohydrates, lipids, or other metabolic pathways in the muscle fibers. The most common disorders are related to glycogen storage problems." With a carnitine deficiency, however, the body lacks a minuscule molecule needed for metabolism. Whether that molecule or an enzyme causes the problem, the result is an inability to extract energy from nutritious meals.

Symptoms and Diagnostic Path

ACUTE PAIN and muscle spasm or cramping often produce the first signs with disproportionate fatigue following a few minutes of EXERCISE. Since most people just assume they are out of shape, a diagnosis may be a long time coming. Then, an exercise test, ELECTROMYOGRAM, muscle biopsy, or other lab work may confirm a diagnosis.

Treatment Options and Outlook

With no specific treatment recommended, therapy must be fitted to the individual, who then takes an active part in lessening the impact of the disease. For example, a person might practice self-awareness to determine what triggers and what eases muscle cramps or pain. Also, foods affect each patient differently, but a physician or nutritionist can discuss the best choices for that particular person.

Risk Factors and Preventive Measures

Overexertion and inadequate meals aggravate the symptoms and sometimes lead to RHABDOMYOLYSIS. A doctor may recommend light exercises, but WEIGHT-BEARING EXERCISE and STRENGTH TRAINING usually prove counterproductive, causing cramps or spasms and, in rare cases, weakened muscles. To maintain mobility and independence, a walker or wheelchair may be needed. However, with a diet and lifestyle designed for the individual, symptoms often remain manageable.

Harati, Y., M.D. "Metabolic Myopathies," Baylor College of Medicine. Available online. URL: http://www.bcm.edu/neurology/research/nmus/nmus3a5.html. Downloaded January 30, 2006.

Muscular Dystrophy Association. "Facts About Metabolic Diseases of Muscle," MDA. Available online. URL: http://www.mdausa.org/publications/fa-metab-qa.html. Downloaded January 30, 2006.

microdiscectomy   This type of DISCECTOMY surgically treats such conditions as a HERNIATED DISC, commonly located in the LUMBAR SPINE. With up-to-date technology, the procedure involves MINIMALLY INVASIVE SURGERY that can sometimes be done in an outpatient clinic but may require an overnight hospital stay.

According to an article posted by Back.com, "Lumbar microdiscectomy is usually recommended only when specific conditions are met. In general, surgery is recommended when a ruptured disc is pinching a spinal nerve root(s) and you have: 1. Leg pain which limits your normal daily activities. 2. Weakness in your leg(s) or feet. 3. Numbness in your extremities. 4. Impaired bowel and/or bladder function."

Procedure

To describe a lumbar microdiscectomy, information from Holy Cross Hospital said, "A microdiscectomy is performed through a very small incision—usually only one to one-and-a-half inches in the lower back. In the procedure, a small portion of the bone over the nerve root and/or disc material from under the nerve root is removed to relieve . . . impingement and create more room for the nerve to heal. Because the procedure leaves nearly all of the joints, ligaments, and muscles intact, it does not change the mechanical structure of the patient's spine."

In a paper presented to the American Academy of Orthopaedic Surgeons, a group of surgeons compared standard equipment traditionally used for lumbar microdiscectomy with a minimally invasive procedure. Both types of surgery use a retractor to hold back muscle in the surgical site, but the differences between those tools will affect the procedure. For instance, "microdiscectomy is typically performed via a small incision utilizing a microscope for enhanced visualization. With the recent interest in minimally invasive surgery, tubular retractors which dilate" or expand "the muscle fibers have become popular in order to minimize the incision length, while achieving the same surgical goals." After reviewing "sixty-two consecutive patients who underwent a total of sixty-five procedures over a 3-year period," the surgeons concluded, "There appears to be no significant difference between the minimally invasive tubular retractors or standard retractors for patients undergoing single-level lumbar microdiscectomy procedures. There may be a trend towards a shorter hospital stay and perhaps a higher rate of persistent symptoms with the use of the tubular retractors, however, it appears that both methods are successful and provide similar clinical results."

Risks and Complications

With a success rate of 90 to 95 percent, microdiscectomy still has the typical surgical risks of bleeding, nerve damage, and infection. Pain will likely continue for a while too.

In an article for eSpine, Dr. Robert Pashman said, "It is normal to have some pain after any operation. After a lumbar microdiscectomy, there may be some leg 'aching' which occurs as the nerve(s) attempts to heal. You also may feel some muscle spasms across your back and down your leg(s). And if there was inflammation in the nerve root, some pain may persist until this inflammation diminishes. You will be given appropriate medication to control your pain, relieve back spasms and reduce inflammation." Besides common occurrences of pain and muscle spasm, Dr. Pashman said, "It is not unusual to feel tired and discouraged for several days following surgery. These feelings may be your body's natural reaction to the cutback of extra hormones it generated during surgery. Although some emotional letdown can be expected, you must not let it get in the way of your recovery."

Outlook and Lifestyle Modifications

In an article for Spine-health, Dr. Peter F. Ullrich Jr. wrote, "Some spine surgeons restrict a patient from bending, lifting, or twisting for the first six weeks following surgery. However, since the patient's back is mechanically the same, it is also reasonable to return to a normal level of functioning immediately following microdiscectomy spine surgery. There have been a couple of reports in the medical literature showing that immediate mobilization (return to normal activity) does not lead to an increase in recurrent lumbar herniated disc."

To assist healing, patients should refrain from smoking. Ample water, SLEEP, NUTRITION, and appropriate EXERCISE provide the healthy lifestyle needed for recovery and also help to avoid future problems with DISCS.

Holy Cross Hospital. "Microdiscectomy." Available online. URL: http://www.holycrosshealth.org/svc_surgery_microdiscectomy.htm. Downloaded January 30, 2006.

Medtronic Sofamor Danek. "Surgical: Lumbar Microdiscectomy," Back.com. Available online. URL: http://www.back.com/treatment-surgical-microdiscectomy.html. Downloaded January 10, 2006.

Pashman, Robert, M.D. "Lumbar Microdiscectomy," eSpine.com. Available online. URL: http://www.espine.com/diagnosis_lm.html. Downloaded January 10, 2006.

Shamie, Arya Nick, M.D., Saman Aboudi, M.D., Larry Khoo, M.D., and Jeffrey C. Wang, M.D. "Lumbar Microdiscectomy Comparing Minimally Invasive Tubular Retractors versus Standard Retractors," Paper No: 185 presented to the American Academy of Orthopaedic Surgeons (AAOS). Available online. URL: http://www.aaos.org/wordhtml/anmt2005/sciprog/185.htm. Last modified December 29, 2004.

Ullrich, Peter F. Jr., M.D. "Microdiscectomy (Microdecompression) Spine Surgery," Spine-health. Available online. URL: http://www.spine-health.com/topics/surg/overview/lumbar/lumb03.html. Downloaded January 30, 2006.

mineral balance Naturally found in the earth, sea, and sky, minerals are inorganic elements that, unlike organic matter, can not respond, reproduce themselves, or get a life. Nevertheless, people need about 17 essential minerals to survive and thrive. Those macro minerals include CALCIUM, MAGNESIUM, PHOSPHORUS, POTASSIUM, silicon, sodium, and sulfur, while trace minerals include chromium, cobalt, copper, iodine, IRON, manganese, molybdenum, selenium, and ZINC. Some consider strontium an essential trace element, too, since it aids bone growth and prevents tooth decay, but its abundance in nature means that most people get enough. Strontium and other semi-essential minerals have yet to be adequately studied, but well-known or not, minerals work to strengthen the VERTEBRAE, support the BACK and SPINE, maintain the acid-alkaline balance in the blood, maintain water balance, assist the production of antibodies, and aid the movement of PARASPINAL MUSCLES.

Since people and animals cannot consume rocks, precious metals, or ore, highly cooperative plant life intervenes. By land, plants sink their roots deep into the earth and extract minerals from the soil, sort of like sipping through a straw. Similarly, sea plants, such as algae, sop up minerals like a sponge or soak themselves in a salt bath and mineral oils from the sea. Whether by land or by sea, these plants provide digestible sources of minerals that people and animals can safely consume and absorb into the body. Fresh water taps into a supply of minerals too, unless distillation or reverse osmosis processing removes those vital elements.

As absorbable forms of minerals arrive each day, bones store such essentials as calcium and phosphorus in reserve, while protein-produced amino acids move along whatever minerals the body needs. Some minerals may be needed more than others, but trace elements or micro minerals, such as iron, have laudable functions too. Generally, a body only needs a trace of trace minerals measured in micrograms, whereas macro minerals, measured in milligrams, remain in macrocosmic demand. For example, the body has a higher need for potassium to put carbohydrates and proteins to good use, while the trace mineral zinc helps the liver to release VITAMIN A. VITAMIN C aids iron absorption, and phosphorus aids the absorption of VITAMIN B-COMPLEX, while VITAMIN D ensures calcium uptake. That same calcium, so demanded by the bones, also helps the muscles to contract, whereas another macro-mineral, magnesium, relaxes those muscular contractions. With the support of other nutrients, minerals smooth the moves of muscles and bones throughout the body, but a mineral imbalance does not.

Risks and Complications

ENVIRONMENTAL INFLUENCES, GENETIC FACTORS, inadequate NUTRITION, various medications, and TENSION put a person at risk for a mineral imbalance. People with food allergies or those who consume large quantities of caffeine or alcohol may also be at higher risk for poor absorption of minerals and other nutrients too.

In patients with chronic kidney conditions, poor absorption thins bones, eventually producing OSTEOPOROSIS. As an article on the National Kidney Foundation Web site explained, "A change occurs in the balance between two important minerals in your body—calcium and phosphorus—leading to loss of calcium from your bones. . . . When your kidneys have stopped working normally, phosphorus may build up in your blood. Too much phosphorus in your blood leads to loss of calcium from your bones, which weakens them over time." In that particular case, a low phosphorus diet, medication, and supplements of calcium and vitamin D may help to restore mineral balance.

More commonly, foods receive an overdose of salt, but excessive sodium can rob bones of calcium. According to an article on a National Institutes of Health Web site, "sodium (and chloride), the components of table salt, increase the calcium requirement by increasing urinary calcium excretion. Individuals with low salt intakes may be able to maintain calcium balance at low calcium intakes, while those with more typical U.S. salt intakes will have higher calcium requirements."

Statistics and Studies

To identify mineral imbalances, The Trichological Society of the United Kingdom studies hair. According to their Web site, "hair mineral analysis is a screening test, which measures the mineral content of your hair. Mineral content of the hair reflects the mineral content of the body's tissues. If a mineral deficiency exists in the hair, it usually indicates a mineral deficiency or excess within the body." For example, "the zinc level is high relative to tissue copper status. A zinc-copper imbalance in conjunction with low copper levels is a strong indicator of a decrease in the role of copper in many functions of metabolism. One of the main functions of copper is its necessity in collagen synthesis. If this profile becomes both severe and chronic, a decrease in collagen synthesis can occur. This can then be an indication to capillary fragility, osteoporosis and premature greying of the hair." Hair color as such does not matter much, but "hair analysis clearly shows individual deficiencies or excesses as well as the presence of toxic metals." Basically, a hair analysis highlights the nutrients needed.

Special Aids and Adaptations

Some patients experience spinal problems from having too little mineral resources and others from too much. To complicate matters more, the recommended daily allowance changes according to age and, sometimes, sex. As a general guideline, Dr. Elson M. Haas wrote, "All the macrominerals are needed in doses of over 100 mg. daily, with sodium requirements somewhere between 2–5 grams, potassium 3–4 grams, phosphorus about 1–2 grams, calcium 1–1.5 grams, and magnesium probably about 0.5–1 gram. The trace minerals are needed in much smaller amounts. To be on the safe side, daily intake of iron and zinc should probably be about 15–30 mg.; manganese about 5–10 mg.; and copper about 2 mg. Other trace minerals, such as chromium, selenium, molybdenum, cobalt, and iodine, are needed in amounts of less than 1 mg. per day."

If a mineral imbalance seems likely, a physician can prescribe diagnostic tests to see which essential elements the body lacks. Then a nutritionist can design a diet adapted to those very specific needs. Although nutritional needs may fluctuate from one person to the next, adaptations can be made for each individual to stay nicely balanced.

Haas, Elson M., M.D. *Staying Healthy with Nutrition.* Berkeley, Calif.: Celestial Arts Publishing, 1992, 160–161, 186.

Kirschmann, Gayla J. and John D. Kirschmann. *Nutrition Almanac,* 4th ed. New York: McGraw-Hill, 1996, 29–30.

National Institutes of Health Osteoporosis and Related Bone Diseases. "Nutrition and the Skeleton: The Role of Calcium and Other Nutrients," NIH ORBD. Available online. URL: http://www.osteo.org/newfile.asp?doc=r708i&doctitle=Nutrition+and+the+Skeleton&doctype=HTML+Fact+Sheet. Downloaded February 1, 2006.

National Kidney Foundation. "Bone Disease in Chronic Kidney Failure." Available online. URL: http://www.kidney.org/atoz/atozItem.cfm?id=49. Downloaded February 1, 2006.

Trichological Society, The. "Hair Mineral Analysis," U.K. Available online. URL: http://www.hairscientists.org/hair-mineral-analysis.htm. Downloaded February 1, 2006.

minimally invasive surgery Not one type of procedure but many, minimally invasive surgery invades the body less than traditional methods. This minimalistic approach also reduces trauma to surrounding tissue, which can be especially important in accelerating recovery after surgery on the BACK or CERVICAL SPINE.

An article posted by Back.com said, "When talking about a minimally invasive surgery, you must consider three factors: scar sizes, muscle dilation vs. stripping, and recovery time. These three factors separate a traditional surgery from a minimally invasive one." While one type procedure may be better at times than another, "the biggest difference between minimally invasive surgeries and traditional surgeries is that of muscle dilation versus muscle stripping. Muscle dilation is achieved by using a series of sequential dilators to separate the fibers of the muscles in your back, making a small tunnel, giving the surgeon a view of your spine through a very small incision. By using these tubes or channel along with a microscope or endoscope the surgeon can access the part of your spine where the problem is, without having to make a long incision along those spinal levels. When performing a traditional surgery, the physician makes an incision along all of the levels of your spine where the problem lies and 'strips' the muscle off of the spine. This muscle stripping, rather than dilation can often play a role in how quickly a patient recovers."

Risks and Complications

As with any SURGERY, minimally invasive procedures can cause bleeding, infection, or nerve damage. Unlike other surgeries though, the surgeon may not be able to see the full picture since the scope of an endoscope, microscope, or other small instrument may limit the view. Also, the skillful use of active chemicals, laser light, balloons, or other tools takes a bit of practice. Therefore, inquiring patients might ask about the experience and success rate a particular surgeon has.

Statistics and Studies

After reviewing the historical perspectives of minimally invasive techniques used on the SPINE, a group of physicians from Stanford University discussed their findings in *Neurosurgical Focus.* According to their report, "Virtually all aspects of the spinal axis can be approached and treated in a minimally invasive approach. . . . With the innovation of better optics and video equipment, retractor and instrumentation systems, image guidance systems, and new biological agents, the majority of traditional 'open' spinal procedures can now be performed in a minimalistic way. For most minimally invasive surgical procedures, however, long-term . . . data are still lacking. In addition, the use of new technology will require a new learning curve that may be discomforting for many surgeons. Special skills may be needed that are beyond those of traditional open surgery."

Special Aids and Adaptations

Minimally invasive surgery adapts technology to surgical techniques. As an article on SpineUniverse explained, "Endoscopic techniques have been used for several decades, but these were exclusively for diagnostic purposes. In the late 1970s and early 1980s, endoscopic techniques were advanced so that both a diagnosis could be made and the disease could be treated. These same endoscopic techniques used in other surgical disciplines have now been advanced to the treatment of spinal disorders." For example, an endoscope may be used during surgery for DEGENERATIVE DISC DISEASE, a FRACTURE, HERNIATED DISC, KYPHOSIS, SCOLIOSIS, or SPINAL TUMOR to "speed recovery, minimize post-operative pain and improve the final outcome."

Cleveland Clinic, The. "Minimally Invasive Endoscopic Spinal Surgery," SpineUniverse. Available online. URL: http://www.spineuniverse.com/displayarticle. php/article2016.html. Last updated June 20, 2005.

Department of Neurological Surgery, University of Pittsburgh. "Minimally Invasive Spine Procedures," Neurological Spine Services Division. Available online. URL: http://www.neurosurgery.pitt.edu/spine/minimal/. Downloaded January 30, 2006.

Medtronic Sofamor Danek. "Minimally Invasive Options," Back.com. Available online. URL: http://www.back. com/articles-minimally_invasive.html?mastbox=yep. Updated February 17, 2005.

Thongtrangan, Issada, M.D., Hoang Le, M.D., Jon Park, M.D., and Daniel H. Kim, M.D. "Minimally Invasive Spinal Surgery: a Historical Perspective," *Neurosurgical Focus* 16, no. 1 (January 2004).

MRI   See MAGNETIC RESONANCE IMAGING.

multiple myeloma   See MYELOMA BONE DISEASE.

muscle cramp or spasm   Involuntarily, muscle contractions tighten the CERVICAL SPINE, knot PARASPINAL MUSCLES in the BACK, or cause a body to twitch. Often, TENSION cramps neck muscles, but faulty POSTURE can too, for instance as a person bends over a book or a workbench. Fatigue, dehydration, and overuse can send muscles into a spasm as can a lack of MINERAL BALANCE. If a muscle fails to relax, the tightness may tie up the RANGE OF MOTION.

Symptoms and Diagnostic Path

Primary symptoms include ACUTE PAIN, which, in the LUMBAR SPINE, may be felt as a BACKACHE or LOW BACK PAIN. In general, tightly knotted muscles can be felt anywhere muscles exist, not only by the pain felt, but by feeling with the fingers and finding a taut area with little give. ATHLETES and others can often self-diagnose the problem, especially if muscle spasms occur after heavy practice or strenuous EXERCISE.

Treatment Options and Outlook

To treat neck spasms, Dr. Pierre Rouzier advised, "If your neck spasm has just occurred, put ice packs on your neck for 20 to 30 minutes three to four times a day." After that initial treatment, "sometimes, especially with recurrent spasms, moist heat can help. Put warm, moist towels on your neck for 20 minutes, or take hot showers or baths." In addition, "you may be able to massage your neck yourself by finding the tight muscles and putting deep pressure on these muscles. You might also get a massage from a friend or therapist." Although MASSAGE THERAPY and TRIGGER POINT THERAPY can help most patients with NECK PAIN, "neck spasms are a common physical symptom caused by stress or depression. Identification of these problems and treatment of them may help considerably with neck spasms." For muscles in general, "spasms are best treated with stretching exercises."

To alleviate the pain of spasms, NONSTEROIDAL ANTI-INFLAMMATORY DRUG (NSAID) THERAPY may help. If muscle cramps continue, medical attention should be sought. In severe cases, MUSCLE RELAXANTS or a SPINAL INJECTION may be needed to relax the contraction.

Dr. Norman L. Epstein addressed "Benztropine for Acute Muscle Spasm in the Emergency Department." According to the article, "Many patients arrive in the emergency department with acute lumbar and cervical muscle spasm . . . that occurs either spontaneously or secondary to nonimpact axial injuries (i.e. lifting and twisting)." For example, a patient might present TORTICOLLIS caused by twisted LIFTING or other awkward movement. To treat these acute spasms in the neck or back, Dr. Epstein said, "My hypothesis was that benztropine, an anticholinergic medication, would reverse the state of muscle spasm and thus provide good pain relief for these patients." Of the eight persons who received that treatment within 24 hours of muscle spasm, "every patient experienced substantial relief and improved range of motion."

Risk Factors and Preventive Measures

In the online article "Muscle Spasms," Dr. Pierre Rouzier recommended, "If you tend to get muscle cramps during exercise, make sure you drink enough fluids. Sports drinks may be very helpful." Also, "proper stretching exercises will help prevent spasms."

Sometimes muscle cramps occur after SURGERY. As Dr. Irwin M. Siegel explained, "Muscle spasm is usually an effort on the part of the body to splint an injured area and prolonged spasm can cause pain in and of itself. Both trauma and interruption of circulation can cause muscle spasm and pain. Sometimes a 'vicious cycle' is set up with pain causing spasm and spasm causing more pain. If the fusion has been successful . . . . , the condition of pain and muscle spasm can be treated by physical therapy, muscle relaxants and the use of an appropriate back support."

In general, however, adequate fresh water, well-balanced NUTRITION, and daily ACTIVITY that includes stretching may prevent future episodes. Warm-ups prior to exercise should also lessen the risk of muscle cramping.

Epstein, Norman L., M.D. "Benztropine for Acute Muscle Spasm in the Emergency Department," *Canadian Medical Association Journal* 164, no. 2 (January 23, 2001): 203–204.

Rouzier, Pierre, M.D., McKesson Provider Technologies. "Muscle Spasms," University of Michigan Health System. Available online. URL: http://www.med.umich. edu/1libr/sma/sma_musspasm_sma.htm. Downloaded February 4, 2006.

———, McKesson Provider Technologies. "Neck Spasms," University of Michigan Health System. Available online. URL: http://www.med.umich.edu/1libr/sma/sma_neckspsm_sma.htm. Last modified April 29, 2005.

Siegel, Irwin M., M.D. "Muscle Spasm From Lumbar Fusion," Muscular Dystrophy Association. Available online. URL: http://www.mdausa.org/experts/question.cfm?id=1870. Downloaded February 4, 2006.

muscle relaxants This type of medication cuts people some slack. Besides releasing TENSION in the PARASPINAL MUSCLES of the BACK, a muscle relaxant eases the stiffness of SPRAINS, STRAINS, and muscle spasm. Muscles loosen up. The person loosens up, and the limber body can then perform therapeutic EXERCISE with greater ease and interest. Often prescribed at the onset of LOW BACK PAIN, this group of drugs provides immediate but temporary treatment to get a person moving again.

Dosage and Potential Side Effects

Spine-health.com provided information on three relaxants commonly used: carisoprodol (Soma), diazepam (Valium), and cyclobenzaprine (Flexeril). For muscle spasm, 350 mg of carisoprodol may be taken every eight hours as needed, but not for long as it can be habit-forming. Diazepam (Valium), which can also be habit-forming, "is usually limited to one to two weeks of use, and the typical dosage is 5–10 mg every six hours as needed to relieve low back pain associated with muscle spasm. . . . Patients should also note that Valium is a depressant and can worsen depression associated with chronic pain." If needed, cyclobenzaprine "can be used on a longer-term basis and actually has a chemical structure related to some antidepressant medications, although it is not an antidepressant. Usually it is prescribed as 10 mg every six hours as needed to relieve low back pain associated with muscle spasm, or it can also be prescribed as 10 mg at night as needed to help with difficulty sleeping." Cyclobenzaprine, however, "can impair mental and physical function."

Besides the side effects unique to each medication and each individual, muscle relaxants should not be taken with alcohol or certain types of medications. The potential for adverse effects increases in patients with allergies to foods or drugs, pregnant or lactating women, young CHILDREN, ELDERLY persons, and patients with chronic medical conditions, such as kidney, liver, or psychiatric disorders.

An article posted by MedlinePlus explained, "Skeletal muscle relaxants act in the central nervous system (CNS) to produce their muscle relaxant effects. Their actions in the CNS may also produce some of their side effects. . . . Skeletal muscle relaxants may cause blurred vision or clumsiness or unsteadiness in some people. They may also cause some people to feel drowsy, dizzy, lightheaded, faint, or less alert than they are normally. *Make sure you know how you react to this medicine before you drive, use machines, or do anything else that could be dangerous if you are dizzy or are not alert, well-coordinated, and able to see well.*"

Statistics and Studies

A group of researchers from Finland reported their concerns about interactions between muscle relaxants and antidepressants. According to the article published in the *Chemist & Druggist,* the anti-depressant "Faverin (fluvoxamine) dramatically increases the blood concentration of Zanaflex (tizanidine)," a muscle relaxant, by an average of 33 times. "This can result in a severe and prolonged fall in blood pressure and enhanced CNS effects."

Instead of mixing medications, researchers from Rutgers University School of Pharmacy split them. Some patients had been advised to divide generic 10 mg tablets in half to get the 5 mg dosage prescribed, so the researchers decided to try this themselves. As *Drug Topics* reported, "Using a tablet splitter and kitchen knives commonly used by patients, three researchers each split 30 tablets, which are not scored, and then weighed the fragments on a spe-cial scale." Instead of getting a 5 mg dosage, however, the hand-carved tablets offered, "anywhere from 50% to 150% of the dose prescribed."

Micromedex, Inc. "Drug Information: Skeletal Muscle Relaxants (Systemic)," MedlinePlus, National Institutes of Health. Available online. URL: http://www.nlm.nih.gov/medlineplus/print/druginfo/uspdi/202523.html. Downloaded January 30, 2006.

Rutgers University School of Pharmacy. "Drug Content of Split Tablets Varies," *Drug Topics* 148, no. 11 (June 7, 2004): 12.

Spine-health.com. "Muscle Relaxants." Available online. URL: http://www.spine-health.com/topics/conserv/overview/med/med04.html. Downloaded January 30, 2006.

Staff. "Drug Interaction Concern," *Chemist & Druggist* (April 10, 2004): 6.

muscle spasm   See MUSCLE CRAMP OR SPASM.

muscular dystrophy (MD)   Usually brought on by GENETIC FACTORS, this group of diseases produces weakness in the skeletal muscles of CHILDREN, primarily boys. As MD progresses, atrophy affects the PARASPINAL MUSCLES, damages POSTURE, and makes daily ACTIVITY or routines increasingly difficult to perform. Eventually, mobility ceases with the quality of life and, ultimately, the life span severely limited.

Symptoms and Diagnostic Path

In discussing the most common form of MD known as Duchenne's muscular dystrophy, information from Cedars-Sinai said, "It generally appears from age three to six years and worsens rapidly. At first, muscle weakness and wasting (atrophy) within the pelvic (hipbone) area occurs followed by similar problems in the shoulder muscles. Eventually, muscle weakness and atrophy affect the trunk and forearms and gradually spread to the major muscles of the body. From 20 to 30 boys of every 100,000 born are affected by Duchenne's muscular dystrophy." Characteristically, symptoms include, "a waddling way of walking, difficulty climbing stairs or rising from sitting and repeated falling. As the disease worsens, other abnormalities may develop, such as curvature of the spine."

Noting similar symptoms, MedlinePlus discussed another type of MD, "Becker's Muscular Dystrophy." As that online article explained, "the pattern of symptom development resembles that of Duchenne's muscular dystrophy, but with a much slower rate of progression. Muscle wasting begins in the legs and pelvis, then progresses to the muscles of the shoulders and neck, followed by loss of arm muscles and respiratory muscles. Calf muscle enlargement (pseudohypertrophy) is quite obvious." Regarding onset, "symptoms usually appear in men at about age 12, but may sometimes begin later. The average age of becoming unable to walk is 25–30."

Besides a family history, medical history, and physical examination, various tests help to confirm the diagnosis. For example, a physician may request a blood test and a muscle biopsy. Usually, an ELECTROMYOGRAM and a NERVE CONDUCTION STUDY will also be prescribed.

Treatment Options and Outlook

Although no cure exists, RESEARCH currently involves options in gene therapy. Meanwhile, physical therapy and therapeutic EXERCISE may ease muscle contractions and minimize CHRONIC PAIN. To manage postural problems, a back brace or other ORTHOTIC device may be prescribed to treat KYPHOSIS, LORDOSIS, and SCOLIOSIS. SURGERY may also be needed to minimize damage to the SPINE.

Generally, treatments include STEROID THERAPY. To discuss this option, Dr. Gregory T. Carter compared two steroids in a question-and-answer column for the Muscular Dystrophy Association (MDA). As reported, "of all of the therapeutic classes of drugs studied in Duchenne muscular dystrophy (DMD), only the corticosteroids, and in particular prednisone and deflazacort, appear to provide, albeit temporary, functional improvement for boys with DMD." However, "based on the available evidence, both prednisone and deflazacort have benefit (and risk). I think the incidence of side effects with prednisone, including weight gain, can be significantly lowered by using pulse therapy (10 days on/10 days off). This essentially reduces the side effects to that of deflazacort. Whether deflazacort actually works better is a question that cannot be succinctly answered based on the studies that have been done to date."

A study from the University of Toronto, Canada, focused on ALENDRONATE as a treatment for the bone-thinning side effects of steroid treatments in boys whose BONE MINERAL DENSITY TESTS scored less than -1.00. As reported in the *Archives of Physical Medicine and Rehabilitation,* "improvement in total body and spine z scores was associated with younger age at baseline." Specifically, "in deflazacort-treated boys, alendronate had a positive effect on BMD z scores; the effect was greatest when given early in the course of disease."

Risk Factors and Preventive Measures

Information from the Loyola University Health System explained, "Muscular dystrophy is a progressive condition that needs life-long management to prevent deformity and complications. Walking and sitting often becomes more difficult as the child grows. Usually by the age of 12, the child needs a wheelchair because the leg muscles are too weak to work."

In addition, inactivity and steroid treatments commonly cause weight gain and deteriorating health. For example, MD patients often experience the adverse effects of too much WEIGHT. While NUTRITION does not cure MD, an individualized diet may help to maintain MINERAL BALANCE and keep body weight within the optimal range for that particular child.

In an overview of preventive measures, the MDA Web site posted "Facts About Duchenne and Becker Muscular Dystrophies (DMD and BMD)." As the article stated, "The impact of DMD and BMD can be minimized significantly by keeping the body as flexible, upright and mobile as possible." For example, RANGE OF MOTION exercises can "delay contractures by keeping tendons from shortening prematurely." However, "it's important that a physical therapist show you how to do range-of-motion exercises correctly. . . . By using all available therapies, patients can prolong their comfort, function and life expectancy."

American Accreditation HealthCare Commission, A.D.A.M. "Becker's Muscular Dystrophy," MedlinePlus. Available online. URL: http://www.nlm.nih.gov/medlineplus/ency/article/000706.htm. Last updated January 6, 2006.

Carter, Gregory T., M.D. "Prednisone or Deflazacort," Ask the Experts, Muscular Dystrophy Association, MDA. Available online. URL: http://www.mdausa.org/experts/question.cfm?id=3050. Downloaded February 6, 2006.

Cedars-Sinai Health System. "Muscular Dystrophy." Available online. URL: http://www.cedars-sinai.edu/3006.html. Downloaded February 1, 2006.

Hawker, G. A., R. Ridout, V. A. Harris, C. C. Chase, L. J. Fielding, and W. D. Bigger. "Alendronate in the Treatment of Low Bone Mass in Steroid-treated Boys with Duchenne's Muscular Dystrophy," *Archives of Physical Medicine and Rehabilitation* 86, no. 2 (February 2005): 284–291.

Loyola University Health System. "Muscular Dystrophy." Available online. URL: http://www.luhs.org/health/topics/nervous/muscular.htm. Last updated January 5, 2005.

Muscular Dystrophy Association. "Facts About Duchenne and Becker Muscular Dystrophies (DMD and BMD)," MDA. Available online. URL: http://www.mdausa.org/publications/fa-dmdbmd-treat.html. Downloaded February 6, 2006.

musculoskeletal disorders In the musculoskeletal system, individual mechanisms of the BACK and SPINE include PARASPINAL MUSCLES, spinal nerves, VERTEBRAE, DISCS, joints, and connective ligaments and tendons. Each of these aspects must work well, or inflammation, ACUTE PAIN, CHRONIC PAIN, muscle spasm, or NERVE COMPRESSION may result. For example, a BACK INJURY, FLEXION-EXTENSION INJURY, RIB INJURY, or other type of SPINAL INJURY, including overuse, can rearrange musculoskeletal components, making the mechanisms downright disorderly. Similarly, SPINAL INFECTIONS can cause temporary disorder, whereas progressive conditions, such as ARTHRITIS, JUVENILE RHEUMATOID ARTHRITIS, MUSCULAR DYSTROPHY, and OSTEOPOROSIS, can subtly disrupt body mechanics throughout the musculoskeletal system.

According to the American College of Rheumatology (ACR), "approximately 1 of 7 patient visits to a primary care provider is prompted by musculoskeletal pain or dysfunction. While many or even most patients with these symptoms have benign, self-limited conditions, arthritis and chronic musculoskeletal disorders are leading causes of disability and work absenteeism, and are occasionally life-threatening. Determining whether the symptom is from local injury or inflammation, a mechanical problem, or a systemic illness will direct subsequent evaluation and management." For example, "musculoskeletal emergencies may present with acute symptoms," whereas "patients with systemic rheumatic diseases, such as rheumatoid arthritis . . . , may have prolonged morning stiffness in multiple symptomatic joints, less stiffness after using their joints, and may have constitutional symptoms (malaise, fever, weight loss) or signs or symptoms of multi-system involvement." Conversely, "individuals with local mechanical problems," such as a muscle SPRAIN or STRAIN, "and osteoarthritis (OA) typically have little morning stiffness, only one or a few symptomatic areas, no pain at rest, worsened symptoms with or after sustained activity, and no symptoms or signs of a systemic illness." The ACR also devised a diagnostic questionnaire for professional assessment, but before seeing a rheumatologist or other doctor, patients might ask such questions of themselves. For instance, "What is hard to do now that you could do before, and how does this affect your daily life?" The answers can help to clarify the symptoms, narrow down the appropriate diagnostic tests, and offer potential solutions too.

Symptoms and Diagnostic Path

During a physical examination, the doctor will attempt to discern whether the source of pain or inflammation arises from a bone, muscle, disc, joint, spinal nerve, or underlying medical condition. Initially, this may be done by testing RANGE OF MOTION during an office visit. Later, outpatient tests, such as X-RAYS or MAGNETIC RESONANCE IMAGING, may be needed to locate or assess damage. In some cases, BONE MINERAL DENSITY TESTS, ELECTROMYOGRAM, or NERVE CONDUCTION STUDY may be recommended. If a patient presents muscle weakness, atrophy, or other symptom of a systemic illness, appropriate tests may then include a blood test, urinalysis, biopsy, or BONE SCAN. As the ACR stated, "The most useful information in evaluating musculoskeletal pain comes from the history and physical examination, with reassessment as necessary. When the diagnosis and proper management are obscure, selective ordering of tests and/or consultation may be the most cost-effective approach."

Treatment Options and Outlook

Both the therapy and the outlook depend on the condition. For instance, a FRACTURE that occurred when a child fell from a tree limb will usually have a better outcome than a VERTEBRAL COMPRESSION FRACTURE arising when an ELDERLY patient simply got out of bed. Both conditions might require a cast or ORTHOTIC device. Both might require SURGERY. Both might involve therapeutic EXERCISE or better forms of NUTRITION. However, the compression fracture would likely necessitate long-term use of medication, such as BISPHOSPHONATES, to slow bone loss. For another example, CHILDREN with progressively weakening muscles may have far different treatment and a more somber outlook than ATHLETES who overexert muscles during game practice.

Risk Factors and Preventive Measures

The immediate medical history of a patient not only offers clues for diagnosing a musculoskeletal disorder but provides information about ongoing risks and preventives. In assessing the most common disorders, a fact sheet from the National Institute for Occupational Safety and Health (NIOSH) included information from the Bureau of Labor Statistics (BLS) on "Work-Related Musculoskeletal Disorders." According to the NIOSH, "musculoskeletal disorders of any cause are among the most prevalent medical problems, affecting 7% of the population and accounting for 14% of physician visits and 19% of hospital stays." Furthermore, "when looking specifically at cases involving days away from work, . . . approximately 32% or 705,800 cases were the result of overexertion or repetitive motion. This figure includes back injuries." For most types of musculoskeletal disorders, ERGONOMIC FACTORS and proper means of LIFTING can often be addressed to prevent recurrence.

A satisfying job may prevent problems too. In an overview of musculoskeletal disorders (MSDs) posted by the NIOSH, Dr. Bruce P. Bernard said, "There is increasing evidence that psychosocial factors related to the job and work environment play a role in the development of work-related MSDs of the upper extremity and back. Though the findings of the studies reviewed are not entirely consistent, they suggest that perceptions of intensified workload, monotonous work, limited job control, low job clarity, and low social support are associated with various work-related MSDs. As some of these factors are seemingly unrelated to physical demands, and a number of studies have found associations even after adjusting for physical demands, the effects of these factors on MSDs may be, in part or entirely, independent of physical factors." In such cases, a job change may help some patients to find a more fitting way to employ their musculoskeletal systems.

American College of Rheumatology Ad Hoc Committee on Clinical Guidelines. "Guidelines for the Initial Evaluation of the Adult Patient with Acute Musculoskeletal Symptoms," *Arthritis & Rheumatism, Official Journal of the American College of Rheumatology* 39, no. 1 (January 1996): 1–8.

Bernard, Bruce P., M.D., editor. "Chapter 7. Work-Related Musculoskeletal Disorders and Psychosocial Factors," The National Institute for Occupational Safety and Health (NIOSH). Available online. URL: http://www.cdc.gov/niosh/ergtxt7.html. Downloaded February 7, 2006.

National Institute for Occupational Safety and Health, The. "Work-Related Musculoskeletal Disorders," NIOSH Facts. Available online. URL: http://www.cdc.gov/niosh/muskdsfs.html. Downloaded February 7, 2006.

myalgia   See PAIN.

myelogram, myelography   More invasive yet sometimes clearer than MAGNETIC RESONANCE IMAGING, this diagnostic test uses X-RAYS to show conditions in the SPINE, SPINAL CORD, and surrounding area. If a doctor needs additional information, a COMPUTED TOMOGRAPHY (CT) SCAN may be performed at the same time.

Procedure

A person must stop eating about eight hours before a myelogram but continue to drink more fluids than usual until about three hours before the test. Prior arrangements also include transportation home from the hospital or outpatient clinic.

To explain the procedure, the Radiological Society of North America (RSNA) said, "Within the spinal canal, the spinal cord and nerve roots are surrounded by a fluid-filled area, the subarachnoid space. This fluid, called cerebrospinal fluid, is confined by the arachnoid membrane and serves to cushion and protect the spinal cord." To guide the placement of the needle, a radiologist uses FLUO-ROSCOPY, which also projects X-ray images onto a monitor. Then, "for myelography, contrast material is injected into the subarachnoid space and x-rays are taken as the contrast flows into different areas. The contrast material outlines areas of the spine that usually are not visible on plain x-rays."

According to Yale New Haven Health, "after the contrast material is injected, you continue lying on your stomach or side while the X-ray pictures are taken. If pictures of your upper back or neck are needed, the contrast material may be moved into those areas by tilting the table or you may be asked to move into different positions. You will be held in position as the table is tilted, and your chin will be placed on a small pillow to keep your neck extended. This prevents the contrast material from entering your head, which can cause headaches or seizures. You need to lie very still to avoid blurring the pictures. Your pulse, breathing rate, and blood pressure may be monitored throughout the test."

The RSNA added, "Myelography itself usually takes 30 to 60 minutes, and a CT scan adds another 30–60 minutes to the total examination time. Some facilities have patients stay in a recovery area for as long as four hours, resting with the head elevated at a 30° to 45° angle. You will be encouraged to take fluids at this time to help eliminate contrast material from your body and prevent headache. You probably will be asked not to engage in strenuous physical activity or bend over for one or two days."

Risks and Complications

Pregnant women, people who have seizures, and patients with certain medical conditions may not be able to take this test. Also, some medications can not be taken within a day or two of a myelogram.

Commonly, patients experience sharp pain from the LUMBAR PUNCTURE or injection into the CERVICAL SPINE. As the contrast dye enters the system, headache or nausea may arise. Some patients have an immediate reaction to the dye, while smokers may get a severe headache after the test. At home, others may get a fever. If the side effects worsen or do not go away in about 24 hours, a doctor should be notified. In rare instances, the test itself can cause ARACHNOIDITIS or other inflammation by invading spinal fluids or membranes.

Outlook and Lifestyle Modifications

If something blocks the flow of the contrast dye, SURGERY may be needed. Commonly, a myelogram detects a SPINAL TUMOR, SPINAL INFECTION, SPINAL STENOSIS, or HERNIATED DISC. Any inflammation in the arachnoid membrane as well as any abnormalities around the spinal cord can also be seen. As the University of Maryland Medical Center Web site said, "A myelogram examination assists your doctor in making a diagnosis. The radiologist interprets the information from the procedure and reports it to your doctor, who in turn will discuss the report with you."

Payne, Kattie. "Myelogram," Yale New Haven Health, Healthwise, Inc. Available online. URL: http://yale newhavenhealth.org/library/healthguide/en-us/ Medicaltests/topic.asp?hwid=hw233057&. Downloaded February 7, 2006.

RadiologyInfo™. "Myelography," Radiological Society of North America, Inc. (RSNA). Available online. URL: http://www.radiologyinfo.org/content/myelography. htm. Last reviewed November 5, 2004.

University of Maryland Medical Center. "Radiology, Myelogram," UMMC. Available online. URL: http:// www.umm.edu/radiology/myelog.htm. Downloaded February 7, 2006.

myeloma bone disease   Sometimes known as multiple myeloma, this primary bone CANCER could be caused by ENVIRONMENTAL INFLUENCES. Higher instances occur among residents of industrialized nations, with approximately 13,500 cases in the United States diagnosed annually. Those statistics mark a 400 percent increase in the last 30 years.

An article posted by the National Institute of Arthritis and Musculoskeletal and Skin Diseases (NIAMS) explained, "Myeloma means, literally, a 'tumor composed of cells normally found in bone marrow.' The majority of patients with myeloma develop destructive bone lesions, also known as osteolytic bone lesions. These lesions occur primarily in the vertebrae, the ribs, the pelvis, and the skull. They occur in the red bone marrow where nests of myeloma cells accumulate," eventually causing bone destruction.

In writing for the Multiple Myeloma Research Foundation, Dr. Sagar Lonial described the progression of this incurable disease: "As tumors grow, they invade the hard outer part of the bone, the solid tissue. In most cases, the myeloma cells spread into the cavities of all the large bones of the body, forming multiple small lesions. This is why the disease is known as 'multiple' myeloma. In some cases, collections of plasma cells arise either within bone or in soft tissues as masses or tumors. These collections are called plasmacytomas, and may represent a more aggressive form of myeloma."

Symptoms and Diagnostic Path

According to the NIAMS, "approximately 70% of myeloma patients experience pain of varying intensity, often in the lower back." Besides LOW BACK PAIN, the sharp onset of ACUTE PAIN may indicate a VERTEBRAL COMPRESSION FRACTURE. In about 30 percent of patients, kidney impairment results in hypercalcemia, which releases too much CALCIUM from the bones into the bloodstream, thereby adding symptoms of thirst, nausea, fatigue, and bone loss. Bone pain or tenderness, fever, and night sweats occur in some patients too.

Diagnostic tools include blood tests, X-RAYS, a BONE SCAN, biopsy, and MAGNETIC RESONANCE IMAGING. Also, BONE MINERAL DENSITY TESTS assess the degree of OSTEOPOROSIS or bone loss that commonly occurs in the ribs, pelvis, skull, and SPINE.

Treatment Options and Outlook

Although no cure exists, a variety of treatments may ease pain and improve quality of life. For example, the Loyola University Health System listed options, such as PAIN RELIEVERS, treatment of FRACTURE, radiation to control pain, chemotherapy, bone marrow transplant, and "alpha interferon—a biological response modifier (a substance that stimulates or improves the ability of the body's immune system to fight disease) that interferes with the division of cancer cells, therefore slowing tumor growth. Interferons are substances normally produced by the body," but they can be produced in a laboratory.

An article on the International Myeloma Foundation (IMF) Web site discussed several treatments appropriate for various types of myeloma. For example, "patients with hypercalcemia due to myeloma usually respond very rapidly to treatment. . . . However, efficacy of steroids in this setting may be due in part to their rapid suppression of myeloma tumor growth."

Risk Factors and Preventive Measures

According to information from the American Academy of Orthopaedic Surgeons, "this disease generally occurs in older adults. Fewer than 3 percent of cases occur in people under the age of 40. Multiple myeloma tends to be more common in men than women. It is twice as common in African Americans as it is in Caucasians," with fewer cases than in either group reported among Asians. GENETIC FACTORS may need to be addressed as well as environmental risks inherent in a particular area, country, and lifestyle.

To investigate how the progression of bone loss in myeloma might be prevented, a group of doctors studied the effects of BISPHOSPHONATES then reported their findings in the *Blood* journal published by The American Society of Hematology. As the article summarized, "Our results suggest that although not useful as a direct therapy to reduce tumor burden in myeloma patients, ibandronate may be extremely useful as an adjunctive therapy for the treatment of the osteolytic component of myeloma disease. Since it is this bone destructive component that causes the most distressing and painful symptoms for the patient, the use of bisphosphonates such as ibandronate in myeloma disease may improve dramatically the quality of life of the patient. However, other treatments, such as chemotherapy, radiotherapy, and marrow transplantation should continue to be the main therapies directed at preventing growth of the myeloma cells."

American Academy of Orthopaedic Surgeons. "Multiple Myeloma/Plasmacytoma," AAOS. Available online. URL: http://orthoinfo.aaos.org/fact/thr_report.cfm?Thread_ID=488&topcategory=Tumors. Downloaded February 8, 2006.

Dallas, Sarah L., I. Ross Garrett, Babatunde O. Oyajobi, Mark R. Dallas, Brendan F. Boyce, Frieder Bauss, Jiri Radl, and Gregory R. Mundy. "Ibandronate Reduces Osteolytic Lesions but Not Tumor Burden in a Murine Model of Myeloma Bone Disease," *Blood*, 93, no. 5 (March 1, 1999): 1,697–1,706.

Lonial, Sagar, M.D. "Intro to Myeloma," Multiple Myeloma Research Foundation, MMRF. Available online. URL: http://www.multiplemyeloma.org/about_myeloma/. Downloaded February 8, 2006.

Loyola University Health System. "Myeloma Bone Disease/Multiple Myeloma." Available online. URL: http://www.luhs.org/health/topics/bone/myeloma.htm. Last reviewed January 5, 2005.

Mundy, Gregory R., M.D. and Babatunde O. Oyajobi. "Myeloma Bone Disease—Update 2003," International Myeloma Foundation, IMF. Available online. URL: http://www.myeloma.org/main.jsp?tab_id=1&type=article&id=1044. Downloaded February 8, 2006.

National Institutes of Health (NIH) Osteoporosis and Related Bone Diseases, National Resource Center, "Myeloma Bone Disease," National Institute of Arthritis and Musculoskeletal and Skin Diseases (NIAMS). Available online. URL: http://www.osteo.org/newfile.asp?doc=r605i&doctitle=Myeloma+Bone+Disease&doctype=HTML+Fact+Sheet. Downloaded February 8, 2006.

myelomeningocele   See SPINA BIFADA.

myofascial release   See ACUPRESSURE, MASSAGE THERAPY, TRIGGER POINT THERAPY.

naproxen In 1976, this NONSTEROIDAL ANTI-INFLAMMATORY DRUG (NSAID) received approval from the Food and Drug Administration (FDA) as both a prescription and an OVER-THE-COUNTER PRODUCT. Best known by such brand names as Aleve or Naprosyn, naproxen acts like any NSAID as a PAIN RELIEVER, fever-reducer, and means of easing inflammation. However, on December 23, 2004, FDA issued this alert: "Based on emerging information, the risk of cardiovascular and cerebrovascular events may increase among patients taking naproxen." Therefore, "FDA recommends patients not exceed the recommended dose" unless a doctor says otherwise. For example, a physician may prescribe a stronger dose of naproxen to treat the CHRONIC PAIN and inflammation of ARTHRITIS, ANKYLOSING SPONDYLITIS, JUVENILE ARTHRITIS, and RHEUMATOID ARTHRITIS.

Dosage and Potential Side Effects

From the start, the FDA advised against the use of naproxen by women in the last three months of pregnancy, people with allergies to ASPIRIN or other NSAIDs, and patients with kidney problems or other serious medical conditions. For most adults though, the FDA recommended, "When taking an over-the-counter naproxen product, 1 tablet (220 mg) should be taken every 8 to 12 hours while symptoms last. You may take 2 tablets within the first hour of symptoms for the first dose. However, you should not exceed 2 tablets (440 mg) in any 8 to 12 hour period or 3 tablets (660 mg) in a 24-hour period."

For CHILDREN, the dosage varies according to body weight. Although a liquid form of naproxen is available, it may not be suitable for a child who has sensitivities to food dyes or artificial flavorings. For patients of all ages, eating a little food and drinking a full glass of water with this medication can help to avoid an upset stomach.

Regarding other potential side effects, Drugs.com cautioned that "naproxen may increase the sensitivity of the skin to sunlight." The Web site also reminded patients to take naproxen for no more than 10 days unless a doctor prescribes differently. Also, "do not crush or chew the extended-release forms of naproxen (e.g., Naprelan, EC Naprosyn, others). Swallow them whole. These are specially formulated to release slowly in the body. Ask your pharmacist if you do not know if you have an extended-release formulation."

Statistics and Studies

As studies of NSAIDs continue, an article in *Medicine & Health* said, "Some of the outside experts on the FDA's NSAID advisory panel suggested that different NSAIDs pose different cardiovascular risks, with the Cox-2's perhaps on the more dangerous end and naproxen . . . perhaps even giving some protection against cardiovascular ills." The acting director of the Office of New Drugs at FDA mentioned a possible "class effect" in NSAIDs, then added, "There may be slight differences between the drugs, or even larger differences, but we don't have enough data to really rank-order these drugs by risk."

Drugs.com™. "Naproxen," Drug Information Online, Micromedex Physicians Desk Reference. Available online. URL: http://www.drugs.com/naproxen.html. Last updated December 1, 2005.

FDA Patient Information Sheet. "Naproxen," Food and Drug Administration. Available online. URL: http://www.fda.gov/cder/drug/InfoSheets/patient/Naproxen-pt.pdf. Downloaded February 8, 2006.

Staff. "FDA Beefs Up NSAID Warnings, Pulls Bextra," *Medicine & Health* 59, no. 13 (April 11, 2005): 1–2.

neck See CERVICAL SPINE.

neck brace See ORTHOTICS.

neck injury See CERVICAL SPINE; SPINAL INJURY.

neck pain Yes, that proverbial pain in the neck can come from dealing with someone who is a pain in the neck, mainly because of the resulting TENSION. More often, neck pain arises from poor POSTURE, DEGENERATIVE DISC DISEASE, SPINAL STENOSIS, or a HERNIATED DISC in the CERVICAL SPINE. In addition, ACUTE PAIN comes in a whiplash as a FLEXION-EXTENSION INJURY causes the neck to exceed its normal RANGE OF MOTION. Although far less dramatic and, usually, much less painful, problems similar to a whiplash can arise with improper LIFTING techniques, poor ERGONOMIC FACTORS, and bad habits, such as cradling a telephone on the shoulder. Forgetting BACKPACK SAFETY or slinging around a heavy shoulder bag can also produce neck pain.

As the American Physical Therapy Association (APTA) advised, "The basic rule is simple: keep your neck in a 'neutral' position whenever possible. In other words, don't bend or hunch your neck forward for long periods. Also, try not to sit in one position for a long time. If you must sit for an extended period, make sure your posture is good: Keep your head in a neutral position, make sure your back is supported, keep your knees slightly lower than your hips, and rest your arms if possible."

Regarding those arms, the APTA said, "Pain in the cervical region can cause arm pain as well as the 'pain in the neck.' Why? In the case of the arms, it's because the nerves that branch out from the neck go all the way down into the arms and into the hands. . . . The uppermost cervical disc connects the top of the spinal column to the base of the skull. The spinal cord, which sends nerve impulses to every part of the body, runs through a canal in the cervical vertebrae and continues all the way down the spine. The cervical nerves spread down into the arms; because of this, arm pain is sometimes traceable to a problem in the neck." This type of problem may begin at a computer station or during SLEEP but can usually be avoided by keeping the SPINE in a neutral position. Doing that, however, may take a bit of practice or a better pillow.

Risks and Complications
Along the same vertebral line, NeuroSurgery.com said, "A muscle spasm, brought on by poor posture, sleeping position, or stress, is the most frequent cause of neck pain. But an aching neck can be a symptom of a more serious problem. Disc degeneration, narrowing of the spinal canal, arthritis and even cancer can cause neck pain. For serious neck problems a primary care physician and often a specialist, such as a neurosurgeon, should be consulted." For example, "cervical disc disorders are typically marked by intermittent neck pain, followed by severe neck and sometimes arm pain. The pain is sufficient to awaken a person from sleep. Irritated nerves also can lead to numbness or weakness in the arm or forearm, tingling in the fingers and coordination problems. Severe nerve impairment or even paralysis can develop if the disorder is left untreated." In addition, "pressure on the spinal cord from a herniated disc or bone spur in the neck can also be a very serious problem. Virtually all of the nerves of the body have to pass through the neck to reach their final destination (arms, chest, abdomen, legs)."

Statistics and Studies
Some studies focus on the effectiveness of ACUPUNCTURE in treating neck pain. For example, one trial studied the outcomes for 124 patients, 18 to 80 years old. As reported in the *Alternative Medicine Review,* "Acupuncture reduced neck pain and produced a . . . significant effect compared with placebo."

From Sweden, another study of neck pain examined out-of-focus eyes. As reported in *Optician,* "People who suffer from back and neck pain following computer use may need their eyes examined." With the help of POSITIVE EMISSION TOMOGRAPHY (PET) SCANS, the researchers, "examined whether eye problems can cause musculoskeletal complaints and vice versa." Apparently, "focusing the lens of the eye requires coordination between various nerve and muscle groups in the eye, neck, and shoulder region." Therefore, "tensing and relaxing the neck, throat, and shoulders affect the eyes," whereas "eye complaints can trigger and/or aggravate muscular aches in the shoulders and/or neck region."

Loosening up can prevent the pain of MUSCULO-SKELETAL DISORDERS anytime but especially as one ages. According to an article in the *Family Practice News*, "most osteoarthritic changes occur between C5 and C6 and between C6 and C7" vertebrae in the cervical spine. "Almost everyone eventually develops osteoarthritis in the neck. On average, 45% of adults aged 40–49 years, 72% of adults aged 50–59 years, and 83% of adults aged 60–75 years have some osteoarthritic changes, but those who keep the neck and shoulders loose with stretching and strengthening exercises don't notice it."

Special Aids and Adaptations

By practicing self-awareness, most people can adapt their movements, thereby reducing incidents of neck pain. For example, a sudden motion, such as abruptly throwing back the head, can press the SPINAL CORD and cause discomfort.

For gentle neck stretches, the *Family Practice News* article suggested, "Stand or sit up straight on a chair, with your feet flat on the floor. Keeping the head level, slowly tuck your chin in toward the back of the head. This movement should give you a bit of a double chin. Hold for 6–8 seconds. Relax. Repeat up to six times."

Information from NeckSurgery.com emphasized neck flexibility, too, but also mentioned "safe and effective abdominal exercises that will help alleviate neck pain." Resting on a floor mat "with your arms crossed in front, bend your knees and keep your feet flat on the floor. Lift your upper back off the floor and lower down." While emphasizing the contraction of abdominal muscles, "you should exhale as you lift up and inhale as you lower down. Go through a series of 10." If getting up and down from a floor mat or padded carpet proves too strenuous, patients can adapt by exercising in bed.

Besides stretching EXERCISE, patients with a CHRONIC PAIN in the neck may be helped by PAIN RELIEVERS, such as ASPIRIN or other NONSTEROIDAL ANTI-INFLAMMATORY DRUG (NSAID), and HEAT THER-APY, such as a warm shower. If those conservative treatments fail, medical tests, such as an X-RAY, MYELOGRAM, or DISCOGRAM, can aid the diagnosis and direct the course of treatment, determining, for example, if an ANTERIOR CERVICAL DISCECTOMY or other type of SURGERY will be needed. According to NeuroSurgery.com, however, "Surgery has its limitations. It can't reverse all the effects of overuse or aging, and it carries risks. Yet it may be the only way to relieve pain, numbness and weakness."

American Physical Therapy Association. "What You Need To Know About Neck Pain," APTA. Available online. URL: http://www.apta.org/AM/Template.cfm?Section=Search &template=/CM/HTMLDisplay.cfm&ContentID=24761. Downloaded February 9, 2006.

Medtronic Sofamor Danek. "Exercises For Neck Pain," NeckSurgery.com. Available online. URL: http://www.neckreference.com/articles-exercise.html. Last updated April 18, 2005.

Nagler, Willibald. "Strength and Flexibility for Older Patients, Part 2," *Family Practice News* 34, no. 23 (December 1, 2004): 52.

NeurosurgeryToday.org. "Neck Pain," American Association of Neurological Surgeons. Available online. URL: http://www.neurosurgerytoday.org/what/patient_e/neck.asp. Downloaded February 9, 2006.

Staff. "Pain in the Neck? Get an Eye Test," *Optician* (July 1, 2005): 1.

White, P., G. Lewith, P. Prescott and J. Conway. "Acupuncture versus Placebo for the Treatment of Chronic Mechanical Neck Pain: a Randomized, Controlled Trial," *Alternative Medicine Review* 10, no. 1 (March 2005): 65.

neck strain   See RHOMBOID MUSCLE STRAIN.

neoplasm   See SPINAL TUMOR.

nerve block   As a diagnostic tool for assessing the BACK or SPINE, a temporary nerve block may be used to locate the precise source of spinal nerve pain before SURGERY is performed. As a treatment to avoid surgery, a nerve block involves the injection of an anesthesia, OPIOIDS FOR PAIN, or a steroid to reduce swelling and inflammation. If a long-term PAIN RELIEVER is used, the patient may experience increased RANGE OF MOTION, thus improving flexibility. This enables the person to resume regular daily ACTIVITY and spine-strengthening EXERCISES that may break a cycle of CHRONIC PAIN.

Information from The Cleveland Clinic discussed common types of nerve blocks: "Trigger point injection—injection (shot) of small amounts of local anesthetic and steroid in the area of the muscle where you have pain or tenderness. Epidural steroid injection—injection of a small amount of steroid medication near nerves in your lower back. Facet joint injection—injection of a small amount of local anesthetic near facet joints (located on the side of your spine, away from the spinal cord). Stellate ganglion block—injection of local anesthetic around a group of nerves (found in the neck area). Lumbar sympathetic block—an injection of local anesthetic around a group of nerves in your lower back (lumbar area). Intercostal nerve block—an injection of local anesthetic in the area between the ribs."

Procedure

A nerve block will seldom be used alone but, more often, as part of a rehabilitation program involving therapeutic exercise, physical therapy, occupational therapy, or some type of COMPLEMENTARY AND ALTERNATIVE MEDICINE (CAM). Each type of nerve block differs slightly, depending on the purpose and location. For instance, some blocks involve a single injection, while others require additional infusions of medication. To guide needle placement, FLUOROSCOPY may also be used.

Risks and Complications

Patients on blood thinners or those with drug allergies should avoid this treatment. Also, a nerve block should not be performed on anyone with a SPINAL INFECTION or other active illness. As a form of PAIN MANAGEMENT, a nerve block aims to calm spinal nerves, but the opposite can happen. Pain may worsen or, worse, permanent numbness can occur at an injection site.

Outlook and Lifestyle Modifications

In the LUMBAR SPINE, an EPIDURAL INJECTION may relieve pain caused by SPINAL STENOSIS or a HER-

NIATED DISC. A nerve block may be used in the THORACIC SPINE and the CERVICAL SPINE too, for instance, to treat the chronic pain of a CERVICOGENIC HEADACHE.

As Dr. Steven Richeimer explained in an article for SpineUniverse, "The occipital nerves travel from the cervical spine in the neck to the back of the head and scalp. These nerves can be damaged by arthritic changes in the cervical spine, by muscle spasm, or by neck injuries. The result can be headaches which typically start in the back of the neck and spread towards the forehead. Occipital nerve blocks with steroids can often help."

Similarly, the article "Nerve Root Block Probes Cervicogenic Headache" in the *Family Practice News* reported on a study of 114 patients, most of whom "were aged 30–50 years and had a history of the headaches for less than 2 years. About half had a history of trauma." Of these, "twenty-one patients improved permanently after the block alone and never required surgery." All of these patients had degenerative conditions "of the cervical spine and were more than 60 years old." With average follow-up at 3.8 years, "70% of the entire cohort of 114 patients achieved complete improvement," with partial improvement noted in another 18%.

Baker, Barbara. "Nerve Root Block Probes Cervicogenic Headache," *Family Practice News* 30, no. 18 (September 15, 2000): 14.

Cleveland Clinic, The. "Nerve Block: Does It Work?" Department of Patient Education and Health Information. Available online. URL: http://www.clevelandclinic.org/health/health-info/docs/0300/0325.asp?index=4417. Downloaded February 10, 2006.

Richeimer, Steven, M.D. "Nerve Blocks: Medication Injections," SpineUniverse. Available online. URL: http://www.spineuniverse.com/displayarticle.php/article1518.html. Last updated June 27, 2005.

nerve compression   Not one disorder but many, nerve compression commonly occurs in the form of carpal tunnel syndrome, but in the VERTEBRAE of the BACK and SPINE, nerve compression can be felt throughout the body. For example, a BRACHIAL PLEXUS INJURY can result from a BIRTH INJURY with compression among the nerves running from the

SPINAL CORD through the CERVICAL SPINE and into the shoulders and arms. Also, trauma or swelling in the neck and shoulders can cause THORACIC OUTLET SYNDROME, which weakens and sometimes numbs upper body muscles down to the fingertips. If injury, overuse, or the effects of WEIGHT weigh too heavily on the lower LUMBAR SPINE, nerve compression may cause pain, tingling, or numbness in the legs.

Symptoms and Diagnostic Path

A diagnostic path starts with a patient history and physical examination, including an evaluation of the person's RANGE OF MOTION. To assess such potential causes as a HERNIATED DISC or SPINAL STENOSIS, imaging tests may begin with X-RAYS. For clear images of the spinal nerves, MAGNETIC RESONANCE IMAGING may be needed, whereas a COMPUTED TOMOGRAPHY (CT) SCAN may best reveal the condition of the spinal canal. If the doctor suspects nerve compression caused by an OSTEOPHYTE or SPINAL TUMOR, a MYELOGRAM may pinpoint the locale.

Treatment Options and Outlook

Besides various forms of PAIN MANAGEMENT, treatments usually include physical therapy, occupational therapy, or therapeutic EXERCISE. Spinal manipulation and other forms of COMPLEMENTARY AND ALTERNATIVE MEDICINE (CAM) may also provide effective options.

For example, a study reported in the *Journal of Vertebral Subluxation Research* considered VERTEBRAL SUBLUXATION. According to the article, "the major variables of compression are the rate of onset, the amount of pressure generated, and the time maintained. Another major variable in the recovery is age. The younger the nerve tissue the better chance for a full recovery." Also, "the garden hose theory or hard bone-soft nerve explanation of vertebral subluxation is considered by some to be archaic but appears to be a valid entity at least in the lower cervical spine. More research is needed to decipher the susceptibility to mild pressure increases throughout the spine."

If conservative treatments fail to alleviate nerve pressure, SURGERY may be needed in about 5 percent of the cases. For instance, such procedures as CERVICAL LAMINAPLASTY and LAMINECTOMY can decompress the pressure on spinal nerves.

Risk Factors and Preventive Measures

According to the North American Spine Society (NASS), "people with cervical" pain and other neck problems "frequently avoid activity. Decreased activity reduces flexibility, strength and cardiovascular endurance." Conversely, "a physical therapy or exercise program usually begins with stretching exercises to restore flexibility to tight muscles in the neck, trunk, arms and legs. You may be asked to stretch frequently to preserve flexibility." Furthermore, "everyday activities will be easier if flexibility, strength and endurance are maintained and increased. Your physical therapist and doctor can tell you how to add a continuing exercise program into your life, either at home using simple equipment or at a fitness facility. . . . For people needing additional assistance, home alterations and safety should be considered. An occupational therapist can provide suggestions for easy performance of everyday tasks such as bathing, dressing and fine motor tasks such as turning keys, opening jars, using phones and computers."

Alderson, R. Scott and George J. Muhs. "The Effects of Mild Compression on Spinal Nerve Roots with Implications for Models of Vertebral Subluxation and the Clinical Effects of Chiropractic Adjustment," *Journal of Vertebral Subluxation Research* 4, no. 2, (May 2001).

Hoyle, Brian Douglas. "Nerve Compression," eNotes.com. Available online. URL: http://health.enotes.com/neurological-disorders-encyclopedia/nerve-compression. Downloaded February 15, 2006.

North American Spine Society. "Cervical Stenosis & Myelopathy," NASS. Available online. URL: http://www.spine.org/articles/cervicalstenosis.cfm. Downloaded February 15, 2006.

nerve conduction study or nerve conduction velocity (NCV) test Used to measure the speed of electrical impulses soaring through the nervous system, this diagnostic tool also assesses spinal nerve damage. Results vary from one area of the body and one person to another, but generally speaking, the faster the nerve conduction, the stronger the nerve.

Procedure

A day or two before a nerve conduction velocity (NCV) test, patients must stop using any MUSCLE RELAXANT and also skin oils or lotion. Fever and heat affect the accuracy of an NCV, too, since a higher body temperature can speed nerve impulses.

To describe the procedure, the St. John's Mercy Health Care Web site said, "A recording electrode will be attached to the skin over the nerve with a special paste and a stimulating electrode will be placed at a known distance away from the recording electrode. The nerve will be stimulated by a mild and brief electrical shock given through the stimulating electrode. You may experience minor discomfort for a few seconds. The stimulation of the nerve and the detected response will be displayed on an oscilloscope (a monitor that displays electrical activity in the form of waves)."

In writing for Yale New Haven Health, R.N. Jan Nissl said, "With the nerve conduction studies, you will feel a brief, burning pain, a tingling sensation, and a twitching of the muscle each time the electrical pulse is applied. It feels similar to the kind of tingling you feel when you rub your feet on the carpet and then touch a metal object. The testing can be quite uncomfortable and makes some people nervous. Keep in mind that only a very low-voltage electrical current is used, and each electrical pulse is very brief (less than a millisecond)."

An NCV may be part of a diagnostic program during hospitalization. When given in an outpatient setting though, the patient may need to curtail regular daily ACTIVITY for the remainder of the day.

Risks and Complications

This test should be postponed for patients with ACUTE PAIN, fever, or an injury to the SPINAL CORD. People who wear a pacemaker or take blood-thinners may not be able to have a nerve conduction study. Otherwise, the electrical voltage used in an NCV should cause no problem or injury.

Outlook and Lifestyle Modifications

Since an NCV evaluates various types of conditions affecting the BACK or SPINE, the outcome affects the outlook. For example, the study may show a need to treat POST-POLIO SYNDROME, SCIATICA, or a HERNIATED DISC.

According to the North Memorial Medical Center, "Nerve damage or disease may still exist despite normal NCV results. This is because other healthy fibers in the same nerve may show a normal reaction time." To evaluate MUSCULOSKELETAL DISORDERS, an NCV may be used in conjunction with an ELECTROMYOGRAM.

McLaughlin, Eileen. "Nerve Conduction Velocity Test," North Memorial Medical Center, Health Encyclopedia. Available online. URL: http://www.northmemorial. com/HealthEncyclopedia/content/1375.asp. Downloaded February 10, 2006.

Nissl, Jan. "Electromyogram (EMG) and Nerve Conduction Studies," Yale New Haven Health. Available online. URL: http://yalenewhavenhealth.org/library/healthguide/en-us/Medicaltests/topic.asp?hwid=hw213 852&. Last updated October 5, 2004.

St. John's Mercy Health Care. "Nerve Conduction Velocity (NCV)," Tests & Procedures. Available online. URL: http://www.stjohnsmercy.org/healthinfo/test/neuro/TP013.asp. Downloaded February 10, 2006.

neuropathy   See CHRONIC BACK PAIN.

neurostimulation   As an option after FAILED BACK SURGERY, this treatment offers an alternative for managing CHRONIC PAIN without increasing medication. For example, neurostimulation can be used to reduce pain in patients with ARACHNOIDITIS and DEGENERATIVE DISC DISEASE.

In describing the concept, Medtronic Pain Therapies said, "Neurostimulation delivers low voltage electrical stimulation to the spinal cord or targeted . . . nerve to block the sensation of pain." This ongoing treatment may be administered through an external device or system. As an internal device though, "the neurostimulation system, implanted in the epidural space, stimulates these pain-inhibiting nerve fibers, masking the sensation of pain with a tingling sensation."

Procedure

The American Pain & Wellness Web site explained, "The trial screening procedure—or test stimulation—consists of a short test stimulation period in the operating room followed by an evaluation period of several days at home. During the evaluation period, you and your doctor determine your response to neurostimulation and your level of pain relief. This trial gives you an opportunity to experience the system and enables the doctor to assess your battery requirements. During the trial screening, your doctor will place a lead in your back to deliver electrical stimulation to the spinal cord. The lead placement is one of the keys to successful results with a neurostimulation system. . . . Typically, you will receive a local anesthetic and mild sedatives to keep you comfortable during the procedure."

Risks and Complications

Neurostimulation can interfere with a pacemaker, whereas MAGNETIC RESONANCE IMAGING and ULTRASOUND THERAPY interfere with neurostimulation. Also, the safety of the treatment has not been studied in INFANTS, CHILDREN, and pregnant women. Adverse events have included increased pain, electrical jolts, and paralysis.

Outlook and Lifestyle Modifications

According to an article posted by The Spine Institute, "because neurostimulation works in the area where pain signals travel, electrical impulses can be directed to cover specific sites where you are feeling pain. Neurostimulation can give effective pain relief and decrease the need for pain medications. In addition, this therapy is non-destructive. Typically, patients who have success with neurostimulation experience a 50% greater reduction in their pain and improved ability to go about daily activities."

American Pain & Wellness. "Spinal Injections/ Procedures, Neurostimulation." Available online. URL: http://www.painandwellness.com/spinal_injections_neurostimulation.html. Downloaded February 10, 2006.
Medtronic Pain Therapies™. "Neurostimulation." Available online. URL: http://www.medtronic.com/neuro/paintherapies/pain_treatment_ladder/neuro stimulation/neuro_neurostimulation.html. Downloaded February 15, 2006.
Spine Institute, The. "Electrical Stimulation," Saint John's Health Center. Available online. URL: http://www.espineinstitute.com/PainMngmt_ElectricalStimulation.htm. Downloaded February 15, 2006.

nonsteroidal anti-inflammatory drug (NSAID) therapy As the name partially implies, an NSAID offers an option to steroids as a treatment for inflammation, fever, and pain. Available as either OVER-THE-COUNTER PRODUCTS or prescription strength drugs, NSAIDs include ASPIRIN, IBUPROFEN, NAPROXEN, and Nabumetone, but not ACETAMINOPHEN since the latter does not ease inflammation.

As the American Academy of Orthopaedic Surgeons (AAOS) explained, "NSAIDs work by preventing an enzyme (a protein that triggers changes in the body) from doing its job. The enzyme is called cyclooxygenase, or COX, and it has two forms. COX-1 protects the stomach lining from harsh acids and digestive chemicals; it also helps maintain kidney function. COX-2 is produced when joints are injured or inflamed." However, "traditional NSAIDs block the actions of both COX-1 and COX-2, which is why they can cause stomach upset and bleeding as well as ease pain and inflammation."

Risks and Complications

By inhibiting the protective action of COX-1, NSAIDs can upset the stomach and even cause internal bleeding. Therefore, ELDERLY persons and patients who have blood-clotting problems or who take other types of blood-thinners should avoid NSAIDs.

According to the December 23, 2004, *FDA Talk Paper*, "The Food and Drug Administration (FDA) today issued a Public Health Advisory summarizing the agency's recent recommendations concerning the use of non-steroidal anti-inflammatory drug products (NSAIDs), including those known as COX-2 selective agents. The public health advisory is an interim measure, pending further review of data that continue to be collected." Furthermore, the FDA announced, "Preliminary results from a long-term clinical trial (up to three years) suggest that long-term use of a non-selective NSAID, naproxen (sold as Aleve, Naprosyn and other trade name and generic products), may be associated with an increased cardiovascular (CV) risk compared to placebo." However, "non-selective NSAIDs are widely used in both over-the-counter (OTC) and prescription settings. As prescription drugs, many are approved for short-term use in the treatment of pain . . . and for longer-term use to treat the signs and symptoms of osteoarthritis and rheumatoid arthritis."

In 2005, *FDA Consumer Magazine* said, "The FDA is asking the manufacturers of all non-prescription NSAIDs sold over the counter (OTC) to revise their labels to include more specific information about potential cardiovascular and gastrointestinal risks and information on the safe use of the drugs. The agency also is asking manufacturers of OTC NSAIDs to include a warning about potential skin reactions."

Statistics and Studies

According to a study reported in *Inflammopharmacology*, "population studies and World Health Organisation (WHO) statistics indicate that 10–50% of individuals suffer from musculoskeletal disorders. Up to 3% will be classified as disabled due to their bone and joint condition, and the majority will suffer from pain. Almost all will require non-steroidal anti-inflammatory drugs (NSAIDs) and other analgesics for their management. The large majority of this population is elderly and, hence, at greater risk of adverse effects to the NSAIDs. The NSAIDs are a necessary choice in pain management because of the integrated role of the cyclo-oxygenase (COX) pathway in the generation of inflammation and in the biochemical recognition of pain. For over 80 years the management of musculoskeletal pain was hampered by NSAID toxicity problems related to the traditional NSAIDs." However, "recent studies have shown that the use of a . . . drug with traditional NSAIDs and with COX-2-selective inhibitors has been shown to significantly reduce GI symptoms. . . . Thus, the traditional NSAIDs have been re-established as the preferred choice in the management of arthritis and musculoskeletal disorders."

Besides easing the CHRONIC PAIN of ARTHRITIS or MUSCULOSKELETAL DISORDERS, NSAIDs alleviate pain in CANCER patients. According to *JAMA, The Journal of the American Medical Association*, "some nonsteroidal anti-inflammatory drugs (NSAIDs) are facing controversy due to their link to increased risk of myocardial infarction and stroke. However, a new study found that long-term daily NSAID use reduced the risk of oral cancer in some smokers but did not increase overall survival thus suggesting

that the value of some of these drugs for certain cancer patients might outweigh the risks."

Special Aids and Adaptations

Patients aid the effectiveness of an NSAID and avoid most of its side effects by having a little food and lots of water with the dosage recommended on the label. Sometimes, a doctor may recommend a higher dose to be used as a PAIN RELIEVER. If an NSAID, such as aspirin, is used to prevent blood clots, however, less is usually more effective as a maintenance dosage since a minimal dose does the job with minimal risk.

American Academy of Orthopaedic Surgeons. "What Are NSAIDs?" AAOS. Available online. URL: http://orthoinfo.aaos.org/fact/thr_report.cfm?Thread_ID=398&topcategory=General%20Information. Downloaded February 15, 2006.

FDA Consumer Magazine. "FDA Announces Changes Affecting the Marketing of Non-Steroidal Anti-Inflammatory Drugs," May–June 2005 issue, U.S. Food and Drug Administration. Available online. URL: http://www.fda.gov/fdac/features/2005/305_nsaid.html. Downloaded February 15, 2006.

FDA Talk Paper. December 23, 2004. "FDA Issues Public Health Advisory Recommending Limited Use of Cox-2 Inhibitors," U.S. Food and Drug Administration. Available online. URL: http://www.fda.gov/bbs/topics/ANSWERS/2004/ANS01336.html. Downloaded February 15, 2006.

Hampton, Tracy. "NSAID Studies Abound in Cancer Research: Drugs May Have Niche in Prevention and Treatment.: (Nonsteroidal Anti-inflammatory Drugs)," *JAMA, The Journal of the American Medical Association* 293, no. 21 (June 1, 2005): 2,579–2,580.

Kean, Walter F. "The Use of NSAIDs in Rheumatic Disorders 2005: a Global Perspective," *Inflammopharmacology* 13, no. 4 (2005): 343–370.

nutrition   Daily nutrition consists of an alphabet of vitamins with trace minerals, such as IRON and ZINC, and essential minerals, such as CALCIUM, MAGNESIUM, PHOSPHORUS, and POTASSIUM, best kept in MINERAL BALANCE. Nutrition also provides life-sustaining proteins, fats, and carbohydrates for BONE BUILDING the BACK and SPINE, energizing cells, overcoming TEN-

SION, combating illness, and repairing hard matter or soft tissue throughout the body.

Diets may be debated, and nutritional needs may be complex, but essentially, nourishment flourishes in simplicity. Basically, the closer a food remains to its natural state, the more nutritious and bone-nurturing it will be. With little or no food processing to strip away nutrients and fiber, natural foods provide the most wholesome source of vitamins, minerals, and trace elements, many of which have not yet been fully studied. Fresh foods also grow naturally free of food colorings, preservatives, and other potentially harmful additives.

As another basic guideline, well-balanced nutrition almost always occurs when a variety of foods has been selected for the week. Typically, those diverse tastes, textures, and colors can be found on the outside walls of a grocery store. Except for grains, which rarely require refrigeration, outer store aisles highlight the basic food groups in colorful displays of fresh fruit, fresh vegetables, dairy products, eggs, fish, and meat. Perhaps weekly, one might encircle the store, aiming for the ultimate goal: Bin there, ate that.

Optimal menu choices will not, of course, be the same for everyone. INFANTS, young CHILDREN, and ELDERLY persons require foods that can easily be digested, whereas active ADOLESCENTS and young to middle-aged adults may need somewhat meatier fare. Temporarily, pregnant women and nursing mothers may need to add an all-natural nutritional supplement to their healthy diets. However, patients with METABOLIC BONE DISEASE or METABOLIC DISEASES OF MUSCLE do not readily absorb nutrients so may need to continue supplements, depending on the advice of their physicians. Also, people with bone loss caused by EATING DISORDERS or bone problems caused by the adverse effects of WEIGHT have special dietary needs that must be met to restore balance. In addition, GENETIC FACTORS and ENVIRONMENTAL INFLUENCES alter the specific needs for a nutrient. For example, a person may require more VITAMIN A, VITAMIN C, and VITAMIN E than commonly needed to boost the immune system. As a memory device, those same three vitamins combine to combat or A. C. E. an illness.

To nourish the back and spine and strengthen bones in general, nutritionists agree on the impor-tance of calcium and VITAMIN D. However, an editorial in the *QJM: An International Journal of Medicine* posed the question, "Nutrition and bone: is there more to it than just calcium and vitamin D?" As the editorial noted, "It is feasible . . . that supplementation of other macro- or micronutri-ents may have value in influencing fracture risk, perhaps especially in those with specific genetic traits. . . . Of even more practical significance would be the opportunity to relate specific food groups to our risk of future fracture, giving a real opportunity for targeted nutritional advice." For example, "potassium is worthy of attention due to its role as a buffer for . . . acid production. . . . Potassium bicarbonate ingestion reduces urinary calcium excretion and improves calcium balance in healthy young adults and can both reduce bone resorption and increase formation in post-menopausal women." Conversely, "an increase in dietary sodium intake leads to an increase in urinary sodium and a consequent increase in urinary calcium loss." Furthermore, "dietary calcium: phosphate ratio may have importance. . . . If this is the case, the habitual consumption of carbonated drinks with their low calcium: phosphate ratio may have detrimental effects which have yet to be fully elucidated."

As the editorial added, "the vitamin-K-dependent proteins . . . are important constituents of bone. . . . Recent evidence has suggested that low intakes of vitamin K are associated with hip fracture in both women and men." Since VITAMIN K counteracts blood-thinners, patients need to amend their menus carefully to avoid foods high in that vitamin. For those who do not need to be wary of eggplant or other sources of K, the editorial suggested, "Rather than focus on individual nutrients, an alternative way of investigating the effect of diet on disease is to study food patterns and food groups. Recently it has been suggested that a diet rich in fruits and vegetables may be associated with higher bone mass, although other food groups have not been examined. Dietary patterns could exert their influence through the nutrients contained in the foods (i.e., vitamins, minerals) or through other components."

Gardeners can check out some components at a local agricultural center or county extension agency, but the presence of PHYTOCHEMICALS, such as antioxidants and PHYTOESTROGENS, may be difficult to ascertain. However, to check out the acid-alkaline balance in the body, most people can do this themselves at home by checking their saliva with litmus paper purchased from a pharmacy. The information can then be used to reassess the diet. For example, if the litmus paper shows high acidity, the person may need to limit the consumption of meat, dairy products, wheat products, and sugars, planning instead a menu of fruits, vegetables, oat products, and wild rice. To replace acid-forming drinks, such as coffee, tea, and colas, a choice glass of filtered water with a squeeze of lime or lemon may help to re-establish a healthy acid-alkaline balance. That particular drink adds active enzymes to the diet too, thus aiding digestion. Fresh fruits and vegetables also bring enzymatic action and healthful phytochemicals to the dinner table unless, of course, preservatives have been added, thus killing the active nutrients. However, a healthier choice of preservative-free dressings can usually be found in a refrigerated case on the outer aisle of a grocery store.

Up and down the aisles and ages, nutrition continues to play a major role in a healthy lifestyle. For example, the article "Nutrition and Aging—Practical Advice for Healthy Eating" in the *Journal of the American Medical Women's Association* said, "The 2005 Dietary Guidelines for Americans emphasize healthy weight: physical activity: choosing a variety of grains, especially whole-grain foods, fruits, and vegetables daily: a diet low in saturated fat, cholesterol, total fat, added sugars, and sodium: and moderate alcohol intake for those who drink." For most age groups, "fruits and vegetables are associated with prevention of major chronic diseases." Furthermore, "new research suggests that fruits and vegetables may protect bone health as well."

Risks and Complications

Eating the most natural foods sounds uncomplicated and risk-free, but that natural state makes them apt to acquire surface bacteria. Like other external contaminants, however, bacteria can usually be washed away with a solution of three parts water and one part vinegar. Vinegar-water can also be used to wipe countertops to avoid contamination during preparation time at home. For natural foods such as grains and ground beef that cannot be surface-washed, thorough cooking eradicates most contaminants.

Besides their concern for food safety, the U.S. Food and Drug Administration (FDA) warned, "approximately 2 percent of adults and about 5 percent of infants and young children in the United States suffer from food allergies." Furthermore, "each year, roughly 30,000 individuals require emergency room treatment and 150 individuals die because of allergic reactions to food." With "eight major foods or food groups—milk, eggs, fish, . . . shellfish, tree nuts, peanuts, wheat, and soybeans" accounting for "90 percent of food allergies," the FDA now requires clear labeling of products containing those ingredients.

While timely emergency treatment may offset a severe allergic response, no cure exists for food allergies. Therefore, infants and young children should be introduced to no more than one new food each week, starting with a mere spoonful. Food-sensitive adults and adolescents must not only avoid foods and ingredients known to produce an adverse reaction, they should make companions and others aware, especially when dining out. At a restaurant, for example, a person who is allergic to peanuts might ask about the ingredients in a salad or dessert but also find out if peanut oil will be used in cooking.

Inquiring minds want to know what they are eating, for safety's sake and also for the overall nutritional content. The FDA helps to satisfy those answers by insisting on product labeling, but food packaging labels do not mention everything of value nor of a potential risk. For example, some dietary supplements, such as calcium, have been proven to aid OSTEOPOROSIS and other conditions involving bone loss, but that does not make calcium tablets the best choice for healthy individuals interested in bone building. HERBAL THERAPY and other supplements, such as GLUCOSAMINE, appear to benefit patients with OSTEOARTHRITIS, but all of the evidence is not yet in. Also, all health supplements are not created equal, which means that some follow higher standards and maintain a stronger potency than others.

Discussing such issues in *The Mount Sinai Journal of Medicine*, Dr. Jeffrey I. Mechanick said, "Creative solutions to clinical problems incorporate . . . qualities that cannot always be scientifically tested. However, the advocacy of unproven therapies, heralded as standards of care or appropriate interventions, cannot be condoned. Such is the case for many of the published indications for dietary supplements . . . and their seemingly widespread recommendation for a host of ailments." When possible, then, one might do well to buy products only from the most reputable companies while continuing to stalk those outer grocery aisles.

Statistics and Studies

Apparently, the majority of teenagers favor the center of the grocery store. According to the National Center for Chronic Disease Prevention and Health Promotion, only 22 percent of the high school students surveyed in 2003 had five or more servings of fruits and vegetables each day. That same year, slightly more than 11 percent of the girls and 22 percent of the boys drank three or more glasses of milk a day. Over 81 percent of teens, however, drank a glass of fruit juice, and over 83 percent ate at least one vegetable.

Regarding adults, a group of researchers from the University of Aberdeen in the United Kingdom (U.K.) studied the typical Western diet then reported, "Low Dietary Potassium Intakes and High Dietary Estimates of . . . Acid Production Are Associated with Low Bone Mineral Density in Premenopausal Women and Increased Markers of Bone Resorption in Postmenopausal Women." That title, which is itself a mouthful, says a lot about the acid-alkaline balance mentioned earlier. As an abstract of the study stated, "The Western diet may be a risk factor for osteoporosis. Excess acid generated from high protein intakes increases calcium excretion and bone resorption. Fruit and vegetable intake could balance this excess acidity by providing alkaline salts of potassium," since that base neutralizes the acid. Thus, the U.K. researchers concluded, "Dietary potassium . . . may exert a modest influence on markers of bone health, which over a lifetime may contribute to a decreased risk of osteoporosis."

In the United States, a group of researchers from Tufts' Jean Mayer USDA Human Nutrition Research Center on Aging investigated "Vitamin B12 Linked to Bone Health vs. Osteoporosis." According to the article by that name in the university publication, *Health & Nutrition Letter*, "Vitamin B12, found in dairy products, meats, poultry and fish as well as in many fortified cereals, may be an important weapon in your battle against osteoporosis." With more than 2,500 men and women participating in the Framingham Osteoporosis Study at Tufts, researchers "found that both men and women with low vitamin B12 levels also averaged lower bone mineral densities than those with higher levels." To be more specific, "the men with low vitamin B12 levels had significantly lower bone density in several areas of the hip, and the women low in B12 had particularly low bone density in the spine."

Special Aids and Adaptations

Patients who do not absorb vitamins well from food sources may need the help of all-natural supplements, in which case a VITAMIN B-COMPLEX will keep B12 in balance with others in the B family. For people with high acidity, fortified cereals higher in oats or other alkaline-producing grains offer a tasty option and provide the daily requirement for other known nutrients. For people with sensitivities to dairy products, soy milk may make cereal more palatable. However, regular milk on fortified cereal offers a reasonably nutritious breakfast or a healthy evening snack with calcium to assist SLEEP.

Good grains can begin a good morning too. At any time of day or night, food choices can be adapted to fit the present person and the present need. For example, after an illness or tiring EXERCISE, people usually need fresh fruits to help detoxify the body. Later in the day, protein helps to rebuild cells. If energy lags mid-day, fresh fruit provides the carbohydrates needed for energy. If hair, skin, or nails feel dry and lifeless, chances are, the bones echo the feeling. In that case, a person might adapt by adding an additional spoon or two of vegetable fat, such as canola or olive oil, each day to lubricate achy joints and transport hormones throughout the body.

Each person differs, yet most people need a variety of foods to assure well-balanced nutrition. Variety also spices life. As an offbeat rule, however, people should be as wary as a finicky toddler whenever food colors clash on a plate. For example, slices of red tomatoes look unappetizing next to a blob of sweet potatoes, but if eaten together, they might taste worse than they look. Conversely, someone who favors only white foods will most likely lack nutrients such as vitamin A or C. However, scientific studies of this artistic interplay of nutrients have yet to be fully performed.

Healthy Youth! "Youth Online: Comprehensive Results," National Center for Chronic Disease Prevention and Health Promotion, CDC. Available online. URL: http://apps.nccd.cdc.gov/yrbss/CategoryQuestions.asp?Cat=5&desc=Dietary%20Behaviors. Last updated September 8, 2004.

Johnson, Mary Ann. "Nutrition and Aging—Practical Advice for Healthy Eating," *Journal of the American Medical Women's Association* 59, no. 4 (2005): 262–269.

Macdonald, H. M., S. A. New, W. D. Fraser, M. K. Campbell, and D. M. Reid. "Low Dietary Potassium Intakes and High Dietary Estimates of Net Endogenous Acid Production Are Associated with Low Bone Mineral Density in Premenopausal Women and Increased Markers of Bone Resorption in Postmenopausal Women," *American Journal of Clinical Nutrition* 81, no. 4 (April 2005): 923–933.

Mechanick, Jeffrey I., M.D. "The Rational Use of Dietary Supplements and Nutraceuticals in Clinical Medicine," *The Mount Sinai Journal of Medicine* 72, no. 3 (May 2005): 161–165.

Reid, D. M., and H. M. Macdonald. "Nutrition and Bone: Is There More to It than Just Calcium and Vitamin D?" *QJM: An International Journal of Medicine* 94, no. 2 (2001): 53–56.

Staff. "Vitamin B12 Linked to Bone Health vs. Osteoporosis," Tufts University *Health & Nutrition Letter* 23, no. 4 (June 2005): 1–2.

U.S. Food and Drug Administration. "Food Allergen Labeling and Consumer Protection Act of 2004 (Title II of Public Law 108–282)," FDA. Available online. URL: http://www.cfsan.fda.gov/~dms/alrgact.html. Downloaded February 18, 2006.

obesity   See WEIGHT, EFFECTS OF.

opiates, opioids for pain   Derived from the opium extracted from poppy, an opiate contains such alkaloids as morphine, codeine, and heroine. Besides this natural source, synthetically produced opioids also provide a narcotic form of PAIN MANAGEMENT. Unlike other PAIN RELIEVERS, though, doctors often hesitate to prescribe these powerful drugs since patients can become addicted to them.

Addressing this concern, an article in *JAOA, The Journal of the American Osteopathic Association,* said, "Administration of opioids for pain control has been shown to be an effective way to improve pain control and quality of life." However, "initial therapy should be with the lowest effective dose possible to minimize pain and medication side effects and to maximize the quality of life." Then, "follow-up visits and continued monitoring is crucial for success and proper management of pain. These visits ensure constant communication, patient coordination, patient support, and opportunities for education and proper adjustments to medication. Visits should be scheduled every 2 weeks for the first 2 to 4 months, then once a month." As the *JAOA* article also pointed out, "understanding the difference between addiction (psychological and deviant behavioral condition) and physical dependence . . . should improve physician comfort levels in prescribing opioid therapy."

InfoFacts from the National Institute on Drug Abuse further explained, "Long-term use also can lead to physical dependence—the body adapts to the presence of the substance and withdrawal symptoms occur if use is reduced abruptly. This can also include tolerance, which means that higher doses of a medication must be taken to obtain the same

initial effects. Note that physical dependence is not the same as addiction—physical dependence can occur even with appropriate long-term use of opioid and other medications," whereas "addiction . . . is defined as compulsive, often uncontrollable drug use in spite of negative consequences."

In "Management Options" for pain, information from the National Library of Medicine offered this assurance: "Opioid tolerance and physiologic dependence are unusual in short term postoperative use. . . . Likewise, psychologic dependence and addiction are extremely unlikely to develop after the use of opioids for acute pain." With morphine providing the standard choice, "opioid analgesics are the cornerstone for management of moderate to severe acute pain," such as the ACUTE PAIN a patient with bone CANCER might experience. Strong narcotics may also be needed to aid recovery after SURGERY, especially when a procedure has been done on a weight-bearing area such as the LUMBAR SPINE or VERTEBRAE. Then, "effective use of these agents facilitates postoperative activities such as coughing, deep breathing exercises, ambulation, and physical therapy." However, "opioid administration is contraindicated when respiratory depression is present (less than 10 breaths per minute)."

Dosage and Potential Side Effects

The most effective dosage for an individual varies according to the type of condition and the level of pain. Although no maximum amount or ceiling has been established for a dosage of this analgesic painkiller, reductions should occur as pain subsides and/or side effects increase. As an online article from the American Medical Association (AMA) explained, "Opioid analgesics do not have an analgesic ceiling effect. Therefore, dose escalation to achieve analgesic effect is limited only by increased incidence of side effects. Because not all persistent pain syndromes respond to opioid therapy, opioid response needs to be assessed through a therapeutic trial." To establish the initial dosage, the AMA said, "Prior to a therapeutic trial, the patient's pain and function must be assessed and/or reassessed to assist in evaluating treatment response. A pain diary can assist in monitoring treatment effect. If the patient's pain does not respond to an opioid trial, it should be stopped and an alternative therapeutic strategy begun. The options include a trial of a different opioid (so-called 'opioid rotation')."

As a memory device for monitoring the most commonly experienced effects, the AMA focused on four *A*'s: Analgesia, Activities, Adverse events, and Aberrant drug-taking behaviors. To summarize, *analgesia* refers to the degree of pain relief as well as any improvement in SLEEP and moods. *Activities* considers whether a patient can carry out normal daily ACTIVITIES, whereas *adverse events* include nausea, constipation, or disruptions in sleep and sexual function. If patients experience *aberrant drug-taking behavior* as a side effect, they typically report losing their supply of narcotics and then demand an early refill.

Statistics and Studies

A brief report in *The Journal of Musculoskeletal Medicine* discussed "the use, effectiveness, and toxicity of opioid analgesics in 230 spine clinic patients for 3 years." With patients "divided into 3 groups: long-term opioid use (3 or more consecutive months), short-term opioid use (3 or fewer months), and no use," the researchers from the Minneapolis Veteran Affairs Medical Center and University of Minnesota found that "use of opioid analgesics reduced the severity of spinal pain significantly in all diagnoses." Furthermore, "adverse effects (e.g., constipation and sedation) were reported by 58% of the opioid-treated patients, but the symptoms were mild. There was no significant increase in the mean daily opioid dose over time."

American Medical Association. "Initiating Opioid Therapy," AMA. Available online. URL: http://www.ama-cmeonline.com/pain_mgmt/module07/06phar/04_02.htm. Downloaded February 22, 2006.

Health Services/Technology Assessment Text. "Management Options," HSTAT, National Library of Medicine. Available online. URL: http://www.ncbi.nlm.nih.gov/books/bv.fcgi?rid=hstat6.section.32282. Downloaded February 23, 2006.

National Institute on Drug Abuse. "NIDA InfoFacts: Prescription Pain and Other Medications," National Institutes of Health (NIH.) Available online. URL: http://www.nida.nih.gov/infofacts/PainMed.html. Downloaded February 22, 2006.

Rasor, Joseph III, and Gerald Harris. "Opioid Use for Moderate to Severe Pain," Supplement 3, *JAOA, The Journal of the American Osteopathic Association* 105, no. 6 (June 2005): 52–57.

Staff. "Opioid Therapy Safe and Effective for Spine Pain," *The Journal of Musculoskeletal Medicine* 22, no. 5 (May 2005): 272.

orthotics   From corsets to neck braces to shoe inserts, orthotic devices aid mobility by stabilizing the VERTEBRAE and correcting POSTURE in the BACK and SPINE. A temporary orthotic may be needed after a FLEXION-EXTENSION INJURY, such as a whiplash, to stabilize the CERVICAL SPINE and avoid further damage to the injured area. With an ongoing condition such as ARTHRITIS that involves CHRONIC PAIN, orthotic SHOES or inserts cushion the feet, equalize posture, and enable a patient to continue daily ACTIVITY. Similarly, bracing can aid mobility in patients who have DEGENERATIVE DISC DISEASE yet limit RANGE OF MOTION in a person with SPINAL STENOSIS.

A neck or back brace may also be used to avoid SURGERY. Often, doctors prescribe various types of back braces for CHILDREN and ADOLESCENTS with SCOLIOSIS to halt deformity during periods of bone growth. As the online article "Adolescent Idiopathic Scoliosis" from the North American Spine Society (NASS) explained, "For patients with curves of 20–40 degrees a brace is used if progression is documented and the patient has substantial growth remaining. Bracing will not correct the curve but might prevent curve progression. Successful use of a brace is dependent on the amount of time the patient wears the brace. The brace is worn until growth is complete and is worn between 16 and 23 hours a day."

When surgery, such as ARTHRODESIS, must be performed, a brace can assist recovery by giving the vertebrae time to fuse. As the NASS article

"Spinal Fusion" said, "In addition to some restrictions in activity, a brace is sometimes used for the early post operative period. There are many types of braces available. Some are very restrictive and are designed to severely limit motion, while others are intended mainly for comfort and to provide some support. The decision to use a brace or not, and the optimal type of brace, depends upon your surgeon's preference and other factors related to your surgery."

Risks and Complications

The availability of numerous OVER-THE-COUNTER PRODUCTS can complicate matters since patients may not select the best orthotic devices for their conditions, thus risking damage to bones and soft tissue. Yet prescription orthotics can be costly, and parents must brace themselves for the possibility that their growing children may refuse to wear the device or slip it off when away from home.

Besides complications that arise from not wearing the prescribed orthotic, patients who use braces risk muscle loss or weakness. An article on The Spine Institute Web site said, "Patients should avoid becoming dependent on the lumbar corsets. If they are used for prolonged periods (weeks and months), the back muscles may begin to weaken and cause a patient to be more prone to reinjury." Nevertheless, lumbar corsets, which can either be rigid or soft, "provide support for the lumbar spine, help reduce the load on back muscles, and are helpful during episodes of acute and chronic low back pain. They are also used for support after spine surgery, such as discectomy, and fusion surgeries." The same could be said for neck bracing too.

To avoid weakening PARASPINAL MUSCLES or neck muscles, patients should ask their doctors about the length of time a brace must be worn. The physician may also prescribe physical therapy and appropriate EXERCISE to help a patient strengthen a specific area, increase overall activity, and lessen the risk of muscle atrophy.

Statistics and Studies

Researchers from Johns Hopkins Children's Center investigated the effectiveness of braces commonly used for scoliosis. According to the report published by *The JHU Gazette*, "in a study of 276 adolescents with the most common form of scoliosis, the overweight were more than twice as likely as those of normal weight to develop worsening curvatures, despite the brace." For about 14 hours daily, each patient wore a back brace that extended from beneath the arms to the hips. In each case, "braces exert their effects on the spine through biomechanical forces, which need to be of sufficient magnitude to create and sustain curve correction." However, adverse effects of WEIGHT caused the patients to "have more and thicker soft tissue and surface area," which compromised the intended effect. Therefore, "almost half of these overweight teens eventually needed corrective surgery."

Special Aids and Adaptations

The ease with which a patient can put on a device helps to ensure that the orthotic will actually be worn. Also, lightweight materials aid comfort, making a patient more apt to wear an orthotic for the prescribed time. Soft braces will usually be more comfortable than hard ones, but each type of brace must be adapted to the present need.

The SpineUniverse article "Spinal Bracing" listed three options: flexible, semi-flexible, and rigid braces. For example, flexible "corsets are used to de-weight spinal structures by increasing abdominal compression." If needed, "rigid stays and inserts can be added to restrict motion and act as a postural reminder." Also, "rigid orthoses are commonly custom fabricated and provide the most support to the area being treated." For instance, "a body jacket . . . controls motion in all planes." Regardless of the type of brace needed, patients should seek a certified orthotist (CO or CPO) to be sure they get the most fitting device.

Collins, Jessica. "Bracing Used for Scoliosis Less Effective in Overweight Teens," Johns Hopkins University, *The JHU Gazette* 33, no. 5 (September 29, 2003).

Falk, David. "Spinal Bracing," SpineUniverse. Available online. URL: http://www.spineuniverse.com/displayarticle.php/article599.html. Last updated October 25, 2005.

North American Spine Society. "Adolescent Idiopathic Scoliosis," NASS. Available online. URL: http://www.spine.org/fsp/prob_action-injury-scoliosis.cfm. Last updated March 3, 2005.

North American Spine Society. "Spinal Fusion," NASS. Available online. URL: http://www.spine.org/fsp/prob_action-surgical-fusion.cfm. Last updated March 3, 2005.

Spine Institute, The. "Body Braces," Saint John's Health Center™. Available online. URL: http://www.espineinstitute.com/Conservative_BodyBraces.htm. Downloaded February 23, 2006.

osteitis deformans Better known as Paget's disease, this progressive bone disorder affects about 3 percent of ELDERLY adults over 60 in the United States. Although the cause of Paget's has not been established, ENVIRONMENTAL INFLUENCES and GENETIC FACTORS may trigger the disease. Any bone can be affected, but evidence of osteitis deformans often appears in the SPINE with white, patchy areas characteristically occurring in the skull, pelvis, and long bones.

As the American Academy of Orthopaedic Surgeons (AAOS) explained, "In normal bone, a process called remodeling takes place every day. Bone is absorbed and then reformed in response to the normal stresses on the skeleton." After osteoclasts absorb old bone cells, the osteoblasts make new bone. However, "in Paget's disease, osteoclasts are more active than osteoblasts. This means there is more bone absorption than normal. The osteoblasts try to keep up by making new bone, but they overreact and make excess bone that is very chaotic. The new bone is abnormally large, is deformed and fits together haphazardly. Normal bone has a tight overlapping structure, like a well-constructed brick wall. Bone afflicted by Paget's disease has an irregular mosaic pattern, as though the bricks were just dumped in place. The end result is bones that are large and dense, but weak and brittle. The bone is prone to fractures, bowing and deformities."

Symptoms and Diagnostic Path

Initially, patients may experience no symptoms whatsoever. Later, bone pain may occur followed by OSTEOARTHRITIS, gradual deformity in the spine, and, in rare cases, CANCER. As the disease progresses, VERTEBRAL COMPRESSION FRACTURE and such POSTURE problems as KYPHOSIS may hinder movements and lessen mobility.

To obtain a diagnosis, X-RAYS show abnormal changes in bone structure, while blood tests or a urinalysis indicate the level of bone turnover. A physician may also request a BONE SCAN and, sometimes, a biopsy.

Treatment Options and Outlook

Doctors often prescribe CALCITONIN or BISPHOSPHONATES to decrease bone loss, while PAIN MANAGEMENT may include ACETAMINOPHEN or NONSTEROIDAL ANTI-INFLAMMATORY DRUG (NSAID) THERAPY. In addition to medications, Holy Cross Hospital listed self-treatments, such as "calcium, usually about 1,000–1,500 mg per day; Adequate exposure to sunshine to promote vitamin D production in the skin (but limit time in the sun to prevent sun burning, wrinkling and aging); Intake of adequate vitamin D, usually about 400 mg per day (more may be needed in older people); Regular exercise to maintain skeletal health, joint mobility, and normal body weight; Avoidance of excess mechanical stress on involved bones; A splint for an area at high risk for fracture." If an ORTHOTIC is needed, patients should discuss the appropriate type of bracing with a doctor.

Risk Factors and Preventive Measures

Since Paget's disease cannot yet be prevented, older patients with a family history of osteitis deformans may need a blood test every two to four years. Adequate EXERCISE and healthful NUTRITION, including supplements of CALCIUM and VITAMIN D, may be helpful. To slow or halt the progression of the disease, new treatments may bring new options. For example, an article posted by News-Medical.net reported a promising study of a drug called zoledronic acid. According to the article, "one 15-minute infusion of zoledronic acid 5 mg generated a therapeutic response in 95% of patients, compared with 75% of patients taking 30 mg/day of oral risedronate, for 60 days. . . . At the six-month follow-up, serum alkaline phosphatase (SAP) levels, a key marker for bone turnover, were normal in 89% of zoledronic acid patients, compared with 56% of risedronate patients."

For those who want to participate in ongoing RESEARCH, the Paget Foundation welcomes contact from patients and also persons with a family history of the disease. Since Paget's more often affects people in northern climates, the URL below provides contact information for The New England Registry for Paget's Disease of Bone.

American Academy of Orthopaedic Surgeons. "Paget's Disease of Bone," AAOS. Available online. URL: http://orthoinfo.aaos.org/fact/thr_report.cfm?Thread_ID=306&topcategory=Tumors. Downloaded February 23, 2006.
Badash, Michelle. "Paget's Disease (Osteitis Deformans)," Holy Cross Hospital. Available online. URL: http://healthychoice.epnet.com/GetContent.asp?siteid=holycross&docid=/dci/pagets. Downloaded February 23, 2006.
News-Medical.net. "First Filing for Zoledronic Acid in Metabolic Bone Disease," *Pharmaceutical News* (May 17, 2004). Available online. URL: http://www.news-medical.net/?id=1628.
Paget Foundation, The. "Patients Needed For Research Study." Available online. URL: http://www.paget.org/page.asp?page=Clinical/main_fr_bottom.asp&title=Patients+Needed+for+Research+Studies. Downloaded February 23, 2006.

osteoarthritis Also known as degenerative joint disease, this most common form of ARTHRITIS often affects the ELDERLY. Normally, cartilage covers the ends of bones, allowing ease in movement, but with osteoarthritis (OA) that protective cartilage wears down until one bone chafes another, causing potentially disabling damage to joints and adjacent bones. However, OA differs from RHEUMATOID ARTHRITIS (RA) in that it typically does not cause the deforming joint inflammation characteristic of RA.

According to the National Institute of Arthritis and Musculoskeletal and Skin Diseases (NIAMS), "osteoarthritis is one of the most frequent causes of physical disability among adults. More than 20 million people in the United States have the disease. By 2030, 20 percent of Americans—about 70 million people—will have passed their 65th birthday and will be at risk for osteoarthritis. Some younger people get osteoarthritis from joint injuries, but osteoarthritis most often occurs in older people. In fact, more than half of the population age 65 or older would show x-ray evidence of osteoarthritis

in at least one joint. Both men and women have the disease. Before age 45, more men than women have osteoarthritis, whereas after age 45, it is more common in women." A FLEXION-EXTENSION INJURY, such as a whiplash or other SPINE INJURY, can also produce the type of joint damage that ultimately leads to OA. Bone spurs or OSTEOPHYTES can have that effect too. As NIAMS explained, "Bits of bone or cartilage can break off and float inside the joint space. This causes more pain and damage."

Symptoms and Diagnostic Path
Over time, degeneration can occur in any joint, but especially in weight-bearing ones in the BACK or SPINE. After EXERCISE or physical exertion, joints may ache or stiffen, typically causing BACKACHE or LOW BACK PAIN. If degeneration occurs in the CERVICAL SPINE, the patient may experience a CERVICOGENIC HEADACHE or NECK PAIN. Movements may cause a crunching sound, yet OA symptoms seldom produce heat or inflammation as arthritis and also rheumatoid arthritis (RA) can do. Similar to both of those rheumatic conditions, however, osteoarthritis may be influenced by GENETIC FACTORS. Therefore, a rheumatologist or other physician may request blood tests and a family history with X-RAYS to assess the affected joints.

Treatment Options and Outlook
If daily ACTIVITY becomes increasingly difficult, a patient may experience depression, anxiety, TENSION, or a sense of powerlessness. With early diagnosis and appropriate treatments though, degeneration may slow down and symptoms may subside.

Usually, therapy begins with ACETAMINOPHEN or other PAIN RELIEVER to keep a patient active during the day yet able to SLEEP at night. Sleep itself can also be therapeutic. To aid rest, the NIAMS said, "Some people feel better when they sleep on a firm mattress or sit using back support pillows. Others find it helps to use heat treatments or to follow an exercise program that strengthens the back and abdominal muscles." To avoid joint strain, these types of exercise can often be done while lying in bed.

In general, HEAT THERAPY and swimming or HYDROTHERAPY help OA patients to limber up without straining their joints. Other forms of COMPLEMENTARY AND ALTERNATIVE MEDICINE such as

ACUPUNCTURE may provide relief too. After reviewing the current literature on that particular CAM option, the Agency for Healthcare Research and Quality (AHRQ) summarized their findings in "Acupuncture for Osteoarthritis:" "Most studies on acupuncture for osteoarthritis do not find a benefit for acupuncture compared to sham acupuncture," done by an untrained acupuncturist. "Researchers hypothesize that this may be because placement of a needle anywhere elicits a physiological response or because the sham sites chosen were actually true acupuncture sites." Another possibility is that the traditional sites, known as meridians, encompass a wider band than originally thought. Regardless, "most studies found a benefit for both acupuncture and sham acupuncture compared to baseline." Although the studies cited did not consider acupuncture the most effective first-line treatment, the AHRQ said "the evidence was probably sufficient to justify the use of acupuncture as a second or third line treatment for a patient who is not responding to conventional management or not tolerating medication or experiencing recurrent pain."

In a similar study of acupuncture as a treatment for osteoarthritis, the New Zealand Ministry of Health reported, "Acupuncture can decrease pain levels in osteoarthritis sufferers compared to no treatment at all. However, this decrease in pain may only be temporary (that is, for four weeks after the end of treatment)." That same report, posted by CAM.org, described minor side effects among "67 in every 1,000 acupuncture visits," with adverse events, such as infection or inadvertent punctures, being "extremely rare."

In summarizing various alternate therapies, the Arthritis Foundation said, "Chiropractic care involves the manipulation and manual adjustment of the spine. Manipulation of some joints may help relieve osteoarthritis pain, but joint manipulation of weak or damaged joints could cause problems. Be sure to tell your chiropractor that your have osteoarthritis and select one that has experience working with people with arthritis." Elsewhere on their Web site, the foundation also mentioned the importance of finding someone experienced in working with OA patients when seeking MASSAGE THERAPY treatments.

NUTRITION comes highly recommended too. As the Arthritis Foundation explained, "Some research has shown that antioxidants in certain vitamins may help ease certain symptoms of osteoarthritis. In general, vitamins from whole foods are believed to be better absorbed by the body than supplements. Vitamin C has been shown to counteract the wearing away of cartilage in animals with OA. In humans, it is associated with decreased OA progression and pain. Vitamin E provides some pain relief to people with OA, however one study showed it was not as effective in easing OA pain in African-American men. Vitamin D may have preventative qualities when it comes to OA. One study found that disease progression was faster in people who had a low intake of the vitamin." To maintain an optimal vitamin and MINERAL BALANCE, patients should not exceed the recommended daily dosage without discussing this with a physician.

Taken as recommended on the product label, HERBAL THERAPY and other supplements may be beneficial too. For example, the *Journal of Inflammation* mentioned the possible benefits of the herb cat's claw in easing OA pain. In addition, the article discussed GLUCOSAMINE, especially when used in combination with chondroitin, a substance found in cartilage and in the basic makeup or matrix of bone. As the article explained, "glucosamine and chondroitin are structural elements of cartilage and matrix. The therapeutic approach centers on the assumption that ingestion of large amounts of these matrix elements will assist in the replacement of the comparable material that is lost as a result of the . . . process associated with inflammation. Recently," however, "it has been suggested that the absorption of oral glucosamine is not sufficient for the chondroitin production and cartilage deposition. There is limited evidence for a direct anti-inflammatory action of glucosamine. Nevertheless by design it is not an approach that influences the disease process directly, but rather is thought to maintain cartilage architecture in the face of ongoing catabolic pathways. Hence, not surprisingly, the onset of action in those individuals for whom it does provide relief is commonly on the order of months after treatment initiation. Studies as to the efficacy of glucosamine and chondroitin have produced variable results suggesting that the benefits of this approach may have limitations."

A 2006 news release from the National Center for Complementary and Alternative Medicine concurred, saying, "In a study published in the *New England Journal of Medicine,* the popular dietary supplement combination of glucosamine plus chondroitin sulfate did not provide significant relief from osteoarthritis pain among all participants. However, a smaller subgroup of study participants with moderate-to-severe pain showed significant relief with the combined supplements."

Risk Factors and Preventive Measures

An article in *The Safety & Health Practitioner* mentioned the risk of OA affecting weight-bearing joints as a person ages. "In addition to ageing, other factors can hasten the development of OA. These include injury to the joints, and excessive weight-bearing, which occurs as a result of obesity." While well-balanced nutrition aids bone health and reduces adverse effects of WEIGHT on the spine, RANGE OF MOTION exercises may limber the affected joints. Exceeding that normal range, however, increases the risk of OA damage, and "prolonged heavy manual work may also have an effect."

Being aware of personal limits and LOAD TOLERANCE may help to avoid OA problems caused by wear and tear. Proper LIFTING techniques offer a preventive too. For families with a history of OA, ENVIRONMENTAL INFLUENCES and a healthy lifestyle may not completely counteract genetic factors. Nevertheless, adequate water intake, a diet rich in fresh fruits and vegetables, limbering exercises, and restful sleep can lessen OA flare-ups and help to prevent further joint damage.

Agency for Healthcare Research and Quality. *Acupuncture for Osteoarthritis.* Rockville, Maryland: AHRQ Technology Assessment, U.S. Department of Health and Human Services booklet, June 17, 2003, p. 6.

Arthritis Foundation. "Alternate Therapies." Available online. URL: http://www.arthritis.org/conditions/diseasecenter/oa/oa_alternatives.asp. Downloaded February 24, 2006.

CAM.org. "Acupuncture for Osteoarthritis," Complementary and Alternative Medicine, New Zealand Ministry of Health. Available online. URL: http://www.cam.org.nz/Treatment%20Methods/Acupuncture/osteoarthritis.htm. Last updated October 20, 2004.

Ide, Chris. "Joint Effort," *The Safety & Health Practitioner* 23, no. 8 (August 2005): 32–34.

Miller, Mark J. S., Komal Mehta, Sameer Kunte, Vidyanand Raut, Jayesh Gala, Ramesh Dhumale, Anil Shukla, Hemant Tupalli, Himanshu Parikh, Paul Bobrowski, and Jayesh Chaudhary. "Early Relief of Osteoarthritis Symptoms with a Natural Mineral Supplement and a Herb-mineral Combination: A Randomized Controlled Trial," *Journal of Inflammation* 2, no. 11 (October 21, 2005). Available online. URL: http://www.journal-inflammation.com/content/2/1/11.

National Center for Complementary and Alternative Medicine. "Efficacy of Glucosamine and Chondroitin Sulfate May Depend on Level of Osteoarthritis Pain," NCCAM, National Institutes of Health. Available online. URL: http://nccam.nih.gov/news/2006/022206.htm. Last modified February 22, 2006.

National Institute of Arthritis and Musculoskeletal and Skin Diseases. "Handout on Health: Osteoarthritis," NIAMS, National Institutes of Health. Available online. URL: http://www.niams.nih.gov/hi/topics/arthritis/oahandout.htm. Downloaded February 25, 2006.

osteogenesis imperfecta Also known as brittle bone disease, osteogenesis imperfecta (OI) occurs when GENETIC FACTORS alter collagen production in the body, thereby weakening bones and causing breakage, even in the womb. INFANTS with severe types of OI may be stillborn or exhibit FRACTURES and BIRTH DEFECTS OF THE SPINE. Milder types of OI may not be apparent until CHILDREN begin to walk, at which time a bone may break from a light fall. In moderate to severe cases, hundreds of fractures may occur over the years, sometimes resulting in skeletal deformities.

To clarify the various levels of severity, the American Academy of Orthopaedic Surgeons (AAOS) defined Type I as the mildest form of OI and Type II the most severe. Although Type II babies seldom survive infancy, Type III cases of OI can also exhibit severe bone deformities and fractures at birth. Of moderate severity, Type IV OI causes bones to fracture easily in children who may be below average height at full growth.

Obviously, parents of children with OI must be especially watchful. However, the AAOS said, "Don't be afraid to touch or hold an infant with OI, but be careful. Never lift a child with OI by holding him or her under the armpits. Do not pull on arms or legs or lift the legs by the ankles to change a diaper. To lift an infant with OI, spread your fingers apart and put one hand between the legs and under the buttocks; place the other hand behind the shoulders, neck and head." The AAOS also suggested, "Select an infant car seat that reclines. It should be easy to place or remove the child in the seat. Consider padding the seat with foam and using a layer of foam between the child and the harness." Similarly, a stroller should be comfortable and large enough to accommodate a cast.

No matter how many precautions a parent takes, bones will break, but as the AAOS advised, "Do not feel guilty if a fracture does occur. Children must develop and fractures will occur no matter how careful you are." Adding to the anguish, parents and other guardians may be falsely accused of child abuse. Because of that possibility, the AAOS counseled, "Always have a letter from your family doctor and a copy of your child's medical records handy."

Symptoms and Diagnostic Path

Depending on the severity, OI symptoms may be present at birth. Besides bone fragility, many patients have a blue or gray tinge to the whites of the eyes. Sensitivity to heat and cold may also be apparent. As the child grows, progressive hearing loss often occurs. Teeth may be brittle. Joints may seem loose and muscle tone lax. Multiple fractures in the SPINE may cause POSTURE problems, short stature, or deformity in the BACK.

A family history, physical examination, X-RAYS, ABSORPTIOMETRY test of bone density, and laboratory tests confirm a diagnosis. However, the Osteogenesis Imperfecta Foundation said, "It is often, though not always, possible to diagnose OI based solely on clinical features. . . . Clinical geneticists can also perform biochemical (collagen) or molecular (DNA) tests that can help confirm a diagnosis of OI in some situations. These tests generally require several weeks before results are known, and approximately 10 to 15 percent of individuals with mild OI who have collagen testing, and approxi-

mately 5 percent of those who have genetic testing, test negative for OI despite having the disorder."

Treatment Options and Outlook

According to the National Institute of Arthritis and Musculoskeletal and Skin Disease (NIAMS), "because there is no cure for OI, its management or treatment currently focuses on minimizing fractures and maximizing mobility and independent function. Aggressive rehabilitation is an important part of treatment for most types of OI. Prolonged immobilization can further weaken bones and lead to muscle loss, weakness, and fracture cycles." For an effective EXERCISE, swimming can be enjoyable with other forms of water activity or HYDROTHERAPY beneficial. For normal daily ACTIVITY though, ORTHOTICS or other protective devices may be needed. To assist BONE BUILDING, such supplements as CALCIUM and VITAMIN D may help, but the overall emphasis should be on providing growing children and ADOLESCENTS with adequate NUTRITION. In some patients, BISPHOSPHONATES may increase bone mass, but the NIAMS cautioned, "There are anecdotal reports of increased bone brittleness and fracture rate after prolonged treatment with bisphosphonates." Children with short stature may respond to medications used to treat GROWTH HORMONE DISORDERS.

For several years, Clinicaltrials.gov has been involved in "Growth Hormone Therapy in Osteogenesis Imperfecta" to find out "how long and how well OI bone will respond to growth stimulation." As this governmental Web site explained, "Growth deficiency is a key feature of severe Osteogenesis Imperfecta (OI) and a frequent feature of mild to moderate forms of the disease. The reason that children with OI are short is not fully understood. We do know that details such as the number of fractures suffered or the type of OI do not fully explain the short stature of OI. Growth patterns have been defined for children with OI Types I, III, and IV." For example, "at about 12 months of age, children with Types III and IV OI demonstrate a predictable plateau of their . . . growth rate. Type IV OI children begin to resume a normal growth rate at about age four to five years, but they will not 'catch up' to a normal height, as they have 'lost' a significant period of growth. The plateau usually continues for children with Type III OI. The reason for this growth plateau is unknown. There have been no studies which evaluate the growth of OI children in this age range. Our previous studies of growth in OI children have begun at age 5 years." In a decade of study, "different medications have been tried to both stimulate growth and improve bone density. Some children have responded to growth hormone (their growth rate increased by at least 50%) and some did not. The majority of children who did respond were Type IV. However, we need to carefully treat and study more children to try to determine which children will benefit from growth hormone medication." Since ongoing RESEARCH will likely remain open, parents may find more options for their child through the Clinicaltrials.gov Web site cited below.

An online OI fact sheet from the National Institutes of Health Osteoporosis and Related Bone Diseases said "the more severe forms of OI are caused by genetic mutations that produce bad structural components (bad fibers) that become part of the skeleton. A major advance in treating OI will be to find a way to prevent the bad fibers from being made in the first place. If this objective could be achieved, the result would be Type I OI, with the person having one normal collagen gene that produces a smaller number of normal collagen fibers instead of defective fibers. Once this goal is accomplished, medicines to stimulate more collagen fiber production from the remaining normal collagen gene might increase bone strength even more."

Risk Factors and Preventive Measures

Sometimes SURGERY may be needed to treat OI. For example, a procedure known as RODDING SURGERY may be performed to insert a rod or stabilizing device into the long bone of a leg or larger vertebrae in the spine. As an article from the Osteogenesis Imperfecta Foundation said, "Babies with severe forms of OI have numerous fractures at birth and repeated fractures over the following months. The fractures are usually treated with splints or casts rather than surgery. Surgery may be needed over the following years if repeated fractures of one or more long bones occur. The timing of surgery depends on the size of the bone," which must be a large enough to accept surgical insertion of a rod. "The bones in OI may be thin and flat, so they may appear wider in diameter on x-ray than they actually are. Children with moderately severe forms of OI also have numerous fractures at birth, but few new fractures until they start to stand and walk, which is when repeated fractures of the upper thigh bone (femur) may occur; at this time, surgery may be required."

American Academy of Orthopaedic Surgeons. "Osteogenesis Imperfecta," AAOS. Available online. URL: http://orthoinfo.aaos.org/fact/thr_report.cfm?Thread_ID=308&topcategory=Children. Downloaded February 27, 2006.

ClinicalTrials.gov. "Growth Hormone Therapy in Osteogenesis Imperfecta," National Institutes of Health (NIH), Department of Health and Human Services. Available online. URL: http://www.clinicaltrials.gov/ct/gui/show/NCT00001305.

National Institute of Arthritis and Musculoskeletal and Skin Disease. "Osteogenesis Imperfecta: A Guide for Nurses," NIAMS, National Institutes of Health. Available online. URL: http://www.niams.nih.gov/bone/hi/osteogenesis/oi_nurse_guide.htm. Downloaded February 27, 2006.

National Institutes of Health Osteoporosis and Related Bone Diseases. "Osteogenesis Imperfecta," NIH Fact Sheets. Available online. URL: http://www.osteo.org/oi.html. Downloaded February 27, 2006.

Osteogenesis Imperfecta Foundation. "Fast Facts on Osteogenesis Imperfecta," NIH Osteoporosis and Related Bone Diseases ~ National Resource Center (ORBD~NRC). Available online. URL: http://www.oif.org/site/PageServer?pagename=FastFacts. Downloaded February 27, 2006.

Smith, Peter, M.D. "OI Issues: Rodding Surgery," Osteogenesis Imperfecta Foundation, National Institutes of Health Osteoporosis and Related Bone Diseases. Available online. URL: http://www.oif.org/site/PageServer?pagename=Rodding. Downloaded February 27, 2006.

osteomalacia   See RICKETS.

osteomyelitis   A bacterial or fungal infection anywhere in the body can circulate through the bloodstream, depositing a problem in the DISCS, SPINE, or other bones and joints. The bacterium *Staphylococcus* *aureus* most often causes infection in the VERTE-BRAE, which, unchecked, can eventually produce a systemic illness.

Symptoms and Diagnostic Path

Characteristic symptoms include a localized BACK-ACHE or gradually increasing LOW BACK PAIN accompanied by fever or chills. If spinal infection arises after SURGERY, oozing or other abnormal discharge may appear at the site of incision. If the patient has not recently undergone a procedure, laboratory tests may be needed to rule out SPINAL TUBERCULO-SIS or to identify the type of bacteria. Also, X-RAY, COMPUTED TOMOGRAPHY SCAN, MAGNETIC RESONANCE IMAGING, or a BONE SCAN can rule out or assess any vertebral damage.

According to an article in the *Southern Medical Journal*, "The diagnosis of . . . vertebral osteomyelitis is sometimes difficult because of nonspecific . . . findings. Early diagnosis and treatment is crucial," especially to prevent neurological involvement of the spinal cord and spinal nerves. "Magnetic resonance imaging (MRI) is considered by some to be a highly specific and sensitive test, even in the early stages of disease. However, no single test can be used to rule out vertebral osteomyelitis. Surgical exploration is warranted in cases in which the clinical suspicion for the disease is high, regardless of multiple negative tests."

Treatment Options and Outlook

To overcome infection and avoid bone damage or vertebral collapse, strong antibiotics must be administered intravenously or orally for several weeks. A back brace, cervical collar, or other ORTHOTIC may be prescribed for vertebral support until the system has re-stabilized. If imaging tests show evidence of bone deterioration, corrective surgery, such as a BONE GRAFT, may be needed.

An article in *Neurosurgical Focus* said, "Nonsurgical therapy is appropriate if neurological signs or symptoms, instability, deformity, or spinal cord compression are absent." If, however, spinal instability, bone abnormalities, or severe nerve pain arise, "surgical decompression, . . . stabilization, and deformity correction are the goals once the decision to perform surgery has been made."

Risk Factors and Preventive Measures

ELDERLY persons, CANCER patients, and people with a weakened immune system remain at high risk for osteomyelitis, but intravenous drug users have the highest risk. In an article for Spine-Health.com, Dr. Alex R. Vaccaro said that most infections in the vertebrae "occur in the lumbar spine because of the blood flow to this region." In the THORACIC SPINE, tuberculosis infections may be apt to occur, while "intravenous drug abusers are more likely to contract an infection of the cervical spine." Although an infection in the LUMBAR SPINE may be the more common occurrence, osteomyelitis in the CERVICAL SPINE or thoracic region can result in paralysis.

In any area of the spine, prompt treatment helps to prevent the progression of KYPHOSIS or other conditions arising from bone damage. An article in *Neurosurgical Focus* stated, "Despite the high frequency of delayed diagnosis, timely intervention with surgery and/or medical therapy can be extremely efficacious. Indications for surgery include intractable pain, progressive vertebral body destruction and/or . . . deformity" similar to severe kyphosis. Surgery may also be needed to ease pressure that interferes with normal neurological function of the spinal nerves. "Surgery is noted by most authors to provide an excellent prognosis overall; in particular it will improve neurological function in a majority of cases."

Acosta, Frank L. Jr., M.D., Cynthia T. Chin, M.D., Alfredo Quiñones-Hinojosa, M.D., Christopher P. Ames, M.D., Philip R. Weinstein, M.D., and Dean Chou, M.D. "Diagnosis and Management of Adult Pyogenic Osteomyelitis of the Cervical Spine," *Neurosurgical Focus* 17, no. 6 (December 2004).

Barnes, Bryan, M.D., Joseph T. Alexander, M.D., and Charles L. Branch Jr., M.D. "Cervical Osteomyelitis: a Brief Review," *Neurosurgical Focus* 17, no. 6 (December 2004).

Mukhopadhyay, Surabhi, M.D., Fredrick Rose, M.D., and Vincent Frechette, M.D. *Southern Medical Journal* 98, no. 2 (February 2005): 226–228.

Vaccaro, Alex R., M.D. "Osteomyelitis, a Spinal Infection," Spine-Health.com. Available online. URL: http://www.spine-health.com/topics/cd/infection/osteomyelitis/os01.html. Downloaded February 24, 2006.

osteopenia This bone-weakening condition occurs when bones in the BACK, SPINE, and body begin to thin. Often, osteopenia precedes OSTEOPOROSIS, a more serious condition of bone loss commonly found in ELDERLY patients.

Symptoms and Diagnostic Path

Patients usually have no indication of bone loss. Therefore, most doctors advise women over 65 and people of both sexes with a family history of bone-thinning conditions to have a BONE MINERAL DENSITY (BMD) TEST, which will provide a number known as a T-score. The results establish a baseline for monitoring a patient in the future and also for comparing the T-score with other people of the same sex and age. The National Osteoporosis Foundation explained, "The difference between your BMD and that of a healthy young adult is referred to as a standard deviation (SD). As outlined in the World Health Organization's diagnostic categories, individuals whose T-score is within one standard deviation of the 'norm' are considered to have normal bone density. Scores below the 'norm' are indicated in negative numbers. For example, a score from -1 to -2.5 SD below the norm indicates low bone mass, or osteopenia, and a score of more than -2.5 SD below the norm is considered a diagnosis of osteoporosis. For most BMD tests, -1 SD equals a 10–12 percent decrease in bone density."

Treatment Options and Outlook

A healthy lifestyle provides the best outlook for most people while offering the least controversial approach. Regarding treatment options, patients and doctors need to discuss their particular preferences, such as whether to begin BISPHOSPHONATES or other medications. However, the outlook provided by BMD tests may be questioned by some. As an article in the *Annals of Internal Medicine* explained, "Bone density measurement remains an important tool in assessing skeletal health, but the determinants of fracture are much more complex and interesting than simply the T-score."

Risk Factors and Preventive Measures

To prevent bone thinning as a person ages, the University of Michigan Health System advised early efforts toward BONE BUILDING. As their online information explained, "Healthy bones develop during childhood. Girls reach 90 percent of their peak bone mass by 18 and boys by 20. Proper diet and exercise can help shore up that bone mass bank. As people reach middle age, they see a gradual decline in bone density. The curve is particularly steep immediately after a woman goes through menopause."

Young people with EATING DISORDERS remain especially at risk for bone loss. Often though, growing CHILDREN and ADOLESCENTS prevent future problems with adequate NUTRITION and regular EXERCISE. Such practices not only establish healthful habits but give the VERTEBRAE and other bones an opportunity to maximize peak bone mass, ultimately becoming strong enough to last a lifetime.

Fawcett, Nicole. "Osteopenia Warns of Dangerous Bone Loss," University of Michigan Health System. Available online. URL: http://www.med.umich.edu/opm/ newspage/2004/hmdensity.htm. Downloaded March 2, 2006.

McClung, Michael R., M.D. "Osteopenia: To Treat or Not To Treat?" *Annals of Internal Medicine* 142, no. 9 (May 3, 2005): 796–797.

National Osteoporosis Foundation. "BMD Testing: What The Numbers Mean," NOF. Available online. URL: http://www.nof.org/osteoporosis/bmdtest.htm. Downloaded March 2, 2006.

osteopetrosis Also called marble bone disease, this uncommon condition causes bones to become very thick and brittle, like marble. Instead of the bone loss that commonly occurs among ELDERLY patients or people with OSTEOPENIA and OSTEOPOROSIS, osteopetrosis causes abnormally high bone density that may be apparent in INFANTS at birth. A less severe form appears in CHILDREN under ten, but the mildest cases occur among 20- to 40-year-old patients.

Regardless of the patient's age, GENETIC FACTORS influence the type and severity of the disease. As information from Osteopetrosis.org explained, "Osteopetrosis is a congenital disease characterized in each of its forms by defective osteoclast function. Osteoclasts are the cells responsible for bone resorption. They are necessary for the formation of bone marrow. In people with osteopetrosis, osteoclasts do not function normally and the cavity for bone marrow does not form. This causes bones that appear dense on x-ray and cannot resist average stressors and therefore break easily. The condition is quite rare; incidences have been reported at 1 in 20,000–500,000" for the most common type of the disorder.

Symptoms and Diagnostic Path

Besides a family history, laboratory tests, and X-RAYS, physicians usually request a BONE MINERAL DENSITY TEST. However, information from Osteopetrosis.org said, "Among the difficulties in diagnosing and being treated for this disease and its symptoms are the realities that there are at least two and as many as five differently recognized types of osteopetrosis."

To complicate a diagnosis more, all symptoms are not immediately apparent but may progress as patients age. For example, the most serious form of malignant infantile osteopetrosis may result in a general failure to thrive. Teeth may not erupt, and motor development may lag, delaying a child's ability to sit, crawl, or walk. Frequent infections occur, too, even for adult patients. Since bones become dense and heavy, this poor bone quality often leads to FRACTURES.

Treatment Options and Outlook

Treatments include STEROID THERAPY and other appropriate medications, depending on the type of osteopetrosis. The National Institutes of Health (NIH) Osteoporosis and Related Bone Diseases said, "The U.S. Food and Drug Administration (FDA) recently approved Actimmune® (Interferon gamma-1b) Injection for delaying the progression of the disease in patients with severe malignant osteopetrosis. Actimmune® is the only therapy approved specifically for the treatment of osteopetrosis. Both adult and pediatric patients may benefit from Actimmune®."

For patients with severe cases, treatment options include bone marrow transplant (BMT). As the NIH explained, "BMT replaces the abnormal osteoclasts, or cells that breakdown bones, with normal cells. This process cures the defect if the transplantation

is successful. The survival rate after BMT in children who have osteopetrosis is 40 to 70 percent depending on how well matched the donor is to the patient. BMT is only used in severely affected patients, because of the high risk of failure with the potential of a fatal outcome."

According to the NIH, "less than 30 percent of all children with the severe malignant infantile form of osteopetrosis survive to their tenth birthday, unless they are treated with BMT or a combination of interferon gamma and calcitriol. Only 10 percent of infants who have blindness and anemia before six months old survive more than one year unless they are successfully treated." However, patients with the adult form of osteopetrosis can expect a normal life span. For this group, "the major complications are fractures and compression of the cranial nerves, or those nerves pertaining to the bones of the head. These complications can lead to blindness, deafness and facial nerve paralysis."

Risk Factors and Preventive Measures

Proper treatment and healthful NUTRITION can increase the quality and, sometimes, the length of life. Patients with severe symptoms or shortened life expectancy may want to expand their treatment options by participating in RESEARCH or CLINICAL TRIALS.

National Institutes of Health Osteoporosis and Related Bone Diseases National Resource Center. "Information for Patients about Osteopetrosis," NIH ORBD-NRC. Available online. URL: http://www.osteo.org/newfile.asp?doc=p117i&doctitle=Osteopetrosis&doctype=HTML+Fact+Sheet. Downloaded March 2, 2006.
Osteopetrosis Web Site. "Osteopetrosis," Osteopetrosis. org. Available online. URL: http://www.osteopetrosis. org/. Downloaded March 2, 2006.

osteophyte   Better known as bone spurs, osteophytes commonly occur in ELDERLY persons or patients with degenerative conditions of the SPINE. GENETIC FACTORS and previous injuries contribute to osteophyte formation too. Despite the name, bone spurs usually form smooth protrusions rather than sharp ones. Yet their presence often causes sharp pain to radiate from a point of origin, which can be anywhere bone is found in the BACK or CERVICAL SPINE, LUMBAR SPINE, and THORACIC SPINE.

Symptoms and Diagnostic Path

Osteophytes often spur episodes of ACUTE PAIN. If a bone spur presses a spinal nerve, symptoms may include numbness or weakness. To show what is going on, imaging tests, such as MAGNETIC RESONANCE IMAGING or COMPUTED TOMOGRAPHY SCAN, provide a clearer picture of the soft tissue and general conditions surrounding each VERTEBRA. For example, imaging may show the osteophyte and also reveal a contributive condition, such as DEGENERATIVE DISC, OSTEOARTHRITIS, or SPINAL STENOSIS.

Treatment Options and Outlook

Therapies address the causative factors as well as an actual osteophyte. Such treatments include NONSTEROIDAL ANTI-INFLAMMATORY DRUG THERAPY, STEROID THERAPY, or, for flare-ups, rest. In some cases, SURGERY, such as LAMINECTOMY, may be needed. As a Spine-Health.com article explained, "Spine surgery for bone spurs becomes necessary if nerve or spinal cord compression is either causing unremitting pain or motor loss is documented on examination." However, "the majority of patients who undergo surgery for bone spurs experience good results, often gaining years of relief and improved quality of life."

Risk Factors and Preventive Measures

In the introduction to "Vertebral Osteophytes: An Experimental Animal Model," the authors said, "Osteophytes are formed as a secondary reactive process to primary degenerative changes of spinal motion segments." In other words, bone spurs occur as a reaction similar, perhaps, to what happens when a badly fitted shoe causes a callous on the foot. As bone spurs form, "the size, shape and location of these osteophytes are, therefore, precisely determined by the nature of the primary instability." Patients with spinal instability may be at greater risk for the development of osteophytes. Nevertheless, some instances may be prevented by BONE BUILDING efforts, including NUTRITION and EXERCISE.

Lee, C. K., M.D., M. Vuono-Hawkins, N. A. Langrana, M. C. Zimmerman, and J. R. Parsons Jr. "Vertebral Osteophytes: An Experimental Animal Model," Research Grant Winners 1990, North American Spine Society. Available online. URL: http://www.spine.org/articles/grantwinners_1990.cfm. Downloaded March 2, 2006.

Schneider, John, M.D. "Bone Spurs (Osteophytes) and Back Pain," Spine-Health.com. Available online. URL: http://www.spine-health.com/topics/cd/spurs/spurs01.html. Downloaded March 2, 2006.

osteoporosis Literally meaning "porous bones," this skeletal condition not only affects bone quality but bone strength. As VERTEBRAE and other bones begin to thin and weaken, the LUMBAR SPINE may encounter more BACKACHES, LOW BACK PAIN, or CHRONIC PAIN in the BACK. These aches and pains typically result from FRACTURES of the SPINE that occur with minimal trauma or a cough or sneeze. The fractures subsequently cause the person to lose height while gaining such POSTURE problems as KYPHOSIS.

Each year over 1.5 million broken bones can be attributed to osteoporosis. While this happens primarily to ELDERLY women, older men encounter bone loss too. In the article "Do Men Get Osteoporosis?" the American Dietary Association reported, "One in every eight men over the age of 50 will suffer a hip fracture because of osteoporosis, according to statistics from Oregon Health Services University. Trouble is, men often are not screened for the disorder until they have their first broken bone."

Similarly, an article in *Rheumatology* said, "About 30% of hip and 33% of vertebral fractures occur in males. The unbalanced focus on osteoporosis prevention as an issue of primarily women's health is therefore unjustified. Factors predisposing to the disease can be identified in up to 77% of male patients with osteoporosis." Therefore, "we propose that the management of middle-aged and elderly men sustaining low traumatic fractures should routinely include a measurement of bone density and referral for medical treatment when indicated. If the diagnosis of low bone mass is missed at the time of fracture presentation, further fractures, perhaps including femur, may ensue."

"The 2004 Surgeon General's Report on Bone Health and Osteoporosis" said that half of all Americans over 50 will have weak bones by the year 2020. "If you are elderly, a broken hip makes you up to four times more likely to die within three months. If you survive, the injury often causes your health to spiral downward. . . . Many others become isolated, depressed, or frightened to leave home because they fear they will fall."

Despite those gloomy statistics, the Surgeon General's Report said, "The good news is that you are never too old or too young to improve your bone health." For instance, the report lauded the benefits of CALCIUM, VITAMIN D, and WEIGHT-BEARING EXERCISE, adding, "When you think of bones, you might imagine a hard, brittle skeleton. In reality, your bones are living organs. They are alive with cells and flowing body fluids. Bones are constantly renewed and grow stronger with a good diet and physical activity."

Information from the National Institutes of Health (NIH) Osteoporosis and Related Bone Diseases National Resource Center further explained, "Throughout your lifetime, old bone is removed (resorption) and new bone is added to the skeleton (formation). During childhood and teenage years, new bone is added faster than old bone is removed. As a result, bones become larger, heavier, and denser. Bone formation continues at a pace faster than resorption until peak bone mass (maximum bone density and strength) is reached around age 30. After age 30, bone resorption slowly begins to exceed bone formation." For white and Asian women in particular, "bone loss is most rapid in the first few years after menopause but persists into the postmenopausal years. Osteoporosis develops when bone resorption occurs too quickly or if replacement occurs too slowly. Osteoporosis is more likely to develop if you did not reach optimal bone mass during your bone building years."

An article published in *Patient Care* explained, "Bone mass in adults is the net result of the progressive bone loss from their peak bone mass, which is accrued between ages 20 and 35. In adolescent males," the effects of such substances as testosterone "achieve a bigger bone size than that found in females . . . , thereby improving their bone mass. Greater . . . bone diameter and larger vertebrae lead to greater bone strength in men. Testosterone also stimulates muscle growth, thereby improving bone

mineral density (BMD)." In both men and women, "osteoporosis results when there is decreased bone formation (common), increased bone resorption or a combination of these 2 conditions."

Symptoms and Diagnostic Path

In discussing what to expect, "Fast Facts" posted by the National Osteoporosis Foundation said, "Osteoporosis is often called a 'silent disease' because bone loss occurs without symptoms. People may not know that they have osteoporosis until their bones become so weak that a sudden strain, bump or fall causes a fracture or a vertebra to collapse. Collapsed vertebrae may initially be felt or seen in the form of severe back pain, loss of height, or spinal deformities such as kyphosis or stooped posture."

To assess bone loss, most physicians prescribe BONE MINERAL DENSITY (BMD) TESTS such as ABSORPTIOMETRY. However, a 2001 report from the Agency for Healthcare Research and Quality (AHRQ) said, "The likelihood of being diagnosed as having osteoporosis also depends on the number of sites tested. Testing in the forearm, hip, spine, or heel will generally identify different groups. A physician cannot say, based only on one of these tests, that the patient 'does not have osteoporosis'." To aid the diagnosis, testing for identifiers or bone markers can help, but the AHRQ cautioned, "No single marker or cluster of markers accurately identified individuals who had osteoporosis, as determined by the results of densitometry" or BMD testing. Therefore, "it is not surprising that agreement between the two tests was poor. Densitometry measures current bone status, whereas markers measure the process of bone turnover."

The health report *Osteoporosis: A Guide to Prevention and Treatment* from the Harvard Medical School said, "Several companies have developed blood and urine tests that indicate the rate at which bone is being formed and destroyed by measuring the markers of bone turnover. While these tests are sometimes used, the information they can provide is limited, and they can't tell you if you are at risk of breaking a bone." For example, "some of these tests measure collagen cross-links—proteins contained in the structural framework of bone, which are released during bone resorption. Others measure alkaline phosphatase and osteocalcin, proteins that are instrumental to bone formation. These tests can indicate high bone turnover, which can be a sign of rapid bone loss. However, they cannot indicate bone mass any more than measurements of metabolic rate can indicate a person's weight. Like metabolism, bone turnover varies from person to person and from time to time. Thus, a turnover rate that may point to bone loss in one person may represent the status quo for another."

Treatment Options and Outlook

Besides the highly recommended options of calcium and other natural sources of NUTRITION such as PHY-TOESTROGENS, two types of therapeutic drugs commonly treat osteoporosis: ANTIRESORPTIVE DRUGS, such as BISPHOSPHONATES and HORMONE REPLACE-MENT THERAPY, and BONE BUILDING drugs, such as PARATHYROID HORMONE (PTH.) These medications do not replace good nutrition, adequate fresh water, and weight-bearing exercise but, rather, complement them. Often, therapeutic drugs improve the overall outlook too. However, a medication proven effective for one patient may not be for another.

According to a report in the *Journal of Bone and Mineral Research,* numerous studies have "investigated the relationship between changes in BMD and fracture risk reduction observed with antiresorptive agents, with inconsistent results." Regarding the lumbar spine, for example, large CLINICAL TRI-ALS showed 6.2 percent increase in BMD in patients who received ALENDRONATE, 5.8 percent increase of BMD with RISEDRONATE, and 2.5 percent with raloxifene. "Despite the differences in BMD response, all three agents were associated with reductions in the risk of vertebral fracture over 3 years." As researchers concluded, "Many factors may influence the outcome . . . , and caution should be used in interpreting the results of such analyses when exploring the relationship between BMD changes and fracture risk reduction with antiresorptive therapy of osteoporosis."

Similarly, an abstract from the *Journal of Women's Health* cautioned, "Great advances have been made in the field of osteoporosis treatment and prevention in recent years that have led to the availability of powerful new drugs. These drugs are viewed by patients and physicians as a major breakthrough in the management of osteoporosis. Unfortunately,

this view has led many to ignore the importance of concurrent calcium supplementation to ensure the maximum benefit from these drugs. . . . As the majority of patients fail to consume the minimum recommended dietary intake of calcium, it is critical to recommend calcium supplements to raise total daily calcium intake to the levels needed to ensure maximum efficacy of osteoporosis treatments. Furthermore, osteoporosis drug labeling should be strengthened to encourage proper use of these drugs in combination with calcium supplements."

The article "Treatment of Osteoporosis: Why, Whom, When and How to Treat" in *The Medical Journal of Australia* stated, "If the aim is to reduce vertebral fractures, then any one of the agents alendronate, risedronate, or raloxifene, or parathyroid hormone, is suitable. However, use of parathyroid hormone is likely to be limited to severe osteoporosis, probably followed by an antiresorptive drug." The article also addressed the issue of when medications should be used: "If drugs were 100% efficacious, 100% safe, and cost-free, and patients were 100% compliant, the answer would be to treat everyone and early. As this is not the case, the most important factor determining whom and when to treat is an individual's absolute risk of fracture. If the risk is 2 per 1,000 women per year, and a drug halves fracture risk, then one event is prevented, one woman will sustain a fracture despite treatment, and 998 who were not going to have a fracture anyhow had treatment. Thus, one fracture is prevented, but 999 women per year are treated without benefit. . . . The imperative to intervene increases with advancing age, lower bone mineral density (BMD) and previous fracture, as each of these contributes independently to fracture risk." In addition, "the risk of further fractures increases threefold to fivefold as the number or severity of prevalent vertebral deformities increases."

An article in *The Journal of Clinical Endocrinology & Metabolism* reported, "One of the most exciting developments in the past year has been the discovery that . . . statins," prescribed to lower cholesterol, may strengthen "bone, thereby potentially reducing the risk of fractures with long-term therapy." Apparently, "studies have suggested that the use of statins is associated with a modest increase in BMD and significant fracture risk reduction on the order of 40–50% for all clinical fractures." Although "it is unclear how this class of drugs reaches the bone and how it affects bone turnover," the article stated, "this is an exciting area of future development, which could offer great potential for patients and physicians. Just as importantly, this class of drugs is certain to open up new research opportunities as investigators begin to unravel the effects of statins on bone and the mechanisms responsible for enhanced bone formation."

Summarizing the most common treatments presently used in the United States, the NIH said, "Currently, estrogen, calcitonin, alendronate, raloxifene, and risedronate are approved by the U. S. Food and Drug Administration (FDA) for the treatment of postmenopausal osteoporosis. Estrogen, alendronate, risedronate, and raloxifene are approved for the prevention of the disease. Alendronate is approved for the treatment of osteoporosis in men. Alendronate and risedronate are approved for use by men and women" with certain types of osteoporosis.

Until recently, surgical treatment for osteoporotic spine fractures was not possible since patients with frail bones could not withstand invasive SURGERY requiring screw and plate fixation of the bone. Now, however, KYPHOPLASTY offers MINIMALLY INVASIVE SURGERY with promising results. Nevertheless, surgery of any kind presents an option to consider only after nonsurgical management has failed.

Risk Factors and Preventive Measures

An article in *Nursing* listed factors that increase the risks for developing osteoporosis or encountering bone loss. For example, a sedentary lifestyle, poor nutrition, excessive alcohol consumption, cigarette smoking, certain medications, and products containing aluminum can deplete bone mass. While ENVIRONMENTAL INFLUENCES can certainly introduce aluminum into the system, OVER-THE-COUNTER PRODUCTS, from baking powder to deodorants, contain that substance along with its potential for a cumulative effect. Therefore, patients do well to read product labels carefully.

People with various medical conditions and medications face increased risks of osteoporosis too. According to an article in *Osteoporosis, Clinical Updates,* "treatment of secondary osteoporosis should be focused on addressing the underlying disease; additional interventions may then be considered." Although "many of these conditions are elusive, often obscured by what appears to be the primary disease," the article said, "virtually every subspecialty in medicine has a disease state or treatment that is associated with or actually causes osteoporosis." For example, poor MINERAL BALANCE brought on by malabsorption may cause bone loss in patients with cystic fibrosis, whereas in prostate CANCER, testosterone deficit may be a cause. Bone loss also occurs in patients with paralysis, liver disease, renal disease, thyroid disease, and other disorders.

Orthopaedic Nursing discussed the risk of bone loss with hormone depletion. According to the article, "the phenomenon of decreased estrogen levels in females as it relates to bone loss is well studied: it must be noted, however, that males also experience a decrease in estrogen . . . secondary to aging, and this can contribute to decreased bone density in males." Interestingly, hormonal depletion did not prove the case in a case cited in the report, but rather GENETIC FACTORS resulted in bone loss.

Genetic factors also incline people of all types and ages toward allergies and such inflammatory diseases as RHEUMATOID ARTHRITIS. Since the glucocorticoids prescribed to treat these conditions often cause secondary osteoporosis, the American College of Rheumatology (ACR) addressed "Recommendations for the Prevention and Treatment of Glucocorticoid-induced Osteoporosis" in their journal, *Arthritis & Rheumatism.* According to the article, "Glucocorticoids alter bone metabolism such that bone formation is reduced and resorption is increased, leading to rapid bone loss after initiation of therapy." Although "a number of antiresorptive agents are available to both prevent and treat glucocorticoid-induced bone loss," the ACR advised "supplementation with calcium and vitamin D at a dosage of 800 IU/day, or an activated form of vitamin D (e.g., alfacalcidiol at 1 g/day or calcitriol at 0.5 g/day), should be offered to all patients receiving glucocorticoids, to restore normal calcium balance. This combination has been shown to maintain bone mass in patients receiving long-term low-to-medium-dose glucocorticoid therapy who have normal levels of . . . hormones. However, while supplementation with calcium and vitamin D alone generally will not prevent bone loss in patients in whom medium-to-high-dose glucocorticoid therapy is being initiated, supplementation with calcium and an activated form of vitamin D will prevent bone loss."

According to the International Osteoporosis Foundation (IOF), "a 10% loss of bone mass in the vertebrae can double the risk of vertebral fractures." Since this places elderly men and women at particularly high risk, the IOF advised, "In the frail elderly, activity to improve balance and confidence may be valuable in fall prevention." For example, "studies have shown that individuals who practice tai chi have a 47% decrease in falls and 25% the hip fracture rate of those who do not and that tai chi can be beneficial for retarding bone loss in weight-bearing bones in early postmenopausal women."

Although many studies focus on older women, CHILDREN or ADOLESCENTS with EATING DISORDERS have a high risk of developing osteoporosis early in life. Conversely, young people who develop healthful habits of nutrition and exercise can bank on their bones being strong in later years. Weight-bearing exercises to build bone mass include competitive sports popular among ATHLETES, such as golf, basketball, gymnastics, and soccer but not swimming. While water sports help patients with joint problems, such as OSTEOARTHRITIS, they do not offer the type of exercise needed to build bone. For older adults who obtain approval from their doctors, such weight-bearing exercises as walking, dancing, and playing tennis can begin slowly then gradually increase to three or four times a week in an ongoing effort to keep bones mobile, healthy, and strong.

Agency for Healthcare Research and Quality. "Osteoporosis in Postmenopausal Women: Diagnosis and Monitoring. Summary, Evidence Report/Technology Assessment: Number 28," AHRQ Publication Number 01-E031, February 2001. Available online. URL: http://www.ahrq.gov/clinic/epcsums/osteosum.htm. Downloaded March 4, 2006.

American College of Rheumatology Ad Hoc Committee on Glucocorticoid-Induced Osteoporosis. "Recommendations for the Prevention and Treatment of Glucocorticoid-Induced Osteoporosis," *Arthritis & Rheumatism*, Official Journal of the American College of Rheumatology 44, no. 7 (July 2001): 1,496–1,503.

American Dietary Association. "Do Men Get Osteoporosis?" Available online. URL: http://www.eatright.org/cps/rde/xchg/ada/hs.xsl/home_4058_ENU_HTML.htm. Posted April 18, 2005.

Delmas, P. D., Zhengqing Li, and Cyrus Cooper. "Relationship Between Changes in Bone Mineral Density and Fracture Risk Reduction With Antiresorptive Drugs: Some Issues With Meta-Analyses," *Journal of Bone and Mineral Research* 19, no. 2 (February 2004): 330–336.

Gaber, T. A.-Z. K., S. Love, and A. J. Crisp. "The High Prevalence of Low Bone Density in Men Aged 55 Yr and Over Presenting with Low Trauma Fractures to an Accident and Emergency Department," *Rheumatology* 42, no. 6 (2003): 807–808.

Hetzell, Carole B. "New Help for Old Bones," *Nursing* 35, no. 5 (May 2005): 20–21.

International Osteoporosis Foundation. "Facts and Statistics about Osteoporosis and Its Impact," IOF. Available online. URL: http://www.osteofound.org/press_centre/fact_sheet.html. Downloaded March 4, 2006.

National Institutes of Health Osteoporosis and Related Bone Diseases National Resource Center. "Osteoporosis Overview," NIH ORBD-NRC. Available online. URL: http://www.osteo.org/osteo.html. Downloaded March 4, 2006.

National Osteoporosis Foundation. "Fast Facts," NOF. Available online. URL: http://www.nof.org/osteoporosis/diseasefacts.htm. Downloaded March 4, 2006.

Office of the Surgeon General. "The 2004 Surgeon General's Report on Bone Health and Osteoporosis," U.S. Department of Health and Human Services. Available online. URL: http://www.surgeongeneral.gov/library/bonehealth/docs/Osteo10sep04.pdf. Downloaded March 3, 2006.

Peer, Kimberly S. and Katherine R. Newsham. "A Case Study on Osteoporosis in a Male Athlete: Looking Beyond the Usual Suspects," *Orthopaedic Nursing* 24, no. 3 (May/June 2005): 193–201.

Rosen, Clifford J. and John P. Bilezikian. "Anabolic Therapy for Osteoporosis," *The Journal of Clinical Endocrinology & Metabolism* 86, no. 3 (2001): 957–964.

Seeman, Ego and John A. Eisman. "Treatment of Osteoporosis: Why, Whom, When and How to Treat," *The Medical Journal of Australia* 180, no. 6 (March 15, 2004): 298–303.

Slovik, David M., M.D., Medical Editor. *Osteoporosis: A Guide to Prevention and Treatment.* Boston, Mass.: Harvard Health Publications, Harvard Medical School, 2005.

Staff. "Men's Health: The Challenge of Osteoporosis in Elderly Men," *Patient Care* 37 (June 2003): 67–70.

Staff, National Osteoporosis Foundation. "The Many Faces Of Secondary Osteoporosis," *Osteoporosis, Clinical Updates* 3, no. 3 (2002): 1–7.

Sunyecz, John Alexander, M.D., Laurel Highlands, M.D., and Steven M. Weisman. "The Role of Calcium in Osteoporosis Drug Therapy," *Journal of Women's Health* 14, no. 2 (March 2005): 180–192.

over-the-counter products   Many health aids for the BACK and SPINE can be purchased without a prescription, providing a variety of over-the-counter (OTC) products. Some of the OTC aids mentioned in this book include medicinal herbs for HERBAL THERAPY, HOMEOPATHIC MEDICINE, NONSTEROIDAL ANTI-INFLAMMATORY DRUGS (NSAIDs), PAIN RELIEVERS, ORTHOTICS, TOPICAL ANALGESICS, and nutritional supplements of vitamins and minerals.

Risks and Complications

OTC products may not come with guarantees, but consumers can be guaranteed problems by not reading labels. Take vitamin supplements, for example, as many people do, and the risks increase with too much of a good thing. With water-soluble vitamins, such as VITAMIN B-COMPLEX or VITAMIN C, the body usually flushes out what is not needed, but VITAMIN A, VITAMIN D, or VITAMIN E hang out with body fat and potentially reach toxic levels. Also, people sometimes decide on their own to take a maintenance dose of 81 mg of ASPIRIN to avoid blood clots, but if the same person takes supplements of blood-clotting VITAMIN K, those two OTC products may wage a battle in the bloodstream.

Product labels give the information needed to make an informed decision, but one little label can not cover each contingency. For example, complications can arise if patients try to speed up the effects of a prescribed medication with homeopathic products or herbs used to treat the same ailment. Nevertheless, a big rule says that no OTC product should be taken for the same condition being treated with pharmaceutical drugs.

To avoid the complications that arise from buying the wrong product or, worse, a dangerous one, the American Osteopathic Association Web site advised, "Read the labels on OTC medication before taking them. Not only does the label provide dosage amounts and frequency, but it also includes warnings about possible drug interactions with other medications, food or health conditions. As an example, many people take decongestants as they battle colds. If these people have high blood pressure, this could mean bad news since this OTC medication may cause blood pressure to rise. . . . Another safety precaution consumers can take is to inform their physicians of all prescription and nonprescription medications that they are currently taking, in order to make it easier for them to spot potential interactions. This includes vitamins as well."

The U.S. Food and Drug Administration (FDA) addressed concerns about adverse interactions that occur when medications overlap. For example, "acetaminophen is an active ingredient found in more than 600 OTC and prescription medicines, such as pain relievers, cough suppressants and cold medications. It is safe and effective when used correctly, but taking too much can lead to liver damage and even death. The risk for liver damage may be increased in people who drink three or more alcoholic beverages per day while using acetaminophen-containing medicines." Inadvertently taking too many NSAIDs produces similar risks. As the FDA said, "NSAIDs are common medications that are used to relieve fever and minor aches and pains. These products can cause stomach bleeding, with an increased risk in consumers who are over 60, are taking prescription blood thinners, are taking steroids, or have a history of stomach bleeding. NSAIDs may also increase the risk of kidney problems in people with pre-existing kidney disease, or who are taking a diuretic."

Special Aids and Adaptations

Many useful orthotic devices, such as corsets or soft cervical collars, can be purchased across the counter to provide temporary support. However, the type of back brace needed for, say, SCOLIOSIS, can not be found without the help of an orthotist or an orthopedist. Similarly, canes or walkers can be purchased over the counter, but advice should first be sought from an occupational therapist, physical therapist, or doctor to determine the correct height and style.

To encourage patients to read OTC product labels thoroughly, the Center for Drug Evaluation and Research (CDER) actually reminded people to put on their glasses! Less obvious perhaps, the CDER Web site shed light on labels, advising consumers to look for the product name, the active ingredients or "therapeutic substances in medicine," the product "category (such as antihistamine, antacid, or cough suppressant)," and the uses, such as the "symptoms or diseases the product will treat or prevent." Consumers especially need to be aware of any warning, such as "when not to use the product, when to stop taking it, when to see a doctor, and possible side effects." Other important information might address proper storage, whereas a list of inactive ingredients commonly includes "substances such as binders, colors, or flavoring." The latter can be particularly important in patients with food allergies or other sensitivities. Also, each OTC product should come with clear directions regarding "how much to take, how to take it, and how long to take it." Adapting to those very specific instructions may ring up the safest use for over-the-counter items.

American Osteopathic Association. "The Use of Over-the-Counter Medicine Is on the Rise," AOA. Available online. URL: http://www.osteopathic.org/index.cfm?PageID=you_otcmed. Downloaded March 4, 2006.

Center for Drug Evaluation and Research. "Over-the-Counter Medicines: What's Right for You?" FDA. Available online. URL: http://www.fda.gov/cder/consumerinfo/WhatsRightForYou.htm. Last updated August 17, 2005.

U.S. Food and Drug Administration. "FDA Launches Campaign on OTC Pain Relief Products," *FDA Consumer Magazine*. March–April 2004. Available online. URL: http://www.fda.gov/fdac/features/2004/204_otc.html. Downloaded March 4, 2006.

oxaprozin   See NONSTEROIDAL ANTI-INFLAMMATORY DRUG THERAPY.

Paget's disease   See OSTEITIS DEFORMANS.

pain   On a scale of one to ten, ACUTE PAIN in the BACK or SPINE often rates high, but acute episodes can also arrive as a dull BACKACHE or nagging CERVICOGENIC HEADACHE. Likewise, CHRONIC PAIN can be intense after a BACK INJURY or FAILED BACK SURGERY but may hover around the low to mid-range in such conditions as ARTHRITIS, OSTEOARTHRITIS, and SPINAL STENOSIS.

To find out what hurts and where, a doctor asks questions, such as when the pain began, how it rates on that scale of one to 10, and what other symptoms have been noticed. Often, the presence or absence of additional symptoms can help to determine an appropriate course of PAIN MANAGEMENT. For example, symptoms of numbness with intermittent but sharp pain radiating from the LUMBAR SPINE may indicate SCIATICA. Specific points of pain, often referred to as trigger points, may point to FIBROMYALGIA or muscle spasms, whereas radiant nerve pain may suggest SPINAL STENOSIS or SPONDYLOLISTHESIS. LOW BACK PAIN accompanied by urinary problems may reveal a kidney disorder. If symptoms include a loss of function in the legs or numbness in the groin, the condition may be diagnosed as CAUDA EQUINA SYNDROME. If so, the condition often requires emergency SURGERY in order to recover spinal nerve function. For fever and acute pain, an antibiotic may be prescribed to eradicate a SPINAL INFECTION or prevent the development of ARACHNOIDITIS.

Regardless of the accompanying symptoms or level of intensity, pain is the main way a body says, "Hello. Can this area please have some attention?" Sometimes that message requires interpretive laboratory tests, X-RAYS or other imaging tests, BONE MINERAL DENSITY TESTS, NERVE CONDUCTION STUDIES, or nerve function tests to identify an underlying medical condition. Tests also clarify the treatment options, from prescription strength PAIN RELIEVERS to ACUPUNCTURE or other forms of COMPLEMENTARY AND ALTERNATIVE MEDICINE to surgery.

Risks and Complications

With or without an underlying disorder, unchecked pain can be physically damaging. Chronically achy DISCS, inflamed joints, muscle STRAIN, or sore VERTEBRAE can cause a person to compensate by favoring that area, thus creating a POSTURE problem. Pain also causes complications by making a person less inclined to perform normal daily ACTIVITY or EXERCISE, so the patient's strength and mobility slowly but steadily decrease. Then PARASPINAL MUSCLE mass declines. Circulation throughout the body diminishes, and pain flares. Worse, an increasingly sedentary lifestyle places the person at a statistically greater risk for developing a serious medical condition.

Statistics and Studies

Natalie Frazin reported on a study linking chronic pain to brain signals. According to that report for The National Institute of Neurological Disorders and Stroke (NINDS), "most studies of chronic pain have focused on signals in the spinal cord and in the peripheral nerves, which carry pain messages from the limbs and other parts of the body to the spinal cord. However, recent studies have suggested that the brain not only receives pain signals from the spinal cord but also undergoes changes in neuronal connections that may permanently strengthen its reactions to those signals. Researchers believe these changes are key to the development of chronic pain." Understanding the changes in brain signals may eventually produce new treatment options.

Another NINDS report, "Low Back Pain Fact Sheet," said, "Nearly everyone at some point has back pain that interferes with work, routine daily activities, or recreation. Americans spend at least $50 billion each year on low back pain, the most common cause of job-related disability and a leading contributor to missed work. Back pain is the second most common neurological ailment in the United States—only headache is more common."

More painful statistics came from the Web site of the American Pain Foundation: "Over 50 million Americans suffer from chronic pain, and nearly 25 million Americans experience acute pain each year due to injuries or surgery." One in three citizens loses over 20 hours of SLEEP each week because of pain, which undoubtedly contributes to the fact that "lost workdays due to pain add up to over 50 million a year." Although the intensity of pain varies with each causality, CANCER pain can be especially severe. As the foundation reported, "An estimated 70% of those with cancer experience significant pain during their illness, yet fewer than half receive adequate treatment for their pain." Reasons vary, of course, but if doctors hesitate to prescribe strong OPIATES or OPIOIDS FOR PAIN when needed, the private fight against cancer pain may succumb to a public fight against drug abuse.

Special Aids and Adaptations

Some types of pain may be avoided as people use proper techniques in LIFTING, remain within their LOAD TOLERANCE, and become aware of ERGONOMIC FACTORS and ENVIRONMENTAL INFLUENCES that trigger painful episodes. Lots of fresh water and well-balanced NUTRITION also help a body to adapt to ever-changing conditions in life. Fitting SHOE CHOICES aid most people, too, for example by encouraging walking and helping the spine to stay in proper alignment.

If good sense and caution do not prevent pain and medical treatments fail to help, BIOFEEDBACK provides yet another option. Also, occupational therapy and physical therapy may help CHILDREN, ADOLESCENTS, and ELDERLY patients. In discussing three common stages of rehabilitation, the American Academy of Physical Medicine and Rehabilitation said, "During the first phase, called the acute phase, physiatrists treat pain and inflammation."

With a diagnosis to guide the treatment, options include MASSAGE THERAPY, ACUPRESSURE, and ULTRASOUND THERAPY. "In the second, or recovery, phase of treatment, flexibility and strength are developed to get the body parts into their proper positions." Then, "the main goal of the third phase of treatment, the maintenance phase, is to minimize recurrence of the problem and to prevent further injury. This often consists of a total body fitness program, designed to maintain body mechanics and increase endurance after the original symptoms have resolved."

American Academy of Physical Medicine and Rehabilitation. "Overview of Neck Pain," AAPM&R. Available online. URL: http://www.aapmr.org/condtreat/pain/neckpain.htm. Downloaded March 6, 2006.

American Pain Foundation. "Fast Facts About Pain." Available online. URL: http://www.painfoundation.org/page.asp?file=Library/FastFacts.htm. Downloaded March 6, 2006.

Frazin, Natalie. "Study Links Chronic Pain to Signals in the Brain," National Institute of Neurological Disorders and Stroke (NINDS.) Available online. URL: http://www.ninds.nih.gov/news_and_events/news_articles/news_article_chronic_pain.htm. Last updated January 25, 2006.

National Institute of Neurological Disorders and Stroke (NINDS.) "Low Back Pain Fact Sheet." Available online. URL: http://www.ninds.nih.gov/disorders/backpain/detail_backpain.htm. Last updated January 25, 2006.

pain management From folk remedies to SURGERY, various types of therapy work to keep pain under control. To manage CHRONIC PAIN, pain management specialists may be consulted. Most often though, pain management begins at home with an ice pack or a hot shower, but the choice of treatments usually depends on the additional symptoms. For instance, if inflammation, swelling, or bruising accompany pain, an appropriate treatment may be an ice pack and ASPIRIN or other NONSTEROIDAL ANTI-INFLAMMATORY DRUG (NSAID) THERAPY. If pain and stiffness occur without inflammation, a hot shower or heating pad may be advisable along with a dose of ACETAMINOPHEN. Whichever PAIN RELIEVER is used, the dose should not exceed what the manufacturer recommends unless a doctor says otherwise. This includes recommended doses for pain-relieving HOMEOPATHIC MEDICINES and HERBAL THERAPY too.

Typically, pain management aims to reduce the discomfort or enable a patient to tolerate pain, but it also focuses on what causes the problem. For example, if ATHLETES succumb to muscle STRAIN or manual laborers exceed their LOAD TOLERANCE, they might reconsider those movements. Similarly, changing the ENVIRONMENTAL INFLUENCES and ERGO-NOMIC FACTORS that trigger pain may bring discernible relief.

Another aspect of pain management addresses mental health or psychological factors. For example, a job may not manufacture pain so much as TENSION, which, in turn, produces episodes of aches and soreness. Dreading work can be a major source of stress, but dreading pain can be too. In the latter case, BIOFEEDBACK may help a patient recognize and, thus, head off conditions leading toward discomfort.

Eventually, most instances of BACK and neck pain resolve themselves in two to four weeks, but CHRONIC PAIN or unexplained pain needs medical treatment. If a fever or other worrisome symptoms arise, the advice of a doctor should be sought immediately. When no other symptoms accompany pain, management may include ACUPRES-SURE, ACUPUNCTURE, COLD THERAPY, HEAT THERAPY, HYDROTHERAPY, MASSAGE THERAPY, ORTHOTICS, SPI-NAL MANIPULATION, STEROID THERAPY, ULTRASOUND THERAPY, or even another SHOE CHOICE. A night of uninterrupted SLEEP can make pain more manageable too.

If home treatments, COMPLEMENTARY AND ALTER-NATIVE MEDICINE (CAM), and allopathic forms of pain management bring no relief, the focus then shifts from pain to rehabilitation. As the director of The National Foundation for the Treatment of Pain explained, "No matter the severity of the underlying pathology, improvement in the physical function of the patient must be the goal in all but the worst cases with multiple failed surgical procedures. The patient can make demonstrable progress in range of motion, and tolerance of activities, with a devoted regimen of hot baths, stretches and other physical therapies. Indeed, relief from pain should be targeted in large part as only a means to making physical therapy possible."

Although uncommon, FAILED BACK SURGERY SYNDROME can produce such unrelenting pain that physical therapy may not be feasible until extreme forms of pain management have begun to take effect. Such treatments may include a NERVE BLOCK, NEUROSTIMULATION, SPINAL INJECTION, or OPIOIDS FOR PAIN, but counseling may also help some patients.

Risks and Complications

An article in the *Lancet* said, "Even early in the course of an episode of low back pain, the reasons why patients might not be recovering are complex and include more than just the pathophysiology of the spine. Psychological distress and misguided beliefs about pain seem to interfere with recovery and raise the risk of chronic disability."

Age raises those risks since ELDERLY patients often experience the added complication of depression. CHILDREN, ADOLESCENTS, and adults with frequent bouts of pain may feel helpless and depressed too. In an article for the American Pain Foundation, Dr. Scott M. Fishman explained, "Depression has an amplifying effect on pain. By decreasing depression, we can de-amplify the sensation of pain, and therefore decrease pain. In my opinion, decreasing depression when it is also present with pain is a very significant intervention for decreasing pain itself and improving the patient's ability to cope with any pain sensations that they have."

Statistics and Studies

Often, the more choices a patient has, the better the outlook. Staying active also improves perspective and provides another form of pain management as does appropriate EXERCISE. An article in the *Annals of Internal Medicine* said, "In chronic low back pain, evidence strongly suggests that exercise is at least as effective as other conservative treatments. Individually designed strengthening or stabilizing programs seem to be effective in health care settings. . . . However, we emphasize that exercise therapy is not the same as advice to stay active, which is a recommended treatment strategy in acute populations."

Unfortunately, all populations may not receive the same quality of treatment. As an article in *The*

Journal of the American Osteopathy Association (JAOA) reported, "Disparities clearly exist in the way in which certain patients receive treatment for their pain. Physicians need to be aware of these problems so they can provide proper care to all their patients, with special attention to racial and ethnic minorities, women, and substance abusers. Only when physicians acknowledge and understand such disparities and barriers can they begin to evaluate and improve on their own practices of pain management."

A patient's anticipation of pain may also contribute to its intensity. According to a report posted online by the National Institute of Neurological Disorders and Stroke, "people with decreased expectations for pain reported less pain. At the same time, activity decreased in areas of the brain important to both sensory and emotional processing of pain. . . . These lower expectations reduced reports of pain by more than 28 percent."

Special Aids and Adaptations

Adequate rest, exercise, NUTRITION, and, sometimes, distractions aid pain reduction. In addition, almost everyone manages pain better if someone else understands what is happening each day. Empathy brings the aid of comfort but also produces creative ideas and workable solutions that can be adapted to fit the individual. This can be particularly important in helping patients deal with pain that does not go away. The Partners Against Pain Web site posted a "Patient Comfort Assessment Guide" developed by Dr. Elizabeth J. Narcessian to help caretakers assess the level of discomfort their partners experience. To start family discussions and also clarify how the patient feels, the assessment offered such questions as, "What time of day is your pain the worst?" and, "What makes your pain better?" By noting relevant symptoms and evaluating the degree to which pain interferes with normal daily ACTIVITY, patients can help their partners understand how to assist in managing and, perhaps, overcoming the discomforts of that day.

Fishman, Scott M., M.D. "Antidepressants for Pain," Pain Question & Answer, American Pain Foundation. Available online. URL: http://www.painfoundation.org/page.asp?file=QandA/Anti-depressants.htm. Downloaded March 11, 2006.

Hay, E. M., R. Mullis, M. Lewis, K. Vohora, C. J. Main, P. Watson, K. S. Dziedzic, J. Sim, C. M. Lowe, and P. R. Croft. "Comparison of Physical Treatments versus a Brief Pain-management Programme for Back Pain in Primary Care: a Randomised Clinical Trial in Physiotherapy," *Lancet* 365, no. 9,476 (June 11, 2005): 2,024–2,030.

Hochman, J. S., M.D. "Essential Considerations in the Treatment of Intractable Pain," The National Foundation for the Treatment of Pain. Available online. URL: http://www.paincare.org/pain_management/essential/factors.html. Downloaded March 11, 2006.

Jones-London, Michelle D., "Expectations of Pain: I Think, Therefore I Am," National Institute of Neurological Disorders and Stroke (NINDS.) Available online. URL: http://www.ninds.nih.gov/news_and_events/news_articles/news_article_pain_perception.htm. Last updated February 15, 2006.

Narcessian, Elizabeth J., M.D. "Patient Comfort Assessment Guide," Partners Against Pain®. Available online. URL: http://www.partnersagainstpain.com/printouts/pcag.pdf. Downloaded March 11, 2006.

Paulson, Margaret III, and Anthony H. Dekker. "Healthcare Disparities in Pain Management," *The Journal of the American Osteopathy Association, JAOA* 105, no. 6, supplement 3 (June 2005): 14–17.

pain relievers As the phrase implies, this form of PAIN MANAGEMENT primarily aims to relieve PAIN. While TOPICAL ANALGESICS may be rubbed onto the skin to reduce muscle soreness, most pain relievers come packaged in caplets, capsules, liquids, or pills to be taken orally. These OVER-THE-COUNTER PRODUCTS (OTC) and prescription strength drugs commonly include ACETAMINOPHEN unless inflammation accompanies the pain. If so, the preferred medication may be ASPIRIN, IBUPROFEN, NAPROXEN, or other NONSTEROIDAL ANTI-INFLAMMATORY DRUG (NSAID).

For CHILDREN and ELDERLY patients, acetaminophen has become the most popular choice of pain relievers. For severe CHRONIC PAIN, a physician may prescribe CYCLOOXYGENASE (COX-2) INHIBITORS, OPIATES or OPIOIDS FOR PAIN, or STEROID THERAPY. However, patients with allergies or sensitivities to medication usually prefer pain relief from HOMEOPATHIC MEDICINES or kitchen herbs. Although studies are still needed to evaluate the effectiveness of homeopathic products and HERBAL THERAPY, people have used willow bark for centuries to relieve pain. Besides lauding that forerunner of aspirin, some people find pain relief with culinary usage of cayenne pepper, ginger, and turmeric. Those choice herbs may or may not eliminate pain, but they do spice foods and conversations about the ancient connections between culinary and medicinal arts.

Risks and Complications

According to the Food and Drug Administration (FDA), "pain reliever and fever reducer drug products have been available for many years without a prescription. These products are safe and effective when used by consumers properly." Nevertheless, "the FDA believes that consumers need to know that pain relievers or fever reducers can cause serious side effects when used improperly. FDA urges people to read the labels of all the OTC medicines they take to know how to take them properly."

Patients would be well advised to read product labels, too, since many OTC medicines include acetaminophen and NSAIDs. If patients take those in addition to a regular dosage of the pure product, they instantly have too much, thus increasing the risk of complications, such as stomach bleeding from an NSAID or liver damage from acetaminophen. In addition, herbal pain relievers should not be taken with any over-the-counter or prescription pain medications.

Opioids often interact with other medications too. As the National Institute on Drug Abuse (NIDA) warned, "opioid medications can affect regions of the brain that mediate what we perceive as pleasure, resulting in the initial euphoria that many opioids produce. They can also produce drowsiness, cause constipation, and, depending upon the amount taken, depress breathing. Taking a large single dose could cause severe respiratory depression or death." To avoid patient addiction and also the complications that arise from rapid withdrawal, "individuals taking prescribed opioid medications should not only be given these medications under appropriate medical supervision, but also should be medically supervised when stopping use in order to reduce or avoid withdrawal symptoms. Symptoms of withdrawal can include restlessness, mus-

cle and bone pain, insomnia, diarrhea, vomiting, cold flashes with goose bumps ('cold turkey'), and involuntary leg movements."

Statistics and Studies

According to the NIDA, "studies have shown that properly managed medical use of opioid analgesic compounds is safe and rarely causes addiction. Taken exactly as prescribed, opioids can be used to manage pain effectively."

Similarly, all pain relievers, including OTC products, must be taken as prescribed. As an article in *Shape* magazine reported, "a study in the journal *Neurology* found that when compared with people who used over-the-counter and/or prescription pain relievers as directed (or didn't use them at all), those who took too much of the drugs were more likely to have chronic migraine headaches, as well as more neck and lower back pain." Also, "a recent survey by the American Gastroenterological Association (AGA) showed that 44 percent of people said they took more than the recommended doses."

Special Aids and Adaptations

In discussing the RESEARCH they sponsor, the National Institute of Neurological Disorders and Stroke (NINDS) said, "Scientists are working to develop potent pain-killing drugs that act on receptors for the chemical acetylcholine. For example, a type of frog native to Ecuador has been found to have a chemical in its skin called epibatidine, derived from the frog's scientific name, Epipedobates tricolor. Although highly toxic, epibatidine is a potent analgesic and, surprisingly, resembles the chemical nicotine found in cigarettes. Also under development are other less toxic compounds that act on acetylcholine receptors and may prove to be more potent than morphine but without its addictive properties."

While new aids continue to become available, some patients have turned to a source of pain relief that may have been used for over 9,000 years. As reported on the University of Maryland Web site, "Capsaicin in cayenne pepper has very powerful pain-relieving properties when applied to the surface of the skin. Laboratory studies have found that capsaicin relieves pain by destroying a chemical known as substance P that normally carries pain messages to the brain. This appears to be true when applied topically," especially for such conditions as RHEUMATOID ARTHRITIS, OSTEOARTHRITIS, BACKACHE, and the pain of an overworked muscle.

Center for Drug Evaluation and Research. "Questions and Answers on Using Over-the-Counter (OTC) Human Drug Products Containing Analgesic/Antipyretic Active Ingredients Safely," Food and Drug Administration (FDA), Department of Health and Human Services. Available online. URL: http://www.fda.gov/cder/drug/analgesics/QandAanalgesics.htm. Created January 22, 2004.

National Institute of Neurological Disorders and Stroke (NINDS.) "Pain: Hope Through Research." Available online. URL: http://www.ninds.nih.gov/disorders/chronic_pain/detail_chronic_pain.htm. Last updated January 25, 2006.

National Institute on Drug Abuse (NIDA.) "NIDA Info-Facts: Prescription Pain and Other Medications," National Institutes of Health, U.S. Department of Health and Human Services. Available online. URL: http://www.nida.nih.gov/Infofacts/Painmed.html. Last updated April 21, 2005.

University of Maryland Medical Center. "Cayenne," Center for Integrative Medicine. Available online. URL: http://www.umm.edu/altmed/ConsHerbs/Cayennech.html. Downloaded September 12, 2006.

paraspinal muscles Up and down the SPINE, pairs of paraspinal muscles attach to either side of the VERTEBRAE, keeping a body upright and moving. If, however, an injury occurs in a DISC, vertebral bone, or connective soft tissue, this group of muscles protectively contracts around the damaged area, causing muscle spasm.

An online article on the Web site All About Back & Neck Pain explained, "Muscles that are in spasm produce too much lactic acid, a waste product from the chemical reaction inside muscle cells. When muscles contract, the small blood vessels traveling through the muscles are pinched off (like a tube pinched between your thumb and finger), which causes a build up of lactic acid. If the muscle cells cannot relax and too much lactic acid builds up, it causes a painful burning sensation." As muscles relax, normal blood flow rinses away the build-up of lactic acid. For that to happen though, a warm

bath, MASSAGE THERAPY, MUSCLE RELAXANT, or restful SLEEP may be needed, and an appropriate change in NUTRITION may restore MINERAL BALANCE.

Risks and Complications
POSTURE problems, such as KYPHOSIS and LORDOSIS, tip musculoskeletal balance, causing CHRONIC PAIN or BACKACHE in the THORACIC SPINE and lumbar region. TENSION in paraspinal muscles can also cause VERTEBRAL SUBLUXATION that throws the spine out of alignment. In addition, a FLEXION-EXTENSION INJURY, such as a whiplash, can misalign the spine and strain the paraspinal muscles.

Statistics and Studies
Researchers from Switzerland studied the effects of SCOLIOSIS on paraspinal muscles then reported in the *European Spine Journal:* "In scoliosis, the spinal musculature is most affected on the concave" or curved-in "side. . . . The muscle adopts a 'faster' . . . profile . . . perhaps consequent to a local change in activity on this side of the spine following progression of the curve. Less marked changes, in the same direction, are also evident on the convex," or rounded, "side; these may be the result of general disuse of the paraspinal muscles associated with the spinal deformity."

According to an article in *Spine,* researchers used ELECTROMYOGRAM to study effects of SPINAL STENOSIS on paraspinal muscles then reported, "Abnormal findings in needle electromyography of the paraspinal muscles were observed in 18 of the 22 (81.8%) examined patients. Abnormal . . . activation of the paraspinal muscles was observed in all the examined patients."

A study in *Radiology* magazine focused on the accuracy of MAGNETIC RESONANCE IMAGING (MRI or MR) used when a neck injury involved paraspinal muscles in the CERVICAL SPINE. The article concluded, "This study shows that contrast-enhanced MR findings in the paraspinal muscles are accurate for diagnosis of cervical root avulsion," or tearing of the spinal nerves in the neck. Apparently, this type of enhancement "demonstrates the abnormality more accurately than do other paraspinal muscle findings."

Special Aids and Adaptations
Paraspinal aids depend on what ails this group of muscles. With a posture problem or whiplash

injury, ORTHOTICS, such as a back brace or neck brace, provide temporary support of the BACK and spine. HEAT THERAPY, HYDROTHERAPY, or massage can often relieve minor aches and ACUTE PAIN as can OVER-THE-COUNTER and prescription strength PAIN RELIEVERS. For other forms of PAIN MANAGEMENT, patients may need to adapt the surrounding ENVIRONMENTAL INFLUENCES and ERGONOMIC FACTORS to fit their needs, rather than trying to adjust themselves to an unhealthy climate or poorly designed chair. For most people, regular daily ACTIVITY and EXERCISES such as STRENGTH TRAINING can build up paraspinal muscles while tearing down some contributive sources of PAIN.

All About Back & Neck Pain. "Paraspinal Muscles," DePuy Spine, Inc. Available online. URL: http://www.allaboutbackpain.com/html/files_links/spine_anatomy_muscle.html. Downloaded March 13, 2006.

Hayashi, Naoto, M.D., Tomohiko Masumoto, M.D., Osamu Abe, M.D., Shigeki Aoki, M.D., Kuni Ohtomo, M.D., and Yasuhito Tajiri, M.D. "Accuracy of Abnormal Paraspinal Muscle Findings on Contrast-enhanced MR Images as Indirect Signs of Unilateral Cervical Root-Avulsion Injury," *Radiology* 223, no. 2 (May 2002): 397–402.

Leinonen, Ville M.D., Sara Maatta, M.D., Simo Taimela, Arto Herno, Markku Kankaanpaa, Juhani Partanen, Osmo Hanninen, and Olavi Airaksinen. "Paraspinal Muscle Denervation, Paradoxically Good Lumbar Endurance, and an Abnormal Flexion-Extension Cycle in Lumbar Spinal Stenosis," *Spine* 28, no. 4 (February 2003): 324–331.

Mannion, A. F., M. Meier, D. Grob, and M. Müntener. "Paraspinal Muscle Fibre Type Alterations Associated with Scoliosis: an Old Problem Revisited with New Evidence," *European Spine Journal* 7, no. 4 (August 1998): 289–293.

parathyroid hormone (PTH)   When working well, the body produces parathyroid hormone (PTH) to maintain MINERAL BALANCE and release an optimal amount of CALCIUM into the bloodstream. Too much or too little PTH inclines the VERTEBRAE to thin with OSTEOPENIA and OSTEOPOROSIS or slant toward other bone disorders, such as RICKETS. Laboratory tests can be used to assess the level of calcium and other minerals in the blood, while BONE MINERAL DENSITY (BMD) TESTS can evaluate the SPINE and other weight-bearing bones. If bone loss has occurred, a synthetic form of PTH may help the body to regulate its BONE BUILDING abilities. Then PTH refers not to the natural hormone, but to the category of anabolic drugs designed to treat bone density problems.

In November 6, 2002, the Food and Drug Administration (FDA) announced the arrival of synthetic PTH, saying, "FDA has approved teriparatide for the treatment of osteoporosis in postmenopausal women who are at high risk for having a fracture. The drug is also approved to increase bone mass in men with . . . osteoporosis who are at high risk for fracture." The first agent officially accepted to stimulate new bone formation, "teriparatide is a portion of human parathyroid hormone (PTH), which is the primary regulator of calcium and phosphate metabolism in bones. Daily injections of teriparatide" delivered in a manner similar to insulin shots "stimulate new bone formation leading to increased bone mineral density."

Prescribed under the brand name Forteo, teriparatide has a different effect on bones from ANTIRESORPTIVE DRUGS, such as BISPHOSPHONATES and CALCITONIN. As explained in an article published in the *Cleveland Clinic Journal of Medicine*, "antiresorptive drugs inhibit osteoclast function, decrease turnover and remodeling, and decrease the remodeling space. . . . Anabolic drugs, in contrast, increase osteoblast and osteoclast function (stimulating osteoblasts more than osteoclasts), increase turnover and remodeling, and increase the remodeling space. Therefore, anabolic drugs may prevent fractures not only by increasing bone mass: they may also change the geometry of bone." In other words, osteoclasts remove old or injured bone tissue, and osteoblasts build new tissue, but for this to produce healthy bone, the math has to be right. Patients who cannot take antiresorptive drugs or those who can but still remain at high risk for FRACTURES may find teriparatide particularly helpful.

Dosage and Potential Side Effects

According to the FDA, "Teriparatide is administered by injection once a day in the thigh or abdomen. The recommended dose is 20 mcg per day." Since growing CHILDREN, ADOLESCENTS, and patients with

OSTEITIS DEFORMANS risk the development of osteosarcoma, teriparatide would not be advisable for them. Pregnant women and patients with CANCER or kidney problems should avoid PTH too. The FDA also warned, "Because the effects of long-term treatment with teriparatide are not known at this time, therapy for more than 2 years is not recommended. . . . Most side effects reported in association with teriparatide in clinical trials were mild and included nausea, dizziness, and leg cramps. During the clinical trials, early discontinuation due to adverse events occurred in 5.6% of patients assigned to placebo and 7.1% of patients taking teriparatide."

Statistics and Studies

While some studies consider whether PTH should be prescribed before or after antiresorptive drug treatment, others focus on combination therapies. An article in *Family Practice News* said, "At 6 months' follow-up, the combination of raloxifene and parathyroid hormone increased bone mineral density over baseline by a mean 6.19% at the lumbar spine . . . as measured by dual x-ray absorptiometry." With bone density again measured by ABSORPTIOMETRY, "by comparison, teriparatide increased lumbar spine density by a mean 5.19%." Additional trials continue, "but the only other previous major study of combination treatment looked at the use of parathyroid hormone with alendronate; it suggested that the addition of alendronate appeared to inhibit the ability of parathyroid hormone to stimulate new bone formation."

Until further RESEARCH has fully determined optimal combinations, patients should discuss with their doctors the advantages and disadvantages relevant to their particular conditions. This especially includes individualizing a program of NUTRITION with appropriate amounts of calcium and VITAMIN D.

Deal, Chad, M.D. and James Gideon, M.D. "Recombinant Human PTH 1-34 (Forteo): An Anabolic Drug for Osteoporosis," *Cleveland Clinic Journal of Medicine* 70, no. 7 (July 2003): 585–601.

Kirn, Timothy F. "Raloxifene, PTH Are Good Osteoporosis Combo: Together, the Two Drugs Could Potentially Maximize the Formation and Minimize the Resorption of Bone," *Family Practice News* 35, no. 3 (February 1, 2005): 58.

U.S. Food and Drug Administration. "FDA Approves Teriparatide To Treat Osteoporosis," *FDA Talk Paper,* November 6, 2002. Available online. URL: http://www.fda.gov/bbs/topics/ANSWERS/2002/ANS01176.html. Downloaded March 14, 2006.

pars defect   See SPONDYLOLISTHESIS.

peak bone mass   See BONE BUILDING.

pediatrics   See CHILDREN, SPINAL CONCERNS FOR.

percutaneous neuromodulation therapy (PNT)
Also known as percutaneous electrical nerve stimulation (PENS), this procedure offers a non-surgical option for treating LOW BACK PAIN (LBP). In addition, researchers from the University of Texas Southwestern Medical Center at Dallas reported on the effects of the treatment in patients with nonradiating pain in the CERVICAL SPINE. Although no long-term benefit has yet been documented, the report in *Anesthesia & Analgesia* did find short-term benefits. As the article said, "Sixty-eight patients received three different nonpharmacologic modalities, namely 'needles only' (neck), local (neck) . . . stimulation, and remote (lower back) . . . stimulation in a random sequence over the course of an 11-wk study period. All treatments were given for 30 min, 3 times per week for 3 wk, with 1 wk 'off' between each modality." The researchers subsequently reported, "We conclude that electrical stimulation" at specific levels produces "greater short-term improvements in pain control, physical activity, and quality of sleep in patients with chronic neck pain."

Procedure

Regardless of the area treated, the word percutaneous in PNT indicates penetration of the skin. Describing this outpatient or office procedure, the Washington State Department of Labor and Industries said, "In a manner similar to electroacupuncture, PNT uses . . . needles positioned in the soft tissues or muscles to stimulate peripheral sensory nerves with electricity." With needles "inserted to a depth of approximately 3 cm" and the electrical frequency alternating between 15 and 30 Hz, "the optimal duration of the electrical stimulation ranges from 30 to 45 minutes." The report also stated, "The Food and Drug Administration (FDA) does not regulate PNT as a therapy. However, the agency does approve for marketing the acupuncture needles and needle electrodes used in the procedure."

Risks and Complications

Patients with ANKYLOSING SPONDYLITIS, CANCER, and other conditions, such as recent SURGERY on the BACK, have been excluded from PNT studies. For those who do try this form of therapy, the level of pain relief varies. Also, insurance programs may not cover the treatment until additional RESEARCH has proven its effectiveness.

Outlook and Lifestyle Modifications

Before trying PNT, patients should exhaust traditional forms of PAIN MANAGEMENT as well as COMPLEMENTARY AND ALTERNATIVE MEDICINE (CAM) therapies. However, PNT offers a viable option for those who want to avoid surgery or be able to undertake a therapeutic course of EXERCISE.

Revord, John P., M.D. "Percutaneous Neuromodulation Therapy (PNT)—a New, Minimally-invasive Treatment for Lower Back Pain," Spine-health. Available online. URL: http://www.spine-health.com/research/pnt/pnt01.html. Downloaded March 15, 2006.

Washington State Department of Labor and Industries, Office of the Medical Director. "Technology Assessment, Percutaneous Neuromodulation Therapy, January 13, 2004." Available online. URL: http://www.lni.wa.gov/ClaimsIns/Files/OMD/PensTa01132004.pdf. Downloaded March 15, 2006.

White, P. F., W. F. Craig, A. S. Vakharia, E. Ghoname, H. E. Ahmed, and M. A. Hamza. "Percutaneous Neuromodulation Therapy: Does the Location of Electrical Stimulation Effect the Acute Analgesic Response?" *Anesthesia & Analgesia* 91, no. 4 (October 2000): 949–954.

peripheral neuropathy A disease or disorder of the spinal nerves is usually classified as a neuropathy, which involves many peripheral possibilities extending from the SPINE. To be more specific, an article in *JAOA, The Journal of the American Osteopathic Association* explained, "The nervous system can be divided into two parts: the central nervous system (CNS), which includes the brain, brainstem, and spinal cord, and the peripheral nervous system (PNS) that consists of the individual cranial, motor, and sensory nerves." Since these peripheral nerves exit either side of the VERTEBRAE, spinal disorders can affect that sensory and motor network, sometimes severely. To assess nerve involvement, the *JAOA* article recommended the advice of a neurologist.

Symptoms and Diagnostic Path

With over 100 types of peripheral neuropathies identified, symptoms vary, but commonly include muscle weakness and sensory disturbances. For example, one patient may lose the protection of pain, feeling nothing with the application of intense heat or a pin prick, while others experience pain with the touch of a bed sheet. Degenerative changes in bone or muscle tone may also occur, interfering with mobility and daily ACTIVITY.

Causalities vary widely, so a diagnosis may be difficult to obtain, but common causes include bone CANCER, ENVIRONMENTAL INFLUENCES, ERGONOMIC FACTORS, FAILED BACK SURGERY, GENETIC FACTORS, deficiencies in MINERAL BALANCE or NUTRITION, SPINAL INFECTION, SPINAL INJURY, and SPINAL TUMORS. Systemic conditions with chronic inflammation or connective tissue damage can produce neuropathies too. Therefore, blood tests may be needed to rule out an underlying medical condition. Other tests, such as a biopsy, ELECTROMYOGRAM, NERVE CONDUCTION STUDY, or nerve function tests, may be prescribed.

Treatment Options and Outlook

Finding and treating the underlying medical cause offers the most promising outlook. Then, a team devoted to PAIN MANAGEMENT can recommend relevant options. For example, if RHEUMATOID ARTHRITIS produces neuropathy, the patient may need to see a rheumatologist and also get referrals for ACUPUNCTURE, BIOFEEDBACK, EXERCISE, MASSAGE THERAPY, occupational therapy, or physical therapy. A patient with neuropathies from an injury or a

POSTURE problem may need referrals from a neurologist for ACUPRESSURE, ORTHOTICS, SPINAL MANIPULATION, or SURGERY. Most patients will also be helped by receiving nutritional counseling.

Risk Factors and Preventive Measures

Patients with inherited types of peripheral neuropathy may be particularly at risk for developing CHRONIC PAIN or numbness. According to the National Institute of Neurological Disorders and Stroke (NINDS), "because specific genetic defects have been identified for only a fraction of the known hereditary neuropathies, the Institute sponsors studies to identify other genetic defects that may cause these conditions. Presymptomatic diagnosis may lead to therapies for preventing nerve damage before it occurs, and gene replacement therapies could be developed to prevent or reduce cumulative nerve damage." Besides that encouraging RESEARCH into peripheral neuropathies, "neuropathic pain is a primary target of NINDS-sponsored studies aimed at developing more effective therapies for symptoms of peripheral neuropathy. Some scientists hope to identify substances that will block the brain chemicals that generate pain signals, while others are investigating the pathways by which pain signals reach the brain."

National Institute of Neurological Disorders and Stroke. "Peripheral Neuropathy Fact Sheet," National Institutes of Health. Available online. URL: http://www.ninds.nih.gov/disorders/peripheralneuropathy/detail_peripheralneuropathy.htm. Last updated January 25, 2006.

Scott, Kevin, M.D. and Milind J. Kothari. "Clinical Practice: Evaluating the Patient with Peripheral Nervous System Complaints," *JAOA, The Journal of the American Osteopathic Association* 105, no. 2 (February 2005): 71–83.

PET scan   See POSITIVE EMISSION TOMOGRAPHY SCAN.

phosphorus   With about 80 percent of this vital mineral stored in the bones and teeth, 10 percent in muscles, and 1 percent in nerves, dietary phosphorus may be in high demand. As the Centers for Disease Control and Prevention (CDC) explained,

"Minerals are involved in a wide range of critical functions in the human body. Calcium, phosphorus, and magnesium are essential in forming and maintaining bones." For example, CALCIUM assists BONE BUILDING and reduces the risk of OSTEOPOROSIS, especially among the ELDERLY. "In addition, calcium plays a role in blood clotting, while phosphorus and magnesium play essential roles in energy metabolism." CDC also said, "The electrolytes sodium and potassium along with calcium, phosphorus, and magnesium play important roles in neural transmission, muscular activity, vascular constriction and dilation, and maintaining normal acid-base balance, osmotic pressure, and normal water balance." Furthermore, "phosphorus, magnesium, copper, and zinc act as components of enzyme systems or cofactors in enzymatic reactions. In addition, phosphorus is a component of nucleotides, nucleic acids, and cell membranes."

Dosage and Potential Side Effects

Well-balanced NUTRITION brings MINERAL BALANCE and offers a sufficient supply of phosphorus, with almonds or other nuts providing some of the best sources. Whole grains, lentils, raisins, and fresh produce, such as asparagus, corn, and cauliflower, have a high content, but chocolate lovers will be glad to know that phosphorus also comes in cocoa. Since the mineral can be found in colas too, heavy-duty soft drink consumption can cause an imbalance.

Should more phosphorus be needed than the diet can provide, supplements can be taken. According to a MedlinePlus article for the National Institutes of Health (NIH), "The National Academy of Sciences has recommended 700mg of phosphorus per day in adults ages 18 years and older, including pregnant or breastfeeding women." For INFANTS, CHILDREN, and ADOLESCENTS, the NIH advised, "The recommended adequate intake in infants 0–6 months-old is 100 mg/ day (additional phosphorus may be added to infant formulas); the recommended adequate intake in infants 7–12 months old is 275mg/ day; the recommended daily intake in children ages 1–3 years-old is 460mg/ day; the recommended daily intake in children ages 4–8 years-old is 500mg/ day; the recommended daily intake in children ages 9–18 years-old is 1,250mg/ day (including pregnant or breastfeeding females)."

Regarding potential side effects, such as toxicity, the NIH warned, "Phosphate salts should . . . be used cautiously in those with impaired kidney function." In general, "excessive intake of phosphates can cause potentially serious or life-threatening toxicity. Intravenous, oral, or rectal/enema phosphates may cause electrolyte disturbances including hypocalcemia (low calcium blood levels), hypomagnesemia (low magnesium blood levels), hyperphosphatemia (high phosphorus blood levels), or hypokalemia (low potassium levels). Calcification of non-skeletal tissues (particularly in the kidneys), severe hypotension (low blood pressure), dehydration, . . . acute kidney failure, or tetany," a nervous disorder, "can occur. Death has been reported in infants or adults with oral, rectal, or intravenous phosphates, particularly in those at increased risk for electrolyte disturbances, and in those receiving more than 45 or 90 milliliters in a 24-hour period." Conversely, some forms of HERBAL THERAPY, STEROID THERAPY, VITAMIN D, or medications may inhibit phosphorus absorption.

Statistics and Studies

The National Institute of Child Health & Human Development posted an online review of medical literature regarding studies of phosphorus supplements for premature infants. According to the review, "supplementation of human milk with minerals (either individually or as one component of a . . . fortifier) has become common practice, based largely on metabolic studies evaluating the composition of human milk and the nutritional requirements of preterm infants." However, "there are insufficient data on supplementation of human milk with calcium and/or phosphorus to make recommendations for practice." This may be worthy of further RESEARCH since the report also said, "Preterm infants are born with low skeletal stores of calcium and phosphorus. Preterm human milk provides insufficient calcium and phosphorus to meet their estimated needs."

Ervin, R. Bethene, Chia-Yih Wang, Jacqueline D. Wright, and Jocelyn Kennedy-Stephenson. "Dietary Intake of Selected Minerals for the United States Population: 1999–2000," U. S. Department of Health and Human Services, Centers for Disease Control and Prevention, Advance Data From Vital and Health Statistics, no. 341 (April 27, 2004). Available online. URL: http://www.fda.gov/ohrms/dockets/dockets/04q0098/04q-0098-let0013-15-Ref-02-Ervin-vol16.pdf. Downloaded March 16, 2006.

Kuschel, C. A. and J. E. Harding. "Calcium and Phosphorus Supplementation of Human Milk for Preterm Infants," National Institute of Child Health & Human Development, National Institutes of Health. Available online. URL: http://www.nichd.nih.gov/cochrane/kuschel7/kuschel.htm. Downloaded March 16, 2006.

MedlinePlus. "Phosphates, Phosphorus," U.S. National Library of Medicine, National Institutes of Health. Available online. URL: http://www.nlm.nih.gov/medlineplus/druginfo/natural/patient-phosphorus.html. Last updated December 13, 2005.

phytochemicals   To squeeze in a quick quiz: Why does a glass of orange juice often offer a better option than a VITAMIN C tablet? Answer: Not only does juice taste better, the real thing has about 170 phytochemicals, including anti-inflammatory properties that may ease ARTHRITIS and other conditions that affect the BACK and SPINE.

"Phyto" means plant, and natural phytochemicals include vitamins, minerals, nutrients, and other protective components such as PHYTOESTROGENS that may assist BONE BUILDING. In addition, phytochemicals pack in antioxidants that RESEARCH has shown to boost the immune system and inhibit CANCER cells.

To aid their appeal, phytochemicals also squeeze in color power. As the article "Phytochemicals: Guardians of Our Health" explained, "Pigments provide a lot of color to our food and enhance the enjoyment of the eating experience. Presently, there are almost 2,000 known plant pigments in our food, including over 800 flavonoids, 450 carotenoids and 150 anthocyanins. These pigments do more than just appeal to our senses; they also protect us from disease." Even on the darkest eggplant or plum, a golden hue indicates the most timely moment to pluck or pick fresh fruit and vegetables.

Dosage and Potential Side Effects

Doctor-prescribed supplements of some phytochemicals may be advisable for INFANTS, ELDERLY patients, pregnant women, and patients with an illness or a medication that interferes with their nutrient uptake. Supplements free of artificial additives then provide the best option when taken according to the recommendations on the label.

Regarding the use of supplements in the general population, information from the American Dietetic Association stated, "The weight of scientific evidence indicates that the optimal approach for achieving a health benefit from the intake of nutrients and other physiologically active constituents is through the consumption of a varied diet that is rich in plant foods. In reality, each vegetable contains numerous different nutrients and phytochemicals—a biologic circumstance that is not currently replicated in pill form. In addition, the assumption that a combination of plant constituents that are naturally occurring is maintained at equivalent levels of biologic activity when extracted, dried, and compacted into pill form is likely unfounded." Nevertheless, "pharmaceutical companies have isolated many food components into supplement form, including allylic sulfides (garlic), isoflavones (soy) . . . , and glycyrrhizin (licorice), to name only a few. In the United States, tens of billions of dollars are spent annually on dietary supplements." However, "supplements can provide nutrients and other physiologically active components in a potentially unbalanced and concentrated form that may be far different from the form used in research studies. Nutrients and other bioactive food components that occur naturally in foods act synergistically with other dietary elements such as fiber to promote health."

Statistics and Studies

The article "Vitamins, Carotenoids, and Phytochemicals" explained, "The results of studies on specific phytochemicals are not necessarily applicable to the vegetables or fruits that harbor small concentrations of these chemicals. Nevertheless, it is obvious that vegetables and fruits are healthful, which is probably due to some balance of phytochemicals, carotenoids, vitamins, fibers, and minerals rather than any single substance. It should be stressed that very little has been proven concerning the benefits of phytochemical supplements sold in health food stores. Furthermore, high concentrations of some of these chemicals may behave like drugs and can be toxic and possibly even contribute to cancer cell growth." The article added, "Most importantly, studies continue to report that the most important health benefits are derived from foods containing important nutrients, not individual supplements." Therefore, ideal NUTRITION will be most likely to flourish with colorful phytochemicals heaped from the garden while appealingly fresh and ready to peel.

American Dietetic Association. "Functional Foods." Available online. URL: http://www.eatright.org/cps/rde/xchg/ada/hs.xsl/advocacy_adap1099_ENU_HTML.htm. Downloaded March 18, 2006.

Craig, Winston J. "Phytochemicals: Guardians of Our Health," Vegetarian Nutrition. Available online. URL: http://www.andrews.edu/NUFS/phyto.html. Downloaded March 18, 2006.

Nidus Information Services, Inc. "Vitamins, Carotenoids, and Phytochemicals." Available online. URL: http://www.reutershealth.com/wellconnected/doc39.html. Downloaded March 18, 2006.

phytoestrogens Literally meaning plant estrogens, phytoestrogens occur naturally in plants. As a form of HERBAL THERAPY and a healthful source of NUTRITION, these plant compounds can assist BONE BUILDING by helping the body to produce its own estrogen. This natural source of estrogen does not have the strength of a prescription and cannot be stored in the body, but phytoestrogens can be readily obtained in a diet flourishing with plant life.

Since phytoestrogens are not a single herb but compounds in any plant with estrogen-producing capabilities, they provide a safe alternative for people who need HORMONE REPLACEMENT THERAPY (HRT) but want to avoid medication. Some herbalists laud black cohosh for HRT purposes, but the herb needs more RESEARCH to substantiate ancient assertions and avoid false claims. Plant estrogens differ, too, in that they offer not an herb capsule, but a dietary choice with the potential of slowing bone loss in post-menopausal women inclined toward OSTEOPENIA or OSTEOPOROSIS. Such a plant-rich diet might also provide a natural nutritional aid for ELDERLY patients with OSTEITIS DEFORMANS or CHILDREN and ADOLESCENTS with bone conditions such as OSTEOGENESIS IMPERFECTA.

Dosage and Potential Side Effects

An online article from the National Institutes of Arthritis and Musculoskeletal and Skin Diseases (NIAMS) explained, "Phytoestrogens consist of more than 20 compounds and can be found in more than 300 plants, such as herbs, grains, and fruits. . . . The three main classes of dietary phytoestrogens are isoflavones, lignans, and coumestans: Isoflavones . . . are primarily found in soy beans and soy products, chickpeas, and other legumes. Lignans . . . are found in oilseeds (primarily flaxseed), cereal bran, legumes, and alcohol (beer and bourbon). Coumestans . . . can be found in alfalfa and clover." As the NIAMS also said, "Most food sources containing these compounds typically include more than one class of phytoestrogens."

With the exception of food allergies, people rarely encounter adverse side effects from consuming whole foods unless, of course, they eat too much. However, supplements in capsules or other forms increase the risk of toxicity. Also, the optimal dosage of phytoestrogen has not been fully ascertained, so patients would do well to proceed with caution, perhaps asking a nutritionist or knowledgeable pharmacist about the safe usage of supplements.

Statistics and Studies

According to the NIAMS, "much of the evidence concerning the potential role of phytoestrogens in bone health is based on animal studies. In fact, soybean protein, soy isoflavones . . . , and coumestrol have all been shown to have a protective effect on bone in animals. . . . In humans, however, the evidence is conflicting. Studies show that compared to Caucasian populations, those in Hong Kong, China, and Japan—where dietary phytoestrogen intakes are high—experience lower rates of hip fracture. Yet, according to the Surgeon General's Report on Bone Health and Osteoporosis, spine fractures are almost as common in Asian women as they are in white women. In addition, reports suggest that Japanese women have a greater risk of sustaining a vertebral fracture than Caucasian women." One might wonder about the difference CALCIUM intake makes, especially since Asian women traditionally avoid dairy products in their regular diets. As NIAMS also said, "Several studies have explored the effects of soy isoflavones on bone health, but results have been mixed, ranging from a modest impact to no effect. Most of these studies have serious limitations, including their short duration and small sample size, making it difficult to fully evaluate the impact of these compounds on bone health."

Studies from the United Kingdom report similarly conflicting results. According to a report from The Institute of Food Science & Technology (IFST), "naturally occurring phytoestrogen sources in the diet, such as soya, may have emerging potential benefits to health. Epidemiological studies suggest that phytoestrogen-containing foods may have a beneficial role in protecting against cancer, osteoporosis, post-menopausal symptoms and cardiovascular disease. There is almost no evidence though to link the effect of phytoestrogen containing foods to phytoestrogens alone. Many other components of soya and linseed are biologically active in various experimental systems and may be responsible for the observed effects in humans."

Besides the high quantities of phytoestrogen found in soy products, IFST listed oat bran, wheat, asparagus, and carrots as containing small amounts. When one considers the VITAMIN A in carrots and healthful fiber in oat bran, one might wonder how long the refrigerator will remain open to inspection before gaining credence as a well-tested way to enjoy a healthier BACK and SPINE.

Institute of Food Science & Technology, The. "Phytoestrogens," IFST: Current Hot Topics. Available online. URL: http://www.ifst.org/hottop34.htm. Downloaded March 17, 2006.

National Institutes of Arthritis and Musculoskeletal and Skin Diseases (NIAMS.) "Phytoestrogens and Bone Health," Health Topics, National Institutes of Health Osteoporosis and Related Bone Diseases, National Resource Center. Available online. URL: http://www.niams.nih.gov/bone/hi/bone_phyto.htm. Downloaded March 17, 2006.

piriformis syndrome Sometimes considered a form of SCIATICA, this condition results from sciatic nerve entrapment in the piriformis muscle in the back of the pelvis as the sciatic nerve passes underneath or sometimes through the muscle. If that muscle gets tight, goes into a muscle spasm, or presses on the spinal nerve, ACUTE PAIN may radiate into the legs and LUMBAR SPINE.

Symptoms and Diagnostic Path

Besides producing symptoms commonly occurring with sciatica, piriformis syndrome may mimic a HERNIATED DISC as patients experience a sharp BACKACHE or LOW BACK PAIN. Daily ACTIVITY may increase discomfort, but sedentary conditions can provoke pain even more. A physical examination of the patient and his or her RANGE OF MOTION may produce a diagnosis. If not, X-RAYS or other imaging tests may help to rule out conditions with similar symptoms.

Treatment Options and Outlook

Treatments usually begin with PAIN MANAGEMENT to ease pain and COLD THERAPY to reduce swelling in the piriformis muscle. Less often, HEAT THERAPY can be applied to ease stiffness. SPINAL MANIPULATION and MASSAGE THERAPY may help some patients, while others need PAIN RELIEVERS, STEROID THERAPY, or various types of SPINAL INJECTIONS. To reduce muscle spasms or muscle cramping, a TRANSCUTANEOUS ELECTRONIC NERVE STIMULATOR (TENS) unit may be used. Most patients will also be helped with therapeutic EXERCISES that involve gentle stretching.

Risk Factors and Preventive Measures

According to the National Institute of Neurological Disorders and Stroke, "the prognosis for most individuals with piriformis syndrome is good. Once symptoms of the disorder are addressed, individuals can usually resume their normal activities. In some cases, exercise regimens may need to be modified in order to reduce the likelihood of recurrence or worsening."

National Institute of Neurological Disorders and Stroke. "NINDS Piriformis Syndrome Information Page," National Institutes of Health. Available online. URL: http://www.ninds.nih.gov/disorders/piriformis_syndrome/piriformis_syndrome.htm. Last updated January 25, 2006.

Revord, John, M.D. "Piriformis Syndrome—Another Irritation to the Sciatic Nerve," Spine-health. Available online. URL: http://www.spine-health.com/topics/cd/piriformis/pir02.html. Downloaded March 8, 2006.

piroxicam   See NONSTEROIDAL ANTI-INFLAMMATORY DRUG THERAPY.

pituitary dwarf   See DWARFISM; GROWTH HORMONE DISORDERS.

polyarticular juvenile rheumatoid arthritis (polyarthritis)   See JUVENILE RHEUMATOID ARTHRITIS.

positron emission tomography (PET) scan   As a radioactive substance in the patient's body emits tiny little particles known as positrons, a monitor shows soft tissue in that person in living color. Brighter may not be better, though, as deepened hues may indicate CANCER or some type of metabolic disease that affects the VERTEBRAE.

To explain how PET works, the Radiological Society of North America (RSNA) Web site said, "Before the examination begins, a radioactive substance is produced in a machine called a cyclotron and attached, or tagged, to a natural body compound, most commonly glucose, but sometimes water or ammonia. Once this substance is administered to the patient, the radioactivity localizes in the appropriate areas of the body and is detected by the PET scanner. . . . Different colors or degrees of brightness on a PET image represent different levels of tissue or organ function. For example, because healthy tissue uses glucose for energy, it accumulates some of the tagged glucose, which will show up on the PET images. However, cancerous tissue, which uses more glucose than normal tissue, will accumulate more of the substance and appear brighter than normal tissue on the PET images. . . . Because PET allows study of body function, it can help physicians detect alterations in biochemical processes that suggest disease before changes in anatomy are apparent with other imaging tests, such as CT or MRI."

Procedure

After receiving a radioactive substance intravenously, the patient quietly waits for an hour or so as the material circulates throughout the body. Then a technician moves the examination table, complete with patient, into a large hole where the equipment records emissions of energy, simultaneously producing images of those emissions onto a screen.

Risks and Complications

As often happens with MAGNETIC RESONANCE IMAGING (MRI), some patients feel claustrophobic during the test. Low radiation exposure presents a very minimal risk, but pregnant women and nursing mothers need to avoid a PET scan if possible. Also, patients with blood sugar problems may find their glucose levels interfere with the test results.

Outlook and Lifestyle Modifications

In an article for SpineUniverse, medical writer Susan Spinasanta said, "The amount of radioactive material injected is . . . quickly broken down by the body and passed within 48 hours. Temporarily increasing fluid intake for a day or two following the test can help facilitate elimination of the tracing substance."

RadiologyInfo.™ "Positron Emission Tomography (PET Imaging)," Radiological Society of North America, Inc. (RSNA.) Available online. URL: http://www.radiologyinfo.org/content/petomography.htm. Last reviewed April 21, 2005.

Spinasanta, Susan. "Nuclear Imaging: PET and SPECT Scans," SpineUniverse. Available online. URL: http://www.spineuniverse.com/displayarticle.php/article231.html. Last updated December 8, 2004.

post-polio syndrome   Commonly known as polio or infantile paralysis, poliomyelitis results from a virally induced neuromuscular disease that once left patients with muscle atrophy or paralysis. An injection developed by Jonas E. Salk in 1955 and an oral polio vaccine produced by Albert B. Sabin in 1962 helped to eradicate polio in the United States. Now, decades later, 100,000 to 200,000 patients who previously had polio have begun to experience a worsening of their condition known as post-polio syndrome (PPS).

Symptoms and Diagnostic Path

Muscle weakness, joint pain, and extreme fatigue characterize post-polio syndrome. Although a rare occurrence, some patients encounter difficulties in swallowing or breathing. Post-polio syndrome may also produce POSTURE disorders, such as SCOLIOSIS. More often, problems arise with SLEEP, muscle spasm, and general performance of normal daily ACTIVITY.

Since symptoms surface many years after the original illness, a medical history will be especially significant. A rheumatologist may then request laboratory tests, while a neurologist may suggest a COMPUTED TOMOGRAPHY (CT) SCAN or MAGNETIC RESONANCE IMAGING to rule out other conditions. However, a previous bout with polio does not necessarily mean a person has post-polio syndrome. Similar symptoms may instead be caused by ARTHRITIS, FIBROMYALGIA, or a degenerative condition of the SPINE.

According to the National Institute of Neurological Disorders and Stroke, "People who had only minimal symptoms from the original attack and subsequently develop PPS will most likely experience only mild PPS symptoms. People originally hit hard by the polio virus, who were left with severe residual weakness, may develop a more severe case of PPS with a greater loss of muscle function, difficulty in swallowing, and more periods of fatigue."

Treatment Options and Outlook

A fact sheet from Post-Polio Health International said, "For diagnosed post-polio syndrome, the current treatment, which must be unique to each individual, is the management of the symptoms. The specific cause(s) of the symptoms need(s) to be identified and treated and/or eliminated. Many times the cause is overuse; however, disuse also can result in new weakness."

Risk Factors and Preventive Measures

Exceeding personal limits, such as engaging in prolonged EXERCISE, can place a patient at greater risk for muscle fatigue or damage. Besides developing self-awareness, preventives include changes in adverse ENVIRONMENTAL INFLUENCES and ERGONOMIC FACTORS. Well-balanced NUTRITION can be supportive too.

National Institute of Neurological Disorders and Stroke. "NINDS Post-Polio Syndrome Information Page,"

National Institutes of Health. Available online. URL: http://www.ninds.nih.gov/disorders/post_polio/post_polio.htm. Last updated March 1, 2006.

Post-Polio Health International. "Polio & Post-Polio Fact Sheet," PH. Available online. URL: http://www.post-polio.org/ipn/fact.html. Last updated November 2, 2005.

posture   Correctly aligned, the inward and outward curves of the CERVICAL SPINE, THORACIC SPINE, and LUMBAR SPINE work together to maintain upright posture and mobility. However, a chronic disorder, such as DEGENERATIVE DISC DISEASE, or an accident, such as a FLEXION-EXTENSION INJURY, can cause the natural curves of the SPINE to straighten out or reverse, thereby producing postural irregularities. For example, KYPHOSIS gives a humpback appearance and LORDOSIS a swayback look. Both types of postural problems characteristically present extreme bowing of a natural curvature, whereas unequal growth on either side of the VERTEBRAE produces the lateral or side-to-side curvature indicative of SCOLIOSIS. Other sources of spinal deformities or a misshapen BACK include ANKYLOSING SPONDYLITIS, BIRTH DEFECTS OF THE SPINE, DWARFISM, aging DISCS in the ELDERLY, poor ERGONOMIC FACTORS, GENETIC FACTORS, OSTEOPOROSIS, POST-POLIO SYNDROME, and VERTEBRAL COMPRESSION FRACTURES, each of which requires differing tests and treatments.

Risks and Complications

Since adequate NUTRITION and MINERAL BALANCE assist BONE BUILDING throughout life, young people with EATING DISORDERS may be particularly at risk for developing permanent posture problems. Slouching may produce temporary problems in growing CHILDREN and ADOLESCENTS, while posture in adults may be temporarily affected by the adverse effects of WEIGHT on the spine, poorly balanced SHOES, or improper back care during PREGNANCY. Unless those conditions resolve themselves, each can permanently affect the ease with which a person remains upright and in spinal balance. If vertebrae stay out of line, BACKACHES, CERVICOGENIC HEADACHES, LOW BACK PAIN, and mobility issues will be more likely to arise.

Statistics and Studies

An online article from *Men's Health* offered these statistics: "The average human head weighs 8 pounds. And if your chin moves forward just 3 inches—as it tends to when you work at a computer—the muscles of your neck, shoulders, and upper back must support the equivalent of 11 pounds. That's a weight-bearing increase of 38 percent—often for hours at a time. Left untreated, the effect of chronic desk slump results in a postural dysfunction that physical therapists call upper-cross syndrome; you know it as rounded shoulders." Also, "if your shoulders are slumped forward for long periods of time, your chest muscles become shortened. That is, since these muscles attach to your upper arms, the distance they need to extend when you slouch is less than when your shoulders are drawn back. Over time, the chest muscles adapt to this position as their natural length, pulling your shoulders forward. As a result, many of the shoulder's stabilizers are overstretched, which makes them weaker."

Special Aids and Adaptations

Minor postural problems may be helped simply by shifting around and changing positions. Some patients, however, need help to do this. For example, INFANTS, infirm patients, and people with OSTEOGENESIS IMPERFECTA (OI) require special care in positioning. As explained by the National Institute of Arthritis and Musculoskeletal and Skin Diseases, "A key method for helping a person with OI maximize strength and function is to encourage him or her to adopt various positions throughout the day or, in the case of an infant or young child, to encourage parents and other caregivers to place the child in different positions. Position changes not only strengthen different muscle groups but also help prevent contractures and malformations that can limit mobility and increase pain. It is important to keep the hips and spine as straight as possible, prevent flattening of the back of the head from lying supine, and promote head-turning in both directions."

After SURGERY that involves a BONE GRAFT, patients can aid their recovery by building up their PARASPINAL MUSCLES and performing EXERCISES that stretch the muscles. Similarly, patients with spinal-fusing conditions such as SPONDYLITIS can establish good postural habits to aid RANGE OF MOTION and flexibility. As an online article from the Spondylitis Association of America (SAA) explained, "People with spondylitis often are painfully aware of the strains imposed by gravity. A vicious pain-poor posture cycle begins because of a tendency to bend over when experiencing pain in the spine, further increasing the amount of strain on the spine." Various forms of PAIN MANAGEMENT, such as NONSTEROIDAL ANTI-INFLAMMATORY DRUG (NSAID) THERAPY, may enable a person to move about more and maintain flexibility. As the association said, most patients can be helped if they "Think Tall." The SAA also advised, "Hold your head in a balanced manner over the trunk in a sitting or standing position. The chin should be horizontal and parallel to the floor, drawn back slightly and centered. Try to stand, walk and sit 'tall' at all times." To do this, some patients may need the aid of a cane or walker, while others may require special ORTHOTIC devices to assist them in remaining upright and on the move.

Gonzalez, Lorenzo. "Are Your Shoulders In a Slump?" *Men's Health.* Available online. URL:http://www.menshealth.com/cda/article.do?site=MensHealth&channel=fitness&category=muscle.building&topic=arms&conitem=98b871957cb98010VgnVCM200000cee793cd____&cm_mmc=AbsDietNL-_-2006_02_06-_-Fitness-_-Are_Your_Shoulders_in_a_Slump? Downloaded March 21, 2006.

National Institute of Arthritis and Musculoskeletal and Skin Diseases. "Therapeutic Strategies for Osteogenesis Imperfecta: A Guide for Physical Therapists and Occupational Therapists," NIAMS, National Institutes of Health. Available online. URL: http://www.niams.nih.gov/bone/hi/osteogenesis/oi_pt_ot_guide.htm. Downloaded March 21, 2006.

Spondylitis Association of America. "Posture." Available online. URL: http://www.spondylitis.org/patient_resources/posture.aspx. Downloaded March 21, 2006.

potassium   Most fresh foods contain this mineral element that helps to maintain overall health and prevent OSTEOPOROSIS and other problems of the BACK and SPINE. Along with CALCIUM and MAGNESIUM, potassium aids the MINERAL BALANCE needed for spinal nerve impulses and normal functioning of PARASPINAL MUSCLES. In conjunction with sodium and chloride, potassium regulates the acid-alkaline balance in the body. Adequate supplies of these minerals and ample WATER strengthen bones and electrify the body with the energy needed for daily ACTIVITY.

The George Mateljan Foundation explained, "Potassium, sodium and chloride comprise the electrolyte family of minerals. Called electrolytes because they conduct electricity when dissolved in water, these minerals work together closely. About 95% of the potassium in the body is stored within cells, while sodium and chloride are predominantly located outside the cell."

Dosage and Potential Side Effects

Natural dietary sources of potassium abound with good NUTRITION, but strenuous EXERCISE and some diuretics can quickly deplete the levels a body needs. A diet centered on fast foods also causes loss of potassium and other nutrients too, which may account for the seemingly epidemic symptoms in this country of muscle weakness, mental confusion, mood swings, and fatigue. Overexertion, nausea, and diarrhea can also result from lowered levels of potassium. However, too much potassium can cause muscle spasms. If those spasms affect cardiac muscle, a heart attack may occur.

Although potassium supplements may be needed temporarily, multivitamin supplements that include minerals but remain free of preservatives and dyes would provide a safer and better-balanced option for regular usage. Better yet would be a diet rich in fresh fruits and vegetables. For those who cannot deal with, say, spinach, similar amounts of potassium occur in lima beans, soybeans, pinto beans, and winter squash. Bananas and cantaloupe have only about half the potassium found in chard or spinach, but cooking greens will drain about half of the mineral, making uncooked fruit a more delectable choice.

Statistics and Studies

According to the American Dietetic Association, "The Institute of Medicine of the National Academies of Science recently issued recommendations for sodium and potassium intake levels, saying healthy adults between 19 and 50 should consume about 1,500 milligrams of sodium per day and 4,700 milligrams of potassium." Not surprisingly, Americans typically consume too much sodium in table salt, canned vegetables, heavily processed foods, and other salty products with too little potassium on the side. To avoid this imbalance, most studies suggest a diet of fresh produce and whole grains as close to their natural state as individual taste buds and tummies can tolerate.

American Dietetic Association. "Are You Getting Enough Potassium? Maybe Not." Available online. URL: http://www.eatright.org/cps/rde/xchg/ada/hs.xsl/home_4149_ENU_HTML.htm. Downloaded March 16, 2006.
———. "Sodium and Potassium: How Much Is Too Much?" Available online. URL: http://www.eatright.org/cps/rde/xchg/ada/hs.xsl/home_4466_ENU_HTML.htm. Downloaded March 16, 2006.
WorldsHealthiestFoods.com. "Potassium," WHF, The George Mateljan Foundation. Available online. URL: http://www.whfoods.com/genpage.php?tname=nutrient&dbid=90. Downloaded March 16, 2006.

Pott's disease   See SPINAL TUBERCULOSIS.

prednisone   See STEROID THERAPY.

pregnancy, back care during   Obvious changes occur during pregnancy with added WEIGHT on the LUMBAR SPINE often causing BACKACHES, LOW BACK PAIN, muscle STRAIN, and, occasionally, POSTURE problems such as LORDOSIS or swayback. Less obviously, hormonal changes and production of new hormones by the placenta enable the musculoskeletal system to accommodate an unborn child. Those hormones not only affect moods but allow the ligaments that hold the pelvic bones together to expand enough for an INFANT to be born. However, the same hormones can also cause the VERTEBRAE to shift and the SPINE to become less stable. As ligaments loosen to allow for expansion, instability may be keenly felt in the SACRAL VERTEBRAE with something akin to SACRO-ILIAC JOINT PAIN SYNDROME.

Risks and Complications
Women with SCOLIOSIS, OSTEOPENIA, OSTEOPOROSIS, DEGENERATIVE DISC DISEASE, or other pre-existing conditions that affect the spine may be at particularly high risk for BACK problems during pregnancy. To assess a serious back condition or a SPINAL INJURY, an X-RAY or other imaging device that uses radiation may be needed. This radiation exposure remains at such a low level that the mother herself will probably not be affected. However, the Centers for Disease Prevention and Control (CDC) studied the risks that tests involving radiation present to a fetus. As the CDC reported, "Because the human embryo or fetus is protected in the uterus, a radiation dose to a fetus tends to be lower than the dose to its mother for most radiation exposure events. However, the human embryo and fetus are particularly sensitive . . . and the health consequences of exposure can be severe, even at radiation doses too low to immediately affect the mother. Such consequences can include growth retardation, malformations, impaired brain function, and cancer." Nevertheless, "beyond about 26 weeks, the fetus is less sensitive to the noncancer health effects of radiation exposure than in any other stage of gestation."

If pregnancy continues beyond normal term, womb crowding can cause BIRTH DEFECTS OF THE SPINE in an otherwise healthy newborn. One risk, for example, includes growth restrictions that increase the likelihood of a BRACHIAL PLEXUS INJURY in the newborn. As the Agency for Healthcare Research and Quality (AHRQ) reported, "Prolonged pregnancy has traditionally been defined as a pregnancy that extends 2 weeks or more beyond the estimated day of confinement, or 42 weeks. Approximately 18 percent of pregnancies in the United States extend beyond 41 weeks, and 7 percent extend beyond 42 weeks."

For the mother, a prolonged pregnancy will be likely to intensify spinal PAIN, but new mothers may be at risk for acquiring new problems too. According to statistics posted by Birthsong Childbirth Education & Support Services, "10% of new moms develop a backache for the first time that lasts at least 6 weeks. Among women who'd had epidurals, the number jumps to 18%. This may be due to poor positioning during birth: women with epidurals may not be able to sense discomfort when they are in a position which is straining muscles, so support people need to pay attention to keeping mom in a comfortable, healthy position."

In addition to those concerns during the birth process, sensitivity to medication can complicate the birth or cause spinal problems for the mother. For example, an EPIDURAL INJECTION to ease labor pain can give birth to an allergic response with the potential for serious complications, such as ARACHNOIDITIS.

Statistics and Studies

An article on the Spine-Health Web site reported, "It is estimated that between 50% and 80% of women experience some form of back pain during their pregnancy, ranging from mild pain associated with specific activities to acute back pain that can become chronic." More specifically, "studies show that low back pain usually occurs between the fifth and seventh month of pregnancy, but can begin as early as eight to twelve weeks into your pregnancy."

Special Aids and Adaptations

While EXERCISE can strengthen PARASPINAL MUSCLES, an ORTHOTIC device may be needed to provide lumbar support throughout the pregnancy. Also, sensible SHOE CHOICES, such as a walking shoe with low heels and padded insole, can provide extra cushioning for the vertebrae, relieve pressure on spinal DISCS, and generally aid vertebral alignment. If exercise proves too painful on the ground, adaptations can be made with HYDROTHERAPY or walking in waist-high water across a swimming pool. As another option to increase daily ACTIVITY and decrease back pain, some women can perform strengthening exercises, such as pelvic tilts and leg raises, while lying in bed.

To aid SLEEP, resting on one side with a pillow between the knees may help to alleviate low back pain. NUTRITION can also be adapted with an emphasis on natural food sources that provide MINERAL BALANCE and ample CALCIUM. A physician may prescribe a natural vitamin and mineral supplement for some pregnant or lactating women, but

in general, a variety of fresh foods and dairy products provides the nutrients needed to sustain both mother and child.

Agency for Healthcare Research and Quality. "Management of Prolonged Pregnancy," *Evidence Report/Technology Assessment:* Number 53. Available online. URL: http://www.ahrq.gov/clinic/epcsums/prolongsum.htm. Downloaded March 22, 2006.

Centers for Disease Control and Prevention. "Prenatal Radiation Exposure: A Fact Sheet for Physicians," CDC, Department of Health and Human Services. Available online. URL: http://www.bt.cdc.gov/radiation/prenatalphysician.asp. Last updated March 23, 2005.

Mehl-Madrona, Lewis, M.D. and Morgan Mehl-Madrona. "Medical Risks of Epidural Anesthesia During Childbirth," Birthsong Childbirth Education & Support Services. Available online. URL: http://onyx-ii.com/birthsong/page.cfm?epidural. Downloaded March 22, 2006.

Montgomery, Stephen P., M.D. and Linda Sawyer. "Back Pain in Pregnancy," Spine-Health.com. Available online. URL: http://www.spine-health.com/topics/cd/pregnancy/preg02.html. Downloaded March 22, 2006.

pressure point   See ACUPRESSURE.

primary hyperparathyroidism   A fact sheet from the National Institutes of Health (NIH) Osteoporosis and Related Bone Diseases explained this hormonal disorder: "Primary hyperparathyroidism is a hormonal problem due to one or more parathyroid glands producing too much parathyroid hormone. Parathyroid glands, four small glands located in the neck near the thyroid gland, keep blood calcium from falling below normal. Rarely, there are more than four of these glands, and they may be in other parts of the neck or in the chest. In 80 to 85 percent of patients with primary hyperparathyroidism, a single gland is affected. In 15 to 20 percent of patients, two or more glands are affected. The affected gland(s) enlarge and produce too much parathyroid hormone. As a result, blood calcium becomes high, bones may lose calcium, and kidneys may excrete too much calcium." According to the NIH, "in the United States, 28 out of 100,000 people develop primary hyperparathyroidism each year. Women outnumber men 3 to 1, and frequency increases with age. In most cases, the cause is unknown," but CANCER, GENETIC FACTORS, and previous exposure to radiation may produce this hormonal imbalance.

Symptoms and Diagnostic Path

Often, bone loss occurs before symptoms present themselves. If too much CALCIUM leaves the bones and flows into the bloodstream, the patient may experience joint pain, muscle weakness, and fatigue. To aid a diagnosis, various laboratory tests can evaluate the MINERAL BALANCE in the body, whereas a BONE MINERAL DENSITY TEST can assess bone loss.

Treatment Options and Outlook

In some instances, SURGERY will be required to remove the affected gland. While BISPHOSPHONATES and HORMONE REPLACEMENT THERAPY cannot correct the causal factor, the drugs may be prescribed to treat or delay the development of secondary OSTEOPOROSIS.

Risk Factors and Preventive Measures

To prevent additional problems from occurring, the NIH recommended, "Patients should drink enough fluid to avoid dehydration, which leads to an increase in blood calcium. To avoid worsening calcium levels, patients should get regular exercise and avoid immobilization. A diet including approximately 1,200 mg of calcium is recommended. Avoiding calcium-containing foods could further stimulate the parathyroid glands." In general, proper NUTRITION, daily ACTIVITY, and EXERCISE offer ongoing BONE BUILDING possibilities.

National Institutes of Health Osteoporosis and Related Bone Diseases. "Information for Patients about Primary Hyperparathyroidism," NIH Fact Sheet. Available online. URL: http://www.osteo.org/newfile.asp?doc=p112i&doctitle=Primary+Hyperparathyroidism&doctype=HTML+Fact+Sheet. Downloaded March 7, 2006.

prolapsed disc   See HERNIATED DISC.

pulled muscle   See STRAIN.

quantitative computed tomography (QCT) This noninvasive BONE MINERAL DENSITY (BMD) TEST offers an alternative to dual X-ray ABSORPTIOMETRY (DEXA or DXA) in assessing bone mass. Although less available and more expensive, quantitative computed tomography (QCT) provides an accurate picture of bone patterns and bone loss. For example, an article in *Osteoporosis International* reported on a study of 64 patients with a SPINAL CORD injury (SCI). Using QCT to measure bone density in the SPINE, "Our results indicate that QCT reveals osteoporosis of the spine after SCI, in contrast to DXA." Therefore, "we postulate that QCT is more valuable for evaluating spinal osteoporosis following SCI than DXA and thus recommend QCT for spinal BMD studies in SCI."

Procedure

Patients can usually keep on street clothing, minus metal and jewelry, for a QCT, which takes about 15 minutes. As the person reclines on a padded table, an imaging device passes over the body and records data, usually from the hips and spine.

Risks and Complications

A QCT requires less radiation than X-RAYS, thus presenting minimal risk of exposure. Also, a QCT requires no injections or contrast dyes that can produce complications in sensitive patients.

Outlook and Lifestyle Modifications

The Journal of Bone and Joint Surgery published a promising outlook from Dr. Brian D. Snyder and associates on predicting FRACTURES with QCT. According to an online summary of the article, "The authors found that standard radiographic criteria . . . were weak predictors of fracture risk, both with regard to sensitivity (28% to 83%) and specificity (6% to 78%). In sharp contrast, all . . . parameters that were obtained with use of quantitative computed tomography were 100% sensitive and were 44% to 89% specific." In addition, the original study mentioned the promising development of equipment intended to eliminate the need for radiation exposure in testing bone density.

Liu, C. C., D. J. Theodorou, S. J. Theodorou, M. P. Andre, D. J. Sartoris, S. M. Szollar, E. M. Martin, and L. J. Deftos. "Quantitative Computed Tomography in the Evaluation of Spinal Osteoporosis Following Spinal Cord Injury," *Osteoporosis International* 11, no. 10 (October 2000): 889–896.

Rimnac, Clare M. "Commentary & Perspective on 'Predicting Fracture Through Benign Skeletal Lesions with Quantitative Computed Tomography' by Brian D. Snyder, MD, PhD, et al.," *The Journal of Bone and Joint Surgery, JBJS,* 88, no. 1 (January 2006): 55–70. Available online. URL: http://www.jbjs.org/Comments/2006/cp_jan06_rimnac.shtml. Downloaded March 21, 2006.

rachischisis   See SPINA BIFIDA.

rachitis   See RICKETS.

radiculitis, radiculopathy   With the words for these inflammatory conditions sometimes used interchangeably, problems begin when fluid leaks from a small tear in an intervertebral DISC or when mechanical pressure in the SPINE irritates the nerve roots in that area. From such tiny points of origin, spinal pain radiates into the arms, head, or legs.

To differentiate between radiculitis and radiculopathy, online information from Nosuffering.com said, "Radiculopathy is radiculitis caused by the nerve root being compressed by a compressed vertebral disk or arthritis. Radiculitis is characterized by pain that seems to radiate from the spine to extend outward to cause symptoms away from the source of the spinal nerve root irritation. The term radiculitis is used when symptoms demonstrate nerve root irritation but x-rays and other radiology show no abnormalities." By contrast, a HERNIATED DISC may bring a definitive bulge that can be seen via X-RAY or other imaging tool.

Symptoms and Diagnostic Path

Sensitivity to touch sometimes characterizes radiculitis, but patients usually experience either numbness or the radiating pain of SCIATICA. A medical history and a physical examination that includes the patient's RANGE OF MOTION may rule out other conditions and help to provide a diagnosis. If soft tissue and spinal nerves need to be evaluated, a neurologist or other physician may request a COMPUTED TOMOGRAPHY SCAN or MAGNETIC RESONANCE IMAGING. More likely, those imaging tests will primarily be used to determine a need for SURGERY.

Treatment Options and Outlook

Treatment usually begins with NONSTEROIDAL ANTI-INFLAMMATORY DRUG (NSAID) THERAPY, physical therapy, and rest. Other nonsurgical options include COMPLEMENTARY AND ALTERNATIVE MEDICINE (CAM) therapies, such as SPINAL MANIPULATION, or allopathic options, such as EPIDURAL INJECTION, INTRADISCAL ELECTROTHERMAL THERAPY, SELECTIVE NERVE ROOT BLOCK, and STEROID THERAPY. If left unchecked, chronic inflammation can produce scarring around the spinal nerves and evoke other problems, such as THORACIC OUTLET SYNDROME.

Risk Factors and Preventive Measures

People who experience a FLEXION-EXTENSION INJURY, such as a whiplash, have increased risk of acquiring this condition. Also, patients with ARTHRITIS, SPINAL STENOSIS, DEGENERATIVE DISC DISEASE, or any disc problem that causes the discs to leak and spinal nerves to inflame may be at higher risk too. Nevertheless, prompt treatment to lessen the damaging effects of ongoing inflammation can lessen the risks.

Medtronic Sofamor Danek. "Radiculopathy," Back.com. Available online. URL: http://www.back.com/symptoms-radiculopathy.html. Last updated February 14, 2005.

Nosuffering.com. "Radiculitis / Radiculopathy." Available online. URL: http://www.nosuffering.com/nosuffering/patient/symptoms/radio.shtml. Downloaded March 24, 2006.

Spinal Injury Foundation. "Chemical Radiculitis," SIF. Available online. URL: http://www.spinalinjuryfoundation.org/101_new/chemical.htm. Downloaded March 24, 2006.

radiofrequency treatment   See FACET NEUROTOMY OR FACET RHIZOTOMY INJECTION.

raloxifene   See SELECTIVE ESTROGEN RECEPTOR MODULATORS (SERMS).

range of motion   The natural flexibility of the SPINE allows versatile movements as the head nods up and down in an affirmative response or turns side to side to negate. In the THORACIC SPINE and LUMBAR SPINE, the normal range of motion can produce a catlike stretch or a backward arch. Shoulders shift and rotate. Hips sway back and forth, and POSTURE can be held upright, assuming the facet joints and DISCS between the VERTEBRAE remain intact and retain their mobility.

The Back.com article "Dynamic Stabilization" said, "Your spine is made up of 24 vertebrae and the connection between each forms a joint, or 'motion segment', with the vertebra above and the vertebra below. These individual motion segments do not provide the same range of motion as elbows and knees, but they work together to allow for forward and backward bending, side-to-side bending and rotation. . . . Movement at a single motion segment is limited to only a few degrees (focal motion), but since motion segments are stacked on top of each other, considerable movement is possible (global motion). And, certain parts of the spine allow for more movement than others. For instance, you may have noticed that the bones in your neck provide more motion than those in your lower back."

Risks and Complications

In the presence of ACUTE PAIN, CHRONIC PAIN, and inflammation, range of motion may decrease unless therapeutic EXERCISE or daily ACTIVITY encourage movement. Often, muscle spasm, SPRAIN, or STRAIN limit flexibility in the PARASPINAL MUSCLES, while a FLEXION-EXTENSION INJURY (whiplash) inhibits natural movement of muscles in the CERVICAL SPINE. Conditions such as ANKYLOSING SPONDYLITIS and SURGERY involving SPINAL FUSION can limit range of motion too. With a SPINAL CORD injury, however, patients cannot exercise spinal muscles and joints without assistance from a therapist or caretaker. Nevertheless, such movements remain necessary to avoid pressure sores and keep the vertebral joints mobile.

Statistics and Studies

Typically, medical technicians measure the range of motion in the spine on a scale of 0 to 10, but researchers from the Netherlands used a more sophisticated approach to study the "Reproducibility of Cervical Range of Motion in Patients with Neck Pain." As reported in *BMC Musculoskeletal Disorders*, "Neck pain is a common musculoskeletal disorder . . . and approximately one-third of all adults will experience neck pain during the course of 1 year. Patients usually receive conservative treatment such as physical therapy or continued care by a General Practitioner (GP). A physical evaluation is often used for both the diagnosis and the evaluation of treatment success in patients with neck pain. One aspect for the physical assessment of the cervical spine is the evaluation of active Range Of Motion (ROM)." Yet, "active cervical ROM is difficult to measure because of compensatory movements, and it is influenced by aging and systemic disorders. Several non-invasive methods for assessing the ROM have been available. . . . For the majority of these instruments the . . . reproducibility has not been tested adequately. Radiography has been proven to be of questionable reproducibility." With a device referred to as the EDI-320 inclinometer, however, the results proved "acceptable, despite slight variations."

Special Aids and Adaptations

To assist patients in performing range of motion exercises, The National Spinal Cord Injury Association (NSCIA) advised, "The exercises should be performed in a smooth motion as quick motions may cause damage to the joints. As the top of each range is reached the position should be held for a count of 10. During rehabilitation the team physical and occupational therapists will provide instructions on how to either perform or instruct others on performing Range of Motion exercises that will best meet your needs." Besides focusing on spinal areas with limited motion, MASSAGE THERAPY may ultimately aid the whole body. As the NSCIA said, "If you were able to trace your nerves you would find that almost every part of your body has a nerve that ends in the foot. Massaging the sole of the foot soothes these nerves and relieves pressure."

Hoving, Jan Lucas, Jan J. M. Pool, Henk van Mameren, Walter J. L. M. Devillé, Willem J. J. Assendelft, Henrica C. W. de Vet, Andrea F. de Winter, Bart W. Koes, and Lex M. Bouter. "Reproducibility of Cervical Range of Motion in Patients with Neck Pain," *BMC Musculoskeletal Disorders* 6, no. 59 (2005). Available online. URL: http://www.biomedcentral.com/1471-2474/6/59. Downloaded March 28, 2006.

Medtronic Sofamor Danek. "Dynamic Stabilization," Back.com. Available online. URL: http://www.back.com/articles-motion_preservation.html. Last updated January 5, 2006.

National Spinal Cord Injury Association, The. "Range of Motion," NSCIA. Available online. URL: http://www.spinalcord.org/html/factsheets/range_of_motion.php. Downloaded March 28, 2006.

reflex sympathetic dystrophy (RSD) syndrome

Also known as Complex Regional Pain Syndrome (CRPS), this condition worsens rather than improves over time. Increased levels of CHRONIC BACK PAIN can be particularly unfortunate for ELDERLY patients and young CHILDREN or ADOLESCENTS perceived as complaining to get attention. Instead, the opposite may be true, as inexplicable but ongoing pain grabs the attention of up to 1.2 million patients of all ages in the United States alone. To make the condition even more insidious, the initial provocation may be as big as a bone FRACTURE or as small as a splinter in the thumb.

A fact sheet from the Reflex Sympathetic Dystrophy Syndrome Association (RSDSA) explained, "RSD is a malfunction of part of the nervous system. Nerves misfire, sending constant pain signals to the brain. RSD develops in response to an event the body regards as traumatic, such as an accident or a medical procedure. This syndrome may follow 5% of all injuries."

Symptoms and Diagnostic Path

Besides moderate to severe pain, RSD/CRPS symptoms characteristically include chronic inflammation, muscle spasms, problems with RANGE OF MOTION, and changes in the nails or skin. Abnormalities in the sympathetic nervous system also occur.

The online article "Clinical Practice Guidelines" posted by the RSDSA explained, "For reasons we do not understand, the sympathetic nervous system seems to assume an abnormal function after an injury. There is no single laboratory test to diagnose RSD/CRPS. Therefore, the physician must assess and document both subjective complaints (medical history) and, if present, objective findings (physical examination), in order to support the diagnosis. There is a natural tendency to rush to the diagnosis of RSD/CRPS with minimal objective findings because early diagnosis is critical. If undiagnosed and untreated, RSD/CRPS can spread to all extremities, making the rehabilitation process a much more difficult one. If diagnosed early, physicians can use mobilization of the affected extremity (physical therapy) and sympathetic nerve blocks to cure or mitigate the disease." The guidelines further stated, "To make the early diagnosis of RSD/CRPS, the practitioner must recognize that some features/manifestations of RSD/CRPS are more characteristic of the syndrome than others, and that the clinical diagnosis is established by piecing each bit of the puzzle together until a clear picture of the disorder emerges. Often the physician needs to rule out other potentially life-threatening disorders that may have clinical features similar to RSD/CRPS, e.g. a blood clot in a leg vein or a breast tumor spreading to lymph glands can cause a swollen, painful extremity. Indeed, RSD/CRPS may be a component part of another disease," such as a HERNIATED DISC.

Treatment Options and Outlook

According to a fact sheet from the National Institute of Neurological Disorders and Stroke, "the prognosis for CRPS varies from person to person. Spontaneous remission from symptoms occurs in certain individuals. Others can have unremitting pain and crippling, irreversible changes in spite of treatment."

To ease inflammation and discomfort, treatment begins with NONSTEROIDAL ANTI-INFLAMMATORY DRUG THERAPY but can escalate to OPIATES or OPIOIDS FOR PAIN. Patients who need additional options may want to investigate the relevant studies posted by ClinicalTrials.gov. At this writing, for example, RESEARCH has begun to assess various medications as well as such COMPLEMENTARY AND ALTERNATIVE MEDICINE treatments as MAGNETIC THERAPY.

Risk Factors and Preventive Measures

Therapeutic EXERCISE, such as swimming, and HYDROTHERAPY may help to keep muscles flexible and bones strong. Daily ACTIVITY and healthful NUTRITION can also be important in preventing muscle wasting or the bone-thinning conditions, such as OSTEOPOROSIS, that sometimes accompany RSD. If symptoms continue to worsen, PAIN MANAGEMENT may include EPIDURAL INJECTION, NERVE BLOCK, OR TRANSCUTANEOUS ELECTRONIC NERVE STIMULATOR (TENS) UNIT.

ClinicalTrials.gov. "Complex Regional Pain Syndrome," list of studies, National Institutes of Health. Available online. URL: http://clinicaltrials.gov/search/term=Complex%20Regional%20Pain%20Syndrome. Downloaded March 28, 2006.

National Institute of Neurological Disorders and Stroke. "NINDS Complex Regional Pain Syndrome Information Page," National Institutes of Health. Available online. URL: http://www.ninds.nih.gov/disorders/reflex_sympathetic_dystrophy/reflex_sympathetic_dystrophy.htm. Last updated March 17, 2006.

Reflex Sympathetic Dystrophy Syndrome Association. "Clinical Practice Guidelines (Second Edition Updated October 15, 2000) for the Diagnosis, Treatment, and Management of Reflex Sympathetic Dystrophy Syndrome (RSD) also Known as Complex Regional Pain Syndrome (CRPS)," RSDSA. Available online. URL: http://www.rsds.org/3/clinical_guidelines/index.html. Downloaded March 28, 2006.

———. "CRPS/RSD Fact Sheet," RSDSA. Available online. URL: http://www.rsds.org/2/fact_fiction/index.html. Downloaded March 28, 2006.

research   In the presence of CHRONIC PAIN, most people want to know "Why?" or "What can be done?" Such questions initiate research too. For example, the research committee of the Orthopaedic Trauma Association (OTA) begins to consider each potential research project by "identifying key questions, recruiting lead investigators, organizing, planning and potentially providing start-up funding for these projects." Typical, perhaps, of the process

involved in research, "the goal is to take advantage of the substantial expertise and experience available in the organization to advance our understanding and to increase the quality of clinical research being performed by the organization."

Besides the many professional associations devoted to spinal health and the BACK, research may begin within a single university or a group of spine centers that pool their resources to investigate a topic. Between 1998 and 2001, for example, a team of physicians from the Hughston Clinic in Columbus, Georgia, the Orthopedic Center of St. Louis, and the Nebraska Spine Center in Omaha studied the effectiveness of BONE MORPHOGENETIC PROTEIN (BMP) in promoting new bone growth in 131 patients requiring ARTHRODESIS in the LUMBAR SPINE. When they had accomplished their goal of inserting BMP into the surgical sites instead of using a BONE GRAFT, the doctors reported their findings in *The Journal of Bone and Joint Surgery:* "The patients in the study group had significantly better outcomes than the control group with regard to the average length of surgery . . . , blood loss . . . , and hospital stay." In addition, "fusion rates were significantly better in the study group."

Other research projects emanate from pharmaceutical companies and government agencies. At this writing, for example, the ClinicalTrials.gov Web site sponsored by the National Institutes of Health listed 26 clinical trials involving the VERTEBRAE, 44 trials involving DISCS, and 103 focusing on the SPINE. Typically, research has a very specific goal or premise. For instance, an initiative from the National Institute of Arthritis and Musculoskeletal and Skin Diseases (NIAMS) questioned the use of important bone markers (BM) as a tool in studying, diagnosing, and effectively treating such conditions as OSTEOARTHRITIS, OSTEOPOROSIS, and RHEUMATOID ARTHRITIS. To clarify the rationale for such a study, the NIAMS said, "BM are likely to be of value in helping identify and classify genetically different patients in clinical trials to ensure uniformity of populations that can then be used to better define change and responses to therapy in relationship to clinical endpoints—such as rate of disease progression." In other words, "BM offer opportunities to more critically define the disease process" among various types of individuals. By better understanding the primary causes and answering relevant questions that concern spinal conditions and their progression, researchers may ultimately find more workable solutions for the back and spine.

Risks and Complications

Ideally, research begins with perceptive questions, but this carries an inherent risk of asking irrelevant ones. Interesting findings can unexpectedly result from a false start as new information surfaces, but researchers prefer to avoid the complications of misspending time, funding, and reputations.

Once a project has been staffed, funded, and approved, the complicated process of screening applicants begins. Even the most willing participants will be turned away if they do not meet the criteria for a particular study, whereas those who do qualify may find the schedule too demanding to continue with the program. Also, some participants will not be selected to try a new medication or treatment but may, instead, be given a placebo, usually without their knowledge. Conversely, patients who do have the opportunity to test a new product or therapy may find the treatment does not keep the condition from worsening. Also, the study itself can encounter risks. If, for example, a patient who receives an experimental drug drops out of the study or dies, this obviously affects that person and his or her family, but it can also hinder the research and complicate results.

Statistics and Studies

Gene therapy often makes stimulating news, but to stimulate the spine, research in this area has been focusing on alternatives to BONE MORPHOGENETIC PROTEIN (BMP) to promote bone growth and speed up spinal fusion. As an article from SpineUniverse reported, "Since 1990, there have been over 300 human gene therapy trials with well over 3,000 patients enrolled, and this number is steadily growing. For terminal systemic disorders such as paralysis or Parkinson's Disease, gene therapy has had limited success; however for localized conditions such as spinal fusion or disc regeneration, gene therapy can be a very powerful and successful tool." For example, "instead of putting a protein into the spine to stimulate fusion," as occurs with bone morphogenetic protein, "surgeons would

instead transfer the gene that codes for that protein into a portion of the spinal tissues, allowing those tissues to produce the protein responsible for bone growth. Although this seems like a complex procedure, it is much less invasive than current spinal fusion methods, which require an open incision, a certain amount of blood loss, pain to the patient and a significant period of healing. Gene therapy has the ability to dramatically change how this surgical procedure is performed." As a practical example and application, this type of gene therapy might be used to repair a SPINAL CORD injury or to treat a disc problem.

The Human Genome Project Information, however, presented a less heartening view. After citing previous setbacks to genetic research, information from their Web site considered other factors, such as procedures needed to handle DNA (deoxyribonucleic acid) that carries each person's genetic information. According to the governmentally sponsored genome project, "before gene therapy can become a permanent cure for any condition, the therapeutic DNA introduced into target cells must remain functional and the cells containing the therapeutic DNA must be long-lived and stable. Problems with integrating therapeutic DNA into the genome and the rapidly dividing nature of many cells prevent gene therapy from achieving any long-term benefits." Consequently, "patients will have to undergo multiple rounds of gene therapy." In addition, "anytime a foreign object is introduced into human tissues, the immune system is designed to attack the invader. The risk of stimulating the immune system in a way that reduces gene therapy effectiveness is always a potential risk. Furthermore, the immune system's enhanced response to invaders it has seen before makes it difficult for gene therapy to be repeated in patients." Although "conditions or disorders that arise from mutations in a single gene are the best candidates for gene therapy," GENETIC FACTORS may not be the only concern. For example, ethical questions arise, such as, "What is normal and what is a disability or disorder, and who decides?" or, "Are disabilities diseases? Do they need to be cured or prevented?" and perhaps the trickiest question, "Does searching for a cure demean the lives of individuals presently affected by disabilities?"

Special Aids and Adaptations

An article in the *AAOS Bulletin* of the American Association of Orthopaedic Surgeons lauded the adaptability of computers in aiding research by gathering and sorting data from various tests and questionnaires, such as "specific outcome questionnaires for each of the major areas of orthopaedic surgery." As the AAOS article explained, "Using the power of the computer and newly developed statistical principles, it is now possible to tailor the test (or questionnaire) to the student (or patient) so that a precise valid score can be obtained using a much smaller set of questions. These methods have been applied to the science of outcomes assessment." At present, "work is underway to develop a state-of-the-art national trauma registry for children and a national total joint registry. Such efforts promise to accelerate the process of clinical research and subsequent improvements." In summarizing their objectives, the AAOS article speaks well for spinal research in general: "Our objectives must be to continue to make the patient's perception of outcome relevant to our clinical decision-making process and to help guide the selection of orthopaedic procedures, devices and pharmaceuticals."

Burkus, J. Kenneth, M.D., Harvinder S. Sandhu, M.D., Matthew F. Gornet, M.D., and Michael C. Longley, M.D. "Use of RHBMP-2 in Combination with Structural Cortical Allografts: Clinical and Radiographic Outcomes in Anterior Lumbar Spinal Surgery," *The Journal of Bone and Joint Surgery* 87, no. 6 (June 2005): 1,205–1,211.

Human Genome Project Information. "Gene Therapy," U.S. Department of Energy Office of Science, Office of Biological and Environmental Research. Available online. URL: http://www.ornl.gov/sci/techresources/Human_Genome/medicine/genetherapy.shtml. Last modified November 18, 2005.

Orthopedic Trauma Association. "OTA Multicenter Research Projects," OTA. Available online. URL: http://www.ota.org/education/multicenter.html. Downloaded March 31, 2006.

Poole, Robin. "NIH White Paper: Biomarkers, the Osteoarthritis Initiative," National Institute of Arthritis and Musculoskeletal and Skin Diseases (NIAMS.) Available online. URL: http://www.niams.nih.gov/ne/oi/oabiomarwhipap.htm. Downloaded March 31, 2006.

Vitale, Michael G., M.D. and Michael W. Keith, M.D. "The Importance of Outcomes Research," American Association of Orthopaedic Surgeons, *AAOS Bulletin.* Available online. URL: http://www2.aaos.org/aaos/archives/bulletin/dec03/fline2.htm. Downloaded March 31, 2006.

Wang, Jeffrey C., M.D. and Mary Claire Walsh. "Gene Therapy: On the Cutting-Edge," SpineUniverse. Available online. URL: http://www.spineuniverse.com/displayarticle.php/article1767.html. Last updated November 23, 2005.

resistance training   This type of EXERCISE relies on hefty opposition from weights. For instance, ATHLETES with spinal concerns may lift barbells to build up the BACK and SPINE or strengthen PARASPINAL MUSCLES, but lugging heavy boxes all day might have the same effect. While other therapeutic exercises rely on gentle stretches to flex the joints or increase the RANGE OF MOTION, resistance training works to increase bone and muscle mass. This does not necessarily mean a heavy duty workout though. With the approval of a doctor and use of safe techniques in LIFTING, hospitalized patients can often perform resistance training exercises from a bed. For example, an ELDERLY patient may be able to handle a short session of raising and lowering a thick magazine or a one- to two-pound dumbbell. Over a course of weeks, the amount of time and the amount of weight or even the number of pages may be gradually increased.

Procedure

The Better Health Channel in Australia did the math for calculating a session of resistance training. According to their Web site, "maximal voluntary contraction (MVC) means the muscle has contracted to the best of its ability. In resistance training, MVC is measured by a formula known as XRM. 'X' refers to the weight that can be lifted x-amount of times before muscle fatigue sets in, and RM means 'repetitive maximum', the number of times the contraction can be performed. The formula 7RM means the person can lift the weight (let's say it's 50 kg) seven times before the muscles are too fatigued to continue. Higher weights mean lower RM—for example, the same person could lift a 65 kg weight perhaps three times. Conversely, lower weights mean higher RM—for example, the person could lift a 35kg weight about 12 times before muscle fatigue set in."

In the United States, the President's Council on Physical Fitness and Sports suggested "an initial starting point consisting of performance of 1 set per exercise (8–10 exercises) for 8–12 repetitions (10–15 for older adults) 2–3 days per week." However, "this initial recommendation has been shown to be effective for progression during the first few months of training, but then benefits can plateau during subsequent months when variation in the program design is minimal." Overall fitness and GENETIC FACTORS, such as body type, also affect individual progress, but in general, a gradual increase in load and variations in the exercise according to the person's particular goals "are critical elements to resistance training programs targeting progression."

Risks and Complications

As the progression of muscle and bone building reaches a plateau, some people get discouraged. Others pump too much weight too hard over too long a session, gaining a muscle spasm for the effort. Overdoing it can also tax muscles and damage joints.

Outlook and Lifestyle Modifications

For healthy adults who engage in resistance training of moderate to high intensity, the American College of Sports Medicine (ACSM) suggested taking one- to two-minute rest periods after each set, especially during novice and intermediate training programs. For the most promising outlook, other types of exercise may be incorporated into the program too. According to an article published in the ACSM journal *Medicine & Science in Sports & Exercise,* "increased physical activity and participation in a comprehensive exercise program incorporating aerobic endurance activities, resistance training, and flexibility exercises has been shown to reduce the risk of several chronic diseases," including LOW BACK PAIN and OSTEOPOROSIS. Furthermore, "resistance training has been shown to be the most effective method for developing musculoskeletal strength, and it is currently prescribed by many major health organizations for improving health and fitness."

Better Health Channel. "Resistance Training," Department of Human Services, State Government of Victoria, Australia. Available online. URL: http://www.betterhealth. vic.gov.au/bhcv2/bhcarticles.nsf/pages/Resistance_ training?OpenDocument. Downloaded April 1, 2006.

Kraemer, William J. and Nicholas A. Ratamess. "Progression and Resistance Training," President's Council on Physical Fitness and Sports, 200 Independence Avenue, S.W., Washington, D.C. 20201, (202) 690-9000, fax (202) 690-5211; *Research Digest* Series 6, no. 3 (September 2005): 1–8.

Kraemer, William J., Kent Adams, Enzo Cafarelli, Gary A. Dudley, Cathryn Dooly, Matthew S. Feigenbaum, Steven J. Fleck, Barry Franklin, Andrew C. Fry, Jay R. Hoffman, Robert U. Newton, Jeffrey Potteiger, Michael H. Stone, Nicholas A. Ratamess, and Travis Triplett-McBride. "American College of Sports Medicine Position Stand on Progression Models in Resistance Training for Healthy Adults," *Medicine & Science in Sports & Exercise* 34, no. 2 (2002): 364–380.

rest   See RICE METHOD; SLEEP.

rhabdomyolysis   This serious disorder occurs as injured muscle tissue releases its contents into the bloodstream, overloading the person's system. Once referred to as crush injury syndrome, the condition can result from direct trauma to skeletal muscles as sometimes encountered by ATHLETES, military trainees, and victims of a vehicular accident or natural disaster. However, over 100 other conditions, such as a SPINAL INFECTION, MUSCULOSKELETAL DISORDER, or bone FRACTURE set too tightly, can also cause rhabdomyolysis. So can excessive consumption of drugs or alcohol as well as too much EXERCISE. A poisonous snakebite and inhalation of carbon monoxide can result in rhabdomyolysis too. In any case, muscle damage on the cellular level sets off rhabdomyolysis in about one of every 10,000 people in the United States.

As explained in an overview posted on the www. rhabdomyolysis.org Web site, "Rhabdomyolysis occurs when an iron-containing pigment found in the skeletal muscle called myoglobin enters the bloodstream. The skeletal muscle releases myoglobin into the bloodstream after the muscle suffers damage. The kidneys attempt to filter the myoglobin out of the bloodstream, but the myoglobin can occlude" or otherwise obstruct "the structures within the kidney, resulting in damage such as . . . kidney failure. The myoglobin then may break down into additional toxic compounds, which can cause further kidney damage and failure. In addition, the dead (necrotic) skeletal muscle can cause large shifts in fluid from the bloodstream into the muscle, which reduces the relative fluid volume of the body and can lead to shock and reduced blood flow to the kidneys."

Symptoms and Diagnostic Path

LOW BACK PAIN, muscle weakness, MUSCLE CRAMPS, and dark urine characterize this disorder. To reach a timely diagnosis, a rheumatologist or other physician will conduct a physical examination, request a medical history, and order the appropriate laboratory tests. An ELECTROMYOGRAM may also be needed.

The IPCS Intox Databank, a medical collective of experts on toxic emergencies and also exposure to toxins, provided this information: "Prolonged muscle weakness is the most frequent complaint following rhabdomyolysis." Spinal nerve disorders can arise, as can severe kidney problems that result in kidney failure. The patient may slip into a coma, but, "in conscious patients, the main complaint may be muscle tenderness, stiffness and cramping, accompanied by weakness and loss of function."

Treatment Options and Outlook

Initial treatments primarily aim to support vital functions of the body. Profuse amounts of filtered WATER may help to cleanse away damaging toxins, but a doctor may prescribe a bicarbonate, a diuretic, or other medication to speed up the body's normal detoxification process. With delayed treatment, kidney failure can become so profound, the patient must go on dialysis to compensate for the work of that vital organ. To avoid a life-threatening problem, some patients require hospitalization to ensure adequate fluid intake and restore MINERAL BALANCE.

Risk Factors and Preventive Measures

To prevent rhabdomyolysis, people should take care to consume adequate amounts of water, especially before and after physical exertion and also when taking any medication, HERBAL THERAPY, or nutritional supplement. Accidents often cannot be prevented, but patients need to be aware of the risks encountered whenever muscle damage and dehydration occur.

An article in *Critical Care Nurse* said, "Understanding rhabdomyolysis requires an awareness of normal intracellular and extracellular distribution of ions and what happens when this precise balance is disrupted." Specifically, "sodium, calcium, chloride, and bicarbonate ions are chiefly extracellular, whereas potassium, magnesium, and phosphate ions are largely intracellular. For the body to function optimally, the relative differences in the concentrations of these ions inside and outside the muscle cells must be preserved." If a crushing blow or other type of injury occurs, "Damage to this essential structure allows intracellular contents to escape and extracellular contents to enter. . . . Where sodium goes, water follows, rapidly swelling the cells." Excessive CALCIUM also enters the muscle cells, causing a further imbalance. With prompt treatment though, "skeletal muscles can recover from episodes of rhabdomyolysis with surprisingly minimal permanent damage, and overall survival after rhabdomyolysis is approximately 77%. When access to aggressive treatment, including hemodialysis, is timely, most deaths are related to patients' other injuries or disease states and are not a direct result of rhabdomyolysis."

Criddle, Laura M. "Rhabdomyolysis Pathophysiology, Recognition, and Management," *Critical Care Nurse* 23, no. 6 (2003): 14–32.

Puppa, T. Della. "Rhabdomyolysis," IPCS Intox Databank. Available online. URL: http://www.intox.org/databank/documents/treat/treate/trt43_e.htm. Downloaded April 1, 2006.

Rhabdomyolysis Kidney Failure and Damage. "Rhabdomylosis: Overview." Available online. URL: http://www.rhabdomyolysis.org/rhabdomyolysis.html. Downloaded April 1, 2006.

rheumatism   This old-fashioned term for any rheumatic disorder may still be used by ELDERLY patients but will rarely be heard from a medical professional. Over 200 conditions with the common denominator of CHRONIC PAIN could be lumped together as rheumatism. Aside from such vague conditions as a BACKACHE or other source of LOW BACK PAIN, specific rheumatic disorders include ARTHRITIS, ANKYLOSING SPONDYLITIS, LUMBAR RADICULOPATHY, FIBROMYALGIA, chronic back pain, OSTEOARTHRITIS, and RHEUMATOID ARTHRITIS. Typically, the first line of PAIN MANAGEMENT involves the use of NONSTEROIDAL ANTI-INFLAMMATORY DRUG (NSAID) THERAPY and, often, HEAT THERAPY. Most patients will also receive healthful benefits from well-balanced NUTRITION and daily ACTIVITY or EXERCISE designed with that person in mind.

rheumatoid arthritis GENETIC FACTORS, ENVIRONMENTAL INFLUENCES, and other provocations, such as a SPINAL INFECTION, can contribute to the development of rheumatoid arthritis (RA). Regardless of the triggering influences, the immune system responds inappropriately, causing the body to attack its own joints in the BACK and other areas of the body. This particular cause of joint inflammation distinguishes RA from similar conditions, such as ARTHRITIS or OSTEOARTHRITIS, the latter of which can result from the joint damage that occurs if the chronic inflammation of RA goes untreated.

Symptoms and Diagnostic Path

CHRONIC PAIN, inflammation, swelling, and stiffness characterize RA and generally reduce the RANGE OF MOTION in the affected joints. In addition to a medical history and physical examination, doctors commonly use X-RAY and laboratory tests to arrive at a diagnosis. Even in patients who have the disease, however, a blood sample does not always show the presence of the rheumatoid factor or antibody that often indicates RA.

Treatment Options and Outlook

The American Academy of Orthopaedic Surgeons said, "Medications used to control RA fall into two categories: those that relieve symptoms and those that have the potential to modify the course of the disease. Often they are used together." ASPIRIN, IBUPROFEN, and other NONSTEROIDAL ANTI-INFLAMMATORY DRUG (NSAID) THERAPY fall into the former category and may be prescribed to ease pain and joint inflammation. Regarding the latter category, "treatment also may include disease-modifying drugs such as methotrexate and sulfasalazine and gold injections. Researchers are also working on biologic agents" or compounds derived from living matter "that can interrupt the progress of the disease. These agents target specific chemicals in the body to prevent them from acting on the joints."

Besides NSAIDs and DISEASE MODIFYING ANTIRHEUMATIC DRUGS (DMARDs), the Center for Drug Evaluation and Research (CDER) reported on CLINICAL TRIALS and RESEARCH aimed toward developing antirheumatic therapies. In considering drug interactions or combination therapies, "a particular concern with biological agents is the development of antibodies . . . resulting in changes in therapeutic benefit over time or following repeated courses of treatment. To address this consideration, it is desirable for sponsors to build into their . . . protocols a coordinated evaluation of drug levels, . . . saturation, antidrug antibodies, and clinical responses. Optimally, these assessments would be conducted at the initiation of therapy and at several time points over the course of therapy."

Protocols may vary from person to person and also between groups of patients. For instance, those with JUVENILE RHEUMATOID ARTHRITIS will be likely to receive treatments that differ from those prescribed for adults. In addition, variations occur in the effectiveness of treatments, such as COLD THERAPY and ULTRASOUND THERAPY. Which treatment to use may depend in part on the primary location of the joint inflammation.

According to The Mount Sinai Medical Center Web site, "For the patient with rheumatoid arthritis, the effects of the arthritis on the cervical spine can vary from minimal symptoms to life threatening pressure on the spinal cord that requires complex surgery to stabilize the spine and reduce the pressure on the spinal cord." For instance, if slippage in the neck VERTEBRAE or SPONDYLOLISTHESIS occurs, the connection between the skull and upper CERVICAL SPINE may become unstable. This condition can cause a CERVICOGENIC HEADACHE or, worse, mobility problems that may indicate potentially dangerous pressure on the SPINAL CORD. If so, ARTHRODESIS may be needed to stabilize the SPINE and prevent further damage.

While some patients need corrective SURGERY, others require only SPINAL MANIPULATION performed by an experienced chiropractor or osteopath to realign the vertebrae gradually. Therapeutic exercise and ORTHOTIC devices, such as a neck brace or corrective SHOES, may help patients too. In addition, COMPLEMENTARY AND ALTERNATIVE MEDICINE therapies may include ACUPUNCTURE, HERBAL THERAPY, HOMEOPATHIC MEDICINE, MAGNETIC THERAPY, and MASSAGE THERAPY. Healthful NUTRITION and doctor-approved EXERCISE also aid the outlook for most patients.

In discussing herbs commonly used for RA treatments, the National Center for Complementary and Alternative Medicine (NCCAM) said, "Three of the . . . botanicals marketed with claims to benefit arthritis pain are: Ginger; Curcumin (a component of the spice turmeric); Boswellia (also called Indian frankincense, made from the resin of a tree that grows in India). . . . A fourth botanical, feverfew, has been used in folk medicine with an intent to treat arthritis, migraine, and other conditions." However, the effectiveness of these treatments has not been proven in scientific studies. Although GLUCOSAMINE may benefit patients with some types of arthritis, that supplement may not be effective in treating RA. Similarly, the omega-6 fatty acid in evening primrose and the omega-3 found in cold water fish may or may not ease joint inflammation. Studies do show, however, that the herb valerian relieves sleep problems often associated with RA, thus improving the quality of life. As the NCCAM Web site said, "Disrupted sleep has been called a common and often neglected symptom of arthritis. A large, nationally representative survey of people over 65 with arthritis in 2000 found that disruption of sleep, among all the disruptions of arthritis, was the main reason that people sought a variety of CAM, self-care, and conventional medical treatments. Valerian has also been taken for other reasons, such as the intent to relieve muscle and joint pain."

Although natural herbs, foods, homeopathic remedies, and supplements may be considered safe or gentle for most people, some patients experience adverse reactions. With caution advised when adding any new treatment, a full glass of WATER should accompany each drug, herb, or supplement, but no herb or homeopathic medicine should be taken for the same condition or symptom for which a drug has been prescribed. For example, the herb valerian should not be taken with a MUSCLE RELAXANT or sedative.

Risk Factors and Preventive Measures

From the Department of Rheumatology at the University of Genova, Italy, a study published in the *International journal of tissue reactions* reported, "Rheumatoid arthritis is an inflammatory joint and systemic disease believed to be of autoimmune origin. Predisposing factors also include genetic factors . . . believed to raise the risk of developing the disease. In rheumatoid arthritis, as in other chronic inflammatory diseases, iron metabolism dysfunction has been observed and attributed to inflammation." In considering the point mutation C282Y, "The aim of this study was to compare the frequency of C282Y in patients with rheumatoid arthritis with that in patients with different forms of spondylarthritis and to correlate these findings with iron metabolism parameters. In the group of patients with rheumatoid arthritis, 2/24 (8.34%) were found to be positive for the C282Y mutation . . . compared with 3/24 (12.5%) of patients with spondylarthritis. In patients with the C282Y mutation, ferritin" or the iron-phosphorus-protein "levels were significantly higher than those in controls; conversely, serum iron levels were higher in patients with spondylarthritis."

Having a tendency toward RA does not mean its inevitability. While no specific preventives have been established, those at risk may be able to prevent flare-ups and slow progression by adapting a healthful lifestyle that includes ample water, good nutrition, limbering exercises, regular daily ACTIVITY, and restorative SLEEP.

American Academy of Orthopaedic Surgeons. "Rheumatoid Arthritis," AAOS. Available online. URL: http://orthoinfo.aaos.org/fact/thr_report.cfm?thread_id=154&topcategory=Arthritis. Downloaded April 3, 2006.

Center for Drug Evaluation and Research. "Guidance for Industry: Clinical Development Programs for Drugs, Devices, and Biological Products for the Treatment of Rheumatoid Arthritis (RA)," CDER, U.S. Food and Drug Administration, Department of Health and

Human Services. Available online. URL: http://www. fda.gov/cder/guidance/1208fnl.htm. Last updated July 5, 2005.

Mount Sinai Medical Center, The. "Rheumatoid Arthritis of the Cervical Spine." Available online. URL: http://www. mountsinai.org/msh/msh_frame.jsp?url=clinical_ services/orthospine_racs.htm. Downloaded April 3, 2006.

National Center for Complementary and Alternative Medicine. "Rheumatoid Arthritis and Complementary and Alternative Medicine," NCCAM, National Institutes of Health. Available online. URL: http://nccam. nih.gov/health/RA/. Last modified March 8, 2006.

Rovetta, G., M. C. Grignolo, L. Buffrini, and P. Monteforte. "Prevalence of C282Y Mutation in Patients with Rheumatoid Arthritis and Spondylarthritis," *International journal of tissue reactions* 24, no. 3 (2002):105–109.

rheumatoid spondylitis See ANKYLOSING SPONDYLITIS.

rhizotomy See FACET NEUROTOMY OR FACET RHIZOTOMY INJECTION.

rhomboid muscle strain From the innermost edges of the shoulder blades, rhomboid muscles connect the shoulders to the upper SPINE. Overextension during EXERCISE or improper LIFTING techniques often cause the muscle spasm or STRAIN typical of this condition. A RIB INJURY can produce rhomboid problems, too, as can stretching too far to reach an overhead object or an overhead tennis shot. More subtly, this condition can occur in CHILDREN and ADOLESCENTS who gradually slouch into habits of poor POSTURE or who fail to practice BACKPACK SAFETY, but all age groups, including ELDERLY patients, can be affected by this type of muscle strain.

Symptoms and Diagnostic Path

A medical history, especially of the events leading to the strain, may be all a doctor needs to confirm a diagnosis. However, contractions in the THORACIC SPINE make this condition discernible through touch as the doctor evaluates muscle tightness during a physical examination. In addition to the telling rigidity of muscles in the BACK, patients typically experience episodes of ACUTE PAIN.

Treatment Options and Outlook

COLD THERAPY, NONSTEROIDAL ANTI-INFLAMMATORY DRUG (NSAID) THERAPY, and MASSAGE THERAPY may minimize the pain, but some patients may need a MUSCLE RELAXANT to aid recovery.

According to an article by Dr. Pierre Rouzier for the University of Michigan Health System, "Recovery time also depends on the severity of the injury. A mild rhomboid strain may recover within a few weeks, whereas a severe injury may take 6 weeks or longer to recover. You need to stop doing the activities that cause pain until your muscle has healed. If you continue doing activities that cause pain, your symptoms will return and it will take longer to recover."

Risk Factors and Preventive Measures

Sensible daily ACTIVITY, adequate WATER intake, NUTRITION with natural sources of CALCIUM, and restful SLEEP help to build BACK muscles, whereas a lack of these habits increases the risk of muscle cramping and strain. Before beginning an exercise program, sedentary persons should seek approval from a doctor. Gentle stretches prior to exercising can warm rhomboid and PARASPINAL MUSCLES and often prevent strain.

Another article from the University of Michigan entitled "Rhomboid Muscle Strain or Spasm Rehabilitation Exercises" offered this exercise: "Thoracic extension: While sitting in a chair, clasp both arms behind your head. Gently arch backward and look up toward the ceiling. Repeat 10 times. Do this several times per day." For thoracic stretches, "Sit on the floor with your legs out straight in front of you. Hold your mid-thighs with your hands. Curl your head and neck toward your belly button. Hold for a count of 15. Repeat 3 times." Patients with CERVICAL SPINE problems might do well to avoid these head curls. To aid and strengthen their back muscles, they might instead use rowing motions with spinal joints in a neutral position, movements slow and steady, and the boat optional.

Clapis, Phyllis and Pierre Rouzier, M.D., for McKesson Provider Technologies. "Rhomboid Muscle Strain or Spasm Rehabilitation Exercises," University of Michigan Health System. Available online. URL: http://www.med.umich.edu/1libr/sma/sma_rhomboid_rex.htm. Downloaded April 4, 2006.

Rouzier, Pierre, M.D., for McKesson Provider Technologies. "Rhomboid Muscle Strain or Spasm," University of Michigan Health System. Available online. URL: http://www.med.umich.edu/1libr/sma/sma_rhomboid_sma.htm. Downloaded April 4, 2006.

rib injury   A fall or blow may FRACTURE a rib, but a heavy cough or a sudden movement in an unnatural position can throw a rib out of alignment. Extending the same arm in a prolonged position, for instance, while using a vacuum cleaner, spraywasher, or weed-eating device, can injure a rib, too, and sometimes cause the additional problem of RHOMBOID MUSCLE STRAIN.

In the online article "What Is a Rib Injury?" University Sports Medicine in Buffalo, New York, explained, "There are 12 ribs on each side of the chest that protect the heart, lungs, and the upper abdominal contents. All of the ribs are attached to the vertebrae (backbone) in the rear. In the front, 10 of them are attached to the sternum (breastbone) by pieces of cartilage. Direct blows to the ribs may bruise or break the ribs or injure the rib cartilage. The ribs may tear away from the cartilage that attaches them to the breastbone. This tearing away from the cartilage is called a costochondral separation."

Symptoms and Diagnostic Path

A rib that pops out of place can press spinal nerves, as VERTEBRAL SUBLUXATION often does in spinal areas, or can cause discomfort similar to a HERNIATED DISC. While ACUTE PAIN and tenderness in the adjacent VERTEBRAE point to a rib injury, some patients may have difficulty breathing.

Besides conducting a physical examination and taking a medical history, the doctor may request X-RAYS to aid a diagnosis, but information from Topcondition.com reported that around 25 percent of rib fractures will not be visible. As the online article advised, "If the possibility of a rib fracture exists, look and feel for deformity and discoloration. If you suspect an underlying injury, the simplest method for diagnosing this is to monitor the breathing of the patient. Labored, difficult breathing or even coughing up blood may indicate damage to the lungs or organs."

Treatment Options and Outlook

Usually, a rib that pops out of alignment can be popped back into place by a chiropractor, osteopath, or sports physician experienced in SPINAL MANIPULATION. With a break or bruising, COLD THERAPY, such as an ice pack kept on for 15 to 20 minutes every two or three hours, and also NONSTEROIDAL ANTI-INFLAMMATORY DRUG (NSAID) THERAPY may ease pain and swelling in the first few days. Commonly, a bruised rib will take about a month to heal and a broken rib about six weeks.

Risk Factors and Preventive Measures

Sedentary persons who suddenly overdo place themselves at risk for a rib injury. Also, ATHLETES involved in contact sports have a higher risk that can be lowered somewhat with protective equipment. Should an injury occur anyway, another risk arises if an athlete returns too soon to practice or to compete in a sports event. If the injured ribs have been taped to keep a body in play, this can complicate matters even more by decreasing lung capacity, thereby putting the patient at risk for overexertion and respiratory ailments.

To strengthen the BACK, ribs, and PARASPINAL MUSCLES, appropriate EXERCISES include RESISTANCE TRAINING and STRENGTH TRAINING. Before and after each session, gentle stretches also help to prevent future injuries by warming up the muscles, especially for those who have been sedentary or previously benched.

Personal Trainer. "The Ribs," Topcondition.com. Available online. URL:http://topcondition.com/members/ribs.htm. Downloaded April 4, 2006.

University Sports Medicine, Buffalo, N.Y. "What Is A Rib Injury?" Available online. URL: http://www.sportsmed.buffalo.edu/info/rib.html. Downloaded April 4, 2006.

ribs   See RIB INJURY; THORACIC SPINE.

RICE method This therapeutic method does not refer to a flavorful grain but a favored pain treatment recommended by most medical professionals. To spell it out, RICE forms the acronym for Rest, Ice, Compression, and Elevation, with each word meaning just what it says. As with any recipe though, RICE involves good timing and appropriately adapting to substitutions, such as any icy item one finds on hand.

Procedure

As suggested by the American Academy of Orthopaedic Surgeons: "Rest: Stop using the injured body part immediately. If you feel pain when you move, this is your body sending a signal to decrease mobility of the injured area. . . . Ice: Apply an ice pack to the injured area, using a towel or cover to protect your skin from frostbite. The more conforming the ice pack the better, in order for the injury to receive maximum exposure to the treatment. . . . Compression: Use a pressure bandage or wrap over the ice pack to help reduce swelling. Never tighten the bandage or wrap to the point of cutting off blood flow. You should not feel pain or a tingly sensation while using compression. . . . Elevation: Raise or prop up the injured area so that it rests above the level of your heart."

Regarding the length of time to apply ice, MamasHealth.com explained, "There are four levels of cold felt by the skin: coldness; a prickly or burning sensation; a feeling of aching pain; and finally a lack of sensation or numbness. When the area feels numb, icing should be discontinued. The skin should return to normal body temperature before icing again. Usually numbness can be achieved in 10 to 20 minutes. Never apply ice for more than 30 minutes at a time or tissue damage may occur." After one to three days of applying RICE at intervals of four to six hours, patients can switch to HEAT THERAPY if inflammation has ceased and no bleeding or bruising occurs. If, however, improvement cannot be seen within a day or so, a doctor should be consulted, Mama says.

Risks and Complications

In discussing common injuries among ATHLETES, the National Institute of Arthritis and Musculoskeletal and Skin Diseases (NIAMS) advised, "Call a doctor when: The injury causes severe pain, swelling, or numbness; You can't put any weight on the area; An old injury hurts or aches; An old injury swells; The joint doesn't feel normal or feels unstable." Otherwise, minor injuries can usually be treated safely with RICE and NONSTEROIDAL ANTI-INFLAMMATORY DRUG THERAPY. Risks of re-injuring an area increase, though, if a patient resumes daily ACTIVITY or EXERCISE too soon.

Outlook and Lifestyle Modifications

To protect the BACK and SPINE from further injury, RESISTANCE TRAINING, STRENGTH TRAINING, and stretching exercises help to build up the PARASPINAL MUSCLES and keep the VERTEBRAE flexible. Good NUTRITION, adequate WATER intake, and regular activities each day provide a promising outlook too. For quick RICE use though, a bag of frozen peas gives about 10 minutes of cooling power before that healthful vegetable converts to a protein-packed meal with, of course, the addition of steamed rice.

National Institute of Arthritis and Musculoskeletal and Skin Diseases. "What Are Sports Injuries? Fast Facts: An Easy-to-Read Series of Publications for the Public," NIAMS, National Institutes of Health. Available online. URL: http://www.niams.nih.gov/hi/topics/sports_injuries/ffsportsinjuries.htm. Downloaded April 4, 2006.

Roach, Louise. "Why R. I. C. E.?" MamasHealth.com.™. Available online. URL: http://www.mamashealth.com/bodyparts/rice.asp. Downloaded April 4, 2006.

rickets Known as osteomalacia in adults, this uncommon bone disease most commonly occurs during stages of rapid growth, sometimes affecting young CHILDREN but very rarely INFANTS or ADOLESCENTS. Primarily caused by a deficiency in VITAMIN D, CALCIUM, or phosphate, rickets can result from poor absorption of nutrients or lack of MINERAL BALANCE. In addition, some medications and toxic ENVIRONMENTAL INFLUENCES produce secondary rickets.

Symptoms and Diagnostic Path

Unlike OSTEOPOROSIS, which can weaken bones without a sound or symptom, rickets may produce

CHRONIC PAIN or tenderness in the BACK, SPINE, and limbs. Muscle spasm, muscle weakness, and poor muscle tone may also occur. Bone growth may slow in young children with some patients gradually developing skeletal deformities similar to SCOLIOSIS and KYPHOSIS. Laboratory tests and X-RAYS usually provide the information needed for a diagnosis, but if not, a bone biopsy may be required.

Treatment Options and Outlook

Natural dietary supplements of vitamins and minerals effectively treat most patients. To prevent skeletal deformity from occurring in children, ORTHOTIC devices may redirect the growth pattern of growing bones. Early bracing often prevents POSTURE problems and permanent disability, but if an orthotic brace proves to be ineffective, SURGERY may improve the overall outlook.

Risk Factors and Preventive Measures

Patients with EATING DISORDERS or GENETIC FACTORS, such as DWARFISM, that affect bone strength may be at higher risk. Risks also increase for sun-sensitive people who have allergies to dairy products, mainly because this lessens the likelihood of their getting adequate calcium and the vitamin D often added to milk. In general though, this condition can usually be prevented with BONE BUILDING principles, appropriate NUTRITION, and about 10 to 15 minutes of daily sunshine with no sunscreen.

Alan, Rick. "Rickets and Osteomalacia," Holy Cross Hospital. Available online. URL: http://healthychoice.epnet.com/GetContent.asp?siteid=holycross&docid=/dci/rickets. Downloaded April 4, 2006.

Ott, Susan, M.D. "Osteomalacia," Osteoporosis and Bone Physiology. Available online. URL: http://courses.washington.edu/bonephys/hypercalU/opmal2.html. Last updated October 10, 2005.

risedronate sodium   Sold under the brand name Actonel, this BISPHOSPHONATE treats bone loss in OSTEOPOROSIS patients and CHILDREN with OSTEOGENESIS IMPERFECTA. Considered to be more potent than either ALENDRONATE or ETIDRONATE, risedronate may prevent VERTEBRAL COMPRESSION FRACTURE and lessen the likelihood of bone FRACTURES in general. The medication can also be used to prevent secondary osteoporosis commonly caused by prolonged use of STEROID THERAPY or other medications that thin bones.

Dosage and Potential Side Effects

Daily doses of 5 mg or weekly doses of 30 to 35 mg slow bone loss and assist BONE BUILDING. However, patients who cannot sit upright for at least a half hour should not take this medication since they must remain in a vertical position after swallowing the drug. As with any bisphosphonate, risedronate can cause digestive problems and can damage the esophagus, but severe side effects seldom occur if patients carefully follow instructions. Most notably, the medication must be taken with a full glass of WATER and an empty stomach. This not only lessens the possibility of serious side effects but allows the medication to be absorbed without interference from other liquids, medications, foods, and minerals.

Statistics and Studies

A recent study hypothesized that ANTIRESORPTIVE DRUGS may lessen bone loss during times of immobility. Since ELDERLY patients often require more frequent or longer hospital stays, especially after SURGERY, researchers thought risedronate would be particularly useful for them. Subsequently, the study on "Hospitalization-related Bone Loss and the Protective Effect of Risedronate" appeared in *Osteoporosis International.* Reporting the outcome for 243 hospitalized patients, the article said that significant loss of bone mineral density occurred in the LUMBAR SPINE, but "in the risedronate-treated participants, all sites exhibited bone gain and there was no significant difference between hospitalized and non-hospitalized participants."

Elsewhere in drug RESEARCH, Doctor's Guide Publishing, Ltd. stated, "In studies of women with postmenopausal osteoporosis, Actonel significantly reduced the risk of new vertebral fractures in just one year. In high-risk patients (greater than or equal to two previous vertebral fractures), Actonel significantly reduced the risk of vertebral fractures by up to 74 percent in just one year (9.8 percent of patients in the control group and only 2.7 percent of patients taking Actonel fractured. . . . Reductions of vertebral fracture risk were seen throughout the three-year study duration." Besides the risedronate, participants received supplements of VITAMIN D and CALCIUM, both of which assist the body in building new bone.

Doctor's Guide Publishing, Ltd. "FDA Approves Actonel (Risedronate) for Osteoporosis." Available online. URL: http://www.pslgroup.com/dg/1cd17e.htm.Downloaded April 4, 2006.

Heaney, R. P., D. J. Valent, and I. P. Barton. "Hospitalization-related Bone Loss and the Protective Effect of Risedronate," *Osteoporosis International* 17, no. 2 (February 2006): 212–217.

rodding surgery This type of SURGERY involves the insertion of a metal rod into a bone, particularly a long bone such as the femur or thighbone. However, rodding surgery can be performed on bones in the BACK, too, for instance, as a treatment for patients with OSTEOGENESIS IMPERFECTA.

Procedure

To describe the procedure, the Osteogenesis Imperfecta Foundation said, "Under general anesthesia, a long bone (e.g., a leg or arm bone) may be cut in one or several places, straightened and 'threaded' onto a metal rod. The surgery generally requires an incision long enough to expose the bone where it is deformed. Alternatively, small incisions can be made at the end of the deformed bone, and the rod may be introduced through the skin and moved through the bone under x-ray guidance. When the bone is acutely fractured, rodding can often be done without opening the fracture site. . . . Rodding does not necessarily *prevent* fractures; the bone may still fracture, but the rod will provide an internal splint that can help keep the bone in alignment."

Risks and Complications

Rods that expand when in place can be used in the larger bones of ADOLESCENTS and older CHILDREN, but small bones in the back and SPINE usually need a nonexpanding rod. With continued bone growth, the nonexpanding rod must eventually be replaced, thus necessitating further surgery. Deformity around a previous site can cause the need for additional rodding surgery too. Since this is major surgery to begin with, each repetition repeats and, perhaps, increases such risks as bleeding or damage to the adjacent nerves and tissue.

Outlook and Lifestyle Modifications

INFANTS with BIRTH DEFECTS OF THE SPINE or BIRTH INJURY TO THE SPINE may be treated with ORTHOTIC devices until rodding becomes the better option. After the procedure, a splint, cast, or orthotic brace will be needed in all age groups for a month or so. When the surgical site has healed, HYDROTHERAPY or therapeutic EXERCISE, such as swimming, may help patients to retain muscle tone and regain mobility.

National Institute of Arthritis and Musculoskeletal and Skin Diseases. "Osteogenesis Imperfecta: A Guide for Nurses," National Institutes of Health. Available online. URL: http://www.niams.nih.gov/bone/hi/osteogenesis/oi_nurse_guide.htm#Rodding. Downloaded April 4, 2006.

Smith, Peter, M.D. "OI Issues: Rodding Surgery," Osteogenesis Imperfecta Foundation. Available online. URL: http://oif.convio.com/site/PageServer?pagename=Rodding. Downloaded April 4, 2006.

ruptured disc See HERNIATED DISC.

S

sacral vertebrae Below the LUMBAR SPINE, five VERTEBRAE fuse together to form the sacrum. On both of the vertical sides of this elongated triangle, the upper portion wings out to connect with the butterfly-shaped pelvic bones, while the lower part extends downward into the COCCYGEAL SPINE, thus suspending the tailbone like a cocoon. This pattern comes with slight variations since CHILDREN and young ADOLESCENTS have a flatter joint surface, whereas men have a narrower, longer sacral triangle than women do. Such subtle variations help to identify the age and sex of human remains, but among the living, these differences make a difference in the SPINE problems that arise.

Risks and Complications

A shorter, broader sacrum places young to middle-aged women at greater risk for developing SACROILIAC JOINT PAIN SYNDROME and varying degrees of LOW BACK PAIN. However, male and female ATHLETES of all ages risk problems if they twist abruptly or exert too much pressure on the sacral vertebrae. Workers who exceed their LOAD TOLERANCE or use improper LIFTING techniques encounter higher risks too. Ironically, sedentary persons also place too much pressure on the sacrum because of prolonged sitting.

Besides the problems of misuse and disuse, an injury can FRACTURE the sacral spine, although this rarely happens. A more likely occurrence might be a VERTEBRAL COMPRESSION FRACTURE in an ELDERLY patient with OSTEOPOROSIS or other condition involving bone loss. INFANTS with BIRTH DEFECTS OF THE SPINE and people who exhibit spinal misalignments, such as SCOLIOSIS, may have problems that eventually affect the sacrum too.

Statistics and Studies

Numerous studies have been done on pelvic tilt or obliquity, but sacral obliquity has not been as well studied or defined. After studying 63 of their own patients who exhibited sacral obliquity, a group of doctors reported for SpineUniverse, "One patient was found to have a traumatic origin. The remainder appear to have a congenital abnormality of varying degrees," indicating an inherited condition. For instance, the sacrum may slant to one side as a patient compensates for an unequal length in the legs. "In some cases, the sacral obliquity had little effect on the spine, but in others the obliquity appears to have . . . lumbar scoliosis of varying degrees."

Special Aids and Adaptations

Sacral tilt or obliquity may require an ORTHOTIC device, such as a shoe insert, to aid balance, compensate for uneven leg lengths, and avoid postural problems. For sedentary persons, ERGONOMIC FACTORS, such as a well-chosen chair, may ease sacral stress. Also, regular EXERCISE and daily ACTIVITY aid flexibility in weight-bearing joints while increasing vertebral strength. Often, a simple exercise can loosen stiff vertebral joints upon awakening or before going to sleep. For example, as the person lies flat on the BACK with knees bent and feet on the mattress, he or she pushes the SPINE into the bed for about five seconds, then relaxes and repeats the process a few times.

Brown, Courtney, M.D., David H. Donaldson, M.D., and John L. Brugman, M.D. "Sacral Obliquity, A Poorly Understood Congenital Anomaly," SpineUniverse. Available online. URL: http://www.spineuniverse.com/displayarticle.php/article2555.html. Last updated April 26, 2005.

Medtronic Sofamor Danek. "Sacral Spine," Back.com. Available online. URL: http://www.back.com/anatomy-sacral.html. Last updated March 25, 2005.

Ullrich, Peter F., M.D. "Sacral Region," Spine-health. Available online. URL: http://www.spine-health.com/topics/anat/a06.html. Last updated August 24, 2004.

sacroiliac joint pain syndrome, sacroiliitis As the SACRAL VERTEBRAE meet the iliac crest of the pelvis, the bones form small sacroiliac joints that bear the full effects of WEIGHT and also daily jolts on the body. Paradoxically, either too little movement or too much can result in joint dysfunction, producing episodes of ACUTE PAIN that feel like SCIATICA or a HERNIATED DISC in the LUMBAR SPINE. Temporary conditions, such as a SPINAL INFECTION, and chronic conditions, such as OSTEOARTHRITIS, can also cause sacroiliac joint pain. If, however, a sacroiliac joint becomes inflamed, the condition will more likely be referred to as sacroiliitis.

Symptoms and Diagnostic Path

Often, radiating pain extends from the lower BACK then branches into one or both legs. If stiffness occurs in the lower SPINE, the RANGE OF MOTION may become limited, but a doctor can check this by giving the patient simple exercises to do during a physical examination. To further aid the diagnosis, an X-RAY, COMPUTED TOMOGRAPHY SCAN, or other imaging test may be requested. If a patient limps in with a fever though, the doctor may suspect sacroiliitis, which can usually be confirmed with a laboratory blood culture.

Treatment Options and Outlook

Conservative treatments for sacroiliac joint pain commonly include COLD THERAPY, NONSTEROIDAL ANTI-INFLAMMATORY DRUG THERAPY, physical therapy, and ULTRASOUND THERAPY. If these prove ineffective, other options include STEROID THERAPY, TRANSCUTANEOUS ELECTRONIC NERVE STIMULATOR (TENS) UNIT therapy, and joint injections with the guidance of FLUOROSCOPY. If needed, a NERVE BLOCK or other type of SPINAL INJECTION may be used, not only to treat pain but to determine its point of origin.

A spinal adjustment by an osteopath or chiropractor can also address sacroiliac pain. Describing this type of treatment, a Spine-health article said, "Chiropractic manipulation of the sacroiliac joint is usually accomplished with the patient lying down on his or her side. More specifically, the knee opposite the side the patient is lying on is flexed and raised toward the patient's chest. The bottom shoulder is positioned forward producing a stretch in the low back and pelvic region." With this very precise positioning, "a low force, high amplitude manipulation is applied by the chiropractor and usually results in an audible release (created by oxygen, nitrogen, and carbon dioxide escaping from the joint). This chiropractic maneuver creates the typical 'crack' often associated with joint manipulation and sounds similar to 'cracking the knuckles',", a procedure that traditionally brings some measure of relief.

Risk Factors and Preventive Measures

Patients with ANKYLOSING SPONDYLITIS, people with POSTURE problems, and ELDERLY patients with ARTHRITIS may be more apt to develop sacroiliac joint pain syndrome. Risks also increase for ATHLETES and young workers who exceed their LOAD TOLERANCE or use improper LIFTING techniques. Conversely, care in lifting can help to prevent episodes of joint pain. As a general preventive, well-designed EXERCISES aid posture, increase PARASPINAL MUSCLE strength, and assist joint mobility.

Malanga, Gerald, M.D. "S-1 Joint Injections to Manage Back Pain," SpineUniverse. Available online.URL: http://www.spineuniverse.com/displayarticle.php/article1858.html. Last updated August 12, 2005.

Medtronic Sofamor Danek. "Inflammatory & Infectious Disorders: Sacroiliitis," Back.com. Available online. URL: http://www.back.com/causes-inflammatory-sacrolitis.html. Last updated March 11, 2005.

Wood, Debra. "Sacroiliac Joint Pain," Holy Cross Hospital. Available online. URL: http://healthychoice.epnet.com/GetContent.asp?siteid=holycross&docid=/dci/sacroiliac. Downloaded April 18, 2006.

Yeomans, Steven G. "What is Sacroiliac Joint Dysfunction?," Spine-health. Available online. URL: http://www.spine-health.com/topics/cd/sjd/sjd01.html. Downloaded April 18, 2006.

SAPHO Syndrome Initially, this acronym stands for Synovitis, Acne, Pustulosis, Hyperostosis, and Osteitis, which basically translates to bone, skin, and joint problems occurring sometime between CHILDHOOD and ELDERLY years. More specifically, synovitis inflames synovial joints producing symptoms akin to ARTHRITIS. Acne and pustulosis involve skin eruptions, while hyperostosis indicates an overgrowth of bone. Similar to SPONDYLITIS, osteitis produces bone inflammation that primarily provokes pain and swelling in the BACK and CERVICAL SPINE.

Symptoms and Diagnostic Path

Bone pain and skin eruptions mark this chronic condition, but specific tests do not. For a diagnosis, a rheumatologist may need to rule out such disorders as ANKYLOSING SPONDYLITIS or JUVENILE ARTHRITIS. As an Orphanet article explained, SAPHO syndrome involves several diseases, so symptoms for each must be considered. "Definite diagnosis can be hard to establish." However, "SAPHO must be suspected when a patient is affected by a . . . skin disease associated with rheumatic pains. If examination shows that the pains are caused by . . . inflammation of bones or joints, the hypothesis tends to be confirmed" unless a fever suggests something else, such as a SPINAL INFECTION.

Treatment Options and Outlook

The team effort of a dermatologist, rheumatologist, and physical or occupational therapist will work toward an effective course of treatment. Symptoms may ease with regular use of NONSTEROIDAL ANTI-INFLAMMATORY DRUG THERAPY, perhaps with STEROID THERAPY prescribed for a limited time. Some patients may be given an antibiotic, but that will usually be an individual option rather than a standard treatment. To protect bone mass, some patients, including children and ADOLESCENTS, may be prescribed CALCITONIN. In any case, each treatment option attempts to alleviate the symptoms of this chronic condition for which no cure exists. On occasion, however, self-healing or remissions may occur.

An article in a 2002 issue of *Rheumatology* said, "The natural history of SAPHO follows a prolonged relapsing and remitting course. As patient numbers have been small, evidence for treatments has been based on anecdotal evidence and small case-control studies. Treatments thought to be of benefit include tetracycline, azithromycin, colchicine and calcitonin. Corticosteroids and non-steroidal anti-inflammatory drugs (NSAIDs) can produce symptomatic improvement but are limited by their potential side-effects in long-term use." Therefore, "we postulated that intravenous disodium pamidronate, a bisphosphonate that reduces bone turnover, would be beneficial in the management of this syndrome as bone biopsies often demonstrate evidence of increased bone turnover, often similar in appearance to Paget's disease, and calcitonin, which reduces the rate of bone turnover, has previously shown benefit." The patient in this case study required an intravenous treatment since she had a preexisting condition of the esophagus that prohibited her taking an oral BISPHOSPHONATE, but "the associated attacks of musculoskeletal pain were dramatically reduced in terms of severity and duration such that, after the three treatments, she was completely pain-free and able to return to work." As the medical researchers concluded, "This case study demonstrates significant and rapid symptomatic benefit from intravenous pamidronate therapy in a woman with SAPHO. It may be that a similar response could be achieved using oral bisphosphonates."

Risk Factors and Preventive Measures

A combination of skin lesions and musculoskeletal disorders affecting the joints and SPINE may not be preventable, but prompt treatment can keep symptoms manageable. A prompt diagnosis may not always be possible though. As an article in *Skeletal Radiology* said, "The diagnosis of SAPHO syndrome is not difficult when the typical" skin lesions or eruptions "are located in characteristic target sites." However, "the diagnosis is more difficult if atypical sites are involved and there is no skin disease."

Earwaker, J. W. and A. Cotton. "SAPHO: Syndrome or Concept? Imaging Findings," *Skeletal Radiology* 32, no. 6 (June 2003): 311–337.

Marshall, H., J. Bromilow, A. L. Thomas and N. K. Arden. "Pamidronate: a Novel Treatment for the SAPHO Syndrome?" *Rheumatology* 41, no. 2 (2002): 231–233.

Schilling, Fritz. "SAPHO Syndrome," Orphanet encyclopedia, January 2003. Available online. URL: http://orphanet.infobiogen.fr/data/patho/GB/uk-sapho.html. Downloaded April 20, 2006.

sarcoma   See CANCER.

Scheuermann's kyphosis   Sometimes referred to as Scheuermann's disease, this developmental type of KYPHOSIS is not a disease but a POSTURE disorder that occurs in growing CHILDREN and ADOLESCENTS, especially boys. According to Holger Scheuermann, the Danish radiologist who discovered the disorder, one side of the SPINE grows faster than the other, producing wedge-shaped VERTEBRAE. Why this happens has not been ascertained, but some scientists credit GENETIC FACTORS while others point to previous injuries or vertebral damage. Regardless, the disorder often produces a HERNIATED DISC, SCHMORL'S NODE, or symptoms similar to DEGENERATIVE DISC DISEASE.

Symptoms and Diagnostic Path

With CHRONIC PAIN as the main warning sign, Scheuermann's manifests itself in a noticeable curvature of the THORACIC SPINE, usually around the T7 to T9 vertebrae. X-RAYS can confirm the condition, but family members may be able to detect the problem early at home. As a Spine-health article said, "Postural roundback can be easily distinguished from Scheuermann's kyphosis by the fact that the deformity goes away when the patient lies down. Typically, patients with true Scheuermann's kyphosis need to sleep on two or three pillows at night to stay comfortable because their deformity remains when they lie down."

Treatment Options and Outlook

If kyphosis reaches or exceeds 40 degrees of curvature, a young patient may be fitted with an ORTHOTIC back brace or individually molded cast. Reporting on a case study in the *Journal of Prosthetics & Orthotics,* a medical team described their method for achieving a proper fit. While reclining, "the patient's hips and knees were kept flexed during the casting in order to attempt to reduce the . . . tilt of the pelvis and specifically, the angle of L5-Sl. We believe that by stabilizing the pelvis in this position and by utilizing the . . . region to apply our primary point of force . . . to 'unbend' the kyphosis, we were able to achieve our results. Also, this technique allowed the patient to achieve good . . . alignment (head over pelvis) using comfortable

levels of force." The patient wore the device for 17 hours a day, and, "after only one month, the in-brace reduction was nearly half that of the original kyphosis. The patient also reported relief of back pain after only one month in the brace."

Risk Factors and Preventive Measures

While bracing will not be effective in adults and older adolescents, patients who still have at least a year or more of growing to do may lose some pain and regain vertebral height with the aid of a well-fitted brace. Timeliness can be especially important since early treatment can sometimes prevent permanent BACK deformity. Patients who have not received this assistance in earlier years of bone growth may be able to strengthen their PARASPINAL MUSCLES through therapeutic EXERCISE. However, anyone with a curvature of 70 degrees or more may need SURGERY involving DISC removal and a BONE GRAFT to straighten and strengthen the spine.

A Spine School article explained, "Surgery for the correction of Scheuermann's kyphosis typically consists of a fusion of the abnormal vertebrae. The operation has two parts—one operation is done on the front of the spine and another on the back of the spine. A posterior-only fusion is rare because of the rigidity of the curves." Some patients may want surgery for cosmetic reasons, but since "the surgery is serious and involves the spine, it generally is not recommended just to improve appearance." The potential surgical complications include injury to the SPINAL CORD, increased pain, and a SPINAL INFECTION. In cases involving an extreme degree of curvature though, the problems caused by the condition may generate more risks than surgery has. For instance, "the disorder can cause decreased lung and cardiac functions. The curve of the spine causes the chest to have less room inside the chest cavity. If the deformity is severe, the chest cannot expand fully when you breathe. Eventually, the heart can be affected by the poor lung function." In such instances, corrective surgery may provide a timely and, possibly, life-saving option.

Gomez, Miguel, M.D., Patrick Flanagan, and Thomas Gavin. "An Alternative Bracing Approach to Scheuermann's Disease: A Case Study," *American Academy* of Orthotists and Prosthetists, *Journal of Prosthetics & Orthotics* 14, no. 3 (2002): 109–112.

MacAfee, Paul, M.D. "Scheuermann's Disease of the Thoracic and Lumbar Spine." Spine-health. Available online. URL: http://www.spine-health.com/topics/cd/scheuermanns/scheu01.html. Downloaded April 20, 2006.

Spine School. "Scheuermann's Kyphosis," SpineUniversity. Available online. URL: http://www.spineuniversity.com/public/spinesub.asp?id=48. Downloaded April 20, 2006.

Schmorl's node   Injuries to the THORACIC SPINE or LUMBAR SPINE combine with the GENETIC FACTORS thought to be responsible for this condition. According to an article for *Dynamic Chiropractor,* "Schmorl's nodes are defined as herniations" or protrusions "of the intervertebral disc through the vertebral end-plate," which is a cartilage-like plate or covering that attaches the DISCS to the VERTEBRAE. Normally, each vertebral end-plate provides nutrients to the whole disc unless herniation disrupts that process, thereby producing nodes as first described in 1927 by the German pathologist Christian G. Schmörl. Active male ADOLESCENTS and ATHLETES most commonly encounter the injuries that trigger this condition. Usually, the nodes cause no problem in adulthood, but their disruptive appearance can cause an affected disc to degenerate at an early age.

Symptoms and Diagnostic Path

Most Schmorl's nodes present no symptoms as such, but BACK pain, stiffness, and tenderness over the affected VERTEBRAE can occur, limiting RANGE OF MOTION. Patients may also show evidence of KYPHOSIS or have muscle spasms in the PARASPINAL MUSCLES. Besides the results of a physical examination, X-RAYS may confirm a diagnosis. If not, a COMPUTED TOMOGRAPHY SCAN or MAGNETIC RESONANCE IMAGING can rule out a SPINAL TUMOR or a HERNIATED DISC.

An article in the *American Journal of Neuroradiology* said, "Schmörl's nodes are typically seen on plain film and CT scans as . . . lesions of varying size contained within the vertebral body at the endplate and . . . in extreme cases may involve most of the vertebral body. . . . Diagnosis of Schmörl's nodes is usually established after late changes have occurred and become visible on plain radiographs or CT scans." However, "in the acute stage, Schmörl's nodes are difficult to diagnose and even to detect, because . . . the herniation has not had time to develop." Although generally occurring in the thoracic or lumbar spine, formations of the nodes have also been reported in the CERVICAL SPINE.

Treatment Options and Outlook

Rest and SPINAL MANIPULATION offer conservative treatment options with daily ACTIVITY gradually resumed. Eventually, most athletes can return to play. Although very uncommon, some patients require SURGERY.

A journal article entitled "Painful Schmorl's Node Treated by Lumbar Interbody Fusion" reported, "Painful Schmorl's node can be diagnosed by discography, which demonstrates an intravertebral disc herniation with . . . back pain. Surgical treatment should be considered in a patient with persistent disabling back pain. When surgical treatment is indicated, eradication of the intervertebral disc including Schmorl's node and . . . fusion are preferable."

Risk Factors and Preventive Measures

A group of doctors from Australia discussed Schmorl's nodes in *Spine.* According to the article, "Seventy . . . spines from cadavers of individuals killed in motor vehicle accidents were examined . . . particularly for the occurrence of acute Schmorl's nodes" in order to "document whether Schmorl's nodes occur acutely as a result of trauma." As the researchers concluded, "Schmorl's nodes do occur acutely as the result of a single traumatic episode, and are almost always associated with other acute spinal injury. The frequency and occurrence of acute Schmorl's nodes in motorcyclists suggest that axial loading," or intense pressure on the spine, "is an important mechanism. Their predominance in the T8-L1 region" of the thoracic and lumbar spine "suggests that this region is particularly susceptible to stress."

Fahey, V., K. Opeskin, M. Silberstein, R. Anderson, and C. Briggs. "The Pathogenesis of Schmorl's Nodes in Relation to Acute Trauma. An Autopsy Study," *Spine* 23, no. 21 (November 1, 1998): 2,272–2,275.

Grivé, Elisenda, Alex Roviraa, Jaume Capelladesa, Antoni Rivasa, and Salvador Pedrazaa. "Radiologic Findings in Two Cases of Acute Schmörl's Nodes," ©1999 American Society of Neuroradiology, *American Journal of Neuroradiology* 20, no. 10 (1999): 1,717–1,721.

Hasegawa, K., A. Ogose, T. Morita, and Y. Hirata. "Painful Schmorl's Node Treated by Lumbar Interbody Fusion," *Spinal cord: the official journal of the International Medical Society of Paraplegia* 42, no. 2 (February 2004): 124–131.

Pate, Deborah. "Schmorl's Nodes," *Dynamic Chiropractic* 9, no. 19 (September 13, 1991). Available online. URL: http://www.chiroweb.com/archives/09/19/16.html. Last modified August 17, 2005.

sciatica A number of disorders, such as a HERNIATED DISC and PIRIFORMIS SYNDROME, can cause sciatic pain, but the condition commonly known as sciatica most often is a symptom. As a single disorder though, sciatica might be more accurately called LUMBAR RADICULOPATHY, which exhibits radiating pain caused by pressure, inflammation, or damage to the sciatic nerve. This large nerve exits the spinal column between the lowest VERTEBRA of the LUMBAR SPINE and the uppermost bone of the SACRAL VERTEBRAE then runs down the middle of each hip and leg. Consequently, sciatica can begin with LOW BACK PAIN or numbness that radiates into one or both legs and feet.

As information from the Sciatica.org Web site explained, "Sciatica arises from injury to the fibers of the sciatic nerve. The injury can occur in one of four places: inside the spinal canal (cauda equina); where bundles of sciatic nerve fibers pass through bony openings in the spine (neuroforamina); in the pelvis (lumbrosacral plexus); where the sciatic nerve exits the pelvis, below the piriformis muscle in the buttock (Piriformis Syndrome), or along the leg."

Symptoms and Diagnostic Path

Danger signs requiring immediate medical attention include lower body weakness and loss of bladder or bowel control. In such cases, a fever may also occur. More commonly, radiant pain, tingling, or numbness accompanies persistent BACK pain. During a physical examination, the doctor may test the RANGE OF MOTION or simply ask the patient to walk across the room. If nerve involvement is suspected, MAGNETIC RESONANCE IMAGING or X-RAYS can be used to locate the source of inflammation.

Treatment Options and Outlook

According to the American Academy of Orthopaedic Surgeons (AAOS), "About 80–90 percent of people with sciatica get better, over time, without surgery. . . . In rare cases, a herniated disk may press on nerves that cause you to lose control of your bladder or bowel. If this happens, you may also have numbness or tingling in your groin or genital area." Like CAUDA EQUINA SYNDROME, "this is an emergency situation that requires surgery." Otherwise, treatments generally include bed rest, NONSTEROIDAL ANTI-INFLAMMATORY DRUG THERAPY, and COLD THERAPY. If no swelling exists, HEAT THERAPY may bring more comfort. The AAOS also said, "Sometimes, your doctor may inject your spine area with a cortisone-like drug. As soon as possible, start physical therapy with stretching exercises to help you resume your physical activities without sciatica pain. To start, your doctor may want you to take short walks."

Risk Factors and Preventive Measures

Regular daily ACTIVITY and EXERCISES to strengthen the PARASPINAL MUSCLES or increase vertebral flexibility may help to avoid sciatic pain. Patients who must sit for long periods of time should move around often, stretch like a cat, and consider supportive ERGONOMIC FACTORS in their choice of chairs. Prompt treatment of DISC problems or a short but healing bed rest may ease sciatica too.

In Vancouver, British Columbia, a group of surgeons considered the impact of surgical delays. After studying 92 patients whose lumbar disc herniation caused sciatica, they reported their findings in the *Journal of Neurosurgery: Spine:* "The only relevant different between our study and others appears to be in the mean time between symptom onset and surgery. The mean of 49 weeks was considerably longer than that in most comparable studies." Yet, despite these surgical delays, "the mean number of days to return to work was 73." Of the patients who did not return to work after recovery, one was a student who needed no employment; three did not respond to a request for information, and one could not find a job.

American Academy of Orthopaedic Surgeons. "Sciatica," AAOS. Available online. URL: http://orthoinfo.aaos. org/fact/thr_report.cfm?Thread_ID=167&topcategory =Spine. Downloaded April 21, 2006.

Fisher, Charles, M.D., Vanessa Noonan, Paul Bishop, M.D., Michael Boyd, M.D., David Fairholm, M.D., Peter Wing, and Marcel Dvorak, M.D. "Outcome Evaluation of the Operative Management of Lumbar Disc Herniation Causing Sciatica," *Journal of Neurosurgery: Spine* 100, no. 4 (April 2004): 317–324.

Sciatica.org. "Frequently Asked Questions," Manhattan Physical Medicine & Rehabilitation. Available online. URL: http://www.sciatica.org/faq.html. Downloaded April 20, 2006.

scoliosis   A sideways curve of the SPINE greater than 10 degrees marks this condition, which may be apparent in INFANTS or gradually appear in growing CHILDREN and ADOLESCENTS. Curves less than 10 degrees are not labeled as scoliosis and are considered normal anatomic variations. However, the spinal development of a baby born with DWARFISM or a BIRTH DEFECT OF THE SPINE needs to be monitored as does the bone growth of a child diagnosed with IDIOPATHIC SCOLIOSIS. Although late onset of scoliosis seldom troubles the BACK of an adult, abnormal curvature can begin with an injury, bone loss, or such conditions as DEGENERATIVE DISC DISEASE, MARFAN SYNDROME, MUSCULOSKELETAL DISORDERS, OSTEOGENESIS IMPERFECTA, OSTEOPOROSIS, RHEUMATOID ARTHRITIS, and VERTEBRAL COMPRESSION FRACTURE.

According to an article posted by the Scoliosis Research Society, "Scoliosis is defined as a side-to-side deviation from the normal frontal axis of the body. Although traditional, this definition is limited since the deformity occurs in varying degrees in all three planes: back-front; side-to-side; top-to-bottom." Therefore, "scoliosis is a descriptive term and not a diagnosis. As such, a search is made for the cause." However, "in more than 80% of the cases, a specific cause is not found and such cases are termed idiopathic, i.e., of undetermined cause. This is particularly so among the type of scoliosis seen in adolescent girls." While GENETIC FACTORS often influence spinal formation, including the particular curvature of the spine, "scoliosis does not come from carrying heavy things, athletic involvement, sleeping/standing postures, or minor lower limb length inequality." If, however, a child with scoliosis slouches or does not practice BACKPACK SAFETY, an existing condition certainly will not improve.

Symptoms and Diagnostic Path

BACKACHE, LOW BACK PAIN, and fatigue frequently accompany scoliosis, along with such visible signs as a tilt to the SACRAL VERTEBRAE or misaligned POSTURE that makes one shoulder noticeably higher than the other. In general though, the location of the curvature affects the overall symptoms.

An article posted online by the National Institute of Arthritis and Musculoskeletal and Skin Diseases (NIAMS) explained, "Doctors group curves of the spine by their location, shape, pattern, and cause. They use this information to decide how best to treat the scoliosis." For example, "to identify a curve's location, doctors find the apex of the curve (the vertebra within the curve that is the most off-center); the location of the apex is the 'location' of the curve." Therefore, a thoracic curvature occurs in the THORACIC SPINE, while a sideways curve in the LUMBAR SPINE will indicate a lumbar curvature. If the apex happens to be at the point where those two portions of the spine come together, a thoracolumbar curve results.

Treatment Options and Outlook

For mild cases with less than a 20-degree curve, SPINAL MANIPULATION may realign the spinal column, but this remains a controversial topic. Many scientific papers have refuted the utility or long-term benefits of this treatment, while patients claim otherwise. Regardless, in between visits to a chiropractor or osteopath, at home EXERCISES may strengthen the PARASPINAL MUSCLES enough to hold the individual vertebrae in place. Growing children and teens with a curvature of 25 to 40 degrees often require an ORTHOTIC cast or brace to prevent further curving of the spine. As the NIAMS said, "Braces can be custom-made or can be made from a prefabricated mold. All must be selected for the specific curve problem and fitted to each patient. . . . To have their intended effect (to keep a curve from getting worse), braces must be worn every day for the full number of hours prescribed by the doctor until the child stops growing."

While a back brace will not correct the spine of an adult, such an orthotic may be beneficial for temporary use, such as to minimize pain during an activity. At any age though, a worsening curve or spinal instability can indicate a need for SURGERY. If so, the type of procedure will depend on the age of the patient, degree of curve, stage of bone development, and causative factor. Commonly, surgery involves spinal fusion, BONE GRAFT, and the implantation of a device designed to stabilize the spine.

Regarding the success of various treatments and improvement in the overall outlook, a retrospective review of 24 cases appeared in *Spine*. According to that report, "The patients were assessed for the amount of correction obtained in the main curve, and for the spontaneous correction of the compensatory curves above and below." With the ages of the patients ranging from 10 to 43 years, "correction of the major curve at follow-up assessment was 54%." Instead of a back or posterior approach, the spinal fusions involved a frontal (anterior) approach with RODDING SURGERY to stabilize approximately two to five vertebral segments. After following up with their patients for an average of 3.6 years, the doctors concluded, "Anterior correction and fusion using solid rod instrumentation constitute effective and safe treatment of thoracolumbar scoliosis. As compared with posterior systems, it provides correction and rebalance of the trunk through a shorter fusion segment."

Risk Factors and Preventive Measures

According to the National Scoliosis Foundation Web site, "The primary age of onset for scoliosis is 10–15 years old, occurring equally among both genders. However, females are eight times more likely to progress to a curve magnitude that requires treatment." Six million people in the United States have scoliosis. "Each year scoliosis patients make more than 600,000 visits to private physician offices, and an estimated 30,000 children are put into a brace for scoliosis, while 38,000 patients undergo spinal fusion surgery." There is no known cure and, for 80 to 85 percent of the cases, no known cause. "Consequently, a scoliosis patient's life is exacerbated by many unknowns and treatments . . . that are often ineffective, invasive, and/or costly. Scoliosis patients also have increased health risks due to frequent x-ray exposure." That exposure poses little risk for most people since the dangers of X-RAYS can usually be kept to a minimum. Nevertheless, exposure may be hazardous for scoliosis patients who frequently require radiographs to monitor the progression of their conditions. In addition, risks may increase for patients who have certain sensitivities or who have cause to question cumulative exposure from ENVIRONMENTAL INFLUENCES.

Information posted online by the Scoliosis Association reported, "Approximately 10% of all teens have some degree of scoliosis. Usually only 1% have severe enough curves to require some kind of medical attention beyond the normal 6 months or yearly observations." Quite likely, X-rays will not be required at each annual or semi-annual checkup, but some type of monitoring will be needed. Sometimes, this can be as simple as noticing a misshapen pattern on a T-shirt.

Since growing teens and children have the highest risk of developing a spinal deformity, awareness and early treatment can often prevent a slight curve from becoming an extreme postural problem. In most cases, good NUTRITION with ample CALCIUM and daily ACTIVITY, such as swimming and rowing, can aid BONE BUILDING and build up spinal health.

Bitan, Fabien D., M.D., Michael G. Neuwirth, M.D., Paul L. Kuflik, M.D., Andrew Casden, M.D., Norman Bloom, M.D., and Sid Siddiqui, M.D. "The Use of Short and Rigid Anterior Instrumentation in the Treatment of Idiopathic Thoracolumbar Scoliosis: A Retrospective Review of 24 Cases," *Spine* 27, no. 14 (July 15, 2002): 1,553–1,557.

National Institute of Arthritis and Musculoskeletal and Skin Diseases. "Questions and Answers about Scoliosis in Children and Adolescents," NIAMS, National Institutes of Health. Available online. URL: http://www.niams.nih.gov/hi/topics/scoliosis/scochild.htm. Downloaded April 21, 2006.

National Scoliosis Foundation. "Information and Support," NSF. Available online. URL: http://www.scoliosis.org/info.php. Downloaded April 21, 2006.

Scoliosis Association, Inc. "Types of Scoliosis." Available online. URL: http://www.scoliosis-assoc.org/default.tpl?PageID=55&cart=11290570424484307&PageName=TYPES%20OF%20SCOLIOSIS&sec_id=55&sec_status=main. Downloaded April 21, 2006.

Scoliosis Research Society. "In Depth Review of Scoliosis: Introduction," SRS. Available online. URL: http://www.srs.org/patients/review/default.asp?page=2. Downloaded April 21, 2006.

secondary osteoporosis Primary OSTEOPOROSIS characteristically results from bone loss in postmenopausal women and ELDERLY patients. For men, CHILDREN, and ADOLESCENTS, secondary osteoporosis may be a likely occurrence since a number of medical conditions and medications, such as STEROID THERAPY, can cause bone mass to decline.

Explaining what typically happens, a fact sheet from the National Institutes of Health (NIH) Osteoporosis and Related Bone Disease National Resource Center said, "As the primary condition, juvenile rheumatoid arthritis provides a good illustration of the possible causes of secondary osteoporosis. In some cases, the disease process itself can cause osteoporosis. For example, some studies have found that children with juvenile rheumatoid arthritis have bone mass that is lower than expected, especially near the joints affected by arthritis. In other cases, medication used to treat the primary disorder may reduce bone mass. For example, drugs such as prednisone, used to treat severe cases of juvenile rheumatoid arthritis, negatively affect bone mass. Finally, some behaviors associated with the primary disorder may lead to bone loss or a reduction in bone formation. For example, a child with juvenile rheumatoid arthritis may avoid physical activity, which is necessary for building and maintaining bone mass, because it may aggravate his or her condition or cause pain."

Risks and Complications

High risks particularly occur for inactive people with active cases of ANKYLOSING SPONDYLITIS, JUVENILE RHEUMATOID ARTHRITIS, MARFAN SYNDROME, OSTEOGENESIS IMPERFECTA, RHEUMATOID ARTHRITIS, RICKETS, and SPINAL CORD injury. Persons with metabolic disorders or medications that interfere with MINERAL BALANCE and NUTRITION also have an especially high risk of developing secondary osteoporosis. In addition, too much dietary IRON and too many colas can interfere with calcium uptake. However, otherwise healthy individuals who consume high quantities of alcohol or drugs or low amounts of CALCIUM, VITAMIN C, VITAMIN D, and other essential nutrients will experience varying degrees of bone loss. Also, males and females with EATING DISORDERS greatly increase their risks of acquiring secondary osteoporosis. In addition, teenage girls and women may incur amenorrhea or the loss of their menstrual cycles. This disruption of the normal hormonal pattern then leads to further loss of bone mass.

Statistics and Studies

According to the NIH, "Individuals with anorexia restrict their dietary intake and experience weight loss and amenorrhea to the extent that their skeletal health is impaired. Low bone mineral density (BMD) is a common feature in anorexia nervosa, and up to two-thirds of affected teens have BMD values more than two standard deviations below the norm."

Regarding studies involving men, an issue of *NIH ORBD-NRC News* posted online by the NIH reported, "The NIH Consensus Development Conference Statement on Osteoporosis Prevention, Diagnosis and Therapy estimates that 30–60 percent of osteoporosis cases in men can be attributed to secondary causes," such as renal disease, CANCER, and problems with PARATHYROID HORMONE (PTH). Treatments vary according to the cause, but for PTH problems, the NIH said, "Researchers in Portland, Oregon, reported on two studies concerning the use of human parathyroid hormone in men with osteoporosis. In one study of 437 men, PTH use was associated with increases in bone mineral density of up to 9 percent at the spine and up to 3 percent at the hip. In a second study of 355 men, PTH decreased the risk of vertebral fractures by more than 80 percent."

Special Aids and Adaptations

A BONE MINERAL DENSITY TEST, such as ABSORPTIOMETRY, assesses bone loss and helps to determine which treatment may be needed. This can be trickier for men since the average T-scores that measure a person's bone mass have been based on data from young women. Also, such treatments as HORMONE REPLACEMENT THERAPY have been well studied in women, but not in men. Nevertheless, some treatments remain the same. For instance, the article

"Osteoporosis in Men: Suspect Secondary Disease First" in the *Cleveland Clinic Journal of Medicine* reported, "Alendronate has been shown to increase skeletal density in men comparably to levels seen in women." Furthermore, "it is now approved for use in men." In addition to that BISPHOSPHONATE, "teriparatide, a parathyroid hormone preparation, is now approved to increase bone mass in men with primary . . . osteoporosis at high risk for fracture." This has particular significance since the article also stated, "Compared with women, men with hip fractures have higher rates of mortality and morbidity. More are institutionalized, and 30% to 50% die within a year of fracture vs. about 20% of women." Although other potential aids, such as CALCITONIN, have not been thoroughly studied in men, "small increases in bone density and a reduction in vertebral fractures were seen in major studies in women."

Other types of BONE BUILDING therapies appropriate for men, women, and children include HERBAL THERAPY, HOMEOPATHIC MEDICINE, and natural forms of nutrition, such as dairy products, fresh fruit, and vegetables. Adequate WATER intake also helps to hydrate bones and body cells, thus minimizing the inflammatory conditions that accelerate bone damage. While some patients cannot avoid some drugs that contribute to bone loss, children and adults who regularly engage in WEIGHT-BEARING EXERCISE, such as jumping rope and running, can continue to build bone strength. Also, calcium needs to be ingested regularly and not just once in a while.

Licata, Angelo, M.D. "Osteoporosis in Men: Suspect Secondary Disease First," *Cleveland Clinic Journal of Medicine* 70, no. 3 (March 2003): 247–254.

National Institutes of Health Osteoporosis and Related Bone Disease National Resource Center, "Juvenile Osteoporosis," NIH ORBD-NRC. Available online. URL: http://www.osteo.org/newfile.asp?doc=r609i. Downloaded April 21, 2006.

National Institutes of Health (NIH) Osteoporosis and Related Bone Diseases (ORBD). "Secondary Osteoporosis," *NIH ORBD~NRC News* 4, no. 1 (December 2001). Available online. URL: http://www.osteo.org/newfile.asp?doc=n401&doctitle=Secondary+Osteoporosis&doctype=HTML+Newsletter. Downloaded April 21, 2006.

selective costimulation modulator See ABATACEPT.

selective endoscopic discectomy (SED) This MINIMALLY INVASIVE SURGERY uses micro-instruments and a minute incision to remove a HERNIATED DISC or DISCS damaged by DEGENERATIVE DISC DISEASE. For some patients, the procedure offers an option other than DISCECTOMY and LAMINECTOMY. The most appropriate treatment option may not be determined, however, until the disc has been located and studied with a DISCOGRAM guided by FLUOROSCOPY.

Procedure

Since the patient must remain awake for this procedure, a local anesthetic will be given to dull the discomfort. Then a thin needle is inserted into the disc space. A slightly larger probe goes into the quarter-inch incision, then with the guidance of a fluoroscope and X-RAYS, the surgeon uses laser to shrink or remove the damaged portion of one or more discs. This out-patient procedure takes about a half hour, but the patient remains in the clinic long enough to be monitored.

Risks and Complications

All spinal SURGERY, including minimally invasive procedures, carries risks of bleeding, nerve damage, or SPINAL INFECTION. In an article for SpineUniverse, Dr. Elliott Gross wrote, "Prior to the procedure, patients are provided with outcome statistics. For example, good to excellent results are expected in 86% of patients if pre-operative pain is primarily low back pain. If the patient's pain was back and leg pain, good to excellent results should approach 92%." For the remaining patients though, CHRONIC PAIN may not subside and may, instead, worsen. Also, this type of surgery will not be the best choice for everyone. Patients with SPINAL STENOSIS, for example, may need open BACK surgery, whereas those with spinal instability may require ARTHRODESIS with a BONE GRAFT.

Outlook and Lifestyle Modifications

Dr. Anthony T. Yeung, who helped to develop selective endoscopic discectomy (SED), discussed the evolution of the procedure in *The Mount Sinai*

Journal of Medicine: "In an attempt to decrease surgical morbidity, the microscope was employed in conjunction with smaller incisions to minimize postoperative trauma to the bone and soft tissue." Of the 500 patients who had been treated at that writing, "most of the cases had a variety of symptomatic disc protrusions, including . . . disc fragments within reach. . . . With the ability to visualize the spinal anatomy in a conscious patient comes the opportunity to diagnose, evaluate, and treat painful conditions."

For most patients, this procedure brings an improved outlook and the means of being sent home with only a tiny bandage to show for the surgery. During the recovery process, patients may need an ice pack to minimize swelling and also NONSTEROIDAL ANTI-INFLAMMATORY DRUG THERAPY to ease pain and inflammation. Within a few days of the procedure though, many patients can return to work.

Gross, Elliott, M.D. "Transforaminal Selective Endoscopic Discectomy™: Recovery, Complications, Procedure and Contraindications," SpineUniverse. Available online. URL: http://www.spineuniverse.com/displayarticle.php/article1420.html. Last updated June 20, 2005.

Yeung, Anthony T., M.D. "The Evolution of Percutaneous Spinal Endoscopy and Discectomy," *The Mount Sinai Journal of Medicine* 67, no. 4 (September 2000): 327–332.

selective estrogen receptor modulators (SERMs)

As the name implies, this treatment modulates the reception of estrogen in the body. The American Medical Association (AMA) had this to say about the SERM raloxifene: "Through its selective interaction with estrogen receptors, raloxifene exerts estrogen agonist action in some target tissues, while acting as an estrogen antagonist in others." With an agonist being for and antagonist against, a SERM can go either way to take needed action. The same principle applies to herbs classified as a tonic in HERBAL THERAPY. Nevertheless, herbals, such as black cohosh and soy supplements, should not be taken in conjunction with a SERM or other drug used for a similar purpose.

In preventing OSTEOPOROSIS in postmenopausal women, raloxifene improves bone density without causing breast tenderness or adding the concerns about CANCER that often accompany HORMONE REPLACEMENT THERAPY (HRT). Indeed, the AMA reported, "investigators found that there was a decreased incidence of breast cancer in the women who took raloxifene for 3 years." Another SERM, tamoxifen, primarily received approval to treat breast cancer, whereas raloxifene was specifically developed and approved to prevent osteoporosis in older women.

Information from the breastcancer.org Web site indicated that CALCITONIN and BISPHOSPHONATES reduce bone loss more than a SERM. Hormone replacement therapy can too, but HRT increases the risk of breast cancer. According to the Web site, "If you've had breast cancer and you need a medicine to build up your bone strength, your doctor will likely recommend an alternative to HRT. Bisphosphonates and SERMs are effective and safer options."

Dosage and Potential Side Effects

Under the brand name EVISTA, raloxifene can be taken as a 60 mg tablet any time of day, with or without food. As the drug manufacturer Eli Lilly and Company advised, "To help you remember to take EVISTA, it may be best to take it at about the same time of the day. Calcium and/or vitamin D may be taken at the same time as EVISTA. If you miss a dose, take it as soon as you remember. However, if it is almost time for your next dose, skip the missed dose and take only your next regularly scheduled dose. Do not take two doses at the same time."

Pregnant women, smokers, and patients with liver problems should not take a SERM. For women in general, potential side effects include hot flashes and blood clots. Since the latter can especially be a problem for patients requiring bed rest or SURGERY, the use of a SERM should be discontinued at least 72 hours before a surgical procedure.

Statistics and Studies

According to the AMA Web site, raloxifene decreases the incidence of VERTEBRAL COMPRESSION FRACTURE by 50 percent. Also, "vertebral fracture reduction is evident at 1 year and is sustained for up to at least 4 years in patients remaining on continuous therapy." However, "when therapy is discontinued, bone turnover returns to its previous state, resulting in bone loss."

A study from the Czech Republic reported on "The Effect of Raloxifene after Discontinuation of Long-term Alendronate Treatment of Postmenopausal Osteoporosis" in the *Journal of Clinical Endocrinology and Metabolism*. According to the abstract, "the aim of this study was to compare bone mineral density (BMD) and biochemical markers of bone turnover in patients receiving long-term alendronate therapy who continued alendronate, were switched to raloxifene, or discontinued antiresorptive therapy" that works with the body's natural bone remodeling cycle. After using ALEN-DRONATE for 43 months to treat 99 women diagnosed with osteoporosis, researchers found, "BMD preservation and increase were most pronounced in patients continuing alendronate." However, "raloxifene treatment, compared with placebo, demonstrated beneficial effects on BMD and bone turnover after discontinuation of long-term alendronate therapy." In addition to SERM therapy, patients received daily supplements of CALCIUM and VITAMIN D, both of which aid BONE BUILDING if taken regularly.

American Medical Association. "Antiresorptive Therapy: Selective Estrogen Receptor Modulators," AMA. Available online. URL: http://www.ama-cmeonline.com/osteo_mgmt/module05/05anti/index.htm. Downloaded April 22, 2006.

breastcancer.org. "Other Bone Medications—SERMs." Available online. URL: http://www.breastcancer.org/bone_serms.html. Downloaded April 22, 2006.

EVISTA.com. "Understanding EVISTA," Eli Lilly and Company. Available online. URL: http://www.evista.com/understand_evista/understand_evista.jsp?reqNavId=1. Downloaded April 22, 2006.

Michalska, D., J. J. Stepan, B. R. Basson, and I. Pavo. "The Effect of Raloxifene after Discontinuation of Long-term Alendronate Treatment of Postmenopausal Osteoporosis," *Journal of Clinical Endocrinology and Metabolism* 91, no. 3 (March 2006): 870–876.

selective nerve root block (SNRB)   This type of NERVE BLOCK does double duty: first, to locate the source of nerve root pain and, second, to relieve it. The procedure effectively treats patients with CHRONIC BACK PAIN that has not been relieved by conservative treatment. As a diagnostic tool, SNRB offers more precision than MAGNETIC RESONANCE IMAGING in locating an inflamed spinal nerve.

Procedure

Before the procedure, patients should avoid PAIN RELIEVERS and discuss other medications or concerns with their doctors. For example, pregnant women need to delay SNRB until a later time.

According to the Spine-health Web site, "in an SNRB, the nerve is approached at the level where it exits the foramen (the hole between the vertebral bodies). The injection is done both with a steroid (an anti-inflammatory medication) and lidocaine (a numbing agent). Fluoroscopy (live x-ray) is used to ensure the medication is delivered to the correct location. If the patient's pain goes away after the injection, it can be inferred that the back pain generator is the specific nerve root that has just been injected. Following the injection, the steroid also helps reduce inflammation around the nerve root."

Risks and Complications

SNRB with FLUOROSCOPY can be more complicated to perform than, say, an EPIDURAL INJECTION. Therefore, patients do well to seek an experienced physician. Reportedly, SNRB carries no risk of springing a leak in spinal fluids since the location of the injection occurs outside the SPINE. However, that same locale houses spinal nerves that may be irritated by the procedure, potentially increasing LOW BACK PAIN. Discomfort may increase for a couple of days, but fever or ACUTE PAIN should be reported promptly.

An article in the *Archives of Physical Medicine and Rehabilitation* reviewed specific "complications and side effects of cervical and lumbosacral selective nerve root injections." At a SPINE clinic in Arizona, 151 patients had 306 selective nerve root injections (SNRI) with follow-ups immediately, then at 1 week and 3 months. According to the study, "there were no major complications, such as death, paralysis, spinal nerve injury, infection, or allergic reaction, during the study. Ninety-one percent of subjects had no side effects during the procedure." Patients who received treatment for locations occurring between the LUMBAR SPINE and SACRAL VERTEBRAE experienced an increase in radicular or radiant nerve pain, such as occurs in SCIATICA. Specifically, their side effects included "increased pain at the injection site (17.1%); increased radicular pain (8.8%); lightheadedness (6.5%); increased spine pain (5.1%); nausea (3.7%); nonspecific headache (1.4%); and vomiting (0.5%)." Patients who received treatments for the CERVICAL SPINE experienced side effects of "increased pain at injection site (22.7%); increased radicular pain (18.2%); lightheadedness (13.6%); increased spine pain (9.1%); nonspecific headache (4.5%); and nausea (3.4%)."

Outlook and Lifestyle Modifications

After SNRB, an ice pack applied four times a day for about ten minutes may relieve pain and swelling. For patients who can take ACETAMINOPHEN, a minimal dose may ease discomfort. To avoid risk of bleeding, a NONSTEROIDAL ANTI-INFLAMMATORY DRUG (NSAID), such as ASPIRIN, should not be taken for at least 36 hours after the procedure.

If needed, SNRB can be repeated up to three times a year. However, patients who experience pain relief do well to increase their daily ACTIVITY, begin a doctor-approved program of EXERCISE, and increase their WATER intake. Similarly, supportive NUTRITION assists spinal health for years to come.

Huston, C. W., C. W. Slipman, and C. Garvin. "Complications and Side Effects of Cervical and Lumbosacral Selective Nerve Root Injections," *Archives of Physical Medicine and Rehabilitation* 86, no. 2 (February 2005): 277–283.
International Spine Intervention Society, Patient Information. "Selective Nerve Root Block," SpineUniverse. Available online. URL: http://www.spineuniverse.com/displayarticle.php/article346.html. Last updated November 16, 2005.
Spine-health.com. "Injections for Back Pain Management." Available online. URL: http://www.spine-health.com/topics/conserv/overview/inj/inj03.html. Downloaded April 8, 2006.

Stanford Interventional Spine Center. "Patient Information and Instructions Following Spinal Injections," Stanford University School of Medicine. Available online. URL: http://isc.stanford.edu/postprocedures_inject.html. Last modified May 25, 2005.

shaken baby syndrome, shaken infant syndrome

Similar to a whiplash, this type of FLEXION-EXTENSION INJURY occurs in a flash as the head snaps forward, then back, damaging the CERVICAL SPINE. In explaining what happens, information from the National Center on Shaken Baby Syndrome said, "The brain rotates within the skull cavity, injuring or destroying brain tissue. When shaking occurs, blood vessels feeding the brain can be torn, leading to bleeding around the brain. Blood pools within the skull, sometimes creating more pressure within the skull and possibly causing additional brain damage. Retinal (back of the eye) bleeding is very common."

Symptoms and Diagnostic Path

Severe cases involve neurological damage and often death. At first, the INFANT becomes unconscious as the central nervous system shuts down, but immediate medical treatment may prevent death or permanent disability. If the child survives, the injuries typically include FRACTURE to the CERVICAL SPINE, damaged VERTEBRAE, and a SPINAL CORD injury that may produce retardation or other neurological symptoms.

Regarding signs of a less severe episode, the National Institute of Neurological Disorders and Stroke (NINDS) said, "Symptoms of shaken baby syndrome include extreme irritability, lethargy, poor feeding, breathing problems, convulsions, vomiting, and pale or bluish skin. Shaken baby injuries usually occur in children younger than 2 years old, but may be seen in children up to the age of 5."

Often, the condition goes unrecognized. In an article for the National Center on Shaken Baby Syndrome, Dr. Carole Jenney wrote, "Not surprisingly, the severely injured children were more likely to be recognized as having head trauma at their first visit to the physician. At the first visit, children who were comatose, whose breathing was compromised, who were seizing or who had facial bruising were more likely to be accurately diagnosed." Especially among babies and young CHILDREN, "non-specific signs such as vomiting, fever and irritability are frequently seen in a myriad of conditions, including many minor illnesses. The difficulty, then, is to be able to tell when these signs and symptoms occurred because of serious head injuries." Early detection is crucial. However, "abusive head trauma was missed significantly more often in children who were Caucasian than in children of minority races, and was more likely missed in families where both parents lived with the child."

Treatment Options and Outlook

Emergency treatments include such life-sustaining efforts as respiratory support and sometimes SURGERY to stop internal bleeding. As the NINDS said, "In comparison with accidental traumatic brain injury in infants, shaken baby injuries have a much worse prognosis. Damage to the retina of the eye can cause blindness. The majority of infants who survive severe shaking will have some form of neurological or mental disability, such as cerebral palsy or mental retardation, which may not be fully apparent before 6 years of age. Children with shaken baby syndrome may require lifelong medical care." To evaluate the damage and establish a prognosis, MAGNETIC RESONANCE IMAGING and a LUMBAR PUNCTURE will usually be required.

Risk Factors and Preventive Measures

An article in the May 2005 issue of *RN* discussed the results of a "simple educational program" tested in 16 hospitals that provide maternity care. "Nurses spoke to parents about the dangers of violently shaking their infant, gave them a one-page brochure, and suggested ways to manage persistent crying. Some parents also viewed a short video." After asking parents to sign a statement showing their understanding and commitment, "Researchers obtained . . . signed statements, which represented about 70% of all births in the region during the study period." Six years prior to the study, "there were 49 cases of shaken baby syndrome in the eight counties, or about 41.5 per 100,000 births. During the 5.5-year study, there were 21 cases, or about 22.2 per 100,000 births. This represented a statistically significant 47% reduction."

The American Association of Neurological Surgeons also offered this potentially life-saving word:

"Shaken baby syndrome is completely preventable. Taking care of a baby can present challenges, especially for first-time parents. However, it is important to remember that it's never acceptable to shake, throw, or hit a baby. The following tips may help prevent abuse: Take a deep breath and count to 10. Take time out and let your baby cry alone. Call someone close to you for emotional support. Call your pediatrician—there may be a medical reason why your baby is crying. Never leave your baby with a caregiver, friend, or family member that you do not trust completely. Always check references carefully before entrusting your baby to a caregiver or daycare center."

Understanding the needs of a baby or young child can ease worries that most new parents experience. Also, the importance of adequate NUTRITION and ample SLEEP for caretakers can not be overstressed. Only a few sleepless nights alters body chemistry, turning a normally patient, loving person into someone with symptoms of psychosis. If support from relatives or friends cannot be found, a parent does well to nap whenever the baby does until restorative rest becomes a family routine.

Bauer, Jeff. "This Nursing Intervention Can Help Prevent Shaken Baby Syndrome," *RN* 68, no. 5 (May 2005): 22.

Jenney, Carole, M.D. "Abusive Head Trauma Can Be Difficult for Physicians to Recognize," National Center on Shaken Baby Syndrome. Available online. URL: http://www.dontshake.com/Subject.aspx?categoryID=12&PageName=MedicalFactsDiagnoseTrauma.htm. Downloaded April 22, 2006.

National Center on Shaken Baby Syndrome. "All About SBS." Available online. URL: http://www.dontshake.com/Subject.aspx?CategoryID=12. Downloaded April 22, 2006.

National Institute of Neurological Disorders and Stroke. "NINDS Shaken Baby Syndrome Information Page," NINDS. Available online. URL: http://www.ninds.nih.gov/disorders/shakenbaby/shakenbaby.htm. Last updated January 25, 2006.

NeurosurgeryToday.org. "Shaken Baby Syndrome," American Association of Neurological Surgeons. Available online. URL: http://www.neurosurgerytoday.org/what/patient_e/shaken.asp. Downloaded April 22, 2006.

shoe choice, spinal effects of   A well-designed shoe not only aids foot motion but helps POSTURE and assists balance in the SPINE. If feet squeeze into too-tight attire, the legs and BACK feel that TENSION. If high heels spike the heel of each foot, natural spinal curvatures curve unnaturally to compensate. If the arch of a shoe does not fit the arch of a foot, SACRAL VERTEBRAE encounter arching pain. If the shoe soles do not stand solely for safety and comfort, intervertebral DISCS receive a soulful slap with each step.

A commercial Web site for Asics America explained normal interactions that occur between body planes and foot motion: "The Sagittal Plane divides the body into left and right halves. The foot motion within this plane is dorsiflexion and plantarflexion." In other words, an imaginary line, drawn from head to toe, shows if the feet go up and down or drag on the ground. Somewhere around the waistline, "the Transverse Plane divides the body into upper and lower halves. The foot motion within this plane is adduction and abduction," which shows if toes turn out or in. Finally, "the Frontal Plane divides the body into front and back halves. The foot motion within this plane is inversion and eversion," which shows if feet tilt toward or away from the body, causing a potential SPRAIN or heel pain either way. Ideally though, a well-designed shoe enables each foot to take a turn contacting the ground, pushing off, going airborne, then returning to the first position. These motions may occur in a fast run, a brisk jog, or a snail-paced walk, but regardless, a fitting shoe helps to ensure the ongoing feat of mobility.

Risks and Complications

Since CHILDREN and young ADOLESCENTS outgrow their shoes quickly, they have increased risks of an improper fit that contributes to musculoskeletal problems. In addressing other concerns, the American Orthopaedic Foot & Ankle Society (AOFAS) said, "Children's feet perspire greatly, and the upper part of their shoes should be made of breathable materials. Leather or canvas allows the foot to breathe. Avoid man made material, such as plastic." Also, "make sure the insole is made of absorbent material. You may want padded insoles. Most children do not need a special arch support.

All toddlers younger than 16 months have flat feet and only fully develop an arch by the age of 6 to 8 years." Poor designs also increase the risks of falls. For instance, "the outer sole provides traction, cushioning, and flexibility to the shoe. Some very sticky and thick outer soles can make young children clumsy and cause falls and should be avoided." The same can be said about appropriate footwear for ELDERLY persons or anyone with a stability problem. For toddlers, "flat outer soles make it easier to begin walking. Older children can wear shoes with heels, but they should not be too high (bigger than one inch) as this can cause the foot to slide forward, cramping the toes against the shoe."

In the online article "Shoes," the American Academy of Orthopaedic Surgeons (AAOS) offered suggestions that may help ATHLETES to lessen the risk of choosing the wrong type of footwear. As the AAOS explained, "The purpose of athletic shoes is to protect the feet from the specific stresses encountered in a given sport and to give the player more traction. A jogging shoe will be designed differently from an aerobics shoe, for example. The differences in design and variations in material, weight, lacing characteristics and other factors among athletic shoes are meant to protect the areas of the feet that encounter the most stress."

To lessen risks of injuries among outdoor workers, the AAOS advised, "Work shoes are also available with varying characteristics, depending on the wearer's occupation. Boots made of thick leather with steel toe boxes can be worn to protect the feet from injury. Boots with varying degrees of traction also are available." For women who work indoors, the AAOS cautioned, "High-heeled, pointed-toe shoes can cause numerous orthopaedic problems, leading to discomfort or injury to the toes, ankles, knees, calves and back. Most high-heeled shoes have a pointed, narrow toe box that crowds the toes and forces them into an unnatural triangular shape. These shoes distribute the body's weight unevenly, placing excess stress on the ball of the foot and on the forefoot." However, "even low-heeled shoes can cause problems if they don't fit well. Years of wearing too-small shoes can lead to permanent deformities." To avoid complications from wearing ill-fitting footwear, the AAOS suggested: "Have your feet measured regularly. Their size may change as you grow older. . . . Don't select a shoe by size alone. A size 10 in one brand or style may be smaller or larger than the same size in another brand or style. Buy the shoe that fits well."

Statistics and Studies

In an article entitled "If the Shoe Fits, Wear It," the AAOS reported, "One in six persons or 43.1 million people in the U.S. have foot problems. Thirty-six percent regard their foot problems as serious enough to warrant medical attention." Although well-made shoes may seem expensive, "the cost of foot surgery to correct foot problems from tight-fitting shoes is $2 billion a year. If time off from work for the surgery and recovery is included, the cost is $3.5 billion."

In an unexpected twist, an AOFAS press release announced, "A recent . . . online survey of over 1,200 runners found that almost two thirds had injuries that they related to their shoes; however, these injuries did not appear to be linked to how much the runners paid for their shoes or whether or not they used an inserted Orthotic device." Interestingly though, "there was no significant difference in incidence of injury between those paying $20 for shoes or those who paid $120." According to the survey, the fit of a shoe carries more weight than the price. Also, the age of a shoe has a bearing on safety. Not only does an older shoe provide the proverbial old shoe comfort, but runners apparently feel more sure-footed too. As the AOFAS said, "All injury types occurred predominantly in shoes less than six months old and in shoes in which the respondents had run less than 300 miles," suggesting that injuries most often occur during the break-in period.

Special Aids and Adaptations

An article in *BioMechanics* discussed how various "In-shoe Interventions Ease Back Pain through Postural Correction." For instance, "heel lifts can correct the amount of pelvic obliquity" or tilt as "determined from the postural radiographs. In our clinics we usually correct the discrepancy in ⅛-inch increments every 10 to 14 days through the use of cork heel lifts. A lift of as much as ½ inch will fit comfortably in most shoes. For correction over ½ inch, the amount of lift needs to be added to the outsole of the shoe. We counsel patients that the added lift may increase pain for a few days as the body adjusts to the changes. A follow-up postural radiograph may be done with the lift in place once the goal height has been achieved or if there is a significant increase in symptoms while the lift height is being increased."

Once an ORTHOTIC has been adjusted, the American Academy of Podiatric Sports Medicine recommended, "If you wear an insert, an orthotic, or an orthotic with a flat insert underneath it, bring these along to the shoe store. And be sure to wear the same type of sock when you are fitted for your shoe as you will wear when participating in your sport." Regardless of the level of daily ACTIVITY or the age of the person, shoes must adapt to the individual, not the other way around. This may not be easy since one foot will usually be larger than the other. If so, the larger size should be purchased with an insert added to accommodate the smaller foot.

Different manufacturers create different designs, but in general, the toe box of the shoe should allow wiggle room. The heel should be snug without raising a blister, and the inner and outer edges or last of the shoe should follow the contour of the foot. No shoe lasts forever, though. As the American Academy of Podiatric Sports Medicine advised, "Make sure you examine and replace your shoes regularly. Most running shoes last for between 350 miles and 500 miles of running. Checking and changing your shoes is one of the best ways to avoid the doctor's office. With a careful training schedule that avoids over training and doing too much, too soon, too quickly and too often, you can reduce your risk . . . markedly. Be sure to check all aspects of your shoe for wear."

American Academy of Orthopaedic Surgeons. "If the Shoe Fits, Wear It," AAOS. Available online. URL: http://orthoinfo.aaos.org/fact/thr_report.cfm?thread_id=104&topcategory=foot. Downloaded April 25, 2006.

———. "Shoes," AAOS. Available online. URL: http://orthoinfo.aaos.org/brochure/thr_report.cfm?Thread_ID=15&topcategory=Foot. Downloaded April 25, 2006.

American Academy of Podiatric Sports Medicine. "Selecting An Athletic Shoe." Available online. URL: http://

www.aapsm.org/fit_shoes.htm. Downloaded April 25, 2006.

American Orthopaedic Foot & Ankle Society. "A Guide To Children's Shoes," AOFAS. Available online. URL: http://www.aofas.org/i4a/pages/index.cfm?pageid= 3290. Downloaded April 25, 2006.

———. "Survey Shows Runners Commonly Experience Shoe Related Injuries: Cost of Shoes Bears Little Relationship to These Injuries," AOFAS. Available online. URL: http://www.aofas.org/i4a/pages/index. cfm?pageid=3284. Downloaded April 25, 2006.

Asics America Corporation. "Cardinal Body Planes." Available online. URL: http://www.asicsamerica.com/ asicstech/cardinal_body_planes.htm. Downloaded April 25, 2006.

Fann, Alice V., M.D. "In-shoe Interventions Ease Back Pain through Postural Correction," *BioMechanics* May 2001, CMP United Business Media. Available online. URL: http:// www.biomech.com/db_area/archives/2001/0105.foot ortho.bio.shtml. Downloaded April 25, 2006.

skeletal dysplasia Sometimes mild, sometimes life-threatening, this group of disorders includes about 200 conditions, such as DWARFISM, OSTEO-GENESIS IMPERFECTA, and some BIRTH DEFECTS OF THE SPINE. Very mild cases may become noticeable in ADOLESCENTS or adults, but most of these disorders become apparent in INFANTS and young CHILDREN. Although causes remain unclear, skeletal dysplasia may result from poor NUTRITION, adverse ENVIRON-MENTAL INFLUENCES, or, more commonly, GENETIC FACTORS involving a gene that affects the formation or quality of cartilage. Ultimately, the defective cartilage alters the shape and strength of spinal joints as well as the development of the BACK, SPINE, and other bones.

The Human Genome in London, England, explained, "The body's scaffolding—the skeleton—grows at a remarkable rate as we transform from a tiny baby into a full-sized adult. Whether we are destined to be tall or short the process is the same: for about 15 years, our bones will lengthen and harden until we reach our full height. Like all tissues of the body, however, bones can be stricken by genetic disease. About one in 4,000 people suffer from skeletal dysplasias, genetic disorders of the skeleton such as brittle bone disease (osteogenesis imperfecta) or dwarfism."

Symptoms and Diagnostic Path

X-RAYS and other imaging tools, such as a COMPUTED TOMOGRAPHY SCAN or MAGNETIC RESONANCE IMAG-ING, will usually be needed to assess bones, joints, and neurological problems such as those caused by compression of the SPINAL CORD. Most patients also exhibit mild to severe POSTURE problems, such as SCOLIOSIS and KYPHOSIS.

In discussing one type of dysplasia, the Greenberg Center for Skeletal Dysplasias at Johns Hopkins said, "Orthopedic problems are common. The joints can be dislocated, especially the shoulder, elbows, hips, and patellae (knee caps). Flexion contractures of knees and shoulders are common. Scoliosis is not present at birth but often is progressive, especially in the early teens. Treatment of the scoliosis includes bracing and occasionally, spinal fusion. Progressive cervical kyphosis can also occur with subluxation of the cervical spine which can result in spinal cord compression."

Treatment Options and Outlook

Skeletal dysplasia frequently produces early onset of OSTEOARTHRITIS, but early treatment may lessen the severity. During formative bone growth, ORTHOTIC devices may help to prevent the progression of curvatures. If a skeletal deformity occurs, a LUMBAR LAMINECTOMY or other type of SURGERY may be needed.

Risk Factors and Preventive Measures

To assess the risk of skeletal dysplasia, genetic counseling includes a prenatal diagnosis during the second trimester of pregnancy. As parents consider their choices, one option includes participation in RESEARCH or CLINICAL TRIALS. In their "Research on Skeletal Dysplasias," for example, the European Skeletal Dysplasia Network has found "identifying groups of proteins associated with specific . . . structures or pathways, and how such patterns are perturbed as a result of pathological changes." Such findings may eventually produce preventives that address and, perhaps, even correct this group of disorders before skeletal defects occur.

European Skeletal Dysplasia Network. "Research on Skeletal Dysplasias." Available online. URL: http://www. esdn.org/research.html. Downloaded April 26, 2006.

Greenberg Center for Skeletal Dysplasias. "Diastrophic Dysplasia," Johns Hopkins Hospital Center for Medical Genetics. Available online. URL: http://www. hopkinsmedicine.org/greenbergcenter/diastrop.htm. Downloaded April 26, 2006.

Human Genome, The. "Growing Pains: Investigating Skeleton Disorders," Wellcome Trust. Available online. URL: http://genome.wellcome.ac.uk/doc%5Fwtd020828. html. Downloaded April 26, 2006.

skeletal fluorosis Caused by ENVIRONMENTAL INFLUENCES, this rare condition can result in skeletal deformities. According to the U.S. National Library of Medicine, "Skeletal fluorosis was first recognized in 1931 among workers processing cryolite," a natural fluoride but also a manufactured ingredient that occurs during the production of aluminum. With extended exposure, "patients may develop bony exostoses," or bony growths on the exterior surface of a bone, as well as "calcified ligaments, kyphosis, and spinal stenosis. Crippling skeletal fluorosis has been reported in workers with fluoride exposures of 20–80 mg/day for 10–20 years."

Symptoms and Diagnostic Path

In the online article entitled "Skeletal Fluorosis," GreenFacts.org said, "The early stages of skeletal fluorosis are characterized by increased bone mass, detectable by x-ray. If very high fluoride intake persists over many years, joint pain and stiffness may result from the skeletal changes."

Besides a patient history and physical examination, X-RAYS can monitor the resultant musculoskeletal conditions, such as KYPHOSIS or SPINAL STENOSIS. If symptoms include muscle wasting or indicate a neurological problem caused by SPINAL CORD compression, additional tests will be needed.

Treatment Options and Outlook

For the best treatment and outlook, an online article by Doctors D. Raja Reddy and Srikanth R. Deme advised, "In all cases of skeletal fluorosis prevention is the aim, since no cure is possible through medi-cal or surgical therapy, especially if it is allowed to develop to the stage when it becomes a crippling disease." Besides safe sources of WATER, "The plane of nutrition appears to play a crucial role in the incidence and severity of fluorosis and hence a balanced diet having adequate calcium and vitamins reduces the toxicity of fluoride."

Risk Factors and Preventive Measures

The article "Scientific Facts on Fluoride" posted by GreenFacts.org said, "In areas of the world with high levels of fluoride naturally present in minerals and water, intake of fluoride from drinking water and foodstuffs is the primary cause for endemic skeletal fluorosis, a crippling disability that affects millions of people in various parts of Africa, China and India. In some regions, the indoor burning of fluoride-rich coal also serves as an important source of fluoride." In the United States, "When drinking water is artificially fluoridated, the 'optimum' level of fluoride, associated with the maximum level of dental caries protection and minimum level of dental fluorosis, is considered to be approximately 1 mg/litre." Dental products increase potential intake, but such amounts remain minimal. However, "at total fluoride intakes of 14 mg/day, there is clear evidence of skeletal fluorosis and an increased risk of bone fractures; at total intake levels above about 6 mg fluoride/day the evidence is suggestive of an increased risk of effects on bone." Therefore, the best preventive comes in being aware of individual intake, prolonged exposure, and personal sensitivities. Healthful NUTRITION emphasizing CALCIUM and the nutrients in fresh fruits and vegetables can also detoxify the body.

GreenFacts.org. "Scientific Facts on Fluoride," GreenFacts™. Available online. URL: http://www.greenfacts. org/fluoride/fluorides-2/99-conclusion.htm#0. Downloaded April 26, 2006.

———. "Skeletal Fluorosis," GreenFacts™. Available online. URL: http://www.greenfacts.org/glossary/pqrs/ skeletal-fluorosis.htm. Downloaded April 26, 2006.

Reddy, D. Raja and Srikanth R. Deme. "Skeletal Fluorosis." Available online. URL: http://www.medvarsity. com/vmu1.2/dmr/dmrdata/cme/fluorosis/Fluorosis. htm. Downloaded April 26, 2006.

U.S. National Library of Medicine. "Skeletal Fluorosis," Haz-Map, National Institutes of Health. Available online. URL: http://hazmap.nlm.nih.gov/cgi-bin/hazmap_generic?tbl=TblDiseases&id=247. Last updated July 20, 2004.

sleep   As a most basic need, rest restores. Restful sleep detoxifies the body, repairs cells, and builds bone tissue, especially when assisted by life-giving NUTRITION and vital amounts of WATER. Adequate rest keeps the mind alert, yet just a night or two of sleep deprivation makes a person physically and mentally unstable. Whether in the form of a catnap or deep rest, each stage of sleep has some measure of recuperative power.

The National Institute of Neurological Disorders and Stroke (NINDS) further explained, "Deep sleep coincides with the release of growth hormone in children and young adults. Many of the body's cells also show increased production and reduced breakdown of proteins during deep sleep. Since proteins are the building blocks needed for cell growth and for repair of damage from factors like stress and ultraviolet rays, deep sleep may truly be 'beauty sleep'." Since sleep requirements change over time, "the amount of sleep each person needs depends on many factors, including age. Infants generally require about 16 hours a day, while teenagers need about 9 hours on average. For most adults, 7 to 8 hours a night appears to be the best amount of sleep, although some people may need as few as 5 hours or as many as 10 hours of sleep each day. Women in the first 3 months of pregnancy often need several more hours of sleep than usual. The amount of sleep a person needs also increases if he or she has been deprived of sleep in previous days. Getting too little sleep creates a 'sleep debt,' which is much like being overdrawn at a bank. Eventually, your body will demand that the debt be repaid."

Risks and Complications

Patients in pain have a greater risk of developing sleep problems. Likewise, patients who have trouble sleeping have an increased risk of pain. As the National Sleep Foundation reported, "a recent study found that about two-thirds of patients with chronic back pain suffered sleep trouble. This same study suggests that disrupted sleep seems to make the pain feel worse. Some pain medication, such as analgesics, may alter sleep patterns and make sleeping more difficult." Alcohol, nicotine, caffeine, antidepressants, and emotional encounters at bedtime increase the likelihood of insomnia, but then ACUTE PAIN, CHRONIC BACK PAIN, BACKACHES, CERVICOGENIC HEADACHES, and LOW BACK PAIN can keep anyone awake.

Statistics and Studies

A study of the effects of ACUPUNCTURE on pain and sleep in *Medical Acupuncture: A Journal for Physicians By Physicians* reported the following results: "Among the 11 patients with low back pain (including 3 with failed back syndrome), 36% (4), 36% (4), and 9% (1) reported significant, moderate, and mild degrees of pain relief, respectively. Nine percent (1), 36.3% (4), and 36.3% (4) reported significant, moderate, and mild degrees of sleep improvement, respectively. In addition, 9% (1), 64% (7), and 9% (1) of patients with low back pain reported significant, moderate, and mild degrees of a sense of improvement in well-being with acupuncture treatment." Regarding the CERVICAL SPINE, "eight patients with chronic neck pain were treated with acupuncture. Seven demonstrated pain relief with acupuncture: 37.5% (3), 37.5% (3), and 12.5% (1) showed significant, moderate, and mild degrees of pain relief, respectively. Five reported sleep improvement: 37.5% (3) and 25% (2) showed a significant and moderate degree of improvement, respectively."

At the National Institutes of Health (NIH), some studies of sleep aids focused on valerian, a form of HERBAL THERAPY. Subsequently, the NIH Office of Dietary Supplements reported, "Although the results of some studies suggest that valerian may be useful for insomnia and other sleep disorders, results of other studies do not. Interpretation of these studies is complicated by the fact the studies had small sample sizes, used different amounts and sources of valerian, measured different outcomes, or did not consider potential bias resulting from high participant withdrawal rates. Overall, the evidence from these trials for the sleep-promoting effects of valerian is inconclusive." Despite a lack of scientific proof, the NIH also said, "Valerian has been used as a medicinal herb since at least the time of ancient Greece and Rome. Its therapeutic uses were described by Hippocrates, and in the 2nd century, Galen prescribed valerian for insomnia." While this ancient treatment may not help some patients, others find the herb relaxing, assuming, of course, that its wet-dog or sweaty-sock smell does not keep a person awake.

Special Aids and Adaptations

As ads often attest, restful sleep begins with a good mattress. This does not refer to price so much as to whether the coils, air, water, or foam cushioning can hold the SPINE in a neutral position. Similarly, pillows should be chosen to keep the neck neutral, so the head tilts neither up nor down. People who sleep on the side often do well with a firm pillow, while BACK sleepers may prefer a medium one. Although stomach sleeping can produce NECK PAIN, this may be avoidable with a down-soft pillow that lays almost flat.

If a comfortable environment does not have the desired effect, comforting forms of MASSAGE THERAPY may sooth INFANTS, CHILDREN, and ELDERLY persons who resist sleep or just have trouble relaxing. For active ADOLESCENTS and adults, daily ACTIVITY or EXERCISE may start a day off right, but evening exercises seldom end well in sleep. HOMEOPATHIC MEDICINE or other temporary sleep aids may help, but adapting a routine conducive to rest provides a better option. For example, poor sleepers might practice techniques to reduce TENSION then wait until a half hour or so before bedtime to take a CALCIUM supplement and a warm bath. For patients with chronic back or joint pain, a PAIN RELIEVER an hour or two before bedtime may ease discomfort in time to catch sight of a few sweet dreams.

Goldberg, Joan Rachel. "Helping Yourself to a Good Night's Sleep," National Sleep Foundation. Available online. URL: http://www.sleepfoundation.org/sleeplibrary/index.php?secid=&id=55. Downloaded April 26, 2006.

Leung, Albert Y., M.D. "Effect of Acupuncture on the Quality of Life in Patients with Chronic Pain: A Prospective Outcome Measure," *Medical Acupuncture: A Journal for Physicians By Physicians* 14, no. 2. Available online. URL: http://www.medicalacupuncture.org/aama_marf/journal/vol14_2/article7.html. Downloaded April 26, 2006.

National Institute of Neurological Disorders and Stroke. "Brain Basics: Understanding Sleep," NINDS, National Institutes of Health. Available online. URL: http://www.ninds.nih.gov/disorders/sleep_apnea/detail_sleep_apnea.htm. Last updated January 25, 2006.

National Sleep Foundation. "Pain and Sleep," Sleep Library. Available online. URL: http://www.sleepfoundation.org/sleeplibrary/index.php?secid=&id=63. Downloaded April 26, 2006.

Office of Dietary Supplements. "Questions and Answers About Valerian for Insomnia and Other Sleep Disorders," National Institutes of Health. Available online. URL: http://ods.od.nih.gov/factsheets/valerian.asp. Downloaded April 26, 2006.

slipped disc   See HERNIATED DISC.

spina bifida   A BIRTH DEFECT OF THE SPINE, spina bifida is often obvious in INFANTS born with an opening in the BACK where none should be. Although spina bifida means cleft spine, not all forms of the disorder may be readily apparent. In explaining the contributive conditions, the Centers for Disease Control and Prevention said, "Neural tube defects (NTDs) are major birth defects of a baby's brain or spine. They happen when the neural tube (that later turns into the brain and spine) doesn't form right, and the baby's brain or spine is damaged. This happens within the first few weeks a woman is pregnant, often before a woman knows that she is pregnant."

According to the Spina Bifida Association (SBA), the three types of spina bifida include occulta, meningocele, and myelomeningocele. Regarding the first and mildest type, the SBA said, "Often called hidden spina bifida, the spinal cord and the nerves are usually normal and there is no opening on the back. In this usually harmless form of spina bifida, there is a small defect or gap in a few of the small bones (vertebrae) that make up the spine. There may be no motor or sensory impairments evident at birth; subtle, progressive neurologic deterioration often becomes evident in later childhood or adulthood. In many instances, spina bifida occulta is so mild that there is no disturbance of spinal function at all. Occulta can be diagnosed at any age." With the meningocele type, "the protective coatings (meninges) come through the open part of the spine like a sac that is pushed out. Cerebrospinal fluid is in the sac and there is usually no nerve damage. Individuals may suffer minor disabilities. New problems can develop later in life." At birth, however, the myelomeningocele type of spina bifida may be more apparent and more severe. "This occurs when the meninges (protective covering of the spinal cord) and spinal nerves come through the open part of the spine. This is the most serious type of spina bifida, which causes nerve damage and more severe disabilities." As the SBA reported, some form of the disorder occurs in the United States in about seven out of every 10,000 births.

Symptoms and Diagnostic Path

A small gap in the VERTEBRAE or an opening in the SPINE alerts a pediatrician. If not, subtle symptoms may appear gradually and include muscle spasm, SCOLIOSIS, or some evidence that the baby experiences spinal discomfort or LOW BACK PAIN.

The American Association of Neurological Surgeons explained, "At birth, the spinal cord is normally located opposite the disc between the first and second lumbar vertebrae in the upper part of the lower back. In a baby with spina bifida, the spinal cord is still attached to the surrounding skin, preventing it from ascending normally, so the spinal cord is low-lying or tethered. Although the skin is separated and closed at birth, the spinal cord stays in the same location after the closure. As the child continues to grow, the spinal cord can become stretched, causing damage and interfering with the blood supply to the spinal cord. This can result in back pain, leg pain, changes in leg strength, progressive or repeated muscle contractions, orthopedic deformities of the legs and scoliosis, and bowel and bladder problems. A definitive diagnosis of a tethered spinal cord is made through diagnostic tests." Releasing a tethered SPINAL CORD often requires SURGERY. "However, since symptoms of tethering can occur during periods of growth, 10 to 20 percent require repeated surgery."

Treatment Options and Outlook

Newborns with severe spina bifida may need surgery within the first hours of life. In less severe cases, babies typically exhibit lower leg move-ments. This normal motion shows they have a good chance of walking when, as young CHILDREN, they reach the mobile stage of their development. Surgery may not be needed for these young patients, but some may require an ORTHOTIC device such as a back brace to slow the progression of a curvature in POSTURE. Others patients may eventually require a walker or wheelchair to achieve mobility.

Risk Factors and Preventive Measures

Spina bifida actually begins in the first month of pregnancy when something hinders normal spinal development. Such malformations can often be prevented if the mother has ample intake of FOLIC ACID or a VITAMIN B-COMPLEX before pregnancy begins. Well-balanced NUTRITION in general also helps a fetus to develop normally, but to be effective, nutrients need to be readily available from the start of life.

Besides obvious physical concerns apparent in infancy or early childhood, older children and ADOLESCENTS with spina bifida may encounter additional problems as they try to adjust. As a fact sheet from the National Dissemination Center for Children with Disabilities said, "Children with myelomeningocele need to learn mobility skills, and often require the aid of crutches, braces, or wheelchairs. It is important that all members of the school team and the parents understand the child's physical capabilities and limitations. Physical disabilities like spina bifida can have profound effects on a child's emotional and social development. To promote personal growth, families and teachers should encourage children, within the limits of safety and health, to be independent and to participate in activities with their nondisabled classmates."

Centers for Disease Control and Prevention. "Folic Acid," CDC, Department of Health and Human Services. Available online. URL: http://www.cdc.gov/ncbddd/folicacid/faqs.htm#spina. Downloaded April 27, 2006.
National Dissemination Center for Children with Disabilities. "Spina Bifida," NICHCY, Fact Sheet 12. Available online. URL: http://www.nichcy.org/pubs/factshe/fs12txt.htm. Downloaded April 27, 2006.
NeurosurgeryToday.org. "Spina Bifida," American Association of Neurological Surgeons. Available online. URL: http://www.neurosurgerytoday.org/what/patient_e/spina.asp. Downloaded April 27, 2006.

Spina Bifida Association. "Are There Different Types of Spina Bifida?," SBA. Available online. URL: http://www.sbaa.org/site/PageServer?pagename=nrc_faqtypesofsb. Downloaded April 27, 2006.

spinal cord   About a foot and a half long at maturity, the spinal cord extends from the skull to the waistline, connecting the brain to the rest of the body as extensions of spinal nerves plug into the areas to which they have been assigned. Normally, the spinal column surrounds and protects the spinal cord and its circuitry of spinal nerves. If, however, the VERTE-BRAE or stabilizing soft tissue endure a severe injury, massive bone loss, or bone-altering disease, such as CANCER, a spinal cord injury (SCI) may result.

Risks and Complications

The National Cancer Institute reported, "Spinal cord compression occurs in 10 to 20 percent of all cancer patients, especially lung, prostate and breast cancer patients. When a tumor spreads to the vertebrae, the spinal cord can be compressed and can cause some patients to lose mobility or bladder control." In such cases, SURGERY may be needed to remove a tumor, ease vertebral pressure, and/or stabilize the spine.

More often, vehicular accidents and severe injuries to ATHLETES cause spinal cord injuries. If damage involves the THORACIC SPINE, paraplegia or paralysis in both legs may result, whereas a CERVICAL SPINE trauma can produce paralysis of the legs, arms, neck, and respiratory system. As information on the Apparelyzed Web site explained, "Quadriplegia / Tetraplegia is when a person has a spinal cord injury above the first thoracic vertebra" so that "paralysis usually affects the cervical spinal nerves resulting in paralysis of all four limbs. In addition to the arms and legs being paralyzed, the abdominal and chest muscles will also be affected resulting in weakened breathing and the inability to properly cough and clear the chest. People with this type of paralysis are referred to as Quadriplegic or Tetraplegic."

A comprehensive article in *Emergency Nurse* explained the biomechanics of various types of spinal cord injury. For example, "the junction between C7 and T1" vertebrae represents "the border between the flexible cervical spine and the rigid thoracic spine, and is the most susceptible to vertebral column damage. This is because, when force is applied to the cervical spine, it is directed downwards because of the latter's flexibility, and is focused on the cervical-thoracic junction. The region must be examined on X-ray therefore before it is given the all-clear." Also, "a similarly important junction exists between T12 and L1, which is between the rigid thoracic and more mobile lumbar regions. This is the second most common site of spinal injury" reported in the United Kingdom.

Statistics and Studies

The National Spinal Cord Injury Association provided these statistics: "Approximately 250,000–400,000 individuals in the United States have spinal cord injuries. Every year, approximately 11,000 people sustain new spinal cord injuries—that's thirty new injuries every day. Most of these people are injured in auto and sports accidents, falls, and industrial mishaps. An estimated 60 percent of these individuals are 30 years old or younger, and the majority of them are men."

The Spinal Cord Injury Information Network further reported, "Persons with tetraplegia have sustained injuries to one of the eight cervical segments of the spinal cord; those with paraplegia have lesions in the thoracic, lumbar, or sacral regions of the spinal cord." However, such injuries do not always bring total paralysis. If some activity or sensations in the muscles continue, the paralysis may be incomplete. "Since 2000, the most frequent neurologic category at discharge of persons reported to the database is incomplete tetraplegia (34.5%), followed by complete paraplegia (23.1%), complete tetraplegia (18.4%), and incomplete paraplegia (17.5%). Less than 1% of persons experienced complete neurologic recovery by hospital discharge. Over time, the percentage of persons with incomplete tetraplegia has increased slightly while both complete paraplegia and complete tetraplegia have decreased slightly." Of the reported cases, "today 88.1% of all persons with SCI who are discharged alive from the system are sent to a private, non-institutional residence (in most cases their homes before injury). Only 5.3% are discharged to nursing homes. The remaining are discharged to hospitals, group living situations or other destinations."

Special Aids and Adaptations

Stem cell RESEARCH may eventually restore damaged spinal cords. As the National Institute of Neurological Disorders and Stroke (NINDS) reported, "For the past 25 years, rehabilitation practices have focused on compensation rather than recovery. Assistive devices have been used to supplement visible functions—mostly intact voluntary movements—but little effort has been directed at understanding and exploiting the nervous system's capacity for retraining. Recent work has greatly enhanced rehabilitation strategies by demonstrating how weight-loading and . . . feedback can lead to recovery of locomotor function."

With new aids on the horizon, effective adaptations may come from outer space. As the NINDS said, "Astronauts exposed to microgravity suffer from physiological alterations that resemble those experienced by patients with SCI, including muscle atrophy, bone loss, disruption of locomotion and coordination, and impairment of functions regulated by the autonomic system. Although astronauts suffer from a mostly reversible and milder degree of the symptoms, the similarities are significant enough to suggest that both areas of research could benefit from each other's findings and therapeutic developments."

Apparelyzed. "Types of Paralysis—Quadriplegia and Paraplegia," Spinal Cord Injury Peer Support. Available online. URL: http://www.apparelyzed.com/paralysis.html. Downloaded April 27, 2006.

National Cancer Institute. "Surgery Helps Relieve Spinal Cord Compression Caused by Metastatic Cancer," National Institutes of Health. Available online. URL: http://www.cancer.gov/clinicaltrials/results/spinal-cord-compression0603. Downloaded April 27, 2006.

National Institute of Neurological Disorders and Stroke. "Functional and Dysfunctional Spinal Circuitry: Role for Rehabilitation and Neural Prostheses," NINDS, National Institutes of Health. Available online. URL: http://www.ninds.nih.gov/news_and_events/proceedings/spinalcircuitrywkshp.htm. Last updated February 9, 2005.

National Spinal Cord Injury Association. "About Spinal Cord Injury," NSCIA. Available online. URL: http://www.spinalcord.org/html/injury.php. Downloaded April 27, 2006.

Sheerin, Fintan. "Spinal Cord Injury: Causation and Pathophysiology," Emergency Nurse 12, no. 9 (February 2005): 29–38.

Spinal Cord Injury Information Network. "SPINAL CORD INJURY Facts and Figures at a Glance," National Spinal Cord Injury Statistical Center (NSCISC.) Available online. URL: http://www.spinalcord.uab.edu/show.asp?durki=21446. Downloaded April 27, 2006.

spinal curvature   See FLAT BACK; KYPHOSIS; LORDOSIS; POSTURE; SCOLIOSIS.

spinal decompression   See LAMINECTOMY, LAMINOTOMY; TRACTION.

spinal fusion   See ARTHRODESIS.

spinal imbalance   See VERTEBRAL SUBLUXATION.

spinal infection   Bacteria or fungus anywhere in the body can invade spinal DISCS and VERTEBRAE, producing an abscess or infection in the SPINE. Such infections can be brought on by an anaerobic microorganism that does not need oxygen to survive or by an aerobic microorganism that must have air. Either way, the American Academy of Orthopaedic Surgeons said, "Disease-carrying bacteria, viruses and parasites that get into the body can destroy healthy tissue, multiply and spread through blood. Infection of skin and other soft tissue can lead to infection of bones (osteomyelitis) and joints (septic arthritis). Without prompt treatment, orthopaedic infections can become chronic."

According to a Spine-surgery.com article, "Infections of the spinal column is a very broad topic and includes those diseases that arise spontaneously and those that are secondary to some inciting event. True infections are uncommon, particularly in the industrialized countries of the world," mainly because of the sanitary conditions that prevent or discourage an invasion of germs. Almost any type of SURGERY, however, carries the risk of infection. For example, "post-operative wound infections range from 1% after a simple discectomy to 6–8% after attempted fusion with hardware."

Symptoms and Diagnostic Path

BACK pain, fever, and stiffness may signal a spinal infection. As a report in the *Southern Medical Journal (SMJ)* stated, "Insidious back pain and signs of spinal cord compression are the most common presenting signs and symptoms; fever is seen in only about 40% of cases of anaerobic infection of the vertebrae or disk space. As for aerobic infection, the lumbar region (43%) was the most commonly involved site of vertebral body or disk involvement. A number of radiographic modalities may identify destructive changes and even gas formation consistent with vertebral body or disk space infection, including plain films, radionuclide bone scanning, Gallium scanning, tomography, CT, and MRI." An X-RAY radiograph, COMPUTED TOMOGRAPHY (CT) SCAN, and MAGNETIC RESONANCE IMAGING (MRI) may all be requested. However, the *SMJ* article said, "Of these, MRI has the most diagnostic accuracy."

Treatment Options and Outlook

The *SMJ* article also advised, "Prolonged courses of . . . antibiotics are generally sufficient for improvement or cure. Relapse is uncommon, and surgical debridement" to remove unhealthy tissue "or drainage of spinal or paraspinal abscesses are occasionally required to optimize outcome."

Risk Factors and Preventive Measures

According to the North American Spine Society, "spinal infections may occur following surgery or spontaneously in patients with certain risk factors. Risk factors for spinal infections include poor nutrition, immune suppression, human immunodeficiency virus (HIV) infection, cancer, diabetes, and obesity." Also, "surgical risk factors include a long surgical time, instrumentation, and re-operations. Infections occur in up to 4% of surgical cases, despite the numerous preventative measures that are taken. The likelihood of an infection increases with the number of operations in an area. Most postoperative infections occur between 3 days and 3 months after the time of surgery." Because of the sanitary precautions found in most hospitals though, a greater risk occurs if a patient with an existing infection in one part of the body needs emergency surgery that exposes the spine or other areas of the body to the contagious cells or tissue.

During or after a spinal infection, CHILDREN may be especially prone to develop DISCITIS. The risk of that or other complications can increase for patients of all ages who have CANCER, RHEUMATOID ARTHRITIS, or other conditions affecting the immune system. To prevent a spinal infection from occurring, even a minor cut, scrape, or scratch should be cleaned, medicated, and watched for signs of oozing, swelling, or redness. Optimal preventives in general include good NUTRITION, ample intake of fresh WATER, adequate SLEEP, and daily ACTIVITY or regular EXERCISE to build up the immune system and maintain overall good health.

American Academy of Orthopaedic Surgeons. "Infections," AAOS. Available online. URL: http://orthoinfo.aaos.org/fact/thr_report.cfm?Thread_ID=260&topcategory=Injury%20Prevention. Downloaded April 28, 2006.

North American Spine Society. "Spinal Infection," NASS. Available online. URL: http://www.spine.org/fsp/prob_action-injury-infection.cfm. Last updated March 3, 2005.

Saeed, Musah U., M.D., Paul Mariani, M.D., Candelaria Martin, M.D., Raymond A. Smego Jr., M.D., Anil Potti, M.D., Robert Tight, M.D., and David Thiege, M.D. "Anaerobic Spondylodiscitis: Case Series and Systematic Review," *Southern Medical Journal* 98, no. 2 (February 2005): 144–148.

Young, Michael J., M.D. and Richard T. Holt, M.D. "Infections of the Spine," Spine-surgery.com. Available online. URL: http://www.spine-surgery.com/Articles/infections.html. Downloaded April 28, 2006.

spinal injection   Several types of spinal injections can be used to confirm a diagnosis, locate a site of vertebral pain or inflammation, and ease discomfort in the SPINE. Usually, the specific type of injection refers to the locale. For instance, an EPIDURAL INJECTION goes into the epidural space around the SPINAL CORD and can be used to treat SCIATICA, SPINAL STENOSIS, or other condition affecting various regions of the spine. A SELECTIVE NERVE ROOT BLOCK goes into inflamed nerves such as those flaring up to protect a HERNIATED DISC. A facet joint injection may treat FACET JOINT DISORDER, while a DISCOGRAM, of course, concerns the DISCS. To treat intense pain and swelling in, say, ARTHRITIS, a CORTICOSTEROID INJECTION may be used, but steroid injections may also be given to keep down spinal cord swelling after a FLEXION-EXTENSION INJURY.

Risks and Complications

Any invasive procedure that pierces the skin carries a risk of infection. Some injections, such as a discogram, require a contrast dye that can cause an allergic reaction. Also, the needle may slip into an area other than the one intended, especially if wielded by the hand of an inexperienced technician.

Statistics and Studies

Radiology published an article based on the study of "Spinal Injection Procedures: Volume, Provider Distribution, and Reimbursement in the U.S. Medicare Population from 1993 to 1999." After reviewing these records, the authors reported, "Despite an overall increase in spinal injection procedure volume and reimbursement . . . , nonradiologists performed most of these procedures. Epidural steroid and facet joint injections had the highest volume and reimbursement during this time period and were performed almost exclusively by nonradiologists (predominantly anesthesiologists). Radiologists performed more discography procedures than did other specialists . . . , but participation decreased each year, while anesthesiologist participation increased; as of 1999, anesthesiologists performed more discography procedures than did radiologists." What difference does this make? Maybe none. However, patients might want to ask their doctors who will perform the injection and what training or experience that person has.

Special Aids and Adaptations

A spinal injection will usually be accompanied by FLUOROSCOPY or X-RAYS. Whether used as a test or a treatment, this outpatient procedure commonly begins with a local anesthetic and ends within 30 minutes or less.

Carrino, J. A., W. B. Morrison, L. Parker, M. E. Schweitzer, D. C. Levin, and J. H. Sunshine. "Spinal Injection Procedures: Volume, Provider Distribution, and Reimbursement in the U.S. Medicare Population from 1993 to 1999," *Radiology* 225, no. 3 (December 2002): 723–731.

International Spine Intervention Society. "About Spinal Injection Procedures . . . ," ISIS. Available online. URL: http://www.spinalinjection.com/a/pes/pes1.htm. Downloaded April 28, 2006.

North American Spine Society. "Spinal Injections," NASS. Available online. URL: http://www.spine.org/articles/injections.cfm. Downloaded April 28, 2006.

spinal injury   Trauma to DISCS and VERTEBRAE can occur anytime or anywhere in the BACK and SPINE. A whiplash may damage the CERVICAL SPINE of a passenger in a car accident, but a similar FLEXION-EXTENSION INJURY can injure an ATHLETE during a contact sport or an INFANT with SHAKEN INFANT SYNDROME. A BIRTH INJURY TO THE SPINE affects a newborn too. In ELDERLY patients, a fall may produce a RIB INJURY or damage the SACRAL VERTEBRAE or COCCYGEAL SPINE, but the same can happen to a child falling off a bicycle. CHILDREN and ADOLESCENTS who forget BACKPACK SAFETY become prone to injuries of the THORACIC SPINE or LUMBAR SPINE, and so do workers who exceed their LOAD TOLERANCE or forget to use safe techniques while LIFTING. Patients with severe bone loss caused by CANCER, OSTEOPOROSIS, or other ongoing conditions may encounter the injury of a VERTEBRAL COMPRESSION FRACTURE simply by walking.

Risks and Complications

According to an article in *The Indian Journal of Radiology and Imaging*, "Management of severe injury to the vertebral column is a frequently encountered problem in a Regional Trauma center. The particular vulnerability of the Cervical Spine has been stressed," since a trauma can potentially produce a FRACTURE, HERNIATED DISC, VERTEBRAL SUBLUXATION, or injury to the SPINAL CORD. Although the spinal cord may show no evidence of damage on an X-RAY, spinal cord injury is "a syndrome of cervical spinal cord trauma, describing post traumatic myelopathy," such as occurs when a trauma produces a spinal cord disease. "The injury is predominantly documented in children, probably due to increased elasticity of pediatric spine. It appears that strain of the cervical spine in any direction can injure the cord. In hyperextension, the cord gets damaged due to compression, while in hyper flexion, . . . injury occurs due to combination of stretching, tethering and vascular compromise" of the blood vessels. In any area of the spine, patients with a preexisting condition, such as SPINAL STENOSIS or ANKYLOSING SPONDYLITIS, may be at higher risk for a spinal injury.

Statistics and Studies

Accidents can happen to anyone, but the damage of one injury may be harder to detect than another. As the article "Initial Assessment of Spinal Trauma" reported, "Some studies of spinal trauma have recorded a missed injury rate as high as 33%. Delayed or missed diagnosis is usually attributed to failure to suspect an injury to the cervical spine, or to inadequate cervical spine radiology and incorrect interpretation of radiographs. An appropriate procedure for the evaluation of the potentially unstable spine must be robust and easy to implement, with a high sensitivity, given the potential importance of such injuries." For example, MAGNETIC RESONANCE IMAGING (MRI) may be needed to evaluate damage to spinal bones, ligaments, and soft tissue. The article also stated, "While it is tempting to focus on the cervical spine, it is important to assess and clear the entire spinal column. The thoracolumbar spine, while more protected, is at risk in major trauma and must be assessed both clinically and radiologically. Additionally, 5% of spinal injuries have a second, possibly non-adjacent, fracture elsewhere in the spine."

Special Aids and Adaptations

A cervical collar or back board provides initial aid in moving a patient with a possible spinal injury. If the trauma involves a whiplash, STEROID THERAPY within a few hours may lessen recovery time. Other types of spinal injuries, however, require other types of SPINAL INJECTIONS. For instance, the Spinal Injury Foundation mentioned a SELECTIVE NERVE ROOT BLOCK as offering good to high results for patients with disc herniation or pressure on the spinal nerves. In the first three months after a whiplash, SPINAL MANIPULATION may be highly effec-

tive, especially for patients with reduced RANGE OF MOTION. If muscle spasms follow an injury, MASSAGE THERAPY may work best. For spinal instability after an accident, ORTHOTICS, such as a neck brace, temporarily aid recovery, but severe instability may require SURGERY. If no bone loss or breakage occurs, ACUPUNCTURE, TRACTION, or a TRANSCUTANEOUS ELECTRONIC NERVE STIMULATOR (TENS) UNIT may reduce the pain.

Brohi, Karim. "Initial Assessment of Spinal Trauma," trauma.org 7:4, April 2002. Available online. URL: http://www.trauma.org/spine/cspine-eval.html. Downloaded April 28, 2006.

Khandelwal, S., G. L. Sharma, U. D. Saxena, P. Sakhi, S. Gopal, and P. Saxena. "Prospective Evaluation of Cervical Spine Injuries by MRI and Assessing Role of MR Findings in Predicting Prognosis," *The Indian Journal of Radiology and Imaging* 14, no. 1 (February 2004): 71–80.

Spinal Injury Foundation. "Patient Resources," SIF. Available online. URL: http://www.spinalinjuryfoundation.org/101_new/treatmen.htm. Downloaded April 28, 2006.

spinal loading   See LOAD TOLERANCE.

spinal manipulation   In this type of COMPLEMENTARY AND ALTERNATIVE MEDICINE (CAM), an osteopath or a chiropractor manually maneuvers the SPINE to realign the VERTEBRAE, relieve spinal pain, and improve RANGE OF MOTION in the spinal joints. Often, a high velocity thrust may be accompanied by a popping sound. Both the sound and the sudden maneuver may be somewhat disconcerting yet capable of correcting VERTEBRAL SUBLUXATION and some curvatures in POSTURE. Other types of spinal manipulation involve a quieter approach, but gentler techniques may require more sessions. To avoid discouragement, patients should ask how many sessions to expect. Regardless of the number of visits and type of technique used, the pain or numbness should lessen during the course of treatment.

Risks and Complications

A spinal correction, such as reestablishing the natural curve of the neck, usually requires several sessions. After each, some soreness may occur as PARASPINAL MUSCLES and vertebral joints readjust to a corrected position. That minor discomfort should soon pass. On very rare occasions, some patients experience nausea or dizziness that may require medical treatment, especially if the adjustment involved the CERVICAL SPINE.

An article in the *Journal of Manipulative and Physiological Therapeutics* reported on the safety of spinal manipulation in treating a lumbar disc herniation in the LUMBAR SPINE. One concern, for instance, was that spinal manipulation of a HERNIATED DISC might cause CAUDA EQUINA SYNDROME (CES.) Statistically though, "an estimate of the risk of spinal manipulation causing a clinically worsened disk herniation or CES in a patient presenting with LDH is calculated from published data to be less than 1 in 3.7 million."

Statistics and Studies

The National Center for Complementary and Alternative Medicine (NCCAM) reported, "Surveys of the U.S. population suggest that between 3 percent and 16 percent of adults receive chiropractic manipulation in a given year, while between 2 percent and 14 percent receive some form of massage therapy. In 1997, U.S. adults made an estimated 192 million visits to chiropractors and 114 million visits to massage therapists. Visits to chiropractors and massage therapists combined represented 50 percent of all visits to CAM practitioners."

Summarizing the effects of spinal manipulation, the NCCAM said, "The most abundant data regarding the possible mechanisms underlying chiropractic manipulation have been derived from studies in animals, especially studies on the ways in which manipulation may affect the nervous system. For example, it has been shown, by means of standard . . . techniques, that spinal manipulation evokes changes in the activity" between nerve cells in the nervous system and paraspinal muscle tissue. "Studies are under way to determine whether input from the paraspinal tissue also modulates pain processing in the spinal cord."

After studying osteopathic manipulative treatment (OMT), researchers reported in *The Journal of the American Osteopathic Association*, "Tissue injury and tissue repair each involve a complex and coordinated set of cellular mechanisms. . . . These increases in cell size and number aid the osteopathic physician in palpating the tissue texture changes." This means that, with a hands-on examination during the palpation process, an osteopath or other physician can feel the cellular changes produced, for instance, by a muscle STRAIN.

A study of military personnel found spinal manipulation "highly effective" when four of five criteria were met. As reported in the *Tufts University Health & Nutrition Letter*, the best results came among patients with LOW BACK PAIN that "lasted less than 16 days," with "no pain below the knee, a willingness to return to normal activities, stiffness in the lower spine, and relatively good rotation in the hips."

Special Aids and Adaptations

The aids of MASSAGE THERAPY, EXERCISE, and adaptation of maneuvers make spinal manipulation even more effective. As the *British Journal of Sports Medicine* reported, "Use of a variety of manual therapy techniques, rather than joint manipulation alone, appears to yield better results." After treating CERVICOGENIC HEADACHES, for example, "at the 12 month follow up, both manual therapy and specific exercise groups had significantly reduced headache frequency and intensity, neck pain, and disability. In this study, manual therapy included both low velocity cervical joint mobilisation techniques and high velocity manipulation techniques."

Dodd, John G., Meadow Maze Good, Tammy L. Nguyen, Andersen I. Grigg, Lyn M. Batia, and Paul R. Standley. "In Vitro Biophysical Strain Model for Understanding Mechanisms of Osteopathic Manipulative Treatment," *JAOA, The Journal of the American Osteopathic Association* 106, no. 3 (March 2006): 157–166.

National Center for Complementary and Alternative Medicine. "Manipulative and Body-Based Practices: An Overview," NCCAM, National Institutes of Health. Available online. URL: http://nccam.nih.gov/health/backgrounds/manipulative.htm. Last modified March 2, 2006.

Oliphant, D. "Safety of Spinal Manipulation in the Treatment of Lumbar Disk Herniations: a Systematic Review and Risk Assessment," *Journal of Manipulative and Physiological Therapeutics* 27, no. 3 (March–April 2004): 197–210.

Sran, M. M. "To Treat or Not to Treat: New Evidence for the Effectiveness of Manual Therapy," *British Journal of Sports Medicine* 2004; 38: 521–525, © 2004 BMJ Publishing Group Ltd. & British Association of Sport and Exercise Medicine. Available online. URL: http://bjsm.bmjjournals.com/cgi/content/full/38/5/521. Downloaded April 29, 2006.

Staff. "Will Spinal Manipulation Help You?" *Tufts University Health & Nutrition Letter* 23, no. 1 (March 2005): 3.

spinal meningitis   See MENINGITIS, MENINGOCOCCAL DISEASE.

spinal muscular atrophy   See WERDNIG-HOFFMAN DISEASE.

spinal stenosis   Through the center of the spinal column, a canal runs the length of the SPINAL CORD and provides its protective housing. If a BIRTH DEFECT OF THE SPINE makes the canal too small to accommodate the spinal cord, this can cause spinal stenosis in INFANTS or CHILDREN. More commonly, progressive changes in the spinal DISCS or VERTEBRAE cause this condition in ELDERLY people, ARTHRITIS patients, or persons with OSTEOPHYTES (bone spurs) obstructing the spinal canal.

The central spinal canal offers only one source of stenosis. As the National Institute of Arthritis and Musculoskeletal and Skin Diseases (NIAMS) explained, "Spinal stenosis is a narrowing of spaces in the spine (backbone) that results in pressure on the spinal cord and/or nerve roots. This disorder usually involves the narrowing of one or more of three areas of the spine: (1) the canal in the center of the column of bones (vertebral or spinal column) through which the spinal cord and nerve roots run, (2) the canals at the base or roots of nerves branching out from the spinal cord, or (3) the openings between vertebrae (bones of the spine) through which nerves leave the spine and go to other parts of the body." Subsequently, "the narrowing may involve a small or large area of the spine."

Symptoms and Diagnostic Path

If stenosis occurs in the CERVICAL SPINE, patients may experience NECK PAIN, CERVICOGENIC HEADACHE, or pain and numbness in the arms and hands. Vertebral slippage or SPONDYLOLISTHESIS may also occur. If stenosis affects the LUMBAR SPINE, symptoms include BACKACHE or LOW BACK PAIN with numbing effects often felt in the legs or lower portion of the body.

During a physical examination, the doctor may test the patient's RANGE OF MOTION. Also, X-RAYS or MAGNETIC RESONANCE IMAGING may be needed to assess the condition, especially if radiating pain suggests pressure on the spinal cord. However, many people with spinal stenosis have no symptoms and need no treatment.

Treatment Options and Outlook

NONSTEROIDAL ANTI-INFLAMMATORY DRUG THERAPY and appropriate EXERCISE to strengthen the BACK and PARASPINAL MUSCLES provide the initial options for treating stenosis. Severe cases may respond to physical therapy, EPIDURAL INJECTION, STEROID THERAPY, SPINAL INJECTION, or SURGERY.

In the article "Cervical Stenosis & Myelopathy," the North American Spine Society (NASS) said, "In mild cases of cervical stenosis with or without myelopathy," which is any disease involving the spinal cord, "nonoperative treatment may be suitable. However, in cases with increasing weakness, pain or the inability to walk, surgical treatment is usually recommended. Surgical options include anterior decompression," which involves frontal entry to relieve the pressure surgically, "and fusion, where the disc and bone material causing spinal cord compression is removed from the front and the spine is stabilized." For example, a LAMINECTOMY may be performed to remove bone spurs or deposits. To stabilize the area, a BONE GRAFT or BONE MORPHOGENETIC PROTEIN may be inserted to speed spinal fusion.

Regarding "The Clinical Syndrome Associated with Lumbar Spinal Stenosis," researchers from the United Kingdom reported, "Claudication-like symptoms may occur not only on walking but also on changing posture. It is our informal observation that some patients may develop radicular symptoms in the legs when standing; it is well known that the lumbar canal may narrow further on erect posture. . . . Furthermore, although claudication is usually defined as pain developing in the legs on walking, almost half of our patients with claudication symptoms complained of either weakness or numbness on walking rather than pain. . . . Pain seems to improve more often than motor weakness." Also, "two factors which correlated with poorer function were complaints of motor weakness in the limbs and significant comorbid disease," the latter of which refers to the coexistence of two potentially deadly diseases.

For patients over 50 whose symptoms ease on bending, a recently developed treatment may offer an improved outlook. As the orthopedic spine surgeon and reviewer of this book Dr. Arya N. Shamie explained, "A new device called the X Stop has been recently approved by the FDA as a minimally invasive treatment for spinal stenosis. The other benefit of the X Stop is that it can be implanted without general anesthesia. X Stop is an interspinous spacer that relieves spinal stenosis by indirectly decompressing the spinal canal." This titanium implant "puts single vertebrae in the flexed position where the spinal nerves have the least amount of pressure on them."

Risk Factors and Preventive Measures

People with bone spurs, OSTEOARTHRITIS, DWARF-ISM, OSTEITIS DEFORMANS, SKELETAL FLUOROSIS, SPINAL TUMOR, or adverse effects of WEIGHT may have a higher risk of developing spinal stenosis. Those with a BACK INJURY or a FLEXION-EXTENSION INJURY have increased risks too. Patients with stenosis in the lower back have a greater risk of CAUDA EQUINA SYNDROME.

The NASS article "Lumbar Spinal Stenosis" stated, "Symptoms of spinal stenosis frequently result in activity avoidance. This results in reduced flexibility, strength and cardiovascular endurance." To avert those risks and prevent flare-ups of pain, "a physical therapy or exercise program usually begins with stretching exercises to restore flexibility to tight muscles. You may be advised to stretch frequently to maintain flexibility gains."

Similarly, the American Academy of Orthopaedic Surgeons advised, "The best way to avoid the symptoms of lumbar spinal stenosis is to stay as physically fit as possible. Regular exercise can improve endurance and keep the muscles that support the spine strong. Avoiding weight gain can decrease the load that the lumbar spine has to carry. Patients should also avoid cigarette smoking. Both the smoke and the nicotine cause the spine to degenerate faster than normal."

Goh, Khean Jin, Wael Khalifa, Philip Anslow, Tom Cadoux-Hudson, and Michael Donaghy. "The Clinical Syndrome Associated with Lumbar Spinal Stenosis," *European Neurology* 52, no. 4 (2004): 242–249.

Lim, Moe R., M.D., Joon Y. Lee, M.D., Alan S. Hilibrand, M.D., John A. Glaser, M.D., and Nancy Fehr. "Lumbar Spinal Stenosis," American Academy of Orthopaedic Surgeons. Available online. URL: http://orthoinfo.aaos. org/fact/thr_report.cfm?Thread_ID=128&topcategory= Spine. Downloaded April 29, 2006.

National Institute of Arthritis and Musculoskeletal and Skin Diseases. "Questions & Answers About Spinal Stenosis," NIAMS, National Institutes of Health. Available online. URL: http://www.niams.nih.gov/ hi/topics/spinalstenosis/spinal_sten.htm. Downloaded April 29, 2006.

North American Spine Society. "Cervical Stenosis & Myelopathy," NASS. Available online. URL: http:// www.spine.org/articles/cervicalstenosis.cfm. Downloaded April 29, 2006.

———. "Lumbar Spinal Stenosis," NASS. Available online. URL: http://www.spine.org/articles/lumbarspinalstenosis.cfm. Downloaded April 29, 2006.

spinal tap   See LUMBAR PUNCTURE.

spinal tuberculosis   Primarily occurring in CHILDREN, ADOLESCENTS, and young adults, tuberculosis can progress from the lungs to other parts of the body, often causing devastating effects on the BACK and SPINE. In Pott's disease, for example, tubercular SPINAL INFECTION in one or more VERTEBRAE can spread to the DISCS, causing OSTEOMYELITIS, SPINAL CORD compression, and bone deformity. Public health precautions and newer drugs eventually reduced outbreaks of this infectious disease in the United States, but developing countries continue to have high incidents of this ancient and contagious disease.

Symptoms and Diagnostic Path

The most common symptoms of BACKACHE and upper or LOW BACK PAIN may be accompanied by fever, fatigue, and muscle weakness. During a physical examination, RANGE OF MOTION tests may spark ACUTE PAIN that subsides when the patient lies down. A diagnosis may be delayed, though, since DEGENERATIVE DISC DISEASE, a HERNIATED DISC, and other conditions produce similar symptoms. X-RAYS will be needed with laboratory tests to confirm the disease. Additional tests, such as a needle biopsy or MAGNETIC RESONANCE IMAGING, can evaluate bone and soft tissue damage.

Treatment Options and Outlook

Multi-drug therapies offer a promising outlook, but such treatments do not begin until the disease has been confirmed. If the patient delays seeking help or some other factor delays a diagnosis, vertebral bones and discs may become damaged or even start to disintegrate.

An online article from the University of Rochester Medical Center said, "Pott's disease (Spinal Tuberculosis) is the most dangerous form of musculoskeletal tuberculosis because it can cause bone destruction, deformity and paraplegia." The latter may occur since the condition commonly involves the THORACIC SPINE, LUMBAR SPINE, and weight-bearing SACRAL VERTEBRAE. "Tuberculosis may spread from that area to adjacent intervertebral discs," progressively causing vertebral collapse and severe POSTURE problems, such as KYPHOSIS. CERVICAL SPINE involvement may also occur, producing SPINAL STENOSIS or, possibly, paralysis. "The spinal canal can be narrowed. . . . Abscesses in the lumbar region may . . . eventually erode into the skin." Also, "neurologic compression occurs in 50% of the cases and includes spinal cord compression with paraplegia . . . and impaired sensation and nerve root pain or cauda equina symptoms. Severe neurologic complications occur in cervical spine tuberculosis. Spine deformity of some degree occurs in almost every patient," which may necessitate SURGERY.

Neurology India published an analysis of a surgical procedure used for 61 patients. According to the review, "anterior spinal instrumentation," which involves a spinal implant and a frontal approach to surgery, "is needed to support the collapsed anterior weight-bearing column of the cervical spine." This not only spared each patient the additional surgery required to obtain a BONE GRAFT, but the method produced better spinal fusion. Also, drug therapy and chemotherapy could continue without interruption, which was crucial since "modern chemotherapy has a significant impact on the natural progression and treatment outcomes in tuberculosis. Tuberculosis infection can be completely cured with adequate treatment."

After studying the progress of patients with spinal tuberculosis who were successfully treated, a group of researchers reported their findings in an article for the *Indian Journal of Tuberculosis*. According to the report, "in the treated patients (cured) the memory response to *M. tuberculosis* antigen is retained," reportedly "even after 10–15 years of treatment."

Risk Factors and Preventive Measures

The July 2004 issue of the *Cleveland Clinical Journal of Medicine* published a comprehensive overview entitled, "Spinal Tuberculosis Deserves a Place on the Radar Screen." According to that article, "Among large immigrant families, one family member might carry active disease and infect other members of the family over time. . . . Similarly, patients who have recently traveled to developing countries, who have visited friends or family members from those areas, or who have a known exposure to someone with tuberculosis also are at higher risk." In the United States and elsewhere, "within cities, the homeless, intravenous drug users, alcoholics, and the chronically ill are at higher risk of contracting active tuberculosis." Risks lessen, however, for patients who have the benefits of preventive measures available through adequate NUTRITION, habits of cleanliness, and prompt medical attention.

Ahsan, Humera, Mashhood-ul-Haque-Qazi, and Per-Lennart Westesson, M.D. "Neuroradiology Case of the Week: Case 117," Radiology, University of Rochester Medical Center. Available online. URL: http://www.urmc.rochester.edu/smd/Rad/neurocases/Neurocase 117.htm. Downloaded May 1, 2006.

"Immune Response to Mycobacterium Tuberculosis Culture Filtrate Antigen in Cured Spinal Tuberculosis Patients and Their Spouses," *Indian Journal of Tuberculosis* 48, no. 1 (2001): 3–6.

McLain, Robert F., M.D. and Carlos Isada, M.D. "Spinal Tuberculosis Deserves a Place on the Radar Screen," *Cleveland Clinical Journal of Medicine* 71, no. 7 (July 2004): 537–549.

Ramani, Premanand S., Alok Sharma, Sunil Jituri, and Dattatraya P. Muzumdar. "Anterior Instrumentation for Cervical Spine Tuberculosis: An Analysis of Surgical Experience with 61 Cases," *Neurology India* 53, no. 1 (March 2005): 83–89.

spinal tumor   Normally, cells reproduce, then begin their individual but cooperative work of building and repairing bones, organs, and soft tissue. If that cellular production goes wild, the new growth finds no place in the body, even if each cell remains harmless or benign. These wayward cells may cluster around DISCS or between VERTEBRAE, forming a primary spinal tumor that does not destroy bone but may put pressure on the SPINAL CORD and nerves. In similar random but rampant events, gangs of unruly cells can become hostile and attack healthy cells to establish a primary CANCER site. Unless stopped, the malignancy may spread, tumultuously producing tumors at secondary sites in the SPINE or other regions of the body.

An information page from the National Institute of Neurological Disorders and Stroke (NINDS) said, "In a small number of individuals, primary tumors may result from specific genetic disease (e.g., neurofibromatosis, tuberous sclerosis) or from exposure to radiation or cancer-causing chemicals." GENETIC FACTORS and ENVIRONMENTAL INFLUENCES may trigger malignant growth, but "the cause of most primary tumors remains a mystery. They are not contagious and, at this time, not preventable."

Symptoms and Diagnostic Path

Depending on the locale, spinal tumors may produce CERVICOGENIC HEADACHE, NECK PAIN, LOW BACK PAIN, or severe BACKACHES that hinder normal daily ACTIVITY and SLEEP. As the North American Spine Society Web site stated, "The symptoms associated with spinal cord tumors may also vary depending on the level of involvement. Cervical (neck) tumors may cause weakness or numbness in the arms or legs. Thoracic (mid-back) and lumbosacral (low-back) tumors may cause weakness or numb-ness in the chest area or legs. Difficulty walking is sometimes a complaint."

A medical history, family history, physical examination, and appropriate diagnostic tests will be needed. For instance, the doctor may order a biopsy to obtain a tissue sample for microscopic assessment of the conditions in the affected cells. Also, the physician may request X-RAY, POSITIVE EMISSION TOMOGRAPHY (PET) SCAN, or other imaging tests. If a benign tumor bears watching or a malignant tumor cannot be removed, MAGNETIC RESONANCE IMAGING (MRI) can be used to detect changes.

Treatment Options and Outlook

An article published in *The Journal of Bone & Joint Surgery* discussed the value of a biopsy in reaching an accurate diagnosis of the specific cancer in order to determine the most appropriate treatment. For instance, chordoma, a rare type of tumor, consists of growths in or around the spine, whereas a plasma-cell tumor involves the cells of such body liquids as blood plasma or lymph. As the article explained, "Depending on the circumstance, treatment based on assumptions of tumor type may lead to under-treatment (e.g., radiation therapy for chordoma, or hormonal treatment for parathyroid cancer) or overtreatment (e.g., corpectomy for plasma-cell tumor)." Also, "biopsy should be considered when a new spinal lesion appears in a patient with a previous or existing malignant lesion. This seems particularly important for patients who have had a lengthy disease-free interval, those who have solitary lesions, those who have low-grade or slowly progressive primary tumors, or those whose lesions have occurred in an atypical manner." In such instances, "needle biopsy would have revealed the true nature of these lesions in each case, without appreciable additional expense or risk." Furthermore, "biopsy should be strongly considered for such patients before initiating definitive . . . care, which usually involves high-dose irradiation or tumor-specific chemotherapy."

In discussing various treatments, the Cervical Spine Research Society (CSRS) said, "Some tumors of the spine may be treatable non-surgically. Treatment options include . . . radiation, . . . radiosurgery, and chemotherapy. Whether the tumor of the spine can be treated with radiation depends on several factors, including the size of tumor and the type of cells the tumor contains. Generally speaking, the smaller the tumor is, the more amenable it is to radiotherapy," which uses high-energy radiation to destroy cancer cells and reduce the tumor. "If the histology" or microscopic study "of the tumor is already known (either by biopsy or because of metastases), and the tumor is radiosensitive," thus responding to radiation, then "radiation therapy may be the only treatment necessary." Radiation can also be combined with SURGERY, such as CERVICAL LAMINAPLASTY, LAMINECTOMY, or VERTEBROPLASTY, "either to shrink the tumor pre-operatively or to treat remaining tumor after surgery. . . . Generally speaking, chemotherapy is reserved for patients with systemic metastases, or as an adjunct to surgical resection of malignant spinal cord tumors."

One rare, and often inoperable, malignant tumor may occur in the remnants of the notochord or rod of cells in unborn INFANTS that normally develops into the spinal vertebrae of the axial or central skeleton. This type of spinal tumor or chordoma can occur in CHILDREN but typically develops in ELDERLY patients, occurring twice as often in men. As the Bonetumor.org Web site explained, "Due to their origin in the notochord, chordomas occur in the mid-line of the axial skeleton. One half of cases occur in the sacrococcygeal region," around the sacrum and coccyx or tailbone, "and one third occur at the base of the skull." If located in the SACRAL VERTEBRAE or upper CERVICAL SPINE, this type of tumor can seldom be removed. For instance, "with sacrococcygeal tumors, sexual function and sphincter control may be compromised after surgery. Radiation is used if complete resection is impossible. Chordomas metastasize to lymph nodes, lungs, liver and bone. Chemotherapy can be used for late stage disease."

Presenting a more hopeful outlook for cancer treatments, the Thomas Jefferson University Hospital in Pennsylvania announced an innovative procedure that wraps radiation around the spine. According to that 2005 news release, "the technology, called shaped beam surgery, relies on sophisticated computers to tailor the shape and intensity of radiation beams to fit the exact size and shape of the tumor—all while sparing healthy tissue. It enables doctors to treat a range of hard-to-reach benign and malignant tumors in the brain and spine they couldn't treat before, often avoiding invasive surgery and speeding the patient's recovery."

As RESEARCH continues in hospitals, universities, and government agencies, researchers aim to find additional treatments and preventives to improve the outlook. For example, the NINDS reported, "Researchers are studying brachytherapy (small radioactive pellets implanted directly into the tumor) and advanced drugs and techniques for chemotherapy and radiation therapy. In gene therapy for brain and spinal cord tumors, scientists insert a gene to make the tumor cells sensitive to certain drugs, to program the cells to self-destruct, or to instruct the cells to manufacture substances to slow their growth. Scientists are also investigating why some genes become cancer-causing. Since tumors are more sensitive to heat than normal tissue, research scientists are testing hyperthermia as a treatment by placing special heat-producing antennae into the tumor region after surgery. In immunotherapy, scientists are looking for ways to duplicate or enhance the body's immune response to fight against brain and spinal cord cancer."

Risk Factors and Preventive Measures

With new possibilities forthcoming, ancient ones provide options too. For instance, the article "Acupuncture in Cancer Treatment" posted by the American Academy of Medical Acupuncture and written by an oncologist said, "Most oncologists have experienced the patients who start vomiting at the thought of their next clinic visit." Besides preventing such nauseating side effects, "acupuncture is effective for control of pain, of local swelling post-operatively, for shortening the resolution of hematoma and tissue swelling and for minimizing use of medications and their attendant side effects. Energetic acupuncture, an approach consisting of the use of needles with electricity and moxibustion (a form of local heating with herbs) imparts a sense of well-being and accelerates patients' recovery. In conjunction with nutritional support, its use is routinely employed in some cancer institutions."

Regarding NUTRITION, an emphasis on fruits, vegetables, grains, and such protective nutrients as VITAMIN A, VITAMIN C, and VITAMIN E can aid recovery, boost energy, and enhance the quality of life.

Some studies even indicate that healthful dietary choices, including ample fresh WATER, may prevent or reduce cancer cells. To avert the spread of an existing malignancy, early detection remains crucial. Therefore, regular medical examinations continue to decrease patient risk and provide optimal measures for stopping the growth of spinal tumors.

Arnold, Paul M., M.D. "Patient Information Sheet on Tumors Involving the Cervical Spine," Cervical Spine Research Society. Available online. URL: http://www.csrs.org/patientinfo/tumors.htm. Downloaded May 2, 2006.

DeGroot, Henry III, M.D. "Chordoma," Bonetumor.org. Available online. URL: http://bonetumor.org/tumors/pages/page101.html. Downloaded May 2, 2006.

Lewandrowski, Kai-Uwe, M.D., Daisure Togawa, M.D., Thomas W. Bauer, M.D., and Robert E. McLain, M.D. "A Role for Vertebral Biopsy in Selected Patients with Known Malignancy," *The Journal of Bone & Joint Surgery*, 87-A, no. 6 (June 2005): 1,348–1,353.

Mak, Eugene, M.D. "Acupuncture in Cancer Treatment," American Academy of Medical Acupuncture. Available online. URL: http://www.medicalacupuncture.org/acu_info/articles/cancertreatment.html. Downloaded May 2, 2006.

National Institute of Neurological Disorders and Stroke. "NINDS Brain and Spinal Tumors Information Page," National Institutes of Health. Available online. URL: http://www.ninds.nih.gov/disorders/brainandspinaltumors/brainandspinaltumors.htm. Last updated March 17, 2006.

North American Spine Society. "Spinal Tumor," NASS. Available online. URL: http://www.spine.org/fsp/prob_action-injury-tumor.cfm. Last updated March 3, 2005.

Thomas Jefferson University Hospital. "Jefferson Neurosurgeons, Radiation Oncologists Wrap Radiation Around Spine to Provide Cancer Pain Relief," News Release, Jefferson Health Systems. Available online. URL: http://www.jeffersonhospital.org/news/2005/article10954.html. Published May 30, 2005.

spine Rings of irregularly shaped VERTEBRAE, gel-cushioning DISCS, muscle-linking tendons, and bone-strapping ligaments come together to form the spine. This stack of components shapes the curvaceous CERVICAL SPINE, THORACIC SPINE, and LUMBAR SPINE then connects with the less flexible bones of the SACRAL VERTEBRAE and COCCYGEAL SPINE. These five regions of the backbone have unique qualities that cooperate to maintain upright POSTURE, protect the SPINAL CORD, and mobilize the body. Even a perfectly designed spine, however, must contend with numerous conditions that oppose the plan, such as GENETIC FACTORS, BIRTH DEFECTS OF THE SPINE, ENVIRONMENTAL INFLUENCES, ERGONOMIC FACTORS, degenerative conditions, and various types of BACK INJURY.

Risks and Complications

Remarkable RANGE OF MOTION also makes the neck susceptible to trauma and NECK PAIN as caused, for instance, by a FLEXION-EXTENSION INJURY. Yet spinal vulnerability increases where the cervical region meets the thoracic spine, mainly because the neck bends easily but connects with an area that does not. Another vulnerable point occurs where the fairly rigid thoracic region meets the highly mobile lumbar spine. Adding to those worries, that thoracolumbar connection encounters the added effects of WEIGHT. Stress on those vertebral joints can be compounded by pounds of body fat. Among CHILDREN and ADOLESCENTS a load of BACK problems occur with the lack of BACKPACK SAFETY. Similarly, adult workers risk exceeding their personal LOAD TOLERANCE in LIFTING heavy or awkward objects.

In ATHLETES, spinal concerns include SPRAIN, STRAIN, or FRACTURE, but anyone who EXERCISES without warming up may be prone to muscle spasm. ELDERLY persons may encounter knotted PARASPINAL MUSCLES too, but aging alone raises the risk of DEGENERATIVE DISC DISEASE and OSTEOPOROSIS. People of all ages, however, gamble with spinal wear-and-tear by wearing SHOES that tear the spine from its proper alignment. Anyone can be plagued with such posture problems as SCOLIOSIS, KYPHOSIS, or LORDOSIS, but prompt treatment, appropriate ORTHOTIC bracing, and sometimes SURGERY may prevent the complications of progressive curvature or spinal deformity.

Statistics and Studies

The American Association of Neurological Surgeons posted an online report of over 530,000 spinal procedures performed in a single year. Of this total, 111,488 patients had ARTHRODESIS or spinal fusion, and 141,620 had a LAMINECTOMY involving one or more discs. Another 14,062 had laminectomies not involving discs, while 85,876 patients had laminectomies to treat SPINAL STENOSIS.

Although some patients require surgery to stabilize the spine, accident victims encounter spinal concerns that extend beyond the hospital or emergency room. According to a study in the February 2006 issue of *The Journal of Trauma*, "reinjury risk is highest soon after injury, but persists for at least 5 years after initial injury. Periodic interventions through 5 years after injury, particularly in certain high-risk groups, might have lasting effects on reinjury rates." Yet the study also said, "any injury to the face, spine, and extremities were associated with a decreased risk of reinjury."

For most people, spine pain occurs in a nontraumatic event such as the common BACKACHE. As the American Academy of Orthopaedic Surgeons reported, "More than 31 million visits were made to physician offices in 2003 because of back problems. . . . Eight out of 10 people will experience back pain at some point in their lives. Low back pain is one of the most frequent problems treated by orthopaedic surgeons."

Special Aids and Adaptations

To help the spine adapt to the loads often placed on it, regular daily ACTIVITY can keep the vertebrae flexible, while WEIGHT-BEARING EXERCISE aids BONE-BUILDING. If bones shift out of place, for instance after a twisted movement or overextended reach, SPINAL MANIPULATION may restore alignment. For achy back muscles, MASSAGE THERAPY, HYDROTHERAPY, COLD THERAPY, and, in the absence of swelling or bleeding, HEAT THERAPY may ease ACUTE PAIN. For CHRONIC BACK PAIN, a first course of treatment often includes NONSTEROIDAL ANTI-INFLAMMATORY DRUG (NSAID) THERAPY, but some people prefer HOMEO-PATHIC MEDICINE or HERB THERAPY to treat inflammation and pain. Each of those special aids are just that though: special aids for a special individual and need. For everyone, however, plenty of fresh WATER, well-balanced NUTRITION, and restful SLEEP can strengthen general health and help the backbone adapt to the special demands of each day.

American Academy of Orthopaedic Surgeons. "The Spine," AAOS. Available online. URL: http://orthoinfo.aaos.org/fact/thr_report.cfm?Thread_ID=91&topcategory=Spine. Downloaded May 3, 2006.

NeurosurgeryToday.org. "AANS National Neurosurgical Statistics Report—1999 Procedural Statistics," American Association of Neurological Surgeons. Available online. URL: http://www.neurosurgerytoday.org/what/stats/spine.asp. Downloaded May 3, 2006.

Worrell, S. S., T. D. Koepsell, D. R. Sabath, L. M. Gentilello, C. N. Mock, and A. B. Nathens. "The Risk of Reinjury in Relation to Time since First Injury: a Retrospective Population-based Study," *The Journal of Trauma* 60, no. 2 (February 2006): 379–384.

spondylitis   See ANKYLOSING SPONDYLITIS.

spondyloepiphyseal dysplasia (SED)   This group of disorders affects the VERTEBRAE and produces abnormal bone growth. The congenital type of spondyloepiphyseal dysplasia (SED) may be quickly apparent in INFANTS with DWARFISM, disproportionately large hands and feet, a barrel chest, and a shortened CERVICAL SPINE. Later, SED tarda, a milder form of SED, may be detected in growing CHILDREN or ADOLESCENTS with short stature or with average height except for a shortened trunk. Although GENETIC FACTORS differ, either type of SED involves a collagen defect and progressive change in the SPINE. However, SED tarda occurs only in males.

Symptoms and Diagnostic Path

X-RAYS confirm the condition in newborns with SED. A characteristic appearance may include flat cheekbones, cleft palate, and skeletal deformity. As POSTURE disorders of SCOLIOSIS, KYPHOSIS, or LORDOSIS worsen, a child may encounter CHRONIC BACK PAIN. Problems in the LUMBAR SPINE may also delay motor development.

According to the Greenberg Center for Skeletal Dysplasias at Johns Hopkins, "Myopia (nearsightedness) is present in 40%. Retinal detachment can occur so careful ophthalmologic follow-up is important to treat small retinal tears. Close ophthalmologic follow-up is important to monitor for retinal problems." To monitor skeletal changes,

MAGNETIC RESONANCE IMAGING and neurological exams may be required, for instance, to assess a potential SPINAL CORD involvement.

An article in *The Indian Journal of Radiology and Imaging* evaluated symptoms in six SED patients then reported, "The first symptoms are usually back pain of a vague pattern, while at a later stage osteoarthritis of the large proximal joints" nearest the source of pain may develop. "In the present series the most common type of presentation was back ache (3 patients), gait abnormalities (2 patients) and pain in the hip and difficulty in walking (1 patient)."

Treatment Options and Outlook

The Genetics Home Reference page posted by the U.S. National Library of Medicine said that in congenital SED, "adult height ranges from 3 feet to just over 4 feet. Abnormal curvature of the spine (kyphoscoliosis and lordosis) becomes more severe during childhood and can cause problems with breathing. Instability of the spinal bones (vertebrae) in the neck may increase the risk of spinal cord damage. Other skeletal features include flattened vertebrae (platyspondyly), an abnormality of the hip joint in which the upper leg bones turn inward (coxa vara), and a foot deformity called a clubfoot."

In cases of skeletal deformity, SURGERY, such as ARTHRODESIS, may be needed to fuse and stabilize the spine. However, persons with bone deformities in the THORACIC SPINE may have poor respiratory function that makes anesthesia inadvisable. Before any surgical procedure, the condition of the neck must also be assessed with care taken to support the VERTEBRAE, especially if SED produces ATLANTO-AXIAL INSTABILITY.

Risk Factors and Preventive Measures

In choosing an appropriate daily ACTIVITY, protective measures should be taken to lessen the risk of head and neck trauma. Since SED carries the risk of early development of ARTHRITIS, DEGENERATIVE DISC DISEASE, and OSTEOARTHRITIS, low-impact EXERCISES can be particularly important, but only as recommended by the primary care physician or therapist. A dietician or nutritionist can suggest supportive NUTRITION, perhaps emphasizing fresh blue-black or red-black fruits that aid the body in producing collagen.

Genetics Home Reference. "Spondyloepiphyseal Dysplasia Congenital," U.S. National Library of Medicine. Available online. URL: http://ghr.nlm.nih.gov/condition=spondyloepiphysealdysplasiacongenita. Published April 28, 2006.

Greenberg Center for Skeletal Dysplasias. "Type II Collagen Conditions," Johns Hopkins Hospital Center for Genetics. Available online. URL: http://www.hopkinsmedicine.org/greenbergcenter/SED.htm. Downloaded May 4, 2006.

Lakhar, B. N. and R. Raphael. "Spondyloepiphyseal Dysplasia: An Evaluation of Six Cases," *The Indian Journal of Radiology and Imaging* 13, no. 2 (May 2003): 199–203.

spondylolisthesis   This spinal condition may occur because of GENETIC FACTORS, SPONDYLOLYSIS, degeneration of the DISCS and SPINE, or an injury brought on by overextension or overuse. As also happens in VERTEBRAL SUBLUXATION, one or more of the spinal VERTEBRAE can become involved as a bone slips out of alignment. Characteristically, this slippage causes the vertebra located above to shift forward, but sometimes backward shifting may occur.

Symptoms and Diagnostic Path

BACKACHES and LOW BACK PAIN may extend into the hips and outer thighs. This dull BACK pain may be accompanied by tightness in the hamstrings and muscle spasms in the calf muscles of the legs. To confirm a diagnosis, a physician will usually request a medical history, physical examination, RANGE OF MOTION tests, and X-RAYS or other imaging tools.

Treatment Options and Outlook

Conservative treatments begin with rest, PAIN RELIEVERS or NONSTEROIDAL ANTI-INFLAMMATORY DRUG THERAPY, and sometimes the temporary use of an ORTHOTIC device. A doctor may also prescribe traditional or COMPLEMENTARY AND ALTERNATIVE MEDICINE, such as COLD THERAPY, HEAT THERAPY, HYDROTHERAPY, MASSAGE THERAPY, SPINAL MANIPULATION, or ULTRASOUND THERAPY. Sometimes SURGERY may be needed to stabilize the spine.

According to an article in *Neurosurgical Focus*, "treatment options for spondylolisthesis are plentiful," with surgical choices ranging from reconstruction during open back surgery to various types of MINIMALLY INVASIVE SURGERY. Also, "in the rapidly evolving field of spinal neurosurgery, . . . techniques have been developed that allow for the placement of . . . screws and interbody devices" between the affected vertebrae. For newer procedures, a long-term outlook has not yet been established. Nevertheless, "there are an assortment of methods that are acceptable for the treatment of spondylolisthesis, which may vary based on the age of the patient, the type of abnormality, and the experience and comfort of the treating surgeon."

Risk Factors and Preventive Measures

Active CHILDREN, ADOLESCENTS, and ATHLETES may be particularly at risk for vertebral slippage. As an article in the March 2006 issue of *Massage Today* explained, "Individuals engaged in certain sports or occupations are particularly susceptible to spondylolisthesis, especially if it involves repetitive flexion and extension of the spine. It is common in gymnastics, rowing, diving, swimming (especially the butterfly), tennis, wrestling, weightlifting and football. An increased incidence also has been identified in loggers and soldiers carrying heavy backpacks. The condition is prevalent in adolescents due to the extremes of physical exertion in athletics and bones that are not fully formed."

Despite those risks, EXERCISE provides an important preventive means of strengthening the PARASPINAL MUSCLES, thus reducing the risk of vertebral slippage. As the North American Spine Society explained, "At first, the exercises you learn may be gentle stretches or posture changes to reduce the back pain or leg symptoms. When you have less pain, more vigorous aerobic exercises (such as stationary bicycling or swimming) combined with strengthening/stretching exercises will likely be used to improve flexibility, strength, endurance, and the ability to return to a more normal lifestyle. Developing your back and stomach muscles will help stabilize your spine and support your body. Exercise instruction should start right away and be modified as recovery progresses."

Heary, Robert F., M.D. "Spondylolisthesis: Introduction and Illustrative Cases," *Neurosurgical Focus* 13, no. 1 (July 2002).

Lowe, Whitney. "Spondylolisthesis: An Elusive Cause of Low Back Pain," *Massage Today* 6, no. 3 (March, 2006).

North American Spine Society. "Adult Isthmic Spondylolisthesis (Slipped Vertebra)," NASS. Available online. URL: http://www.spine.org/articles/spondylolisthesis.cfm. Downloaded May 4, 2006.

spondylolysis This type of stress FRACTURE may result from exceeding LOAD TOLERANCE or receiving repeated trauma to the SPINE. Most often, the break involves the L5 VERTEBRA of the LUMBAR SPINE with most incidents occurring in males. Among older women and ELDERLY patients, spondylolysis may not result from stress so much as degenerative conditions such as OSTEOARTHRITIS. That type of the condition may involve the CERVICAL SPINE, THORACIC SPINE, or lumbar region and affect the intervertebral DISCS, possibly causing FACET JOINT DISORDER.

With SPONDYLOLISTHESIS, vertebral shifting may also be involved. To explain the difference between that condition and spondylolysis, the Spine Institute of New York said, "Spondylolisthesis . . . most commonly occurs in the lowest lumbar vertebra on the bony ring formed by the pedicle and lamina bones, which protects the spinal cord and spinal nerves. The bone is weakest in an area called the 'pars interarticularis,' which joins the upper and lower joints. This pars defect or fracture is called spondylolysis and is believed to be a stress fracture that results from repeated strain on a bone. At first, the body can heal the damage produced by strain on the bone. However, if repeated strains occur faster than the body can respond, the bone will eventually fracture. If the pars is fractured, the condition is called spondylolysis."

Symptoms and Diagnostic Path

While NECK PAIN indicates involvement of the cervical spine, lumbar spondylolysis produces LOW BACK PAIN. In the upper back, CHRONIC BACK PAIN suggests thoracic spine involvement. Regardless of the spinal region, the diagnostic path includes a medical history, physical examination, and X-RAYS or other type of imaging tests.

Treatment Options and Outlook

According to the American Academy of Orthopaedic Surgeons (AAOS), "initial treatment for spondylolysis is always conservative. The individual should take a break from the activities until symptoms go away, as they often do. Anti-inflammatory medications such as ibuprofen may help reduce back pain. Occasionally, a back brace and physical therapy may be recommended."

Risk Factors and Preventive Measures

To explain the ongoing risks, the Mount Sinai Medical Center said, "Pinched or irritated nerves produce compressive symptoms. This occurs in spondylolysis when a lump of tissue forms around the crack—where the body tries to heal the stress fracture. The lump can cause pressure on the spinal nerves where they leave the spinal canal." In such instances, "pressure on the nerve can produce pain that radiates down to the foot. It can also cause numbness in the foot and weakness in the muscles supplied by the nerve."

Simply resting the area provides opportunity for the spine to heal, especially if the person has the NUTRITION, WATER, and SLEEP needed for restoration. As the AAOS said, "In most cases, activities can be resumed gradually and there will be few complications or recurrences. Stretching and strengthening exercises for the back and abnormal muscles can help prevent future recurrences of pain."

American Academy of Orthopaedic Surgeons. "Spondylolysis and Spondylolisthesis," AAOS. Available online. URL: http://orthoinfo.aaos.org/fact/thr_report.cfm?Thread_ID=155&topcategory=Spine. Downloaded May 5, 2006.

Mount Sinai Medical Center, The. "Spondylolysis and Spondylolisthesis." Available online. URL: http://www.mountsinai.org/msh/msh_frame.jsp?url=clinical_services/orthospine_spondylolysis.htm. Downloaded May 5, 2006.

Spine Institute of New York. "Spondylolisthesis," Beth Israel Medical Center. Available online. URL: http://www.spineinstituteny.com/conditions/spondylolisthesis.html. Downloaded May 5, 2006.

sports injury   See ATHLETES, SPINAL CONCERNS OF; SPINAL INJURY.

sprain   A fall, a twisting motion, or a blow to the body can quickly cause a vertebral joint to get out of joint. Bones sometimes pop back into place without medical treatment, but they might not. Either way, a sudden, sharp movement can stretch, tear, or put a hurt on the surrounding ligaments.

Symptoms and Diagnostic Path

ACUTE PAIN, swelling, and, occasionally, bruising characterize a sprain, but similar symptoms can occur with a STRAIN or muscle tearing. If a sprain affects joint function, the RANGE OF MOTION will be limited.

In explaining the three types of sprains, the National Institute of Arthritis and Musculoskeletal and Skin Diseases (NIAMS) said, "In general, a grade I or mild sprain is caused by overstretching or slight tearing of the ligaments with no joint instability." A mild sprain can often be treated at home, but a grade II or III sprain may require an X-RAY to rule out a FRACTURE. As the NIAMS said, "A grade II or moderate sprain is caused by further, but still incomplete, tearing of the ligament and is characterized by bruising, moderate pain, and swelling. A person with a moderate sprain usually has more difficulty putting weight on the affected joint and experiences some loss of function." By contrast, "people who sustain a grade III or severe sprain completely tear or rupture a ligament. Pain, swelling, and bruising are usually severe, and the patient is unable to put weight on the joint." In such cases, MAGNETIC RESONANCE IMAGING may be needed to assess the damage.

Treatment Options and Outlook

Initially, the RICE METHOD of rest, ice, compression, and elevation reduces swelling with the addition of NONSTEROIDAL ANTI-INFLAMMATORY DRUG THERAPY to ease BACK pain. A moderate sprain may require the temporary use of an ORTHOTIC brace for the NECK or back to minimize movement during recovery. If a ligament has been completely torn, however, restorative SURGERY will often be required.

When LOW BACK PAIN and muscle spasms involve stress but no tearing of the ligaments, the American Association of Neurological Surgeons said, "The pain is worsened by activities and bed rest is an absolute necessity for a short period of time—one to three days." Assuming there is no lower body weakness, "the pain is typically limited to five to ten days and does not involve either leg." During this time, however, "patients are typically bent over and unable to straighten up or maintain a normal posture. Any particular activity is impossible, including sitting, standing, walking, driving, etc."

If a sprain involves the CERVICAL SPINE, the American Academy of Orthopaedic Surgeons said, "Usually, neck sprains, like other sprains, will gradually heal, given time and appropriate treatment. You may have to wear a soft cervical collar to help support the head and relieve pressure on the neck so the ligaments have time to heal." If the sprain resulted from a FLEXION-EXTENSION INJURY, other treatment options include MASSAGE THERAPY, TRACTION, or ULTRASOUND THERAPY.

Risk Factors and Preventive Measures

Too much WEIGHT adversely affects the LUMBAR SPINE, yet good NUTRITION can keep down body pounds and aid all regions of the back. Also, adequate WATER intake and warm-ups before EXERCISE can keep the vertebral ligaments flexible and better able to stretch. With the approval of a doctor, daily ACTIVITY to limber up and exercises to strengthen the PARASPINAL MUSCLES can gradually be increased to improve health and lower the risk of future injuries.

American Academy of Orthopaedic Surgeons. "Neck Sprain," AAOS. Available online. URL: http://orthoinfo. aaos.org/fact/thr_report.cfm?Thread_ID=141&topcategory=Neck. Downloaded May 5, 2006.

National Institute of Arthritis and Musculoskeletal and Skin Diseases. "Questions and Answers About Sprains and Strains," NIAMS, National Institutes of Health. Available online. URL: http://www.niams.nih.gov/hi/topics/strain_sprain/strain_sprain.htm. Downloaded May 5, 2006.

NeurosurgeryToday.org. "Sprain and Strain," American Association of Neurological Surgeons. Available online. URL: http://www.neurosurgerytoday.org/what/patient_e/sprain.asp. Downloaded May 5, 2006.

steroid therapy Cortisone-like medicines stem from the cortisone-like hormones the body pro-

duces to ease pain, swelling, itching, and inflammation. For instance, an insect bite, food allergen, or inflammatory condition in the vertebral joints may trigger a reaction that pumps up natural cortisone production. If that natural response fails to relieve the symptoms, then mild drugs, such as antihistamines and NONSTEROIDAL ANTI-INFLAMMATORY DRUG THERAPY, may initially be prescribed. A severe reaction would, of course, require emergency medical treatment. Otherwise, a condition that becomes too intense or too prolonged for the body to handle on its own may need other types of medication. In such cases, the patient may be given synthetic cortisone, prednisone, or other form of steroid therapy to be taken orally or by injection.

Risks and Complications

In an article for SpineUniverse, Dr. Gerald Malanga wrote, "In the setting of acute low back pain with radiculopathy," which has a pattern of pain and numbness in muscles supplied by the same nerve root, "oral corticosteroids are typically prescribed in a quick tapering fashion over one week." However, "multiple adverse effects have been associated with prolonged steroid use, including" suppression of the immune system, SECONDARY OSTEOPOROSIS, psychoses, gastric ulcers, electrolyte disturbances, "and impaired wound healing. . . . The severity of these complications correlates with the dosage, duration of use, and the potency of the steroid prescribed."

Extended use of steroids may occur, for example, in treating RHEUMATOID ARTHRITIS (RA) or JUVENILE RHEUMATOID ARTHRITIS, which then incurs the risk of bone loss. Other risks involved in steroid therapy include muscle weakness, impaired growth in CHILDREN and ADOLESCENTS, swings in blood pressure and moods, SLEEP problems, and dry or brittle bones, including the VERTEBRAE. Also, steroid therapy may produce the complication of sudden WEIGHT gain with adverse effects.

"Your Child and Prednisone" explained how steroid therapy can negatively affect the immune system. According to the article, "normally, the body makes approximately 25 mg of cortisol per day. When 'stressed' the body may make over 100 mg. (Stress in this sense means trauma, such as major surgery, broken bones, or a major illness.) Prednisone has roughly five times the potency of cortisol, so 5 mg of prednisone is like 25 mg of cortisol." This effectively combats inflammation. However, prednisone also "inhibits immune cells that kill other cells, and it inhibits the secretion of substances (cytokines) which tend to 'rev up' the immune system. The result is that all inflammatory processes are slowed and weakened," thereby slowing the natural immune system.

Statistics and Studies

An article published in *Pain Medicine* reported, "The only rationale for intra-articular steroids" (injected between the spinal joints) "appears to be the expectation that they should work. The most commonly used indication has been back pain, for which no specific diagnosis has been made. When the results of observational studies are pooled, they paint a picture of impressive immediate responses, but a rapid decay of outcomes by three and six months. Initial responses, however, are dissonant with the literature from controlled studies of the prevalence of lumbar . . . joint pain. Moreover, controlled trials have shown that there is no attributable effect to the injection of steroids."

An article in the *BMJ Journal* reviewed a study of the effectiveness of EPIDURAL INJECTION in treating LOW BACK PAIN then reported, "Epidural injection therapy has not yet been shown to be effective, nor has it been shown to be ineffective. Side effects are relatively minor, and a tendency exists towards an outcome favouring injection therapy. On the basis of our longstanding clinical experience we suggest that epidural steroid injection may have a role in specific clinical situations. Low back pain that has not resolved within three months leads to greater long term morbidity. Epidural injection therapy may provide a useful adjunct to recovery in patients whose symptoms have extended beyond three months." However, "the evidence for and against epidural steroid injection should be clearly explained to allow patients to make an informed choice regarding their treatment."

In October 2004, the American College of Rheumatology (ACR) issued a press release that reported "between 35 percent and 45 percent of patients with rheumatoid arthritis currently use prednisone," a type of steroid therapy. Prior to that announcement, a two and a half year study compared the effects of prednisone to those of biologic drugs prepared from living organisms and, consequently, less likely to cause toxicity or allergic reactions in most patients. As the ACR reported, "While participants who used biologic drugs were 30 percent more likely to get pneumonia, those on prednisone were 170 percent more likely. Therefore prednisone, the corticosteroid most often prescribed to treat inflammation, poses a much larger risk."

Special Aids and Adaptations

Before beginning long-term use of steroids, various forms of COMPLEMENTARY AND ALTERNATIVE MEDICINE (CAM) may offer workable options. Although many CAM therapies have not been proven effective, they have seldom been proven ineffective. Also, each patient responds differently to ACUPUNCTURE, HERBAL THERAPY, and HOMEOPATHIC MEDICINE. Almost everyone, though, can benefit from natural aids, such as ample WATER intake, well-balanced NUTRITION, and some type of daily ACTIVITY. Besides those natural aids, short-term steroid therapy may be just what the doctor orders to ease pain and inflammation long enough to adapt to a long-range course of appropriate EXERCISE.

American College of Rheumatology. "Prednisone May Prove to Be a High Risk Factor for Pneumonia in Patients with Rheumatoid Arthritis," Press Release October 17, 2004. Available online. URL: http://www.rheumatology.org/press/2004/wolfe_pneumonia.asp. Downloaded May 5, 2006.

Bogduk, N. "A Narrative Review of Intra-articular Corticosteroid Injections for Low Back Pain," *Pain Medicine* 6, no. 4 (July–August 2005): 287–296.

Malanga, Gerald, M.D. "Corticosteroids in the Treatment of Acute Low Back Pain," SpineUniverse. Available online. URL: http://www.spineuniverse.com/display-article.php/article1835.html. Last updated February 13, 2006.

Punch, Jeffrey D., M.D. "Your Child and Prednisone," C.L.A.S.S., Children's Liver Association for Support Services. Available online. URL: http://www.classkids.org/library/pred.htm. Downloaded May 5, 2006.

Samanta, Ash and Jo Samanta. "Is Epidural Injection of Steroids Effective for Low Back Pain?" *BMJ Journal* (June 2004). Available online. URL: http://bmj.bmjjournals.com/cgi/content/full/328/7455/1509. Downloaded May 5, 2006.

Still's disease   See JUVENILE RHEUMATOID ARTHRITIS.

stinger   See BRACHIAL PLEXUS INJURY.

strain   TENSION, improper LIFTING techniques, and sudden movements can strain PARASPINAL MUSCLES to the limit. Too far can stress muscle tissue in the BACK and connective tendons too.

To differentiate between a strain and a ligament-stretched SPRAIN, the National Institute of Arthritis and Musculoskeletal and Skin Diseases (NIAMS) said, "A strain is an injury to either a muscle or a tendon (fibrous cords of tissue that connect muscle to bone). Depending on the severity of the injury, a strain may be a simple overstretch of the muscle or tendon, or it can result from a partial or complete tear."

Symptoms and Diagnostic Path

As the NIAMS Web site said, "A strain is caused by twisting or pulling a muscle or tendon. Strains can be acute or chronic. An acute strain is associated with a recent trauma or injury; it also can occur after improperly lifting heavy objects or overstressing the muscles. Chronic strains are usually the result of overuse: prolonged, repetitive movement of the muscles and tendons." ACUTE PAIN, BACKACHE, and muscle spasms may indicate a muscle strain, but the same symptoms can occur with other causes of LOW BACK PAIN. To find out what precipitated the event, a doctor will request a medical history in addition to performing a physical examination.

Treatment Options and Outlook

The RICE METHOD of rest, ice, compression, and elevation often offers the first option of home treatment. In discussing ATHLETES with muscle strain, the North American Spine Society (NASS) said, "Initial treatment may require a period of rest, removing the athlete from sports participation. Treatments may include medication and special exercise. Ice can be used along with pain medications, which should be used sparingly. In addition, other measures to control pain and restore motion are commonly used. Initially, ice and medications such as nonsteroidal anti-inflammatories can be used. For persistent symptoms, particularly those associated with muscle spasm, heat may also be very helpful." Besides applying COLD THERAPY followed by HEAT THERAPY, the NASS suggested slowly beginning "sport-specific exercises that mimic activities of athletic competition. . . . It is also always important to evaluate and correct poor technique and mechanics that may have predisposed the athlete to the initial injury."

Risk Factors and Preventive Measures

The American Academy of Orthopaedic Surgeons (AAOS) warned, "People at risk for the injury have a history of sprains and strains, are overweight, and are in poor physical condition." Among athletes, those who engage in sports that involve jumping or twisting have a higher risk of muscle strain. In addition, "inadequate rest breaks during intensive training precipitates a strain."

If muscle strain immobilizes a person for two weeks or more, muscles may weaken. Therefore, when swelling and intense pain have subsided, a doctor may advise gradually increasing daily ACTIVITY and conditioning EXERCISE.

American Academy of Orthopaedic Surgeons. "Sprains and Strains," AAOS. Available online. URL: http://orthoinfo.aaos.org/fact/thr_report.cfm?Thread_ID=45&topcategory=General%20Information. Downloaded May 5, 2006.

National Institute of Arthritis and Musculoskeletal and Skin Diseases. "Questions and Answers About Sprains and Strains," NIAMS, National Institutes of Health. Available online. URL: http://www.niams.nih.gov/hi/topics/strain_sprain/strain_sprain.htm. Downloaded May 5, 2006.

North American Spine Society. "Treatment of the Young Athlete," NASS. Available online. URL: http://www.spine.org/articles/young_athlete.cfm. Downloaded May 5, 2006.

strength training   Typically, strength training combines a variety of EXERCISES, such as weight lifting, WEIGHT-BEARING EXERCISE, stair-climbing, and other activities designed to increase balance, strengthen PARASPINAL MUSCLES, support POSTURE, and aid BONE BUILDING. Energy, endurance, overall muscle tone, and mental outlook may also improve. Generally, active CHILDREN and ADOLESCENTS seldom need strength training, but people of any age with musculoskeletal problems often do. Frail patients and ELDERLY persons might begin with a simple movement, such as getting up and down from a sturdy chair. The next step might be holding on to that chair or a waist-high handrail while standing on one foot then the other for a few seconds at a time.

As the American College of Sports Medicine (ACSM) explained, "Strength conditioning is generally defined as training in which the resistance against which a muscle generates force is progressively increased over time. . . . Strength conditioning results in an increase in muscle size, and this increase in size is largely the result of an increase in contractile protein content." However, "it is clear that when the intensity of the exercise is low, only modest increases in strength are achieved by older subjects." Nevertheless, "a number of studies have demonstrated that, given an adequate training stimulus, older men and women show similar or greater strength gains compared with young individuals as a result of resistance training." Indeed, "two to threefold increases in muscle strength can be accomplished in a relatively short period of time (3–4 mo.) in fibers recruited during training in this age population."

Risks and Complications

Strength training may not be for everyone, however. As the Exercise and Physical Fitness Web page from Georgia State University pointed out, "If you feel your body is not ready for strength training for any reason, talk to your physician." Risks increase for those with "any cardiovascular disease including chest pains at rest or exertion; family history of coronary heart disease before the age of 55; high cholesterol . . . ; abnormal ECG, or cardiac arrhythmias; smoking; chronic hypertension; extreme obesity; any chronic muscular or joint problem; currently pregnant, or within 3 months of delivery; recent surgery; arthritis; diabetes; asthma; years of a sedentary lifestyle."

To avoid complications, people who exceed their optimal WEIGHT and also patients with ARTHRITIS, OSTEOARTHRITIS, DISC problems, or any condition involving bone loss need the advice of a doctor on the particular course of exercise best suited to their needs. For instance, a normally sedentary person might start weight lifting with a can of vegetables in either hand before proceeding to one-pound dumbbells. Or a doctor might recommend leg lifts for a person whose LUMBAR SPINE prohibits stair-climbing. A list of potential recommendations could go on for pages, but everyone can lower the risk of muscle SPRAIN and STRAIN by warming up with gentle stretches.

Statistics and Studies

According to the North American Spine Society (NASS), "recent studies have shown that even 90- to 100-year-old nursing home residents can benefit from a regular program of strength building exercises." For instance, "strength training can help improve balance—a key issue for the elderly who are at risk for falls. Particularly, hip muscle strength reduces the risk of a fall. If you can't rise out of a chair without using your hands, you need to strengthen your hip muscles." Such movements not only help patients to avoid FRACTURES, the NASS said, "Studies show that people who exercise regularly enjoy a higher quality of life and increased mental alertness. Even patients who have minor mental impairments after a stroke have shown small improvements in thinking with exercise."

Similarly, information from the Centers for Disease Control and Prevention (CDC) said, "Scientific research has shown that exercise can slow the physiological aging clock. . . . Studies have shown that lifting weights two or three times a week increases strength by building muscle mass and bone density." In addition, "one 12-month study conducted on postmenopausal women at Tufts University demonstrated 1% gains in hip and spine bone density, 75% increases in strength and 13% increases in dynamic balance with just two days per week of progressive strength training."

Special Aids and Adaptations

For those who have not been active for a while, the CDC recommended beginning with squats and wall pushups for a couple of weeks. Then, to improve balance and increase strength, proceed to the next step of step-ups on a low stair. As the CDC explained, "With your feet flat and toes facing forward, put your right foot on the first step. Holding the handrail for balance, to a count of two, straighten your right leg to lift up your left leg slowly until it reaches the first step. As you're lifting yourself up, make sure that your right knee stays straight and does not move forward past your ankle. Let your left foot tap the first step near your right foot. Pause. Then, using your right leg to support your weight, to a count of four, slowly lower your left foot back to the floor. Repeat 10 times with the right leg and 10 times with the left leg for one set. Rest for one to two minutes. Then complete a second set of 10 repetitions with each leg."

Not only does strength training aid muscle strength and balance, this type of exercise can help a person adapt to the aging process. As the ACSM said, "Strength training helps offset the loss in muscle mass and strength typically associated with normal aging. Additional benefits from regular exercise include improved bone health and, thus, reduction in risk for osteoporosis; improved postural stability, thereby reducing the risk of falling and associated injuries and fractures; and increased flexibility and range of motion. While not as abundant, the evidence also suggests that involvement in regular exercise can also provide a number of psychological benefits related to preserved cognitive function, alleviation of depression symptoms and behavior, and an improved concept of personal control and self-efficacy."

Centers for Disease Control and Prevention. "Growing Stronger—Strength Training for Older Adults: Introduction," Department of Health and Human Services. Available online. URL: http://www.cdc.gov/nccdphp/dnpa/physical/growing_stronger/why.htm. Last reviewed March 22, 2006.

Doyle, J. Andrew. "Strength Training Main Page," The Exercise and Physical Fitness Web Page, Department of Kinesiology and Health at Georgia State University. Available online. URL: http://www2.gsu.edu/~wwwfit/strength.html. Downloaded May 6, 2006.

Mazzeo, Robert S., Peter Cavanagh, William J. Evans, Maria Fiatarone, James Hagberg, Edward McAuley, and Jill Startzell. "Exercise and Physical Activity for Older Adults," Position Stand, American College of Sports Medicine. Available online. URL: http://www.acsm.org/Content/NavigationMenu/Research/Roundtables_Specialty_Conf/PastRoundtables/Exercise_for_Older_Adults.htm. Downloaded May 6, 2006.

North American Spine Society. "Strength Training for the Elderly," NASS. Available online. URL: http://www.spine.org/articles/elderlyexercise.cfm. Downloaded May 6, 2006.

stretching   See EXERCISE.

strontium ranelate   By stimulating new bone growth and decreasing bone resorption, this medical compound aids BONE BUILDING, reduces FRACTURE risks, and affects bone strength in a manner similar to CALCIUM.

Dosage and Potential Side Effects

Most patients tolerate strontium ranelate (SR) well, with minimal side effects similar to those found in a placebo. Regarding the dosage, an article in *Osteoporosis International* reported on a study that aimed to find out the minimum amount of the medication that could be used to optimal effect in preventing and treating OSTEOPOROSIS. According to those findings, "the minimum dose at which SR is effective in preventing bone loss in early postmenopausal non-osteoporotic women and in the treatment of postmenopausal osteoporosis is 1 g/day and 2 g/day, respectively."

Statistics and Studies

After studying "The Effects of Strontium Ranelate on the Risk of Vertebral Fracture in Women with Postmenopausal Osteoporosis," a group of doctors reported in the January 2004 issue of *The New England Journal of Medicine*, "New vertebral fractures occurred in fewer patients in the strontium ranelate group than in the placebo group, with a risk reduction of 49 percent in the first year of treatment and 41 percent during the three-year study period. . . . Strontium ranelate increased bone mineral density at month 36 by 14.4 percent at the lumbar spine."

Similarly, a study published in *Arthritis News* reported, "Concurrently, spinal and non-spinal fractures were reduced by 32 percent and 31 percent, respectively, in the subgroup of elderly women, ages 80 and older. Strontium ranelate appeared to both increase bone formation and decrease bone density loss in the majority of patients, demonstrating a good bone and general safety response."

On June 5, 2006, the Medical News Today Web site announced, "In previous clinical trials strontium ranelate has proven effective in preventing fractures for up to three years. But according to new data presented today . . . that window of opportunity can now be extended to at least five years."

American College of Rheumatology. "Medication Shows Promising Results For Reducing Fracture Risks For Osteoporosis Patients," *Arthritis News,* Press Release, October 17, 2004. Available online. URL: http://www.rheumatology.org/press/2004/reginster_strontium_ranelate.asp. Downloaded May 6, 2006.

Medical News Today. "The Strength Of Strontium Ranelate—Protects Bones For At Least Five Years, Remodels Bone Architecture," Orthopedic News, June 5, 2006. Available online. URL: http://www.medical-newstoday.com/medicalnews.php?newsid=44627. Downloaded September 15, 2006.

Meunier, Pierre J., M.D., Christian Roux, M.D., Ego Seeman, M.D., Sergio Ortolani, M.D., Janusz E. Badurski, M.D., Tim D. Spector, M.D., Jorge Cannata, M.D., Adam Balogh, M.D., Ernst-Martin Lemmel, M.D., Stig Pors-Nielsen, M.D., Reni Rizzoli, M.D., Harry K. Genant, M.D., and Jean-Yves Reginster, M.D. "The Effects of Strontium Ranelate on the Risk of Vertebral Fracture in Women with Postmenopausal Osteoporosis," Massachusetts Medical Society, *The New England Journal of Medicine* 350, no. 5 (January 29, 2004): 459–468.

Reginster, J. Y. and P. J. Meunier. "Strontium Ranelate Phase 2 Dose-ranging Studies: PREVOS and STRATOS Studies," *Osteoporosis International* 14, Supplement 3 (2003): S56–65.

subluxation   See VERTEBRAL SUBLUXATION.

sulindac   See NONSTEROIDAL ANTI-INFLAMMATORY DRUG THERAPY.

surgery   From MINIMALLY INVASIVE SURGERY to open BACK procedures, many surgical options address the SPINE. Yet, with the rare exception of a trauma or such emergency conditions as CAUDA EQUINA SYNDROME, surgery seldom provides the first course of treatment.

Initially, most conditions ease with rest, PAIN RELIEVERS, various forms of COMPLEMENTARY AND ALTERNATIVE MEDICINE, prescription medications, and treatments such as a SPINAL INJECTION. If CHRONIC BACK PAIN or NECK PAIN continue, surgical options often relieve SPINAL CORD compression, correct a spinal deformity, or stabilize the VERTEBRAE. For instance, a DISC may be replaced or an instrument inserted into a bone, such as occurs in RODDING SURGERY. If a surgeon must work in a minute area, FLUOROSCOPY, X-RAYS, and other special tools provide surgical assistance. Commonly, spine surgery includes ARTHRODESIS, BONE GRAFT, and BONE MORPHOGENETIC PROTEIN to speed fusion in the CERVICAL SPINE, THORACIC SPINE, or LUMBAR SPINE.

The American Academy of Orthopaedic Surgeons (AAOS) Web site discussed how to define surgical sites with precision. According to the information, "Location documents which area of the spine is being worked on: cervical (C1-C7), thoracic (T1-T12), lumbar (L1-L5) or sacral (S1-S4)." This may sound simple enough, but each spinal region has its own set of nerves, needs, and medical experts. "Confusion arises when there is crossover of anatomic regions, such as a multiple level arthrodesis of T10-L2."

While coding information may be somewhat subject to interpretation, two surgical paths remain clear. "Although," the AAOS explained, "there are several different approaches to the spine, the two most common are anterior and posterior." With anterior meaning the front and posterior the back, "both have sub-approaches that could be considered." For example, "the posterior approach to the cervical spine is via the lamina," which involves LAMINECTOMY. Once those variations have been considered, "the next key issue is the pathology of the vertebral area being worked on." For instance, "is the medical indication related to disc, spinal stenosis, scoliosis, or some other condition? Once the pathology is identified, the real coding can take place." Then, "the next question is: what is being done to correct that pathology—discectomy, decompression, corpectomy, arthrodesis or a combination of these procedures?" Whether a DISCECTOMY, CORPECTOMY, or something else entirely, numerous procedures have been developed to address specific spinal needs.

Risks and Complications

With continuous improvements in tools and techniques, an unexpected risk comes from a lack of surgical experience in performing a new procedure or using newly purchased equipment. Patients can decrease that risk by inquiring into the training of a surgeon and the number of similar procedures he or she has previously performed. Candidates for surgery should also ask about each aspect of a procedure, including the expected rate of success and time of recovery. This realistic approach lowers the risk of false expectations and better prepares a patient to cooperate fully in his or her own healing.

In the online article "Having Surgery? What You Need To Know," the Agency for Healthcare Research and Quality (AHRQ) advised, "Ask your surgeon what you will gain by having the operation." Also, "ask how long the benefits will last. For some procedures, it is not unusual for the benefits to last for a short time only. You may need a second operation at a later date. For other procedures, the benefits may last a lifetime." Besides suggesting pertinent questions, the AHRQ reminded patients that "all operations have some risk. This is why you need to weigh the benefits of the operation against the risks of complications or side effects. . . . Typical complications are infection, too much bleeding, reaction to anesthesia, or accidental injury. Some people have a greater risk of complications because of other medical conditions."

Surgical risks may increase for INFANTS, CHILDREN, ADOLESCENTS, ELDERLY persons, and frail patients of any age. Lifestyle issues can also affect the surgical outcome. For instance, the AAOS considered the effects that smoking may have on healing, then reported, "In a study on spinal fusions in the lower back, the success rate was 80 to 85 percent for patients who never smoked or who quit smoking after their surgery. The success rate dropped to under 73 percent for smokers." Surgical risks also increase for patients adversely affected by WEIGHT, whether from obesity or from the weight loss and bone loss that typically occur with EATING DISORDERS.

The article "Fit for Surgery . . . " in *The Surgeon, Journal of the Royal Colleges of Surgeons of Edinburgh and Ireland* warned that "the causes of infectious surgical complications are . . . dependent to an extent on the primary surgical pathology, and the type and magnitude of the operation. Nevertheless, there is growing evidence that traumatic and surgical insult is associated with a period of relative immune suppression, which may expose patients to subsequent risk of infection." Adequate NUTRITION may help surgical patients to boost their immune systems and, thereby, overcome the risk of postoperative infections. However, the article reported that "malnutrition is common among hospitalised patients and in the community, while patients' nutritional status often declines during hospital stay." Therefore, "where pre-operative malnutrition is severe, surgery may need to be delayed for two to three weeks while the patient undergoes further nutritional assessment. . . . If malnutrition is only mild to moderate, then surgery should go ahead as planned."

Statistics and Studies

In considering the effects of nutrition, the article entitled "Nutrition and the Surgical Patient: Triumphs and Challenges" published in *The Surgeon, Journal of the Royal Colleges of Surgeons of Edinburgh and Ireland* stated, "A more significant development for understanding the scientific basis of the role of nutrients in the surgical patient had been occurring, particularly during the last ten years. There has been an understanding that specific nutrients could have an effect on a variety of metabolic, immune and inflammatory processes, if taken in amounts that were considered to be in excess of the normal physiological requirements. A term that has been used to describe this is nutritional pharmacology and when focused on the immune system, has been termed immunonutrition. . . . As our understanding has increased, it is clear that many different nutrients will modulate these processes, but with respect to clinical practice, the emphasis has been on the amino acids arginine and glutamine, fatty acids, ribonucleotides and certain trace elements.

While these effects in the laboratory and in experimental animal models clearly have a potential for benefit in a variety of disease states in man, the provision of a single nutrient has had limited benefit in terms of affecting clinical outcomes. Perhaps the exception is glutamine, as a recent analysis of 14 trials of glutamine supplementation (in a variety of disease states) demonstrated possible benefits. Glutamine supplementation reduced the likelihood of patients having infectious complications and, in surgical patients, there was also a benefit in terms of a reduction in hospital stay." Although further RESEARCH will be needed, "it has become evident that nutrients do exert many actions through a variety of intracellular pathways and by direct interactions with genes." Therefore, "the understanding of the role of nutrition in the surgical patient has led to major developments in the nutritional support of patients undergoing surgery. Reductions in morbidity by ensuring that patients receive optimal nutritional support can be achieved. Furthermore, the use of nutrients to modify immune, inflammatory and metabolic processes also offers new possibilities for reducing morbidity following major surgery."

Special Aids and Adaptations

While nutritional support undoubtedly aids both pre- and postoperative patients, culinary odors may not. Indeed, smells, sights, sounds, and other sources of sensory stimulation can have a nauseating effect. Some patients also feel nauseated as an adverse reaction to the anesthesia or other medication. Regardless of the triggering factor, vomiting can hinder healing by disturbing the MINERAL BALANCE in the body and depleting the WATER needed to repair tissue on the cellular level.

According to the article "Managing Nausea and Vomiting" published in *Critical Care Nurse*, "the use of supplemental oxygen has been shown to decrease the occurrence of postoperative nausea and vomiting. Also, the restriction of oral intake until the return of bowel function after surgery has been used for decades to decrease the occurrence of postoperative nausea and vomiting." Anti-nausea medication may also be prescribed. However, "nausea is a complex response. . . . No single pharmacological agent is available that blocks all the receptors that trigger nausea or elicit vomiting. . . . Therefore,

the choice of drugs should be individualized to each patient's needs."

The same article also mentioned the postoperative aid of using ACUPUNCTURE above the wrist and below the knee to lessen nausea and vomiting. More commonly, other post-operative aids usually include bland food and stomach-settling cold liquids such as ginger ale. Ginger also offers an HERBAL THERAPY traditionally used but scientifically unproven to ease nausea. However, a doctor should be consulted before adapting the diet, since some herbs interfere with medicines and blood flow. For example, a hefty amount of garlic can thin the blood and cause a queasy stomach to heave.

A more productive aid to recovery may come from basking in the sun. An article entitled "The Effect of Sunlight on Postoperative Analgesic Medication Use: a Prospective Study of Patients Undergoing Spinal Surgery" in *Psychosomatic Medicine* said, "The exposure postoperatively of patients who have undergone spinal surgery to increased amounts of natural sunlight during their hospital recovery period may result in decreased stress, pain, analgesic medication use, and pain medication costs." Apparently, successful recovery from surgery can be aided, not only by looking on the bright side, but by actually sunning there.

Agency for Healthcare Research and Quality. "Having Surgery? What You Need To Know," AHRQ, U.S. Department of Health and Human Services. Available online. URL: http://www.ahrq.gov/consumer/surgery/surgery.htm. Downloaded May 9, 2006.

American Academy of Orthopaedic Surgeons. "Surgery and Smoking," AAOS. Available online. URL: http://orthoinfo.aaos.org/fact/thr_report.cfm?Thread_ID=324&topcategory=General%20Information. Downloaded May 9, 2006.

Garrett, Kitty, Kayo Tsuruta, Shirley Walker, Sharon Jackson, and Michelle Sweat. "Managing Nausea and Vomiting," *Critical Care Nurse* 23, no. 1 (2003): 31–50.

Haralson, Robert H. III, M.D. and Margie Scalley Vaught. "Coding Spinal Procedures," American Academy of Orthopaedic Surgeons. Available online. URL: http://www.aaos.org/wordhtml/bulletin/aug04/code.htm. Downloaded May 9, 2006.

Heys, S. D., A. C. Schofield, K. W. J. Wahle, and M. Garcia-Caballero. "Nutrition and the Surgical Patient: Triumphs and Challenges," *The Surgeon, Journal of the Royal Colleges of Surgeons of Edinburgh and Ireland* 3, no. 3 (June 2003): 139–144.

Walch, J. M., B. S. Rabin, R. Day, J. N. Williams, K. Choi, and J. D. Kang. "The Effect of Sunlight on Postoperative Analgesic Medication Use: a Prospective Study of Patients Undergoing Spinal Surgery," *Psychosomatic Medicine* 67, no. 1 (January–February 2005): 156–163.

Windsor, A., M. Braga, R. Martindale, P. Buenos, R. Tepaske, L. Kraehenbuehl, and A. Weimann. "Fit for Surgery: An Expert Panel Review on Optimising Patients Prior to Surgery, with a Particular Focus on Nutrition," *The Surgeon, Journal of the Royal Colleges of Surgeons of Edinburgh and Ireland* 2, no. 6 (December 2004): 315–319.

sway back or swayback   See LORDOSIS.

synovial cyst   Similar to a ganglion cyst in the wrist, this benign growth commonly appears in a facet joint between the VERTEBRAE, but not on the SPINAL CORD as happens with the type of cyst that produces SYRINGOMYELIA. A synovial cyst can cause spinal nerve compression as can a HERNIATED DISC, but the difference is that a cyst usually presses from above, whereas a bulging DISC pushes from beneath an affected nerve. Any of the above conditions can also produce CHRONIC BACK PAIN.

Symptoms and Diagnostic Path

The location of a cyst determines the area of discomfort, but LOW BACK PAIN often occurs with or without the radiant pain of RADICULOPATHY. Since a synovial cyst induces symptoms similar to SPINAL STENOSIS and other conditions of the SPINE, an MRI (MAGNETIC RESONANCE IMAGING) will be needed to assess the cyst and surrounding area.

Treatment Options and Outlook

An article in the *Journal of Manipulative and Physiological Therapeutics* reported on two cases involving cysts in the LUMBAR SPINE where both patients received SPINAL MANIPULATION without any ill effects. As reported, "this treatment may be an initial conservative treatment option for synovial cysts with careful patient monitoring for progressive neurologic deficit" or nerve involvement "which would necessitate surgery."

In a 2005 issue of the *Southern Medical Journal,* another report on lumbar cysts said, "Early recognition and treatment helps prevent complications and leads to improved outcome, whereas preoperative diagnosis allows more precise surgical planning, thus diminishing the risks inherent to surgery." Before considering SURGERY though, "conservative treatment is preferred if the cyst wall is not calcified and symptoms show gradual decrease." Some cysts may resolve on their own. If not, STEROID THERAPY may be tried. Then, "injections of corticosteroids epidurally or into the corresponding facet joint may reduce the inflammatory process and resolve symptoms in up to 70% of patients, but is only temporarily effective. In cases of intractable pain and significant clinical symptomatology that persists despite conservative methods, surgical excision remains a safe and definitive treatment." In that event, "the surgical approach requires a wide exposure to provide access to the lesion and the adjacent neural structures, and to enable careful dissection while protecting important structures."

Risk Factors and Preventive Measures

An article in *Radiology* said, "In the lumbar spine, ganglion cysts are thought to be the result of degenerative changes" in the associated ligaments such as "occur in conjunction with hypermobility associated with degenerative disk disease, degenerative spondylolisthesis, and subluxation of the facet joints." Also, "lumbar facet joint synovial cysts are most frequent at the L4–5 level" of the vertebrae. In addition, "osteoarthritis of the adjacent facet joint is usually present and severe, and low-grade degenerative spondylolisthesis also is a frequent finding in these patients." Therefore, early treatment of DEGENERATIVE DISC DISEASE, OSTEOARTHRITIS, SPONDYLOLISTHESIS, and other underlying conditions may help to prevent cyst formation.

Bureau, Nathalie J., M.D., Phoebe A. Kaplan, M.D., and Robert G. Dussault, M.D. "Lumbar Facet Joint Synovial Cyst: Percutaneous Treatment with Steroid Injections and Distention—Clinical and Imaging Follow-up in 12 Patients," *Radiology* 221, no.1 (October 2001): 179–181.

Cox, J. M. and J. M. Cox II. "Chiropractic Treatment of Lumbar Spine Synovial Cysts: a Report of Two Cases," *Journal of Manipulative and Physiological Therapeutics* 28, no. 2 (February 2005): 143–149.

Kouyialis, Andreas T., M. D., Efstathios J. Boviatsis, M.D., Stefanos Korfias, M.D., and Damianos E. Sakas, M.D. "Lumbar Synovial Cyst as a Cause of Low Back Pain and Acute Radiculopathy: A Case Report," *Southern Medical Journal* 98, no. 2 (February 2005): 223–225.

syringomyelia (SM)   A cyst on the SPINAL CORD produces this disorder. Initially, a fall, trauma, or GENETIC FACTOR causes cyst formation, yet years may go by before syringomyelia (SM) develops enough to be noticed.

The American Syringomyelia Alliance Project explained, "For reasons that are only now being understood, cerebrospinal fluid enters the spinal cord, forming a cavity known as a syrinx. (Doctors sometimes use other words such as cyst, hydromyelia or syringohydromyelia.) This syrinx often expands and elongates over time, destroying the center of the spinal cord." Typically, "this malformation occurs during fetal development and is characterized by downward displacement of the lower part of the brain . . . beneath the foramen magnum, into the cervical spinal canal. This displacement blocks the normal flow of cerebrospinal fluid. When normal flow is obstructed, a syrinx can then form in the spinal cord." Although a cyst can develop secondarily to other conditions, such as ARACHNOIDITIS, SPINAL TUMOR, or MENINGOCOCCAL DISEASE, SM is most often, "related to a congenital malformation involving the hindbrain (cerebellum) called a Chiari I Malformation, named after the physician who first described it." Nevertheless, "not all patients with Chiari Malformations will develop a syrinx."

Symptoms and Diagnostic Path

Depending on the spinal region involved, symptoms may include CERVICOGENIC HEADACHE, NECK PAIN, BACKACHE, LOW BACK PAIN, weakness in the PARASPINAL MUSCLES, or stiffness in the VERTEBRAE. Pain may also extend from the BACK or neck into the limbs, sometimes causing numbness or sensitivity to climatic changes. Besides a medical history and physical examination, the physician may request MAGNETIC RESONANCE IMAGING (MRI) to assess the spinal cord, vertebral bones, and soft tissue, including the brain.

Treatment Options and Outlook

Some patients require no treatment; others must simply curtail any daily ACTIVITY that aggravates the symptoms. Still other patients require SURGERY. As a fact sheet from the National Institute of Neurological Disorders and Stroke (NINDS) explained, "The main goal of surgery is to provide more space for the cerebellum (Chiari malformation) at the base of the skull and upper neck, without entering the brain or spinal cord. This results in flattening or disappearance of the primary cavity. If a tumor is causing syringomyelia, removal of the tumor is the treatment of choice and almost always eliminates the syrinx." For some patients, "it may be necessary to drain the syrinx, which can be accomplished using a catheter, drainage tubes, and valves. This system is also known as a shunt."

Risk Factors and Preventive Measures

According to the NINDS Web site, "the decision to use a shunt requires extensive discussion between doctor and patient, as this procedure carries with it the risk of injury to the spinal cord, infection, blockage, or hemorrhage and may not necessarily work for all patients."

More options, however, may become available as RESEARCH continues to decrease the risks and increase the diagnostic tools and preventive measures used for SM. For instance, the NINDS reported, "A new technology known as dynamic MRI allows investigators to view spinal fluid pulsating within the syrinx . . . , and other diagnostic tests," such as a COMPUTED TOMOGRAPHY SCAN, "have also improved greatly with the availability of new, non-toxic, contrast dyes. Patients can expect even better techniques to become available in the future from the research efforts of scientists today."

American Syringomyelia Alliance Project, Inc. "What Is Syringomyelia?" ASAP. Available online. URL: http://www.asap.org/syringomyelia.html. Downloaded May 8, 2006.
National Institute of Neurological Disorders and Stroke. "Syringomyelia Fact Sheet," NINDS, National Institutes of Health. Available online. URL: http://www.ninds.nih.gov/disorders/syringomyelia/detail_syringomyelia.htm. Last updated May 4, 2006.

tailbone See COCCYGEAL SPINE.

tension Stresses can tighten PARASPINAL MUS-CLES, stiffen vertebral joints, and make the BACK as unyielding as a shield. This tightening often produces BACKACHE, CHRONIC BACK PAIN, LOW BACK PAIN, and CERVICOGENIC HEADACHES. With or without muscle spasms, tension can limit the RANGE OF MOTION, making an uptight person even more prone to injury. Ultimately, this lack of ease can lead to *dis*ease, but between that state and wellness, a taut body loses snap.

An article entitled "The Stress of Life" in *The Chiropractic Journal* explained, "Health is much more than the absence of symptoms. There is a long, grey area between the two extremes. . . . Our goal should not be to treat disease, but to prevent it." However, "to prevent disease you must know what is normal and be able not just to see the deviations from normal, but also recognize what stresses are challenging the body to remain within normal limits. . . . Obviously, the intent of the body's response to stress is to permit the person to perform far more strenuous physical activity than would otherwise be possible. . . . To do this the body kicks off an immediate hormonal cascade to switch from glucose to fat as the primary source of fuel for energy production. This involves the release of epinephrine," a hormone that constricts blood vessels. "The sympathetic system is also strongly activated in many emotional states."

Risks and Complications

An article posted online by the American Medical Women's Association (AMWA) said, "Too much stress also affects your immune system, weakening it and making you more susceptible to colds, coughs, and infections. It has been traced as the culprit in flare-ups of arthritis and asthma." With active women at high risk, the AMWA further stated, "Even women who sense their own need to slow down are programmed toward over-commitment because they feel guilty about not being able to be everything to everyone in their lives. Time spent alone or nurturing their own mental and physical well-being might be construed as selfish, so they push even harder on all fronts—home, work, and social." In addition, "sociologists speculate that many women today may be disadvantaged because they have incorporated a male standard for achievement in the work world with an old-fashioned female standard for perfection at home."

Statistics and Studies

An online brochure posted by the National Institute for Occupational Safety and Health Web site reported, "In the past 20 years, many studies have looked at the relationship between job stress and a variety of ailments. Mood and sleep disturbances, upset stomach and headache, and disturbed relationships with family and friends are examples of stress-related problems that are quick to develop and are commonly seen in these studies. These early signs of job stress are usually easy to recognize. But the effects of job stress on chronic diseases are more difficult to see because chronic diseases take a long time to develop and can be influenced by many factors other than stress. Nonetheless, evidence is rapidly accumulating to suggest that stress plays an important role in several types of chronic health problems—especially cardiovascular disease, musculoskeletal disorders, and psychological disorders."

According to the National Center for Complementary and Alternative Medicine (NCCAM), "mind-body interventions constitute a major portion of the overall use of CAM by the public. In 2002, five relaxation techniques and imagery, biofeedback, and hypnosis, taken together, were used by more than 30 percent of the adult U.S. population. Prayer was used by more than 50 percent of the population. . . . Mind-body interventions have also been applied to various types of pain. Clinical trials indicate that these interventions may be a particularly effective adjunct in the management of arthritis, with reductions in pain maintained for up to 4 years and reductions in the number of physician visits." RESEARCH has also focused on relaxation therapies, such as music, to prepare patients for SURGERY. As the NCCAM said, "Initial randomized controlled trials . . . found that subjects receiving the mind-body intervention recovered more quickly and spent fewer days in the hospital."

Special Aids and Adaptations
Recovering goals and values may aid people during times of mental stress. To aid musculoskeletal tension, hands-on treatments such as MASSAGE THERAPY, TRIGGER POINT THERAPY, SPINAL MANIPULATION, ACUPRESSURE, or ACUPUNCTURE commonly require more than one session. For example, the American Academy of Medical Acupuncture said, "Typically, a patient will find relief after an average of 12 to 15 sessions depending on the severity of the problem. A typical session, which most patients find painless, lasts from 30 minutes to one hour."

To relieve NECK PAIN produced by tension in the CERVICAL SPINE, the North American Spine Society (NASS) suggested, "Nod your head slowly forward, bringing your chin toward your chest. Repeat five times. Turn your head from side to side very slowly until you can align your chin with your shoulder. Repeat five times. Tilt your head slowly from side to side, bringing your ear over your shoulder." To loosen the THORACIC SPINE, "Roll your shoulders forward, then backward in a circle. Do this for 10–15 seconds to start. Begin with little circles and progress to large circles. Do this several times during the day to relieve tension. These are good if you spend a lot of time at a computer." Similarly, backward bending EXERCISES stretch the LUMBAR SPINE. As the NASS said, "This is especially good if you've been sitting at a desk. Stand up, placing hands on the top of buttocks, just below the waist. Keep your feet shoulder width apart with your toes turned slightly out. Bend your head, then shoulders, then back backward, letting hips go slightly forward for balance. Slowly return to standing. Repeat 10 times."

For overall tension relief, the AMWA suggested, "First, it is necessary to change your behavior so you can slow the emotional pace of your life. Second, learn how to turn off your general adaptation reflex. You can do this by using exercise and relaxation techniques." Well-balanced NUTRITION, enjoyable daily ACTIVITY, and restful SLEEP also help people to readjust their tension settings and adapt to a life of ease.

American Academy of Medical Acupuncture. "Doctors Pinpoint A Solution To Stress-Related Aches And Pains," AAMA. Available online. URL: http://www.medicalacupuncture.org/acu_info/pressrelease/aches.html. Downloaded May 10, 2006.

American Medical Women's Association. "Stress: How Stress Affects You," AMWA. Available online. URL: http://www.amwa-doc.org/index.cfm?objectid=F0CF89D7-D567-0B25-5A03B3F538A94048. Downloaded May 9, 2006.

Loomis, Howard. "The Stress of Life," *The Chiropractic Journal*, A Publication of the World Chiropractic Alliance, May 2005. Available online. URL: http://www.worldchiropracticalliance.org/tcj/2005/may/loomis.htm. Downloaded May 10, 2006.

National Center for Complementary and Alternative Medicine. "Mind-Body Medicine: An Overview," NCCAM, National Institutes of Health. Available online. URL: http://nccam.nih.gov/health/backgrounds/mindbody.htm. Last modified March 2, 2006.

National Institute for Occupational Safety and Health. "NIOSH Safety and Health Topic: Stress at Work," Centers for Disease Prevention and Control, DHHS (NIOSH) Publication No. 99–101. Available online. URL: http://www.cdc.gov/niosh/stresswk.html. Downloaded May 10, 2006.

North American Spine Society. "Stretching/Flexibility Exercises," NASS. Available online. URL: http://www.spine.org/fsp/maintenance-exercise-flexibility.cfm. Last updated March 3, 2005.

teriparatide   See PARATHYROID HORMONE (PTH).

thoracic laminectomy See LAMINECTOMY, LAMINOTOMY.

thoracic outlet syndrome According to the National Institutes of Neurological Disorders and Stroke (NINDS), "Thoracic outlet syndrome (TOS) consists of a group of distinct disorders that affect the nerves in the brachial plexus (nerves that pass into the arms from the neck) and various nerves and blood vessels between the base of the neck and axilla (armpit). For the most part, these disorders have very little in common except the site of occurrence. The disorders are complex, somewhat confusing, and poorly defined, each with various signs and symptoms of the upper limb." Causes also vary from GENETIC FACTORS and BIRTH DEFECTS OF THE SPINE to poor POSTURE, trauma, and FLEXION-EXTENSION INJURY. A BRACHIAL PLEXUS INJURY may be a precipitating factor in TOS too.

Symptoms and Diagnostic Path

An article from the American Pain Foundation said, "The most common symptoms of this disease include pain, coldness, weakness and numbness of the arm and hand, as well as possibly a drooping shoulder. The affected arm and hand may also feel a tingling-type sensation. The majority of patients who have a diagnosis of thoracic outlet syndrome only have the neurological (or nerve related) symptoms described above. Only five percent have vascular (or vein related) symptoms as evidenced by problems with blood flow in the arm and hand, such as swelling, discoloration and/or bulging of the veins."

The most commonly associated anatomic finding with TOS is a cervical rib, diagnosed when the seventh (lowest and final) cervical vertebra has a rib association visible on X-RAY. This extra rib can put pressure on the brachial plexus, thus resulting in the arm symptoms associated with the diagnosis of TOS. With no conclusive tests though, a doctor may first rule out such conditions as FIBROMYALGIA, REFLEX SYMPATHETIC DYSTROPHY SYNDROME, or DEGENERATIVE DISC DISEASE.

Treatment Options and Outlook

NONSTEROIDAL ANTI-INFLAMMATORY DRUG THERAPY can ease pain and inflammation, while physical therapy and EXERCISES increase RANGE OF MOTION and strengthen the PARASPINAL MUSCLES. Although rarely done, SURGERY may be needed to remove a portion of bone or soft tissue hindering the spinal nerves.

Risk Factors and Preventive Measures

To prevent flare-ups, the American Academy of Orthopaedic Surgeons (AAOS) advised, "If you have symptoms of TOS, avoid carrying heavy bags over your shoulder because this depresses the collarbone and increases pressure on the thoracic outlet. You could also do some simple exercises to keep your shoulder muscles strong. Here are four that you can try; do 10 repetitions of each exercise twice daily. 1. Corner Stretch: Stand in a corner (about one foot away from the corner) with your hands at shoulder height, one on each wall. Lean into the corner until you feel a gentle stretch across your chest. Hold for 5 seconds. 2. Neck Stretch: Put your left hand on your head, and your right hand behind your back. Pull your head toward your left shoulder until you feel a gentle stretch on the right side of your neck. Hold for 5 seconds. Switch hand positions and repeat the exercise in the opposite direction. 3. Shoulder Rolls: Shrug your shoulders up, back, and then down in a circular motion. 4. Neck Retraction: Pull your head straight back, keeping your jaw level. Hold for 5 seconds." However, AAOS also cautioned, "As with any exercise program, if you start to hurt—stop!"

American Academy of Orthopaedic Surgeons. "Thoracic Outlet Syndrome," AAOS. Available online. URL: http://orthoinfo.aaos.org/fact/thr_report.cfm?Thread_ID=206&topcategory=Shoulder. Downloaded May 10, 2006.

Fishman, Scott M., M.D. "Pain Question & Answer: Thoracic Outlet Syndrome," American Pain Foundation. Available online. URL: http://www.painfoundation.org/page.asp?file=QandA/Thoracic.htm. Downloaded May 10, 2006.

National Institutes of Neurological Disorders and Stroke. "NINDS Thoracic Outlet Syndrome Information Page," National Institutes of Health. Available online. URL: http://www.ninds.nih.gov/disorders/thoracic/thoracic.htm. Last updated January 25, 2006.

thoracic spine   Located between the flexible CER-VICAL SPINE and mobile LUMBAR SPINE, the thoracic spine requires less RANGE OF MOTION for its protective role. As explained by the North American Spine Society, "The main function of the thoracic spine is to protect the organs of the chest, especially the heart and lungs. There are 12 thoracic vertebrae with one rib attached on each side, to create a thoracic cage, which protects the internal organs of the chest." As a mark of POSTURE, "the thoracic spine has a normal kyphosis, or 'C' curve," but abnormal KYPHOSIS and SCOLIOSIS can also occur.

Risks and Complications

A lot rides on the upper BACK of the thoracic spine. For example, CHILDREN and ADOLESCENTS may forget BACKPACK SAFETY, or workers may overload the thoracic VERTEBRAE while LIFTING heavy objects. Such excesses can cause upper back pain or even a FRACTURE. With no provocation though, ELDERLY patients with OSTEOPOROSIS and children with OSTEOGENESIS IMPERFECTA or other conditions of bone loss may develop a VERTEBRAL COMPRESSION FRACTURE in the thoracic spine.

More often, pain radiates from other regions of the SPINE. As an article on the Spine-health Web site explained, "Because there is little motion and a great deal of stability throughout the upper back (thoracic spine), this section of the spine does not tend to develop common spinal disorders" such as a HERNIATED DISC or SPINAL STENOSIS. Those conditions "are exceedingly rare in the upper back," yet pain elsewhere may be felt in the thoracic region.

Statistics and Studies

The American Academy of Orthopaedic Surgeons summarized data presented in various studies: "Fracture of one or more parts of the spinal column (vertebrae) of the middle (thoracic) or lower (lumbar) back is a serious injury usually caused by high-energy trauma like a car crash, fall, sports accident or act of violence (i.e., gunshot wound). Males experience the injury four times more often than females do. The spinal cord may be injured depending on the severity of the fracture."

Special Aids and Adaptations

ATHLETES need the aid of well-maintained equipment to protect the upper back. In general,

therapeutic aids include SPINAL MANIPULATION, ACU-PUNCTURE, MASSAGE THERAPY, TRIGGER POINT THER-APY, HYDROTHERAPY, and EXERCISE to strength the PARASPINAL MUSCLES. For postural problems in the upper back, an ORTHOTIC brace may reduce progression, but with a severe curvature, SURGERY, such as THORACOPLASTY, may be needed.

American Academy of Orthopaedic Surgeons. "Fracture of the Thoracic and Lumbar Spine," AAOS. Available online. URL: http://orthoinfo.aaos.org/fact/thr_report.cfm?Thread_ID=299&topcategory=Spine. Downloaded May 10, 2006.

North American Spine Society. "Definition of Parts and What They Do," NASS. Available online. URL: http://www.spine.org/fsp/anatomy-functions.cfm. Last updated March 8, 2005.

Sellers, J. Talbot. "All about Upper Back Pain," Spine-health. Available online. URL: http://www.spine-health.com/topics/cd/pain/upperback1.html. Downloaded May 10, 2006.

thoracoplasty   This type of SURGERY commonly focuses on the rib deformity present with SCOLIO-SIS in the upper BACK or THORACIC SPINE. Although primarily performed for cosmetic reasons, thoracoplasty may address some rib deformities or BIRTH DEFECTS of the chest wall that hinder breathing. Therefore, the procedure will often be used to treat INFANTS, CHILDREN, and growing ADOLESCENTS.

Procedure

The iScoliosis.com Web site explained, "Thoracoplasty involves the surgical removal (resection) of rib segments. More specifically, this surgical procedure involves shortening certain ribs in the thoracic or chest area. The surgeon determines which ribs to shorten based on which ones (1) are prominent, and (2) are not expected to be reduced by correction of the curvature. The surgeon determines how much to shorten the ribs based on the nature of the patient's curve and the severity of the rib hump. A shortened rib, once it has completely healed, is as strong as the original rib." Since the removed portion of bone can also provide a BONE GRAFT for other types of spinal surgery involving the spine, thoracoplasty may be scheduled prior to another surgical event. Sometimes that may not be possible. Also, "some patients elect to have a thoracoplasty performed after they have recovered from their spinal surgery. For patients who choose to undergo the thoracoplasty as a separate procedure, the hospital stay is usually 5 to 7 days; and the recovery time is around 2 to 3 months. In contrast, performing a thoracoplasty during spinal surgery does not prolong the patient's recovery period."

Risks and Complications

Without thoracoplasty, unbalanced growth in the SPINE may continue, yet surgery offers no guarantees. As an article in *The Journal of Bone and Joint Surgery* said, "Early surgical stabilization of the curve in patients with congenital scoliosis is based on the concept that a short straight spine is better than a long crooked one." Generally, "normal thoracic volume depends on adequate height of the thorax from growth of the thoracic spine and on adequate thoracic width and depth from growth of the rib cage. Normal thoracic function in a child depends on intact diaphragmatic function for the primary breathing mechanism and on normal rib motion for the secondary breathing mechanism." Conversely, "abnormalities in thoracic volume or function may result in thoracic insufficiency syndrome, which is the inability of the thorax to support normal respiration or lung growth." Such complications can be fatal.

Outlook and Lifestyle Modifications

In general, thoracoplasty provides a good outlook. As the National Scoliosis Foundation reported, "For moderately severe deformities, the procedure appears to result in a significantly greater improvement in a patient's overall appearance, though it will not result in perfect symmetry. The procedure also relieves pain that may be associated with a rib hump, such as when an individual leans up against a chair."

Campbell, Robert M. Jr., M.D. and Anna K. Hell-Vocke, M.D. "Growth of the Thoracic Spine in Congenital Scoliosis after Expansion Thoracoplasty," *The Journal of Bone and Joint Surgery, Inc.,* 85, no. 3 (March 2003): 409–420.

Medtronic Sofamor Danek. "Surgical: Thoracoplasty," Treatment Options, iScoliosis.com. Available online. URL: http://www.iscoliosis.com/treatment-surgical-thoracoplasty.html. Last updated December 27, 2005.

National Scoliosis Foundation. "Rib Thoracoplasty," NSF. Available online. URL: http://www.scoliosis.org/resources/medicalupdates/ribthoracoplasty.php. Downloaded May 10, 2006.

topical analgesic   Whether in a cream, salve, gel, or spray, this type of PAIN RELIEVER works on the surface. As *Arthritis Today's Drug Guide 2005* explained, "Capsaicin works by blocking the transmission of a pain-relaying substance, called substance P, to the brain." Conversely, "substances, such as menthol, oil of wintergreen, camphor, eucalyptus oil and turpentine oil, . . . fool pain by creating a feeling of cold or heat over sore muscles," while salicylates provide "compounds that inhibit pain and inflammation by seeping through the skin."

Bandolier also discussed topical salicylates or NONSTEROIDAL ANTI-INFLAMMATORY DRUGS (NSAIDs), saying, "Topical NSAIDs for pain relief remain one of the more controversial subjects in analgesic practice. In some parts of the world their use is regarded as sensible, with adequate evidence for their use. In other parts of the world they are regarded as little more than placebo, with any effect due just to the rubbing."

Dosage and Potential Side Effects

Each analgesic has a different approach and dosage. For instance, the article "Topical Capsaicin for Chronic Pain" said, "For osteoarthritis, treatment is with 0.025% cream, four times daily." However, "estimates of efficacy are low, and adverse event rates high." Therefore, "topical capsaicin is an unlikely first or even second choice for treatment, but will help some people."

Statistics and Studies

An article entitled "Topical Salicylate for Acute and Chronic Pain" reported, "Three placebo controlled trials (one of low validity) had information from 182 patients. The mean percentage of patients with at least 50% pain relief was 67% with topical salicylate and was 18% with placebo." Furthermore, "local adverse events and withdrawals were generally rare," but patients with sensitive skin need to be especially wary.

A *BMJ* editorial cautioned "that topical nonsteroidal anti-inflammatory drugs were superior to placebo in reducing pain and improving function over a fortnight, but that these effects were lost after four weeks had elapsed. The authors conclude that little evidence exists to support the long term use of topical non-steroidal anti-inflammatory drugs in osteoarthritis and suggest that current recommendations be revised. Most of the randomised controlled trials included in the review were of short duration (two weeks or less) and not a single study extended beyond one month."

Arthritis Foundation. "Rub It On: Topical Analgesics," *Arthritis Today's Drug Guide 2005.* Available online. URL: http://www.arthritis.org/conditions/DrugGuide/rubiton.asp. Downloaded May 12, 2006.

Bandolier. "Topical Analgesics Introduction." Available online. URL: http://www.jr2.ox.ac.uk/bandolier/booth/painpag/topical/Topintro.html. Downloaded May 12, 2006.

————. "Topical Capsaicin for Chronic Pain." Available online. URL: http://www.jr2.ox.ac.uk/bandolier/booth/painpag/topical/topcap.html. Downloaded May 12, 2006.

————. "Topical Salicylate for Acute and Chronic Pain." Available online. URL: http://www.jr2.ox.ac.uk/bandolier/booth/painpag/topical/toprube.html. Downloaded May 12, 2006.

Cooper, Cyrus and Kelsey M. Jordan. "Topical NSAIDs in Osteoarthritis," *BMJ* 329, no. 7 (August 2004): 304–305.

torticollis Also known as wryneck or twisted neck, this condition may be apparent in INFANTS and young CHILDREN who hold their heads to one side. For some, this can result from a BIRTH INJURY, but womb crowding may be a more likely cause. Regardless, muscles on one side of the CERVICAL SPINE tighten, tilting the chin toward the opposite shoulder.

Torticollis can also appear in adults, for instance after a FLEXION-EXTENSION INJURY or as a side effect of medications. In some instances, GENETIC FACTORS may be involved. As the eMedicineHealth.com Web site explained, "When the disorder occurs in people with a family history, it is referred to as spasmodic torticollis. The characteristic twisting of the neck is initially spasmodic and begins between ages 31–50

years. If you leave the condition untreated, it likely will become permanent."

Symptoms and Diagnostic Path

Besides slanted POSTURE, torticollis can produce muscle spasm and limit RANGE OF MOTION. If a lump appears on the neck of a newborn, this may slowly disappear. However, severe cases of torticollis may result in a misshapen BACK. To assess the condition, a physical examination and X-RAYS will usually be needed.

Treatment Options and Outlook

Regarding newborns, the American Academy of Orthopaedic Surgeons (AAOS) advised, "The initial treatment consists of a series of exercises that must be done several times a day. The physician may refer you to a physical therapist, but most of the time, the parents will be doing the exercises with the child, turning and bending the child's head to stretch the muscle." The AAOS also said, "Placing toys and other objects in positions where the infant has to turn the head to see them encourages the infant to stretch the muscle. So does carrying the infant in a side-lying position, with the face away from you."

For adults who develop torticollis, NONSTEROIDAL ANTI-INFLAMMATORY DRUG THERAPY and MUSCLE RELAXANTS may be prescribed. Also, MASSAGE THERAPY, TRIGGER POINT THERAPY, or special therapeutic EXERCISES may be recommended.

Risk Factors and Preventive Measures

Although a rare occurrence, what first appears to be torticollis could be something else. For example, the eMedicineHealth.com article advised that "anyone who experiences spasms of the neck muscles involved with swallowing or breathing or symptoms that might involve the central nervous system should be evaluated." Since mobility problems or difficulty in speaking may indicate SPINAL CORD involvement, a COMPUTED TOMOGRAPHY SCAN may be needed. For most patients, though, neck stiffness eventually eases with proper treatment.

American Academy of Orthopaedic Surgeons. "Congenital Torticollis (Twisted Neck)," AAOS. Available online. URL: http://orthoinfo.aaos.org/fact/thr_report.cfm?Thread_ID=259&topcategory=Neck. Downloaded May 12, 2006.

Kulkarni, Rick, M.D. and David Geffen. "Torticollis," eMedicineHealth.com. Available online. URL: http://www.emedicinehealth.com/torticollis/article_em.htm. Downloaded May 13, 2006.

traction   With weights and pulleys stretching the SPINE, this treatment may look more torturous than therapeutic. Nevertheless, traction can often relieve muscle spasm and pain caused by OSTEOARTHRITIS, FACET JOINT DISORDER, a HERNIATED DISC, DEGENERATIVE DISC DISEASE, and other conditions that exert pressure on the VERTEBRAE.

Procedure

Explaining the procedure, the National Institute of Arthritis and Musculoskeletal and Skin Diseases (NIAMS) said, "Traction involves using pulleys and weights to stretch the back. The rationale behind traction is to pull the vertebrae apart to allow a bulging disc to slip back into place. Some people experience pain relief while in traction, but that relief is usually temporary."

With a strapping device secured around the skull or CERVICAL SPINE, a pulley exerts tension for several minutes to, sometimes, several hours. This pulling effect may be intermittent or continuous, but either way, the amount of weight used should remain within 10 percent of the patient's body weight.

Risks and Complications

According to the NIAMS, "once traction is released, the stretch is not sustained and back pain is likely to return." This does not render traction invalid but merely reminds patients that, as happens with a PAIN RELIEVER, the treatment does not cure an underlying problem. Using italics for emphasis, the NIAMS added, *"There is no scientific evidence that traction provides any long-term benefits for people with back pain."*

Generally, traction relieves a pressing, albeit, temporary condition. This treatment would be inappropriate, however, for spinal concerns during PREGNANCY or for OSTEOGENESIS IMPERFECTA, OSTEOPOROSIS, and other conditions of bone loss. For a SPRAIN, STRAIN, or FRACTURE, traction could be a wrenching experience.

Outlook and Lifestyle Modifications

For some spinal conditions, traction does improve the overall outlook. For instance, an article on the SpineUniverse Web site said, "There are a number of medically accepted uses for spinal traction, which include the mobilization of soft tissues or joints, decompression of pinched nerve roots, and reduction of herniated intervertebral disks. Currently, the most important use of traction is for the management of cervical spine instability. Instability is defined as damage to the cervical spinal column, either through trauma or disease, resulting in a potential for shifting/malunion of fractured bones prior to healing or abnormal movement of the injured region with a likelihood of additional neurological damage. Traction is an extremely effective means of realigning a cervical spinal dislocation and providing stabilization for these types of cervical spine injury."

National Institute of Arthritis and Musculoskeletal and Skin Diseases. "Handout on Health: Back Pain," NIAMS, National Institutes of Health. Available online. URL: http://www.niams.nih.gov/hi/topics/pain/backpain.htm. Downloaded May 13, 2006.

Traynelis, Vincent C., M.D. "Spinal Traction," SpineUniverse. Available online. URL: http://www.spineuniverse.com/displayarticle.php/article1478.html. Last updated November 22, 2005.

transcutaneous electronic nerve stimulator (TENS) unit   As its name suggests, a transcutaneous electronic nerve stimulator (TENS) unit electronically sends stimulation across, through, and beyond the skin, distracting spinal nerve pain with soothing pulses. This treatment may be used to ease chronic symptoms of OSTEOARTHRITIS, RHEUMATOID ARTHRITIS, SCIATICA, and FLEXION-EXTENSION INJURY.

Procedure

With electrodes placed on or near the point of pain, a unit about the size of a deck of cards transmits electronic pulses along the spinal nerves. If desired, the patient can adjust the location and frequency with each treatment. As an article on the Spine-health Web site explained, "High frequency stimulation, sometimes called 'conventional', is tolerable for hours, but the resultant pain relief lasts for a shorter period of time. Low-frequency stimulation, sometimes called 'acupuncture-like', is more uncomfortable and tolerable for only 20–30 minutes, but the resultant pain relief lasts longer."

Usually patients attach and operate a TENS unit themselves. However, an article in *Academic Emergency Medicine* said, "Patients with acute low back pain may require emergency transport because of pain and immobilization." In such cases, "TENS was found to be effective and rapid in reducing pain during emergency transport of patients with acute low back pain and should be considered due to its ease of use and lack of side effects in the study population."

Risks and Complications

While TENS can aid LOW BACK PAIN, it does not treat spinal concerns during PREGNANCY, nor should it be used for patients with a pacemaker. If a doctor approves TENS use, the person should follow instructions, make adjustments as needed, and give the treatment a chance to take effect.

Outlook and Lifestyle Modifications

Patients may have no say in pain, but they can control TENS treatment. Some may be helped for days with a half-hour session. Others need more time. Either way, patients often feel in control of their lives again. In addition, TENS encourages the body's production of natural chemicals, such as endorphins, that ease pain and foster a sense of well-being.

Bertalanffy, Alexander, M.D, Alexander Kober, M.D., Petra Bertalanffy, M.D., Burkhard Gustorff, M.D., Odette Gore, M.D., Sharam Adel, M.D., and Klaus Hoerauf, M.D. "Transcutaneous Electrical Nerve Stimulation Reduces Acute Low Back Pain during Emergency Transport," *Academic Emergency Medicine* 12, no. 7 (2005): 607–611.

Revord, John, M.D. "Transcutaneous Electrical Nerve Stimulators (TENS)," Spine-health. Available online. URL: http://www.spine-health.com/topics/conserv/electro/el02.html. Downloaded May 13, 2006.

trigger point therapy When something hurts, a natural inclination is to hold or press the achy area, so for thousands of years, people have instinctively cradled or pressed into pain. Trained practitioners

do this to full effect, but anyone can apply trigger point therapy by gently rubbing or pressing and releasing a painful site. While those knotted PARASPINAL MUSCLES in the back of the BACK may be hard to reach, the curved end of a walking cane makes a useful device for lightly pressing, releasing, and untethering the tightness up and down the SPINE.

More akin to MASSAGE THERAPY than ACUPRESSURE, trigger point therapy provides an effective treatment for FIBROMYALGIA, TENSION, or muscle spasm. With great care taken, of course, this therapy can even treat an INFANT who experienced a mild BIRTH INJURY TO THE SPINE, but not a FRACTURE. Growing CHILDREN and ADOLESCENTS with POSTURE problems may also be helped by trigger point therapy.

Procedure

An article posted on the Fibromyalgia Symptoms Web site identified trigger points and their treatment. As the article explained, "Active trigger points cause pain when you press them. They do not refer pain to other parts of the body." Likewise, "latent trigger points also cause pain when they are pressed. However, they can also result in pain in other areas of your body. For instance, a trigger point in your neck may cause you to feel pain in your back." To explain a typical procedure, the article said, "During trigger point therapy, your practitioner will exert pressure on your trigger points by using her fingers, knuckles, or elbows. This pressure is maintained for about 10 seconds and then released. Pressure is then reapplied in a pumping action for a further 30 seconds. After treatment, your muscles are stretched and lengthened to enhance flexibility."

Risks and Complications

Too much pressure on a knotted muscle can produce bruising in anyone, but for patients with OSTEOPOROSIS or other conditions of bone loss, that same pressure could result in VERTEBRAL COMPRESSION FRACTURE. This therapy would also be ill-advised for patients with DEGENERATIVE DISC DISEASE, HERNIATED DISC, or any degenerative disorder of the musculoskeletal system.

Outlook and Lifestyle Modifications

Trigger point therapy often improves circulation and RANGE OF MOTION, enabling patients to increase daily ACTIVITY and begin therapeutic EXERCISE to relax spinal muscles. Dietary modifications include increasing WATER and CALCIUM-rich foods to avoid future episodes of muscle knotting. According to MamasHealth. com, "the purpose of trigger point therapy is to eliminate pain and to re-educate the muscles into pain-free habits. After several treatments, the swelling and stiffness of neuromuscular pain is reduced, range of motion is increased, tension is relieved, and circulation, flexibility and coordination are improved."

Fibromyalgia Symptoms. "Trigger Point Therapy," Hearth-stone Communications, Ltd. Available online. URL: http://www.fibromyalgia-symptoms.org/fibromyalgia_trigger_therapy.html. Downloaded May 15, 2006.

MamasHealth.com. "Trigger Point Therapy." Available online. URL: http://www.mamashealth.com/massage/trigger.asp. Downloaded May 15, 2006.

tuberculosis   See SPINAL TUBERCULOSIS.

Turner syndrome   See DWARFISM.

ultrasound therapy Whether used to diagnose a musculoskeletal problem or take care of one, this treatment sends waves of sound resonating beneath the skin. As a diagnostic tool, ultrasound assesses damage to tendons and ligaments after a SPRAIN or STRAIN. Therapeutically, the treatment relieves pain, inflammation, and muscle spasm, and, in the process, a patient's RANGE OF MOTION may also improve.

Procedure

The Radiological Society of North America described a typical procedure for using ultrasound as a diagnostic tool: "The patient is positioned on an examination table that can tilt and move. A clear gel is applied to the area that will be examined. Since the sound waves cannot penetrate air, the gel helps the transducer make a secure contact and eliminates air pockets between the transducer and skin. The radiologist then pressures the transducer firmly against the skin and sweeps it back and forth to image the area of interest, reviewing the images on the monitor and capturing 'snapshots' as required."

Risks and Complications

Painless and noninvasive, ultrasound has no known risks. Unlike X-RAY, the equipment involves no radiation, but X-rays or MAGNETIC RESONANCE IMAGING (MRI) will better assess a bone FRACTURE. For patients with pacemakers though, ultrasound can be used when an MRI cannot.

Outlook and Lifestyle Modifications

An article in *Sports Medicine* reported, "A new direction for ultrasound therapy has been revealed by recent research demonstrating a beneficial effect of ultrasound on injured bone. During fresh fracture repair, ultrasound reduced healing times by between 30 and 38%. When applied to non-united fractures, it stimulated union in 86% of cases. These benefits were generated using low-intensity . . . pulsed ultrasound," or LIPUS. "Although currently developed for the intervention of bone injuries, LIPUS has the potential to be used on tissues and conditions more commonly encountered in sports medicine. These include injuries to ligament, tendon, muscle and cartilage."

Explaining how ultrasound has potential healing effects, a SpineUniverse article said, "As the probe glides over the skin's surface, sound waves penetrate the skin's surface causing soft tissues to vibrate creating deep heat. In turn, the heat induces vasodilation: drawing blood into the target tissues. Increased blood flow delivers needed oxygen and nutrients, and removes cell wastes."

Davis, Dana L. and Susan Spinasanta. "Ultrasound: A Common Treatment Used in Physical Therapy," SpineUniverse. Available online. URL: http://www.spineuniverse.com/displayarticle.php/article1495.html. Last updated July 24, 2005.

Radiological Society of North America, Inc. "Ultrasound-Musculoskeletal," *RadiologyInfo* ™. Available online. URL: http://www.radiologyinfo.org/pdf/musculous.pdf. Downloaded May 13, 2006.

Warden, S. J. "A New Direction for Ultrasound Therapy in Sports Medicine," *Sports Medicine* 33, no. 2 (2003): 95–107.

upper back pain See THORACIC SPINE.

vertebrae   From the neck to the tailbone, about 33 irregularly shaped bones stack up as the spinal column. Seven smaller vertebrae comprise the CERVICAL SPINE, but the size increases in the 12 bones of the THORACIC SPINE. The largest vertebrae, however, occur in the LUMBAR SPINE and fused SACRAL VERTEBRAE before tapering into the COCCYGEAL SPINE. Those posterior regions hold the WEIGHT of the body yet lack the gel-filled DISCS that cushion upper vertebrae and aid RANGE OF MOTION.

In the article "Definition of Parts and What They Do," the North American Spine Society (NASS) explained, "Each individual vertebra has unique features depending on the region in which it is found. Every vertebra, regardless of location, has three basic functional parts: 1) the drum-shaped vertebral body, designed to bear weight and withstand compression or loading; 2) the posterior (backside) arch, made of the lamina, pedicles, and facet joints; and 3) the transverse processes, to which muscles attach. . . . The pedicle is a paired, strong, tubular bony structure made of hard cortical bone on the outside and cancellous bone on the inside. Each pedicle comes out of the side of the vertebral body and projects to the back. Pedicles act as the lateral (side) walls of the bony spinal canal that protects the spinal cord and cauda equina, or nerve roots in the lumbar region. There is also a space created between the facet joints and pedicles of one vertebral body and the next, called the intervertebral foramen, through which the spinal nerves branch out to the rest of your body." Also, "the lamina are shingle-like plates of bone coming from the pedicles to arch over the nerves and join at the midline. . . . As the lamina come together at the back of the spinal column, they join to form the spinous process, the bony part of the spine that you can feel at the midline when you rub your back."

Risks and Complications

In considering the typical risks in the life of a vertebra, an article on the Spine-health Web site said, "Fifty percent of flexion (bending forward) occurs at the hips, and fifty percent occurs at the lower spine (lower back). The motion is divided between the five motion segments in the lower back, although a disproportionate amount of the motion is at L4–L5 (lumbar segment 4 and 5) and L3–L4 (lumbar segment 3 and 4). Consequently, these two segments of the lower back are the most likely to break down with degeneration. As these segments break down they can become unstable with an excess of motion creating low back pain." With trauma though, the cervical spine may be more likely to feel the effects of a FLEXION-EXTENSION INJURY.

Besides having a higher risk of injuries, ELDERLY persons and patients with OSTEOPOROSIS may sustain VERTEBRAL COMPRESSION FRACTURE and subsequent POSTURE disorders, such as KYPHOSIS. However, the same could be said for CHILDREN and ADOLESCENTS with EATING DISORDERS, whereas the spinal concerns of ATHLETES reflect those of aging patients with FACET JOINT DISORDER. Whether from wearing, tearing, or daring, vertebral damage can also produce SPINAL STENOSIS and spinal nerve compression, either of which can cause ACUTE PAIN to radiate from head to toe. More worrisome, vertebral injuries, collapsing bone, and spinal instability can affect the SPINAL CORD, producing severe pain or paralysis.

Statistics and Studies

To find a relatively easy and inexpensive way to stabilize the spine, researchers studied the therapeutic use of a large ball. According to the report published in the *Journal of Strength and Conditioning Research*, "Stability ball training (SBT) is believed to improve spinal stability (SS) and could reduce the risk of back pain in sedentary individuals." Therefore, "the purpose of this study was to examine the effects of SBT on SS. Twenty sedentary individuals were randomly assigned to either an experimental group that performed SBT twice per week for 10 weeks or to a control group." With significant improvement shown in the experimental group, the researchers concluded that "this type of programming might be beneficial to individuals who spend a good deal of time sitting (i.e., in corporate fitness programs) or for individuals who are prone to back pain and have been cleared to exercise."

Special Aids and Adaptations

Although GENETIC FACTORS affect the spinal column, adaptations can be made in daily ACTIVITY and ENVIRONMENTAL INFLUENCES to aid the back and spine. For example, WEIGHT-BEARING EXERCISE, well-balanced NUTRITION, ample WATER, and other BONE BUILDING efforts help to keep the vertebrae strong.

Carter, J. M., W. C. Beam, S. G. McMahan, M. L. Barr, and L. E. Brown. "The Effects of Stability Ball Training on Spinal Stability in Sedentary Individuals," *Journal of Strength and Conditioning Research* 20, no. 2 (May 2006): 429–435.

North American Spine Society. "Definition of Parts and What They Do," NASS. Available online. URL: http://www.spine.org/fsp/anatomy-functions.cfm. Last updated March 8, 2005.

Ullrich, Peter F. Jr., M.D. "Vertebrae in the Cervical, Thoracic and Lumbar Spine," Spine-health. Available online. URL: http://www.spine-health.com/topics/anat/a02.html. Downloaded May 13, 2006.

vertebral compression fracture This spontaneous type of FRACTURE in the VERTEBRAE can be caused by RICKETS, CANCER, OSTEOGENESIS IMPERFECTA, OSTEOPENIA, or other conditions of bone loss. However, the most common cause of compression fractures is OSTEOPOROSIS. As the Spine Institute of New York explained, "Bending forward, for example, can be enough to cause a 'crush fracture' in a weakened vertebra. This type of fracture causes the loss of body height and a humped back (kyphosis), especially in elderly women." In severe cases, coughing or rolling out of bed can cause a bone to break.

Symptoms and Diagnostic Path

Some patients experience mild discomfort requiring no treatment. Others have ongoing breaks that destabilize the SPINE and greatly reduce height. A medical history, physical examination, and X-RAYS can confirm a diagnosis, but if symptoms include numbness in the arms or legs, tests may also include a MYELOGRAM and a COMPUTED TOMOGRAPHY SCAN to evaluate SPINAL CORD involvement.

An article on the Spine-health Web site discussed the loss of height, both as a symptom and as a diagnostic tool: "As the vertebrae cave in, each vertebra tends to lose at least 15–20% of its height." This spinal reduction "changes the musculature in the back and can cause pain from muscle fatigue that can continue after the bone fracture has healed." Besides CHRONIC BACK PAIN, another telling sign may be a bulging abdomen or pot belly. "As the vertebral fractures cause the patient's spine to shrink in height, his or her abdominal contents are compressed into less vertical space. As a result, the abdomen can bulge out, causing clothes not to fit properly and an appearance of gaining weight, even though the patient has not put on weight."

Treatment Options and Outlook

To ease the pain of a vertebral compression fracture, medications vary from such PAIN RELIEVERS as NONSTEROIDAL ANTI-INFLAMMATORY DRUG THERAPY to OPIOIDS FOR PAIN relief. Other options range widely from no treatment at all to ORTHOTIC bracing of the THORACIC SPINE to spine-stabilizing SURGERY. If patients experience significant loss of height, the minimally invasive procedure of VERTEBROPLASTY can stabilize the spine, relieve pain, and correct POSTURE deformities, such as KYPHOSIS.

Risk Factors and Preventive Measures

Growing CHILDREN and ADOLESCENTS with EATING DISORDERS, post-menopausal women, and ELDERLY patients over 65 have the high risks of fractures caused by bone loss. With BONE MINERAL DENSITY TESTS to monitor progress every year or two, many patients prevent recurring fractures through such BONE BUILDING efforts as WEIGHT-BEARING EXERCISE,

healthful NUTRITION, and medications, such as CAL-
CITONIN or BISPHOSPHONATES.

Boden, Scott, M.D. "Symptoms of a Vertebral Fracture,"
Spine-health.com. Available online. URL: http://www.
spine-health.com/topics/cd/fracture/fracture02.html.
Posted May 11, 2005.

Kim, David H., M.D., Jeffrey S. Silber, M.D., and Todd
J. Albert, M.D. "Chapter 46: Osteoporotic Vertebral
Compression Fractures, ICL 52," abstract posted by
the American Academy of Orthopaedic Surgeons.
Available online. URL: http://www5.aaos.org/oko/
vb/search/display_all/icl/icl52/52-46.cfm?browse_
source=http://www5.aaos.org/oko/vb/Browse/ICL/
52/v52s7.cfm. Downloaded May 13, 2006.

Spine Institute of New York. "Compression Fracture," Beth
Israel Medical Center. Available online. URL: http://
www.spineinstituteny.com/conditions/compression.
html. Downloaded May 13, 2006.

vertebral subluxation   In chiropractic terminology, subluxation indicates shifting in the VERTEBRAE
just short of a DISLOCATED VERTEBRA or spinal joint.
For instance, INFANTS may encounter vertebral shifts
from undue pressure on the SPINE during a difficult
birth. Besides this potential BIRTH INJURY TO THE SPINE,
growing CHILDREN and ADOLESCENTS may be prone
to spinal misalignment caused by ill-fitting SHOES or
lack of BACKPACK SAFETY. In addition, biomechanical
changes in POSTURE or an external influence, such as
ERGONOMIC FACTORS or a FLEXION-EXTENSION INJURY,
can cause misalignment of the spine. Although a
flexion-extension injury commonly produces a
whiplash in the CERVICAL SPINE, subluxation of the
THORACIC SPINE can occur when an ATHLETE overex-
tends while reaching for a ball or an ELDERLY person
pops a rib while weeding a garden. In the LUMBAR
SPINE, a saggy mattress might cause subluxation and
interrupt SLEEP at almost any age.

Symptoms and Diagnostic Path

Depending on the cause and location, symptoms
may include ACUTE PAIN, LOW BACK PAIN, muscle
fatigue, CERVICOGENIC HEADACHE, and reduced
RANGE OF MOTION. As chiropractor Rick Swartzburg
explained, "Most recently, the term vertebral subluxation complex has been utilized to help patients
understand that it is more than just a bone out of
place that is causing the improper vertebral joint
function, but rather a series of complex changes
occurring. These changes include stiffening of joint
mobility from scar tissue formation, lack of circulation within the joint structure, tightening response
of the tiny vertebral muscles, and pressure build
up around the nerve roots. A vertebral subluxation
complex may cause further imbalance in the muscles and lead to spasm and tearing of the fibers,"
such as occurs with a muscle SPRAIN or STRAIN.

Treatment Options and Outlook

SPINAL MANIPULATION offers the first course of treatment. To promote healing, physical therapy, MAS-
SAGE THERAPY, ULTRASOUND THERAPY, or other type
of COMPLEMENTARY AND ALTERNATE MEDICINE may be
useful too.

Risk Factors and Preventive Measures

To prevent further episodes, EXERCISE to strengthen
the PARASPINAL MUSCLES can be particularly helpful
in keeping a spine in line. Not only does this lower
the risk of vertebral subluxation, it may affect organ
health too. For example, a study of 925 patients
considered the "Correlation between Organ Dys-
functions and Vertebral Displacements," and found
"impulses to the heart are conveyed from segments
T1 to T5" of the thoracic vertebrae "and segments
C3 and C4 . . ." vertebrae of the cervical spine. To
determine the effects of subluxation on other areas
of the body, further RESEARCH might focus on "a
study involving a large patient population . . . with
ECGs before and after treatment."

Fysh, Peter. "Spinal Subluxations in Children," *Dynamic
Chiropractic* 13, no. 2 (January 16, 1995). Available
online. URL: http://www.chiroweb.com/archives/
13/02/21.html. Downloaded May 13, 2006.

Sickesz, M., M.D. "Correlation between Organ Dysfunc-
tions and Vertebral Displacements." Available online.
URL: http://www.orthomanual-medicine.com/tekst2.
html. Downloaded May 13, 2006.

Swartzburg, Rick. "Vertebral Subluxation Complex,"
#1 Back Pain Site. Available online. URL: http://
www.1backpain.com/backvertebralsubluxation.htm#A
ll%20About%20Your%20Condition%20and%20How
%20to%20Approach%20Treatment. Downloaded May
13, 2006.

vertebroplasty In this minimally invasive procedure, the surgeon injects a type of bone cement into VERTEBRAE that have collapsed from VERTEBRAL COMPRESSION FRACTURES caused by OSTEOPOROSIS or other conditions of bone loss. In about 10 minutes, the cement solidifies harder than bone, fusing fragments and relieving CHRONIC BACK PAIN.

Procedure

According to the North American Spine Society (NASS), "after a diagnosis of the compression fracture has been made through an MRI or CT scan, the patient lies prone and is sedated with a mild anesthetic. Under the guidance of an imaging technique called C-arm fluoroscopy, the physician injects a cement-like mixture (polymethylmethacrylate) into the vertebra. The entire process takes one to two hours, although the actual injection usually takes only about 10 minutes. The cement mixture hardens in about half an hour and after a short recovery period the patient is sent home."

Risks and Complications

The NASS reported, "Percutaneous vertebroplasty is relatively new and long-term results are not known. Patients who have one vertebral fracture are five times more likely to get another adjacent to the damaged one; therefore steps should be taken to limit the effects of osteoporosis. Although complications appear to be less than 1%, percutaneous vertebroplasty can cause infection, bleeding or embolism if the cement mixture gets into the blood stream and passes through the heart and lungs."

An article in *The Journal of Supportive Oncology* listed contraindications for vertebroplasty as including DISCITIS, OSTEOMYELITIS, and "inability of the patient to lie prone for the duration of the procedure." Comparing vertebroplasty to KYPHOPLASTY, the article reported, "Although an increase in vertebral body height has been seen with vertebroplasty alone, kyphoplasty results in significantly greater height restoration (97%) than vertebroplasty (30%.)" Furthermore, "both treatments increase the strength of the vertebral body, but only kyphoplasty restores stiffness," which may help patients to increase their LOAD TOLERANCE.

Outlook and Lifestyle Modifications

According to the Radiological Society of North America, "vertebroplasty is often performed on patients too elderly or frail to tolerate open spinal surgery, or with bones too weak for surgical spinal repair. Patients with vertebral damage due to a malignant tumor may sometimes benefit from vertebroplasty. In rare cases, it can be used in younger patients whose osteoporosis is caused by long-term steroid treatment or a metabolic disorder. Typically, vertebroplasty is recommended after simpler treatments—such as bedrest, a back brace or pain medication—have been ineffective, or once medications have begun to cause other problems, such as stomach ulcers. Vertebroplasty can be performed right away in patients who have severe pain requiring hospitalization or conditions limiting bedrest and medications." After the procedure, "about 75 percent of patients regain lost mobility and become more active, which helps combat osteoporosis. After vertebroplasty, patients who had been immobile can get out of bed, reducing their risk of pneumonia. Increased activity builds more muscle strength, further encouraging mobility."

Halpin, Ryan J., Bernard R. Bendok, M.D., and John C. Liu, M.D. "Minimally Invasive Treatments for Spinal Metastases: Vertebroplasty, Kyphoplasty, and Radiofrequency Ablation," *The Journal of Supportive Oncology* 2, no. 4 (July/August 2004): 339–355.

North American Spine Society. "Percutaneous Vertebral Augmentation," NASS. Available online. URL: http://www.spine.org/articles/NT_Percu_Vert_Aug.cfm. Downloaded May 15, 2006.

RadiologyInfo ™. "Vertebroplasty," Radiological Society of North America. Available online. URL: http://www.radiologyinfo.org/content/interventional/vertebro.htm. Last reviewed September 1, 2005.

vitamin A This family of compounds strengthens bones and body cells but is commonly known as a visual aid. For instance, beta-carotene readily converts into vitamin A, aiding eyes and vision as claimed by the parents intent on getting their CHILDREN to eat their carrots. While many dark orange or green vegetables contain beta-carotene, another precursor of vitamin A, retinol, can be found in cod liver oil or meat. As the Linus Pauling Institute said, "Different dietary sources of vitamin A have different potencies. For example, beta-carotene is less easily absorbed than retinol and must be converted . . . by the body."

Since vitamin A is fat-soluble, this nutrient can be stored in body fat cells for future needs. That same trait, however, makes it easy to accumulate too much vitamin A, which, in excess, can lower bone mineral density. Either too much or too little vitamin A can also result in BIRTH DEFECTS. Although a well-balanced diet rarely needs supplements, a doctor may recommend a specific dosage to treat a specific concern. Otherwise, a multi-vitamin usually works well, but good NUTRITION works better.

Statistics and Studies

According to the Office of Dietary Supplements, "researchers are now examining a potential new risk factor for osteoporosis: an excess intake of vitamin A. Animal, human, and laboratory research suggests an association between greater vitamin A intake and weaker bones. Worldwide, the highest incidence of osteoporosis occurs in northern Europe, a population with a high intake of vitamin A. However, decreased biosynthesis of vitamin D associated with lower levels of sun exposure in this population may also contribute to this finding."

Higdon, Jane. "Vitamin A," Linus Pauling Institute, Oregon State University. Available online. URL: http://lpi.oregonstate.edu/infocenter/vitamins/vitaminA/index.html. Downloaded May 15, 2006.
Office of Dietary Supplements. "Dietary Supplement Fact Sheet: Vitamin A and Carotenoids," National Institutes of Health. Available online. URL: http://ods.od.nih.gov/factsheets/vitamina.asp. Downloaded May 15, 2006.

vitamin B-complex   This family of eight vitamins includes thiamine (B1), riboflavin (B2), niacin (B3), pyridoxine (B6), FOLIC ACID (B9), cyanocobalamin (B12), pantothenic acid, and biotin. While each B has a unique chemistry and unique influence on the body, each is water soluble. This means the body washes away the excess, yet too much at once can irritate nerves, especially if Bs have been taken separately. Conversely, inadequate intake can result in BIRTH DEFECTS OF THE SPINE, fatigue, or spinal nerve irritation. Since B vitamins may help to ease TENSION, these nutrients can have therapeutic value in such conditions as REFLEX SYMPATHETIC DYSTROPHY and FIBROMYALGIA.

If B supplements are needed to treat a bone, SPINE, or nerve condition, they should not be taken individually unless a doctor prescribes otherwise. Debates about B continue, for instance on their value in treating neurological conditions. As the Agency for Healthcare Research and Quality reported, "B vitamin supplementation may be of value for neurocognitive function, but the evidence is inconclusive." For general use, a multi-vitamin supplement containing 100 percent of the daily requirement for each B vitamin would be preferable to products favoring one B over another. Even more favorable would be well-balanced NUTRITION with such natural food sources as shellfish, eggs, dairy products, and fortified grain products of cereal or bread.

Agency for Healthcare Research and Quality. "B Vitamins and Berries and Age-Related Neurodegenerative Disorders," AHRQ. Available online. URL: http://www.ahrq.gov/clinic/tp/berrytp.htm#Report. Downloaded May 15, 2006.

vitamin C   Also known as ascorbic acid, this water-soluble vitamin occurs naturally in citrus fruits, but strawberries and uncooked red or green peppers pack more C punch. Not only does this nutrient protect the immune system, but vitamin C may help a body to lose WEIGHT.

Dosage and Potential Side Effects

Information from the Linus Pauling Institute Web site advised, "In the U.S., the recommended dietary allowance (RDA) for vitamin C was recently revised upward from 60 mg daily for men and women. The RDA continues to be based primarily on the prevention of deficiency disease, rather than the prevention of chronic disease and the promotion of optimum health. The recommended intake for smokers is 35 mg/day higher than for nonsmokers, because smokers are under increased . . . stress from the toxins in cigarette smoke and generally have lower blood levels of vitamin C." Although adequate intake has not been established for INFANTS, the dosage for CHILDREN gradually increases from an RDA of 15 mg at age one to 75 mg during ADOLESCENT years.

Statistics and Studies

A 2006 issue of *The Annals of Nutrition and Metabolism* published these recent findings from Switzerland: "A large number of randomized controlled intervention trials with intakes of up to 1 g of vitamin C and up to 30 mg of zinc are available. These trials document that adequate intakes of vitamin C and zinc . . . shorten the duration of respiratory tract infections including the common cold." In addition, "vitamin C contributes to maintaining the . . . integrity of cells and thereby protects them . . . in the inflammatory response." With more RESEARCH needed, vitamin C may prove similarly useful in easing inflammation that occurs in such conditions as ARTHRITIS. Also, "vitamin C concentrations . . . rapidly decline during infections and stress," thus indicating the need for more C in times of TENSION.

Higdon, Jane. "Vitamin C," Linus Pauling Institute, Oregon State University. Available online. URL: http://lpi. oregonstate.edu/infocenter/vitamins/vitaminC/index. html. Downloaded May 15, 2006.

Wintergerst, Eva S., Silvia Maggini, and Dietrich H. Hornig. "Immune-Enhancing Role of Vitamin C and Zinc and Effect on Clinical Conditions," *Annals of Nutrition and Metabolism, European Journal of Nutrition, Metabolic Diseases, and Dietetics* 50, no. 2 (2006): 85–94.

vitamin D With a well-deserved reputation for aiding CALCIUM uptake, this fat-soluble vitamin aids BONE BUILDING and prevents RICKETS. Recent RESEARCH indicates vitamin D regulates cellular activity and may boost the immune system too.

Dosage and Potential Side Effects

Fortified dairy products provide an excellent food source but may cause an allergic response, particularly in INFANTS with lactose intolerance. For older CHILDREN, ADOLESCENTS, and adults, yogurt provides a good source without aggravating allergies. Better yet would be brief daily ACTIVITY in the sun.

A fact sheet from the Office of Dietary Supplements explained, "UV rays from the sun trigger vitamin D synthesis in skin." However, "season, geographic latitude, time of day, cloud cover, smog, and sunscreen affect UV ray exposure and vitamin D synthesis. For example, sunlight exposure from November through February in Boston is insufficient to produce significant vitamin D synthesis in the skin. Complete cloud cover halves the energy of UV rays, and shade reduces it by 60%." Also, "sunscreens with a sun protection factor (SPF) of 8 or greater will block UV rays that produce vitamin D." Therefore, "an initial exposure to sunlight (10–15 minutes) allows adequate time for Vitamin D synthesis and should be followed by application of a sunscreen with an SPF of at least 15 to protect the skin. Ten to fifteen minutes of sun exposure at least two times per week to the face, arms, hands, or back without sunscreen is usually sufficient to provide adequate vitamin D," but "it is very important for individuals with limited sun exposure to include good sources of vitamin D in their diet." Besides dairy products, natural sources include eggs and cold water fish. For babies, "the American Academy of Pediatrics . . . recommends a daily supplement of 200 IU vitamin D for breastfed infants beginning within the first 2 months of life unless they are weaned to receive at least 500 ml (about 2 cups) per day of vitamin D-fortified formula. Children and adolescents who are not routinely exposed to sunlight and do not consume at least 2 8-fluid ounce servings of vitamin D-fortified milk per day are also at higher risk of vitamin D deficiency and may need a dietary supplement containing 200 IU vitamin D." Because vitamin D is fat-soluble, however, excess amounts can quickly accumulate in the body, causing the person to experience a toxic reaction. Then, "vitamin D toxicity can cause nausea, vomiting, poor appetite, constipation, weakness, and weight loss. It can also raise blood levels of calcium, causing mental status changes such as confusion. High blood levels of calcium also can cause heart rhythm abnormalities."

To keep D in perspective, an article in *The Journal of Steroid Biochemistry and Molecular Biology* said, "Actual toxicity is not seen below serum 25OHD values of 250nmol/L," which means "a value that would be produced only at continuing oral intakes in excess of 10,000IU (250microg)/day." The article also summarized the importance of vitamin D in "optimizing intestinal calcium absorption" and minimizing risks of FRACTURE in ELDERLY patients with OSTEOPOROSIS.

Heaney, R. P. "The Vitamin D Requirement in Health and Disease," *The Journal of Steroid Biochemistry and Molecular Biology* 97, no. 1–2 (October 2005): 13–22.

Office of Dietary Supplements. "Dietary Supplement Fact Sheet: Vitamin D," National Institutes of Health. Available online. URL: http://ods.od.nih.gov/factsheets/vitamind.asp. Downloaded May 15, 2006.

vitamin E   According to a fact sheet from the Office of Dietary Supplements, "vitamin E is a fat-soluble vitamin that exists in eight different forms. Each form has its own biological activity, which is the measure of potency or functional use in the body." However, "alpha-tocopherol (α-tocopherol) is the name of the most active form of vitamin E in humans. It is also a powerful biological antioxidant. Vitamin E in supplements is usually sold as alpha-tocopheryl acetate, a form that protects its ability to function as an antioxidant. The synthetic form is labeled 'D, L' while the natural form is labeled 'D'. The synthetic form is only half as active as the natural form."

Dosage and Potential Side Effects

Natural sources can be found in wheat germ, vegetable oils, and nuts, but packaged products seldom list available amounts. Also, people on a low-fat diet may not get enough vitamin E. Since the body stores this vitamin in fat, however, too much E may accumulate. Therefore, the previously mentioned Fact Sheet advised that "the Food and Nutrition Board of the Institute of Medicine has set an upper tolerable intake level (UL) for vitamin E at 1,000 mg (1,500 IU) for any form of supplementary alpha-tocopherol per day. Based for the most part on the result of animal studies, the Board decided that because vitamin E can act as an anticoagulant and may increase the risk of bleeding problems this UL is the highest dose unlikely to result in bleeding problems." Although upper limits have not been established for INFANTS, CHILDREN under three

should not exceed 200 mg, while 800 mg is the maximum for ADOLESCENTS.

Statistics and Studies

According to the Linus Pauling Institute, "a recent meta-analysis that combined the results of 19 clinical trials of vitamin E supplementation for various diseases . . . reported that adults who took supplements of 400 IU/day or more were 6% more likely to die from any cause than those who did not take vitamin E supplements. However, further breakdown of the risk by vitamin E dose and adjustment for other vitamin and mineral supplements revealed that the increased risk of death was statistically significant only at a dose of 2,000 IU/day, which is higher than the UL for adults."

Higdon, Jane. "Vitamin E," Linus Pauling Institute, Oregon State University. Available online. URL: http://lpi.oregonstate.edu/infocenter/vitamins/vitaminE/index.html. Downloaded May 15, 2006.

Office of Dietary Supplements. "Dietary Supplement Fact Sheet: Vitamin E," National Institutes of Health. Available online. URL: http://ods.od.nih.gov/factsheets/vitamine.asp. Downloaded May 15, 2006.

vitamin K   Primarily known for its ability to clot the blood, this nutrient also aids bone health. As occurs with other fat-soluble vitamins, the body stores vitamin K but not in significant amounts. Therefore, most people need to replenish K each day through their choices in NUTRITION.

Dosage and Potential Side Effects

Multivitamins contain various amounts of vitamin K, with the highest numbers usually found in supplements labeled or lauded as bone supplements. Reading product labels is particularly important for patients who take blood-thinning medications. More subtle conflicts also occur among natural food sources where the highest amounts of K arrive in such dark green leafy vegetables as kale or collard greens. Lesser amounts occur next in broccoli, lettuce, and asparagus. For those determined to eat their spinach, the U.S. Department of Agriculture showed that a cup of raw spinach has half again as much vitamin K as a cup of raw broccoli. However, a cup of cooked collard greens, kale, or spinach that has been previously frozen contains almost five times as much vitamin K as a cup of cooked broccoli.

Statistics and Studies

Information from the Linus Pauling Institute reported, "The discovery of vitamin K-dependent proteins in bone has led to research on the role of vitamin K in maintaining bone health." For instance, "osteocalcin, a bone-related protein that circulates in the blood, has been shown to be a sensitive marker of bone formation." Nevertheless, "in the absence of long-term intervention studies using nutritionally optimal doses of vitamin K, evidence of a relationship between vitamin K nutritional sta-

tus and bone health in adults is considered weak. Further investigation is required to determine the physiological function of vitamin K-dependent proteins in bone and the mechanisms by which vitamin K affects bone health and osteoporotic fracture risk."

Higdon, Jane. "Vitamin K," Linus Pauling Institute, Oregon State University. Available online. URL: http://lpi.oregonstate.edu/infocenter/vitamins/vitaminK/index.html. Downloaded May 16, 2006.

U.S. Department of Agriculture. "USDA National Nutrient Database for Standard Reference, Release 18, Vitamin K . . . ," USDA. Available online. URL: http://www.nal.usda.gov/fnic/foodcomp/Data/SR18/nutrlist/sr18a430.pdf. Downloaded May 16, 2006.

water and spine health With water as vital to the body as air, everybody needs daily hydration to survive. Indeed, a *Boston Globe* article reported, "An average adult body is 50 to 65 percent water—that's roughly 45 quarts." Generally, "men are more watery than women. A man's body is 60 to 65 percent water, compared to 50 to 60 percent for a woman." Apparently, this occurs because men have more muscle mass, but "water content differs throughout the body. Blood is made up of 83 percent water, bones are 22 percent water, and muscle is 75 percent water." Those numbers increase in value, though, as "water plays several crucial roles in the body. It helps regulate temperature, carries nutrients and oxygen, and removes waste. It also cushions joints and organs." However, strenuous EXERCISE, climatic changes, and illness reduce water content. Also, "planes are especially drying. It's estimated that you can lose up to two pounds of water during a three-hour flight. . . . By the time you notice the symptoms of dehydration—dry mouth, dark urine, lightheadedness—you're already very dehydrated."

To avoid dehydration, the American Dietetic Association (ADA) recommended consuming eight cups of liquids a day, with more fluids added during heightened daily ACTIVITY or hot weather. This does not have to be water only though. Juice and other healthful drinks count, as do fruits and vegetables with high water content. For instance, the ADA listed a half-cup of lettuce as containing 95 percent water, a half-cup of watermelon 92 percent, and a medium apple 84 percent.

Risks and Complications

While raw fruits and veggies may themselves sip up the adverse effects of such ENVIRONMENTAL INFLUENCES as bug sprays, they generally provide an unpolluted water source that could be crucial for survivors of a disaster, natural or otherwise. Usually though, tap water has been well-treated to treat a body well. If, however, a person has a sensitivity to fluorides or other additives, charcoal filtering devices may be useful. To remove worrisome microbes, distillation does the job, but this process also removes CALCIUM, MAGNESIUM, and other nutrients needed for MINERAL BALANCE.

Along that flow of thought, the World Health Organization (WHO) reported, "Drinking-water may be contaminated by a range of chemical, microbial and physical hazards that could pose risks to health if they are present at high levels. Examples of chemical hazards include lead, arsenic and benzene. Microbial hazards include bacteria, viruses and parasites, such as *Vibrio cholerae, hepatitis A virus,* and *Crytosporidium parvum,* respectively. Physical hazards include glass chips and metal fragments. Because of the large number of possible hazards in drinking-water, the development of standards for drinking-water requires significant resources and expertise." Bottling standards may be high, but "contrary to this, some substances may prove more difficult to manage in bottled than tap water. This is generally because bottled water is stored for longer periods and at higher temperatures than water distributed in piped distribution systems. Control of materials used in containers and closures for bottled waters is, therefore, of special concern. In addition, some micro-organisms, which are normally of little or no public health significance, may grow to higher levels in bottled waters. This growth appears to occur less frequently in gasified water and in water bottled in glass containers compared to still water and water bottled in plastic containers. However, the public health significance of this remains little understood, especially for vulnerable individuals, such as infants and children, pregnant women, immuno-compromised individuals and the elderly. In regard to infants, as bottled water is not sterile, it should be disinfected—for example, by boiling for one minute—prior to its use in the preparation of infant formula."

Statistics and Studies

Researchers from the University of Texas studied "The Influence of Water Removal on the Strength and Toughness of Cortical Bone," which involves the hard outer layer or protective bone surface. According to the report in the *Journal of Biomechanics*, "bone strength increased with a 5% loss of water by weight . . . ," but "with water loss exceeding 9% . . . , strength actually decreased." Also, "stiffness . . . increased with an increase in water loss. . . . Therefore, we speculate that loss of water in the collagen phase decreases the toughness of bone, whereas loss of water associated with the mineral phase decreases both bone strength and toughness."

When dry bones become stiff and brittle, the BACK and SPINE gradually feel those changes, but a dry body in general exhibits the sort of changes often associated with disease. Indeed, a 2003 Nobel Prize resulted from RESEARCH into those changes, which can now be detected and monitored with MAGNETIC RESONANCE IMAGING (MRI). As the Nobelprize.org Web site explained, water molecules contain oxygen with twice as much hydrogen that act "as microscopic compass needles. When the body is exposed to a strong magnetic field, the . . . hydrogen atoms are directed into order—stand 'at attention.'" With waves pulsing from an MRI, "the small differences in the oscillations . . . are detected. By advanced computer processing, it is possible to build up a three-dimensional image that reflects the chemical structure of the tissue, including differences in the water content and in movements of the water molecules. This results in a very detailed image of tissues and organs in the investigated area of the body." Such a finding can have enormous impact in diagnosing and monitoring musculoskeletal conditions, because "in many diseases the . . . process results in changes of the water content, and this is reflected in the MR image."

American Dietetic Association. "Water, Water Everywhere. How Much Should You Drink?" ADA, January 17, 2005 Release. Available online. URL: http://www.eatright.org/cps/rde/xchg/ada/hs.xsl/media_3173_ENU_HTML.htm. Downloaded May 16, 2006.

Mansfield, D. A. "What Percentage of the Human Body Is Water, and How Is This Determined?" *The Boston Globe.* Available online. URL: http://www.boston.com/globe/search/stories/health/how_and_why/011298.htm. Downloaded May 16, 2006.

Nobelprize.org. "Press Release: The 2003 Nobel Prize in Physiology or Medicine," The Official Web site of the Nobel Foundation. Available online. URL: http://nobelprize.org/medicine/laureates/2003/press.html. Last updated November 8, 2004.

Nyman, J. S., A. Roy, X. Shen, R. L. Acuna, J. H. Tyler, and X. Wang. "The Influence of Water Removal on the Strength and Toughness of Cortical Bone," *Journal of Biomechanics* 39, no. 5 (2006): 931–938.

World Health Organization. "Bottled Drinking Water," WHO media centre. Available online. URL: http://www.who.int/mediacentre/factsheets/fs256/en/. Downloaded May 16, 2006.

weight-bearing exercise   To define this special type of EXERCISE, the American Academy of Orthopaedic Surgeons (AAOS) said, "Weight-bearing describes any activity you do on your feet that works your bones and muscles against gravity. Bone is living tissue that constantly breaks down and reforms. When you do regular weight-bearing exercise, your bone adapts to the impact of weight and pull of muscle by building more cells and becoming stronger." Although swimming can be ideal for patients with OSTEOARTHRITIS or DEGENERATIVE DISC DISEASE to move around without stressing their joints, the water bears the weight rather than the body. Similarly, riding a bicycle provides a healthful daily ACTIVITY, but then bike tires, not bones, bear the body weight. Therefore, the AAOS suggested such BONE BUILDING activities as ball playing, hiking, skiing, or pushing a lawn mower. For indoor adventures, weight-bearing exercises include weight lifting, dancing, bowling, stair climbing, and taking a long walk in an enclosed mall.

Risks and Complications

Weight-bearing exercise may be ill-advised for some people, such as ELDERLY patients with OSTEOPOROSIS and CHILDREN with OSTEOGENESIS IMPERFECTA or severe POSTURE problems. When the consent of a doctor has been obtained, each session should begin with warm-ups to avoid risk of muscle STRAIN or SPRAIN. Also, dehydration can cause muscle spasm, so WATER intake should proportionately increase. Adequate SLEEP before exercising can help to prevent injuries too.

Perhaps the greatest risk comes when people refrain from exercise. As the National Institute of Arthritis and Musculoskeletal and Skin Diseases (NIAMS) explained, "While weight-bearing activities contribute to the development and maintenance of bone mass, weightlessness and immobility can result in bone loss." For instance, "Astronauts exposed to the microgravity of space experience significant bone loss, leaving their bones weak and less able to support the body's weight and movement upon return to Earth."

Statistics and Studies

According to the NIAMS, "in general, healthy people who undergo prolonged periods of bed rest or immobilization can regain bone mass when they resume weight-bearing activities. Studies suggest that there is a good chance to fully recover the lost bone if the immobilization period is limited to 5 to 10 weeks. Additionally, even brief intervals of weight-bearing activity during periods of limited mobility or bed rest can help lessen bone loss." Conversely, "those who cannot resume weight-bearing exercise are at significant risk for osteoporosis." Therefore, "researchers are investigating ways for this population to protect bone mass. Until scientists know more, the best advice is to reduce or eliminate other risk factors for osteoporosis, such as smoking and excessive alcohol consumption, and to eat a diet rich in calcium and vitamin D. Taking an osteoporosis medication may also be an option to minimize bone loss."

Special Aids and Adaptations

To adapt the musculoskeletal system gradually to an optimal amount of weight-bearing exercise, the AAOS recommended, "You should exercise for at least 30 minutes a day, four or more days a week. Besides improving bone strength, regular exercise also increases muscle strength, improves coordination and balance and leads to better overall health. To sustain the bone strengthening benefit of weight-bearing activity, you must increase the intensity, duration and amount of stress applied to bone over time."

Similarly, the online article "Fitness and Bone Health" said, "Weight-bearing activities improve bone health for many reasons. First, weight-bearing exercise appears to stimulate bone formation. Second, it strengthens muscles that in turn pull or tug on bones. This action keeps bones strong. And third, physical activity improves your strength, balance, and coordination—all of which help reduce your risk of falls and bone injuries." Well-balanced NUTRITION with natural forms of CALCIUM aid these endeavors too.

American Academy of Orthopaedic Surgeons. "Weight-Bearing Exercise for Girls and Young Women," AAOS. Available online. URL: http://orthoinfo.aaos.org/fact/thr_report.cfm?Thread_ID=328&topcategory=Women. Downloaded May 17, 2006.

Fitness Jumpsite ™, The. "Fitness and Bone Health." Available online. URL: http://www.primusweb.com/fitnesspartner/library/activity/bonehlth.htm. Downloaded May 17, 2006.

National Institute of Arthritis and Musculoskeletal and Skin Diseases. "Bed Rest and Immobilization: Risk Factors for Bone Loss," NIAMS. Available online. URL: http://www.niams.nih.gov/bone/hi/bed_rest.htm. Downloaded May 17, 2006.

weight, effects of   With over 60 million Americans exceeding their optimal body weight, the media has often focused on health consequences such as heart disease. In 2005, however, the North American Spine Society (NASS) began its own campaign, called "Take a Load off Your Back!" to educate the public. As the NASS Web site reported, this educational effort intends "to focus widespread attention on the debilitating effects of obesity on Americans' spines." With SPINE problems "up nearly 67 percent from just five years ago," NASS conducted a survey of spine care professionals and found that "44 percent of the patients they see are considered obese."

Risks and Complications

According to the NASS survey, "the three most common diagnoses in obese patients include degenerative disc disease, which includes wear and tear of the disc itself; spondylolisthesis, which is a slippage" of the VERTEBRAE "in the lower back from wear and tear; and a disc rupture or herniation. Obese patients are also at an increased risk of developing spondylolysis, a fracture in the vertebrae, and spinal stenosis, which is narrowing of the spinal canal."

While older adults and ELDERLY patients may carry a heftier risk of developing SPINAL STENOSIS, SPONDYLOLISTHESIS, or DEGENERATIVE DISC DISEASE, teenagers often crave slimness. If this desire carries too much weight in their lives, risks greatly increase for developing EATING DISORDERS. However, a more common risk occurs when a person of any age snacks on packaged foods or continuously craves sedentary pursuits, such as impulse eating.

Statistics and Studies

As reported by the *Child Health News,* one of the largest studies ever conducted of ADOLESCENTS assessed NUTRITION and daily ACTIVITY then found "lack of vigorous physical activity is the main contributor to obesity in adolescents ages 11 to 15. . . . In analyzing dietary factors, the researchers found that fiber intake, and not fat calories, was most closely related to an individual's weight. While the percentage of calories consumed from fat did not differ significantly between a group of normal-weight adolescents and those identified as being at-risk for obesity, or already overweight, the normal-weight adolescents consistently reported higher intake of fibrous foods such as whole grains, fruits and vegetables, as compared to the at-risk and overweight children."

Special Aids and Adaptations

A *Nutrition Journal* article reported "childhood obesity has reached epidemic levels in developed countries. Twenty-five percent of children in the U.S. are overweight and 11% are obese. About 70% of obese adolescents grow up to become obese adults." To aid CHILDREN in adapting a healthier lifestyle, "a number of potential effective plans can be implemented to target built environment, physical activity, and diet. These strategies can be initiated at home and in preschool institutions, schools or after-school care services as natural setting for influencing the diet and physical activity and at home and work for adults." For instance, "increases in sports participation and/or physical education time would need policy-based changes at both school and education sector levels. Similarly, increases in active modes of transport to and from school (walking, cycling, and public transport) would require policy changes at the school and local government levels, as well as support from parents and the community. In some communities a variety of such programs have been implemented e.g. road crossings, 'walking bus', and designated safe walking and cycling routes."

For persons of all ages, the U.S. Food and Drug Administration advised, "To lose weight safely and keep it off requires long-term changes in daily eating and exercise habits. Many experts recommend a goal of losing about a pound a week. A modest reduction of 500 calories per day will achieve this goal, since a total reduction of 3,500 calories is required to lose a pound of fat. An important way to lower your calorie intake is to learn and practice healthy eating habits."

A healthy habit of BONE BUILDING commonly includes CALCIUM, which also aids weight loss. As the article "The Role of Dairy Foods in Weight Management" reported in the *Journal of the American College of Nutrition,* "Dietary calcium appears to play a pivotal role in the regulation of energy metabolism and obesity risk. High calcium diets attenuate body fat accumulation and weight gain during periods of over-consumption of an energy-dense diet and . . . increase fat breakdown and preserve metabolism during caloric restriction, thereby markedly accelerating weight and fat loss." While calcium supplements may carry weight in strengthening bone, whey sways a body toward milk and dairy products with three servings recommended per day.

VITAMIN C may also be key. In another issue of the *Journal of the American College of Nutrition,* an article entitled "Strategies for Healthy Weight Loss: From Vitamin C to the Glycemic Response" said,

"Individuals with adequate vitamin C status oxidize 30% more fat during a moderate exercise bout than individuals with low vitamin C status; thus, vitamin C depleted individuals may be more resistant to fat mass loss." Besides that nutrient, "food choices can impact post-meal satiety and hunger. . . . High-protein foods promote . . . greater satiety as compared to high-carbohydrate, low-fat foods; thus, diet regimens high in protein foods may improve diet compliance and diet effectiveness." Also, "vinegar and peanut ingestion can reduce the glycemic effect of a meal, a phenomenon that has been related to satiety and reduced food consumption." With that in mind, a teaspoon of vinegar in WATER at meals may help to keep down pounds.

Dehghan, Mahshid, Noori Akhtar-Danesh, and Anwar T. Merchant. "Childhood Obesity, Prevalence and Prevention," *Nutrition Journal* 4, no. 24 (September 2005). Available online. URL: http://www.nutritionj. com/content/4/1/24. Downloaded May 16, 2006.

Johnston, Carol S. "Strategies for Healthy Weight Loss: From Vitamin C to the Glycemic Response," *Journal of the American College of Nutrition* 24, no. 3 (2005): 158–165.

News-Medical.Net. "Lack of Vigorous Physical Activity Is the Main Contributor to Obesity in Adolescents Ages 11 to 15," *Child Health News*, published April 6, 2004. Available online. URL: http://www.news-medical.net/ ?id=331. Downloaded May 16, 2006.

North American Spine Society. "North American Spine Society Unveils 2005 Patient Education Campaign— Take a Load Off Your Back!" NASS. Available online. URL: http://www.spine.org/fsp/sh05.cfm. Last updated June 28, 2005.

U.S. Food and Drug Administration. "The Facts About Weight Loss Products and Programs," FDA. Available online. URL: http://www.cfsan.fda.gov/~dms/wgtloss. html. Downloaded May 16, 2006.

Zemel, Michael B. "The Role of Dairy Foods in Weight Management," *Journal of the American College of Nutrition* 24, no. 90006 (2005): 537S–546S.

Werdnig-Hoffman disease Also known as Spinal Muscular Atrophy (SMA), this rare disorder usually begins in INFANTS then progressively worsens. In addressing the GENETIC FACTORS involved in this condition, the SMA Support Web site explained, "SMA is a muscular disease passed on genetically to children by their parents. . . . It is a 'Recessive' genetic disease, meaning that BOTH parents must carry a copy of the recessive SMA gene. There is only a 25% chance each pregnancy of the child having SMA and a 75% chance each pregnancy that the child will be healthy. One out of 40 people is a carrier of this recessive gene." Gradually, "SMA affects a child's muscular development, and the severity depends on what 'type' of SMA the child has. There are four 'Types' of SMA, Type 1, 2, 3 & 4. . . . Type 4 is the least severe, affecting adults."

Symptoms and Diagnostic Path

According to the National Organization for Rare Disorders (NORD), "approximately 80% of SMA falls into the severe category (SMA1). Infants with SMA1 experience severe weakness before 6 months of age, and the patient never achieves the ability to sit independently when placed. Muscle weakness, lack of motor development and poor muscle tone are the major clinical manifestations of SMA1. . . . Muscle weakness occurs on both sides of the body and the ocular muscles are not affected."

Regarding other types, information from the SMA Support Web site said, "Type 2 children are diagnosed before 2 years of age, usually more like 15 months. These children are usually able to be in a sitting position without support, but often can not get there by themselves. They can sometimes crawl with bracing and therapy, and on occasion may stand with braces. . . . They will usually never walk." Type 3 symptoms may begin in very young CHILDREN or ADOLESCENTS. "In the beginning these children are able to stand and walk but usually have difficulty doing so. They typically have a normal lifespan; however, as with all forms of SMA, weakness gets progressively worse and they usually will be wheelchair bound." Type 4 begins in adults "around age 35. They also usually have a normal lifespan; though, as with all forms of SMA, weakness gets progressively worse." At any age though, intelligence is not affected, so caretakers must take care to treat the person in an age-appropriate manner. To confirm the diagnosis, a blood test, ELECTROMYOGRAM, and biopsy will usually be required.

Treatment Options and Outlook

Regarding the overall prognosis, the NORD advised, "most affected children die before 2 years of age but survival may be dependent on the degree of respiratory function." Conversely, "for infants who appear to have normal development for several months prior to the onset of muscle weakness, the disorder may tend to have a more slowly progressive course."

Treatments primarily aim to make patients comfortable, but active therapies may include occupational therapy, speech therapy, HYDROTHERAPY, and therapeutic EXERCISE to aid breathing and muscle movement. Parents should also discuss the best course of NUTRITION with the pediatrician or a dietician who specializes in child care.

Risk Factors and Preventive Measures

Because of the genetic factors involved, the National Institute of Neurological Disorders and Stroke (NINDS) advised prospective parents to get genetic counseling. The NINDS also reported, "Researchers have found the specific gene that, when mutated, causes SMA. Several animal models of the disease have been developed as well as tests that can determine SMA gene function. This allows scientists to screen drugs that may be useful in treating SMA."

National Institute of Neurological Disorders and Stroke. "NINDS Spinal Muscular Atrophy Information Page," National Institutes of Health. Available online. URL: http://www.ninds.nih.gov/disorders/sma/sma.htm. Last updated January 25, 2006.

National Organization for Rare Disorders. "Werdnig-Hoffman Disease," NORD. Available online. URL: http://www.rarediseases.org/search/rdbdetail_abstract.html?disname=Werdnig%20Hoffman%20Disease. Downloaded May 17, 2006.

SMA Support, Inc. "About SMA," Spinal Muscular Atrophy. Available online. URL: http://www.smasupport.com/sma_main_page.htm. Downloaded May 17, 2006.

whiplash   See FLEXION-EXTENSION INJURY.

wryneck   See TORTICOLLIS.

X-ray Also known as a radiograph, this diagnostic tool utilizes electromagnetic waves to produce internal images of the body onto film. X-rays especially help to detect problems in teeth, bones, VERTEBRAE, and the musculoskeletal system. To assess soft tissue, a COMPUTED TOMOGRAPHY (CT or CAT) SCAN or MAGNETIC RESONANCE IMAGING (MRI) will usually be preferred.

Procedure

With all jewelry and metal objects removed, patients either lie down or stand in various positions as a technician takes two or three views of an area. To avoid blurring the picture, the patient must remain completely still for a few seconds as each X-ray is taken.

Risks and Complications

INFANTS, very young CHILDREN, ELDERLY persons, and pregnant women may be sensitive to X-rays, but for most patients, the risk of radiation exposure remains minimal. Risks increase for those who have had numerous X-rays in a short time or who have been subjected to adverse ENVIRONMENTAL INFLUENCES involving radiation. This excessive exposure can cause complications, such as nausea or hair loss, and increase the risk of CANCER.

Outlook and Lifestyle Modifications

Radiographs help to detect various disorders of the SPINE, from a bone FRACTURE to an OSTEOPHYTE to a SPINAL TUMOR. X-rays can also monitor bone loss in an ongoing condition, such as OSTEOPOROSIS or OSTEOGENESIS IMPERFECTA, and evaluate curve progression in such POSTURE problems as SCOLIOSIS, LORDOSIS, or KYPHOSIS. Whether used as a diagnostic tool or a monitoring device, X-rays provide the information needed to determine an appropriate course of treatment.

Radiological Society of North America, Inc. "X-Ray," RSNA. Available online. URL: http://www.radiologyinfo.org/glossary/glossary1.cfm?sTerm=X. Downloaded May 17, 2006.

Spine Institute of New York. "X-Ray," Beth Israel Medical Center. Available online. URL: http://www.spineinstituteny.com/conditions/xray.html. Downloaded May 17, 2006.

Z

zinc This essential mineral can be found in many foods and almost every cell of the body. According to the Office of Dietary Supplements, "zinc . . . stimulates the activity of approximately 100 enzymes, which are substances that promote biochemical reactions in your body. Zinc supports a healthy immune system, is needed for wound healing, helps maintain your sense of taste and smell, and is needed for DNA synthesis." In addition, zinc aids bone development in growing INFANTS, CHILDREN, and ADOLESCENTS.

Dosage and Potential Side Effects

Baked beans, fortified cereals, and most meats, including shellfish, offer forms of NUTRITION high in zinc. Vegetarians and people who consume large quantities of alcohol may develop a zinc deficiency as may children with growth deficiencies. Such instances require zinc supplements, but excessive doses can alter MINERAL BALANCE.

For babies six months to three years, the Recommended Daily Allowance (RDA) is 3 mg. For children four to eight, the RDA is 5 mg. The RDA of 8 mg for children 8 to 13 increases to 11 mg for male adolescents and adults. Pregnant teenagers need a higher amount of 13 mg, but women 19 and older need 11 mg during pregnancy and 12 mg during lactation. Otherwise, RDA for women remains around 8 mg.

Statistics and Studies

The Office of Dietary Supplements reported, "Some researchers have questioned the effect of iron fortification on absorption of other nutrients, including zinc. Fortification of foods with iron does not significantly affect zinc absorption. However, large amounts of iron in supplements (greater than 25 mg) may decrease zinc absorption, as can iron in solutions. Taking iron supplements between meals will help decrease its effect on zinc absorption."

In other RESEARCH involving zinc, "a study of over 100 employees of the Cleveland Clinic indicated that zinc lozenges decreased the duration of colds by one-half, although no differences were seen in how long fevers lasted or the level of muscle aches." Still other studies showed "when zinc supplements are given to individuals with low zinc levels, the numbers of T-cell lymphocytes circulating in the blood increase and the ability of lymphocytes to fight infection improves."

National Agricultural Library. "USDA National Nutrient Database for Standard Reference, Release 18," U.S. Department of Agriculture. Available online. URL: http://www.nal.usda.gov/fnic/foodcomp/Data/SR18/nutrlist/sr18a309.pdf. Downloaded May 17, 2006.

Office of Dietary Supplements. "Zinc," National Institutes of Health. Available online. URL: http://ods.od.nih.gov/factsheets/cc/zinc.html. Downloaded May 17, 2006.

APPENDIXES

Appendix I: National and International Organizations for the Back and Spine

Appendix II: Related Organizations

Appendix III: Other Relevant Web Sites

Appendix IV: Internet Journals and Magazines

APPENDIX I
NATIONAL AND INTERNATIONAL ORGANIZATIONS FOR THE BACK AND SPINE

Adolescent Scoliosis Society
of North America
P.O. Box 1178
Rocky Mount, NC 27802-1178
(252) 754-8268 (fax)
JMOSTE84@aol.com
http://www.teenscolinet.org/

American Back Society
2647 International Boulevard, Suite 401
Oakland, CA 94601
(510) 536-1812 (fax)
info@americanbacksoc.org
http://www.americanbacksoc.org/

American Society of Spine Radiology
2210 Midwest Road, Suite 207
Oak Brook, IL 60523-8205
(630) 574-0220 ext. 226
(630) 574-0661 (fax)
kcammarata@asnr.org
http://www.theassr.org/

American Spinal Injury Association - ASIA
2020 Peachtree Road, NW
Atlanta, GA 30309-1402
(404) 355-9772
(404) 355-1826 (fax)
http://www.asia-spinalinjury.org/

Bone and Joint Decade
The Bone and Joint Decade Secretariat
Department of Orthopaedics
University Hospital
221 85 Lund
Sweden

+46 46 17 71 67 (fax)
bjd@ort.lu.se
http://www.boneandjointdecade.org/

Cervical Spine Research Society
6300 North River Road, Suite 727
Rosemont, IL 60018-4226
(847) 698-1628
(847) 823-0536 (fax)
http://www.csrs.org/

The International Society for the Study
of the Lumbar Spine
2075 Bayview Avenue
Room MG323
Toronto, Ontario, Canada, M4N 3M5
(4l6) 480-4833
(4l6) 480-6055 (fax)
http://www.issls.org/

The International Spine Intervention Society
(ISIS)
5 Ash Avenue
Kentfield, CA 94904-1504
(888) 255-0005 or (415) 457-ISIS (4747)
(415) 457-3495 fax
http://www.spinalinjection.com/a/

Model Spinal Cord Injury Center System
(MSCIS) Dissemination Center
TIRR, B-107
1333 Moursund
Houston, TX 77030-3405
(713) 797-5971
(713) 797-5982 (fax)
http://www.mscisdisseminationcenter.org/

National Scoliosis Foundation
5 Cabot Place
Stoughton, MA 02072
(800) 673-6922 or (800) NSF-MYBACK
(781) 341-8333 (fax)
nsf@scoliosis.org
http://www.scoliosis.org/

**National Spinal Cord Injury Association
(NSCIA)**
6701 Democracy Boulevard
Suite 300-9
Bethesda, MD 20817
(800) 962-9629
(301) 881-9817 (fax)
info@spinalcord.org
http://www.spinalcord.org/

North American Spine Society
22 Calendar Court, 2nd Floor
LaGrange, IL 60525
(877) 774-6337
info@spine.org
http://www.spine.org/

The Scoliosis Association, Inc.
P.O. Box 811705
Boca Raton, FL 33481
(561) 994-4435
(561) 994-2455 (fax)
http://www.scoliosis-assoc.org/

Scoliosis Research Society (SRS)
555 East Wells Street
Suite 1100
Milwaukee, WI 53202-3823
(414) 289-9107
(414) 276-3349 (fax)
info@srs.org
http://www.srs.org/

Spina Bifida Association of America
4590 MacArthur Boulevard, NW
Suite 250
Washington, DC 20007-4226
(800) 621-3141 or (202) 944-3285
sbaa@sbaa.org
http://www.sbaa.org

Spinal Cord Injury Informational Network
UAB Model SCI System
Office of Research Services
619 19th Street South, SRC 529
Birmingham, AL 35249-7330
(205) 934-3283
sciweb@uab.edu
http://www.spinalcord.uab.edu/

Spinal Injury Foundation (SIF)
11080 Circle Point Road
Suite 140
Westminster, CO 80020
(866) 5-SPINE-5 or (866) 577-4635
(303) 429-6373 (fax)
http://www.spinalinjuryfoundation.org/

Spine-health.com
123 West Madison Street
Suite 1450
Chicago, IL 60602
admin@spine-health.com
http://spine-health.com/

UCLA Spine Center
1245 16th Street, Suite 202
Santa Monica, CA 90404
(310) 440-2999
http://www.espinecare.com/

APPENDIX II
RELATED ORGANIZATIONS

Agency for Healthcare Research and Quality
U.S. Department of Health and Human Services
540 Gaither Road, Suite 2000
Rockville, MD 20850
(301) 427-1364
http://www.ahrq.gov/

AMC Cancer Research Center
1600 Pierce Street
Denver, CO 80214
(800) 321-1557 or (303) 233-6501
http://www.amc.org/

American Academy of Family Physicians (AAFP)
P.O. Box 11210
Shawnee Mission, KS 66207-1210
(800) 274-2237 or (913) 906-6000
fp@aafp.org
http://www.aafp.org/

American Academy of Medical Acupuncture (AAMA)
4929 Wilshire Boulevard, Suite 428
Los Angeles, CA 90010
(323) 937-5514
JDOWDEN@prodigy.net
http://www.medicalacupuncture.org/

American Academy of Orthopaedic Surgeons (AAOS)
6300 North River Road
Rosemont, IL 60018-4262
(847) 823-7186 or (800) 346-AAOS
(847) 823-8125 (fax)
pemr@aaos.org
http://www.aaos.org/

American Academy of Pain Management
13947 Mono Way #A
Sonora, CA 95370
(209) 533-9744

(209) 533-9750 (fax)
aapm@aapainmanage.org
http://www.aapainmanage.org/

American Academy of Pediatrics (AAP)
National Headquarters
141 Northwest Point Boulevard
Elk Grove Village, IL 60007-1098
(847) 434-4000
(847) 434-8000 (fax)
http://www.aap.org/

American Academy of Physical Medicine & Rehabilitation (AAPM & R)
330 North Wabash Avenue, Suite 2500
Chicago, IL 60611-3604
(312) 464-9700
(312) 464-0227 (fax)
info@aapmr.org
http://www.aapmr.org/

American Chiropractic Association (ACA)
1701 Clarendon Boulevard
Arlington, VA 22209
(703) 276-8800
(703) 243-2593 (fax)
memberinfo@acatoday.org
http://www.amerchiro.org/

American College of Sports Medicine (ACSM)
P.O. Box 1440
Indianapolis, IN 46206-1440
(317) 637-9200, ext. 138
(317) 634-7817 (fax)
http://www.acsm.org/index.asp

American Dietetic Association (ADA)
120 South Riverside Plaza, Suite 2000
Chicago, IL 60606-6995
(800) 877-1600
http://www.eatright.org

American Geriatrics Society (AGS)
The Empire State Building
350 Fifth Avenue, Suite 801
New York, NY 10118
(212) 308-1414
(212) 832-8646 (fax)
info@americangeriatrics.org
http://www.americangeriatrics.org/

American Massage Therapy Association (AMTA)
500 Davis Street, Suite 900
Evanston, IL 60201
(877) 905-2700 or (847) 864-0123
(847) 864-1178 (fax)
info@amtamassage.org
http://www.amtamassage.org/

American Medical Association (AMA)
515 North State Street
Chicago, IL 60610
(800) 621-8335
http://www.ama-assn.org/

American Occupational Therapy Association (AOTA)
4720 Montgomery Lane
P.O. Box 31220
Bethesda, MD 20824-1220
(800) 377-8555 or (301) 652-2682
(301) 652-7711 (fax)
educate@aota.org
http://www.aota.org/

American Osteopathic Foundation (AOF)
142 East Ontario Street
Chicago, IL 60611
(800) 621-1773, ext. 8234, 8230, 8232, 8233 or
    (312) 202-8234
(312) 202-8216 (fax)
info@aof-foundation.org
http://www.aof-foundation.org/

American Pain Foundation (APF)
201 North Charles Street, Suite 710
Baltimore, MD 21201-4111
(888) 615-PAIN (7246)
info@painfoundation.org
http://www.painfoundation.org/

American Pain Society (APS)
4700 West Lake Avenue
Glenview, IL 60025
(847) 375-4715
(877) 734-8758 (fax)
info@ampainsoc.org
http://www.ampainsoc.org/

American Physical Therapy Association (APTA)
1111 North Fairfax Street
Alexandria, VA 22314-1488
(800) 999-APTA (2782) or
    (703) 684-APTA (2782)
(703) 684-7343 (fax)
http://www.apta.org/

Arthritis Foundation
P.O. Box 7669
Atlanta, GA 30357-0669
(800) 568-4045 or (404) 872-7100
help@arthritis.org.
http://www.arthritis.org/

Arthritis Research Institute of America
300 South Duncan Avenue, Suite 188
Clearwater, FL 33755
(727) 461-4054
(727) 449-9227 (fax)
info@preventarthritis.org
http://www.preventarthritis.org/

CureSearch
National Childhood Cancer Foundation
4600 East West Highway, Suite 600
Bethesda, MD 20814-3457
(800) 458-6223
info@curesearch.org
http://www.curesearch.org

International Myeloma Foundation
12650 Riverside Drive, Suite 206
North Hollywood, CA 91607-3421
(800) 452-2873 (U.S. and Canada)
(818) 487-7455 (elsewhere)
(818) 487-7454 (fax)
TheIMF@myeloma.org
http://www.myeloma.org

March of Dimes Birth Defects Foundation
1275 Mamaroneck Avenue
White Plains, NY 10605

(914) 997-4488
http://www.marchofdimes.com/

National Cancer Institute (NCI)

NCI Public Inquiries Office
6116 Executive Boulevard
Room 3036A
Bethesda, MD 20892-8322
(800) 4-CANCER or (800) 422-6237
cancergovstaff@mail.nih.gov
http://www.cancer.gov/

National Center for Complementary and Alternative Medicine (NCCAM)

NCCAM Clearinghouse
P.O. Box 7923
Gaithersburg, MD 20898-7923
(888) 644-6226
(866) 464-3615 (for hearing impaired)
(301) 519-3153 (international number)
(866) 464-3616 (fax)
info@nccam.nih.gov
http://nccam.nih.gov/

National Chronic Fatigue and Fibromyalgia Association (NCFSFA)

P.O. Box 18426
Kansas City, MO 64133
(816) 313-2000
information@ncfsfa.org
http://www.ncfsfa.org/

National Chronic Pain Outreach Association (NCPOA)

P.O. Box 274
Millboro, VA 24460
(540) 862-9437
(540) 862-9485 (fax)
http://www.chronicpain.org/

National Fibromyalgia Association (NFA)

2200 North Glassell Street, Suite A
Orange, CA 92865
(714) 921-0150
(714) 921-6920 (fax)
nfanurse@comcast.net
http://www.fmaware.org/

National Foundation for the Treatment of Pain

P.O. Box 70045

Houston, TX 77270-0045
(713) 862-9332
(713) 862-9346 (fax)
http://www.paincare.org/

National Institutes of Health (NIH)

9000 Rockville Pike
Bethesda, MD 20892
(301) 496-4000
NIHinfo@od.nih.gov
http://www.nih.gov/

National Institutes of Health: Osteoporosis and Related Bone Diseases

2 AMS Circle
Bethesda, MD 20892-3676
(800)-624-BONE or (202) 223-0344
(202) 293-2356 (fax)
http://www.niams.nih.gov/bone

National Osteoporosis Foundation (NOF)

1232 22nd Street NW
Washington, DC 20037-1292
(202) 223-2226
(202) 223-2237 (fax)
http://www.nof.org/

National Pain Foundation (NPF)

300 East Hampden Avenue, Suite 100
Englewood, CO 80113
aardrup@nationalpainfoundation.org
http://www.nationalpainfoundation.org/

Osteogenesis Imperfecta Foundation

804 West Diamond Avenue, Suite 210
Gaithersburg, MD 20878
(800) 981-BONE (2663) or (301) 947-0083
(301) 947-0456 (fax)
bonelink@oif.org
http://www.oif.org/

The Paget Foundation

120 Wall Street, Suite 1602
New York, NY 10005-4001
(800) 23-PAGET or (212) 509-5335
(212) 509-8492 (fax)
Pagetfdn@aol.com
http://www.paget.org/

The President's Council on Physical Fitness and Sports (PCPFS)

Department W, Room 738-H

200 Independence Avenue, SW
Washington, D.C. 20201-0004
(202) 690-9000
(202) 690-5211 (fax)
http://www.fitness.gov/

Reflex Sympathetic Dystrophy Syndrome Association (RSDSA)

P.O. Box 502
Milford, CT 06460
(203) 877-3790 or (877) 662-7737 (toll free)
(203) 882-8362 (fax)
info@rsds.org
http://www.rsds.org

Spondylitis Association of America

P.O. Box 5872
Sherman Oaks, CA 91413
(800) 777-8189 or (818) 981-1616
info@spondylitis.org
http://www.spondylitis.org/

U.S. Department of Health and Human Services

200 Independence Ave., SW
Washington, DC 20201
(877) 696-6775 or (202) 619-0257
http://www.hhs.gov/

APPENDIX III
OTHER RELEVANT WEB SITES

The following sources do not provide full contact information. Depending on the staff or location, you may find a mail or e-mail address but no phone number or a phone number may be given with no address. Sites with pop-ups were not included, but that does not guarantee that none have since been added.

Agency for Toxic Substances and Disease Registry (ATSDR)
(404) 498-0110 or (888) 422-8737 (toll free)
(404) 498-0093 (fax)
http://www.atsdr.cdc.gov/

The Alternative Medicine Homepage
University of Pittsburgh
Pittsburgh, PA
http://www.pitt.edu/~cbw/altm.html

Beth Israel Medical Center
Department of Pain Medicine and Palliative Care
First Avenue at 16th Street
New York, NY 10003
(877) 620-9999
http://www.stoppain.org/

Cancer Information Service
(800) 4-CANCER (6237)
http://cis.nci.nih.gov/

healthfinder ®
P.O. Box 1133
Washington, DC 20013-1133
http://www.healthfinder.gov/

Mayo Clinic
http://www.mayoclinic.com/

National Center on Birth Defects and Developmental Disabilities
bddi@cdc.gov
http://www.cdc.gov/ncbddd/

The Rosenthal Center for Complementary and Alternative Medicine
Columbia University
http://www.rosenthal.hs.columbia.edu/CAM.html

Touch Research Institutes
Miami, FL
info@touchresearch.com
http://www.touchresearch.com/

SpineUniverse
http://www.spineuniverse.com/

APPENDIX IV
INTERNET JOURNALS AND MAGAZINES

The U.S. National Institutes of Health (NIH) offers a digital archive of biomedical and life sciences journals with free Internet access to articles through their Web site, http://www.pubmedcentral.nih.gov/. As with other online journals, additional contact information, such as a mail or e-mail address, may not be included on the Web site.

Arthritis Research and Therapy
http://arthritis-research.com/

BMC Musculoskeletal Disorders (published by BioMed Central)
http://www.biomedcentral.com/bmcmusculoskeletdisord

BMJ - British Medical Journal
http://bmj.bmjjournals.com/

Dartmouth Medicine
http://dartmed.dartmouth.edu

JAOA - Journal of the American Osteopathic Association
http://www.jaoa.org/

Journal of Neurosurgery: Spine
http://www.thejns-net.org/

Massage Therapy Journal (published by the American Massage Therapy Association)
http://www.amtamassage.org/journal/home.html

Mount Sinai Journal of Medicine
http://www.mssm.edu/msjournal/back.shtml

Nutrition & Metabolism
http://www.nutritionandmetabolism.com/

Nutrition Journal
http://www.nutritionj.com/

Spine Surgery
http://www.spine-surgery.com/

TCJ - The Chiropractic Journal
http://www.worldchiropracticalliance.org/tcj/

BIBLIOGRAPHY

PRIMARY REFERENCES

Baggaley, Ann, ed. *Human Body.* New York: Dorling Kindersley Publishing, Inc., 2001.

Balch, James F., M.D., and Phyllis A. Balch. *Prescription for Nutritional Healing,* 2d ed. Garden City Park, N.Y.: Avery Publishing Group, 1997.

Beers, Mark H., M.D., et al., eds. *The Merck Manual of Medical Information, Second Home Edition.* Whitehouse Station, N.J.: Merck Research Laboratories, 2003.

Brueninger, Cynthia C., and Pat Wittig, eds. *Diseases,* 3rd ed. Springhouse, Pa.: Springhouse Corporation, 2001.

Carroll, Stephen, M.D., and Tony Smith. *The Complete Family Guide To Healthy Living.* New York: Dorling Kindersley Publishing Inc., 1995.

Cassell, Dana K., and Noel Rose, M.D. *The Encyclopedia of Autoimmune Diseases.* New York: Facts On File, Inc., 2003.

Holmes, H. Nancy, et al., eds. *Handbook of Signs & Symptoms,* 3rd ed. Ambler, Pa.: Lippincott Williams & Wilkins, 2006.

Kunz, Jeffrey R. M., M.D., ed. *The American Medical Association Family Medical Guide.* New York: Random House, 1982.

Patton, Kevin, and Gary Thibodeau, et al., eds. *Mosby's Handbook of Anatomy and Physiology.* St. Louis, Mo.: Mosby, Inc., 2000.

Rothenberg, Mikel A., M.D., and Charles F. Chapman. *Dictionary of Medical Terms for the Nonmedical Person,* 3rd ed. Hauppauge, N.Y.: Barron's Educational Series, Inc., 1994.

Segen, Joseph C., M.D., and Joseph Stauffer. *The Patient's Guide to Medical Tests.* New York: Facts On File, Inc., 1998.

Thibodeau, Gary A., and Kevin T. Patton. *Structure & Function of the Body,* 10th ed. St. Louis, Mo.: Mosby-Year Book, Inc., 1997.

Thomas, Clayton, M.D., et al., eds. *Taber's Cyclopedic Medical Dictionary, Edition 18.* Philadelphia, Pa.: F.A. Davis Company, 1997.

BIRTH DEFECTS

Wynbrandt, James, and Mark D. Ludman, M.D. *The Encyclopedia of Genetic Disorders and Birth Defects,* 2d ed. New York: Facts On File, Inc., 2000.

BONE CANCER

Altman, Robert, and Michael J. Sarg, M.D. *The Cancer Dictionary,* Rev. Ed. New York: Facts On File, Inc., 2002.

COMPLEMENTARY AND ALTERNATIVE MEDICINE (CAM)

Bestic, Liz. *A Guide to Natural Home Remedies.* Bath, U.K.: Parragon Publishing, 2002.

Buchman, Dian Dincin. *Herbal Medicine.* Avenel, N.J.: Wings Books, 1996.

Fetrow, Charles W., and Juan R. Avila. *The Complete Guide to Herbal Medicines.* New York: Pocket Books, 2000.

Fleming, Thomas R., et al., eds. *PDR for Herbal Medicines.* Montvale, N.J.: Medical Economics Company, Inc., 1998.

Gach, Michael Reed. *Acupressure's Potent Points: A Guide to Self-Care for Common Ailments.* New York: Bantam Books, 1990.

Graedon, Joe, and Teresa Graedon. *The People's Pharmacy Guide to Home and Herbal Remedies.* New York: St. Martin's Press, 2001.

Harrold, Fiona. *The Complete Body Massage.* New York: Sterling Publishing Company, Inc., 1992.

Mowrey, Daniel B. *Herbal Tonic Therapies.* Avenel, N.J.: Wings Books, 1996.

Murray, Michael T., and Joseph E. Pizzorno. *Encyclopedia of Natural Medicine.* Rocklin, Calif.: Prima Publishing, 1991.

Tenney, Louise, M. H. *Today's Herbal Health,* 3rd ed. Provo, Utah: Woodland Books, 1992.

Tkac, Debora, et al., eds. *The Doctors Book of Home Remedies.* Emmaus, Pa.: Rodale Press, Inc., 1990.

Wagner, Edward M., M.D., with Sylvia Goldfarb. *How to Stay Out of the Doctor's Office.* New York: Instant Improvement, Inc., 1993.

Whorton, James C. *Nature Cures: The History of Alternative Medicine in America.* New York: Oxford University Press, 2002.

NUTRITION

Cassell, Dana K. *Food for Thought: The Sourcebook for Obesity and Eating Disorders.* New York: Checkmark Books, 2000.

Cassell, Dana K., and David H. Gleaves. *Encyclopedia of Obesity and Eating Disorders,* 2d ed. New York: Facts On File, Inc., 2000.

Cheraskin, E., M.D., D.M.D.; W. M. Ringsdorf, Jr., D.M.D.; and J. W. Clark. *Diet and Disease.* New Canaan, Conn.: Keats Publishing, Inc., 1995.

Colbin, Annemarie. *Food and Healing.* New York: Ballantine Books, 1996.

Haas, Elson M., M.D. *Staying Healthy with Nutrition.* Berkeley, Calif.: Celestial Arts Publishing, 1992.

Harris, Ben Charles. *Better Health with Culinary Herbs.* New York: Weathervane Books, 1971.

———. *Kitchen Medicines.* Barre, Mass.: Barre Publishers, 1968.

Hausman, Patricia, and Judith Benn Hurley. *The Healing Foods.* Emmaus, Pa.: Rodale Press, 1989.

Kirschmann, Gayla J., and John D. Kirschmann. *Nutrition Almanac,* 4th ed. New York: McGraw-Hill, 1996.

OSTEOPOROSIS

Nelson, Miriam E., with Sarah Wernick. *Strong Women, Strong Bones.* New York: G. P. Putnam's Sons, 1999.

PAIN MANAGEMENT

D'Orazio, Brian P. *Low Back Pain Handbook.* Woburn, Mass.: Butterworth-Heinemann, 1999.

Griffith, H. Winter, M.D., et al. *1999 Edition Complete Guide to Prescription and Nonprescription Drugs.* New York: Perigee Books, 1998.

Melnik, Michael. *Understanding Your Back Injury.* Rockville, Md.: The American Occupational Therapy Association, Inc., 1994.

Sifton, David W., ed. *The PDR ® Pocket Guide to Prescription Drugs,* ™, 5th ed. New York: Pocket Books, 2002.

INDEX

A

abatacept **1**
absorptiometry **1–3,** 43, 136, 204, 217, 254
acetaminophen **3–4,** 9, 30, 195, 213, 214, 258
acromegaly disorders 112–113
activity, daily **4–6**
  backache 28
  bone building 39
  bone graft 42
  cervical foraminal stenosis 53
  cervical spine 57
  cold therapy 66
  corticosteroid injection 71
  discectomy 77
  DISH 75
  dwarfism 83
  elderly, spinal concerns of 86
  exercise 94
  FBSS 99
  fractures 108
  genetic factors, genomics 110
  herbal therapy 118
  herniated disc 119
  iron 133
  juvenile spondyloarthritis 139
  laminectomy 143
  low back pain 148
  lumbar spinal fusion 153
  lumbar spine 155
  MBD 165
  MD 172
  muscle cramp/spasm 171
  NCV test 184
  nerve block 182
  opiates 192
  orthotics 192

osteoarthritis 195
osteogenesis imperfecta 198
paraspinal muscles 216
peripheral neuropathy 218
post-polio syndrome 224
potassium 226
pregnancy, back care during 228
primary hyperparathyroidism 229
range of motion 232
rheumatism 239
rheumatoid arthritis 240
rhomboid muscle strain 241
RICE method 243
RSD syndrome 234
sacral vertebrae 246
Schmorl's node 250
sciatica 251
scoliosis 253
SED 280
shoe choice, spinal effects of 261
sleep 265
SM 292
SNRB 258
spinal infection 269
spinal tumor 276
spine 279
sprain 283
steroid therapy 284
strain 285
tension 294
trigger point therapy 300
vertebrae 304
water and spine health 311
weight, effects of 314
weight-bearing exercise 312
Actonel 37

acupressure **6–7,** 300
acupuncture **7–8**
  acupressure 6
  arthritis 19
  neck pain 180
  sleep 264
  spinal tumor 277
  surgery 290
acute back pain **8–9**
  backache 28
  back injury 29
  children, spinal concerns for 61
  chronic back pain 63
  costotransverse joint injections 71
  dislocated vertebra 81
  facet joint disorder 97
  herniated disc 118
  ibuprofen 126
  juvenile osteoporosis 136
  laminectomy 143
  low back pain 148
  muscle cramp/spasm 170
  musculoskeletal disorders 174
  myeloma bone disease 177
  NCV test 184
  neck pain 180
  opiates 191
  osteophyte 203
  paraspinal muscles 216
  piriformis syndrome 223
  range of motion 232
  rhomboid muscle strain 241
  rib injury 242
  sacroiliac joint pain syndrome 247
  SNRB 257

acute back pain *(continued)*
  spinal tuberculosis 275
  spine 279
  sprain 282
  strain 285
Adam's forward bend test 127
addiction 191–192
adolescents, spinal concerns for
  10–11
  antiresorptive drug 15
  backache 28
  backpack safety **31–32**
  birth defects of the spine 35
  eating disorders, bone loss
    caused by 85
  exercise 94
  folate 105
  GH disorders 112
  herniated disc 119
  idiopathic scoliosis 126
  juvenile arthritis 135
  juvenile osteoporosis 136
  juvenile rheumatoid arthritis
    137
  kyphosis 141
  lifting 144
  lordosis 147
  low back pain 148
  lumbar spine 154
  magnesium 157
  Marfan syndrome 160
  nutrition 187, 189
  orthotics 192
  osteopenia 201
  osteoporosis 207
  pain management 212
  phosphorus 219
  posture 225
  PTH 216–217
  rhomboid muscle strain 241
  rodding surgery 245
  RSD syndrome 233
  sacral vertebrae 246
  SAPHO Syndrome 248
  Scheuermann's kyphosis
    249
  Schmorl's node 250
  scoliosis 252
  secondary osteoporosis 254
  SED 279

shoe choice, spinal effects of
  260
skeletal dysplasia 262
sleep 265
spina bifida 266
spinal tuberculosis 274
spine 278
spondylolisthesis 281
steroid therapy 283
strength training 286
surgery 289
thoracoplasty 296
vitamin C 308
vitamin D 308
vitamin E 309
weight, effects of 314
Werdnig-Hoffman disease 315
Advil 126
African Americans 157
Agency for Toxic Substances and
  Disease Registry (ATSDR) 89
alcohol 89–90, 168
alendronate **11–12**
  bisphosphonates 37, 38
  juvenile osteoporosis 137
  MD 173
  osteoporosis 205
  PTH 217
  SERMs 257
Aleve (naproxen) 179, 185
alfacalcidol 206
alkaline phosphatase (ALP) 123
allergies 111, 163, 213. *See also*
  food allergies
alpha interferon 177
alpha-tocopheryl acetate 309
alternative medicine. *See* complementary and alternative medicine
aluminum 89, 206
analgesic painkiller 191–192
ankylosing spondylitis **13–14**. *See
  also* juvenile spondyloarthritis
  arthritis 18
  CES 52
  DMARD 80
  juvenile spondyloarthritis 138
  PNT 218
  posture 225–226
  SAPHO Syndrome 248
  spinal injury 271

anorexia nervosa (AN) 84–85, 254
anterior cervical discectomy **14–
  15,** 55, 59, 181
antihistamines 116
antiresorptive drugs **15–16**
  alendronate **11–12**
  bisphosphonates **37–38**
  calcitonin 48
  risedronate sodium **244–245**
  SERMs **256–257**
arachnoiditis **16–18,** 151, 184,
  228
arms 180
arnica 120
arthritis **18–20**. *See also*
  osteoarthritis; rheumatoid
  arthritis
  acetaminophen 3
  acute back pain 8
  ankylosing spondylitis 13
  aspirin 21, 22
  costotransverse joint
    injections 71
  COX-2 inhibitors 72
  DISH 75
  fibrous dysplasia 102
  gold salt treatment **111–112**
  herbal therapy 117
  hydrotherapy 122
  juvenile arthritis 135
  juvenile rheumatoid arthritis
    137
  juvenile spondyloarthritis
    138–139
  magnetic therapy 158, 159
  musculoskeletal disorders
    174
  NSAID therapy 186
  orthotics 192
  osteoarthritis **195–197**
  phytochemicals 220
  post-polio syndrome 224
  rheumatoid arthritis 239
  SAPHO Syndrome 248
  spinal stenosis 273
  strength training 286
arthrodesis vi, **20–21**
  arthritis 19
  birth defects of the spine 35
  bone graft 41

cervical radiculopathy 55
corpectomy **69–70**
CSM 59
disc replacement 80
dwarfism 82
FBSS 99
laminectomy 142
lumbar spinal fusion **152–154**
orthotics 192
rheumatoid arthritis 239
SED 255, 280
spine 279
artificial spinal disc 79
ascorbic acid. *See* vitamin C
aspirin **21–22**
EMG 88
epidural injection 91
herbal therapy 116
ibuprofen 126
naproxen 179
NSAID therapy 185
over-the-counter products 208
athletes, spinal concerns of **22–25**
exercise 94
female athlete triad **99–100**
flexion-extension injury 104
fractures 106
lumbar spine 154
muscle cramp/spasm 170
musculoskeletal disorders 175
osteoporosis 207
resistance training 236
rhabdomyolysis 237
rib injury 242
RICE method 243
sacral vertebrae 246
sacroiliac joint pain syndrome
247
Schmorl's node 250
shoe choice, spinal effects of
260
spinal cord 267
spine 278
spondylolisthesis 281
strain 285
thoracic spine 296
atlantoaxial instability **25–26,**
280
auranofin (Ridaura) 112
aurothioglucose (Solganal) 112

autoimmune disorders 240
autopsy 163
azathioprine 80, 81

B

back **27–28**
backache **28–29**. *See also specific
forms of back pain, e.g.:* acute back
pain
acupressure 6
acupuncture 7
ergonomic factors 91
exercise 94
herbal therapy 116
homeopathic medicine 120
ibuprofen 126
low back pain **147–150**
lumbar spine 154
medical tests 163
muscle cramp/spasm 170
osteoarthritis 195
paraspinal muscles 215
piriformis syndrome 223
pregnancy, back care during
227
rheumatism 239
scoliosis 252
spinal stenosis 273
spinal tuberculosis 275
spine 279
spondylolisthesis 280
strain 285
back belt 144
back brace 160, 192, 193
back injury **29–31**
backpack safety **31–33**
backache 28
herniated disc 119
low back pain 148
lumbar spine 154
rhomboid muscle strain 241
scoliosis 252
spine 278
thoracic spine 296
vertebral subluxation 305
bacterial meningitis 164
Becker's muscular dystrophy 173
bed rest v, 9
benztropine 24, 171

beta blockers 160
beta-carotene 306
binge-eating 84
biofeedback **33–34,** 212
biopsy 162
birth defects of the spine **34–36**
atlantoaxial instability 26
dislocated vertebra 82
dwarfism 82
flat back 102
folate 105
infant massage therapy 130
infants, spinal concerns for
130
lordosis 146–147
lumbar spine 154
osteogenesis imperfecta 197
pregnancy, back care during
227
rodding surgery 245
sacral vertebrae 246
scoliosis 252
spina bifida **265–267**
spinal stenosis 273
thoracoplasty 296
vitamin B-complex 307
birth injury to the spine **36–37**
children, spinal concerns for
61
infant massage therapy 130
infants, spinal concerns for
130
rodding surgery 245
torticollis 298
trigger point therapy 300
vertebral subluxation 305
bisphosphonates **37–38**
alendronate **11–12**
antiresorptive drug 15
cancer 51
etidronate **93**
female athlete triad 100
fibrous dysplasia 102
ibandronate **125**
juvenile osteoporosis 137
musculoskeletal disorders
175
myeloma bone disease 177
osteitis deformans 194
osteogenesis imperfecta 198

bisphosphonates *(continued)*
    PTH 216
    risedronate sodium **244–245**
    SAPHO Syndrome 248
    secondary osteoporosis 255
    SERMs 256
black walnut 116
blood test 162–163
BM (bone markers) 234–235
BMD. *See* bone mineral density
BMP. *See* bone morphogenetic
  protein
BMT (bone marrow transplant)
  202
bone break. *See* fractures
bone building **38–41**
    absorptiometry 2
    acetaminophen 3
    activity, daily 5
    antiresorptive drugs 15
    bisphosphonates 38
    bone graft 42
    calcitonin 48
    calcium 49
    cervical radiculopathy 55
    cervical spine 57
    children, spinal concerns for
      61
    coccygeal spine 66
    etidronate **93**
    FBSS 99
    female athlete triad 100
    HRT **121–122**
    ibandronate **125**
    iron 133
    juvenile osteoporosis 137
    lumbar spine 154
    nutrition 186
    osteogenesis imperfecta 198
    osteopenia 201
    osteophyte 203
    osteoporosis 205
    phytochemicals 220
    phytoestrogens 221
    posture 225
    primary hyperparathyroidism
      229
    PTH 216
    resistance training 236
    rickets 244

risedronate sodium **244–245**
scoliosis 253
secondary osteoporosis 255
SERMs 257
spine 279
strontium ranelate **287–288**
vertebrae 304
vertebral compression fracture
  304–305
vitamin D 308
vitamin K **309–310**
weight-bearing exercise
  312–313
bone graft **41–42**
    anterior cervical discectomy
      14
    arthrodesis 20
    cervical radiculopathy 55
    cervical spondylosis 58
    corpectomy 69
    CSM 59
    disc replacement 80
    flat back 103
    lumbar spinal fusion 152–153
    osteomyelitis 200
    posture 225
    research 234
    Scheuermann's kyphosis 249
    scoliosis 253
    SED 255
    spinal stenosis 273
    spinal tuberculosis 275
    thoracoplasty 296
bone loss 4, 84–85, 144, 168. *See
  also* osteoporosis
bone markers (BM) 234–235
bone marrow 177
bone marrow transplant (BMT)
  202
bone mineral density (BMD) 16,
  189, 254
bone mineral density (BMD) tests
  42–44
    absorptiometry 1
    alendronate 12
    antiresorptive drugs 16
    bisphosphonates 38
    bone building 39
    CAT scan 69
    eating disorders, bone loss
      caused by 85

female athlete triad 99
HRT 121
juvenile osteoporosis 136
magnesium 157
MBD 165
MD 173
medical tests 162, 163
myeloma bone disease 177
osteopenia 201
osteopetrosis 202
osteoporosis 204
primary hyperparathyroidism
  229
PTH 216
QCT **230**
secondary osteoporosis 254
vertebral compression fracture
  304
bone morphogenetic protein
  (BMP) **44–45**
    arthrodesis 20
    bone graft 42
    CSM 59
    lumbar spinal fusion 152
    research 234, 235
    spinal stenosis 273
bone scan **46,** 162, 194
bone spur. *See* osteophyte
Boniva 37
boswellia 240
botanicals. *See* herbal therapy
bottled water 311–312
braces. *See* orthotics
brachial plexus injury **46–47,**
  182–183, 227
brachytherapy 277
bradycardia 114
brain 258
brain matter, loss of 148
brittle bone disease. *See*
  osteogenesis imperfecta
bulimia 84–85

C

caffeine 168
calcitonin **48**
    antiresorptive drug 15
    antiresorptive drugs 15
    osteitis deformans 194

PTH 216
SAPHO Syndrome 248
secondary osteoporosis 255
SERMs 256
calcitriol 206
calcium **48–49**
  absorptiometry 2
  adolescents, spinal concerns
    for 10
  alendronate 12
  bone building 39–40
  calcitonin 48
  cervical spine 57
  children, spinal concerns for
    61
  elderly, spinal concerns of 86
  environmental influences 89
  FBSS 99
  female athlete triad 100
  infants, spinal concerns for
    130
  iron 133
  juvenile osteoporosis 137
  magnesium 156
  mineral balance 168, 169
  myeloma bone disease 177
  nutrition 187, 189
  osteitis deformans 194
  osteoporosis 204, 206–207
  phytoestrogens 222
  potassium 226
  pregnancy, back care during
    228
  primary hyperparathyroidism
    228–229
  PTH 216
  rhabdomyolysis 237
  rhomboid muscle strain 241
  rickets 243
  scoliosis 253
  secondary osteoporosis 254
  SERMs 257
  skeletal fluorosis 263
  sleep 265
  trigger point therapy 301
  vitamin D 308
  weight, effects of 314
  weight-bearing exercise 313
CAM. *See* complementary and
  alternative medicine

cancer **50–52**
  bisphosphonates 37–38
  environmental influences 89
  epidural injection 91
  kyphoplasty 140
  kyphosis 141
  low back pain 148
  medical tests 162
  myeloma bone disease **176–
    178**
  NSAID therapy 186
  opiates 191
  osteitis deformans 194
  osteomyelitis 200
  osteoporosis 206
  pain 211
  PET scan 223
  phytochemicals 220
  PNT 218
  primary hyperparathyroidism
    229
  PTH 217
  secondary osteoporosis 254
  SERMs 256
  spinal cord 267
  spinal infection 269
  spinal tumor **276–278**
capsaicin 214–215, 297
capsicum (cayenne pepper) 29,
  214–215
cardiovascular (CV) events 72
carisoprodol (Soma) 171
carpal tunnel syndrome 181
car seats, infant 130–131
cauda equina syndrome (CES)
  52–53
  acute back pain 9
  herniated disc 118
  laminectomy 143
  low back pain 149
  lumbar spine 154
  sciatica 251
  spinal manipulation 272
  spinal stenosis 274
cayenne pepper. *See* capsicum
Celebrex (celecoxib) 18, 72
cerebellum 292
cervical foraminal stenosis
  53–54
cervical laminaplasty **54,** 183

cervical laminectomy. *See*
  laminectomy
cervical radiculopathy 25, **55,** 90
cervical spine xii–xiii, **56–58**
  anterior cervical discectomy
    14
  arthrodesis 20
  athletes, spinal concerns of
    23
  atlantoaxial instability **25–26**
  birth injury to the spine 36
  brachial plexus injury 46
  CAM 67
  cervical foraminal stenosis 53
  cervical radiculopathy 55
  cervical spondylosis 58
  corpectomy 69
  corticosteroid injection 70–71
  CSM 59
  DISH 75
  dwarfism 82
  flexion-extension injury 103
  foraminotomy 106
  heart, effects of the spine on
    the 114
  herniated disc 118
  infants, spinal concerns for
    131
  laminectomy 142
  lifting 144
  massage therapy 160
  meningitis, meningococcal
    disease 164
  minimally invasive surgery
    169
  myelogram 176
  nerve block 182
  nerve compression 183
  orthotics 192
  osteoarthritis 195
  osteomyelitis 200
  paraspinal muscles 215
  PNT 217
  posture 225
  range of motion 232
  rheumatoid arthritis 239
  rhomboid muscle strain 241
  SAPHO Syndrome 248
  Schmorl's node 250
  SED 279

cervical spine *(continued)*
   shaken baby syndrome 258
   sleep 264
   SNRB 258
   spinal cord 267
   spinal manipulation 272
   spinal stenosis 273
   spinal tuberculosis 275
   spinal tumor 277
   spondylolysis 281
   sprain 283
   surgery 288
   tension 294
   torticollis 298
   traction 299
   vertebral subluxation 305
cervical spondylosis 55, **58–59,** 74
cervical spondylotic myelopathy
  (CSM) **59–60**
cervicogenic headache **60–61**
   cervical spondylosis 58
   flexion-extension injury 103
   nerve block 182
   osteoarthritis 195
   rheumatoid arthritis 239
   spinal manipulation 272
   spinal stenosis 273
CES. *See* cauda equina syndrome
ch'i. *See* qi
children, spinal concerns for **61–
63**. *See also* adolescents, spinal
  concerns for; infant entries;
  juvenile entries
   absorptiometry 2
   activity, daily **4–6**
   alendronate 12
   antiresorptive drug 15
   aspirin 21
   atlantoaxial instability 25–26
   backache 28
   backpack safety **31–32**
   birth defects of the spine
     34–35
   birth injury to the spine **36–37**
   BMD tests 43
   bone building 38
   calcitonin 48
   calcium 49
   cervical spine 57
   discitis 77

dwarfism 82
eating disorders, bone loss
  caused by 85
exercise 94
folate 105
fractures 106
GH disorders **112–113**
gold salt treatment 112
herbal therapy 117
herniated disc 119
hydrotherapy 122
idiopathic scoliosis 126
kyphosis 141
lifting 144
lordosis 147
low back pain 148
lumbar spine 154
magnesium 156–157
Marfan syndrome 160
massage therapy 161
MD **172–174**
muscle relaxants 172
musculoskeletal disorders 175
naproxen 179
neurostimulation 185
nutrition 187
orthotics 192
osteogenesis imperfecta
  197–199
osteopenia 201
osteopetrosis **201–202**
osteoporosis 207
pain management 212
pain relievers 213
phosphorus 219
posture 225
PTH 216–217
rhomboid muscle strain 241
rickets 243
risedronate sodium 244
rodding surgery 245
RSD syndrome 233
sacral vertebrae 246
SAPHO Syndrome 248
Scheuermann's kyphosis 249
scoliosis 252
secondary osteoporosis 254
SED 279
shaken baby syndrome **258–
259**

shoe choice, spinal effects of
  260
skeletal dysplasia 262
sleep 265
spina bifida 266
spinal infection 269
spinal stenosis 273
spinal tuberculosis 274
spinal tumor 277
spine 278
spondylolisthesis 281
steroid therapy 283–284
strength training 286
surgery 289
thoracoplasty 296
torticollis 298
vertebrae 303
vitamin C 308
vitamin D 308
vitamin E 309
weight, effects of 314
Werdnig-Hoffman disease
  315–316
chiropractic ix, 67–68, 114, 196,
  305
chlorophyll 156
chloroquine. *See*
  hydroxychloroquine/
  chloroquine
chocolate 156
chondroitin 196–197
chondroitin sulfate 110–111
chordoma 277
chronic back pain **63–64**
   acute back pain 8
   arachnoiditis 17
   aspirin 22
   backache 28
   cancer 51
   children, spinal concerns for 61
   costotransverse joint
     injections 71
   discectomy 77
   discogram 78
   DMARD 80
   elderly, spinal concerns of 86
   epidural injection 90
   facet joint disorder 97
   FBSS 98
   flat back 102

flexion-extension injury 103
GH disorders 112
homeopathic medicine 120
ibuprofen 126
intrathecal spinal pump 132
juvenile arthritis 135
juvenile osteoporosis 136
juvenile spondyloarthritis 139
magnetic therapy 158
massage therapy 160
MBD 165
medical tests 162
musculoskeletal disorders 174
naproxen 179
nerve block 182
neurostimulation 184
orthotics 192
pain management 211–212
pain relievers 213–214
paraspinal muscles 215
peripheral neuropathy 219
range of motion 232
research 234
rheumatism 238
rheumatoid arthritis 239
rickets 244
RSD syndrome 233
Scheuermann's kyphosis 249
SED 255, 279
SNRB 257
spine 279
spondylolysis 281
surgery 288
synovial cyst 291
vertebral compression fracture 304
vertebroplasty 306
clinical trials 12, 51, **64–65,** 159, 202, 262
clotting 21
coccydynia **65,** 66
coccygeal spine **65–66,** 246, 278
cold therapy **66–67**
acute back pain 9
arthritis 19
backache 28
back injury 30
brachial plexus injury 47
CAM 67

cervical radiculopathy 55
coccydynia 65
costotransverse joint injections 71
flexion-extension injury 103
laminectomy 143
rib injury 242
sciatica 251
strain 285
collagen 168
complementary and alternative medicine (CAM) **67–68**
acupressure **6–7**
acupuncture **7–8**
acute back pain 9
arthritis 18–19
backache **28–29**
biofeedback **33–34**
cancer 51
children, spinal concerns for 62
fibromyalgia 101
heat therapy **115–116**
herbal therapy **116–118**
homeopathic medicine **119–121**
hydrotherapy **122–123**
infant massage therapy **129–130**
juvenile arthritis 135
magnetic therapy **158–159**
massage therapy **160–162**
nerve compression 183
osteoarthritis 195–196
PNT 218
rheumatoid arthritis 240
RSD syndrome 234
spinal manipulation **271–273**
steroid therapy 284
trigger point therapy **300–301**
ultrasound therapy **302**
Complex Regional Pain Syndrome (CRPS). *See* reflex sympathetic dystrophy syndrome
computed tomography/ computerized axial tomography (CT/CAT) scan **68–69**
ankylosing spondylitis 13
cervical spine 56
discogram 78

image-guided surgery 128
medical tests 162
sacroiliac joint pain syndrome 247
copper 168
corpectomy **69–70**
corticosteroid injection 19, **70–71,** 173, 270
costotransverse and costovertebral joint injections **71**
coumestans 222
COX, COX-1, COX-2. *See* cyclooxygenase entries
CSM (cervical spondylotic myelopathy) **59–60**
CT/CAT scan. *See* computed tomography/computerized axial tomography scan
curcumin 117, 240
curvature of the spine
flat back **102–103**
idiopathic scoliosis **126–128**
kyphosis **140–141**
lordosis **146–147**
posture **225–226**
Scheuermann's kyphosis **249–250**
scoliosis **252–254**
SED **279–280**
CV (cardiovascular) events 72
cyclobenzaprine (Flexeril) 171–172
cyclooxygenase (COX) 72, 185
cyclooxygenase (COX-1) 185
cyclooxygenase (COX-1) inhibitors 22, 72
cyclooxygenase (COX-2) inhibitors 18, 21, **72–73**
cyclooxygenase (COX-2) selective agents 185, 186
cyst 291–292

D

deflazacort 173
degenerative disc disease vi, **74–75**
arthritis 19
discogram 78
hydrotherapy 122
IDET 131

degenerative disc disease *(continued)*
  lifting 144
  neurostimulation 184
  orthotics 192
  SED 255
  spine 278
  synovial cyst 291
  weight, effects of 314
depression 212
devil's claw 19, 117
DEXA. *See* dual energy X-ray
  absorptiometry
diagnostic tests. *See* medical tests
  for conditions affecting the back
  and spine
diazepam (Valium) 171
diet. *See* nutrition
dietary supplements. *See*
  supplements
diffuse idiopathic skeletal
  hyperostosis (DISH) **75**
disc (disk) **75–76**
  CAT scan 69
  cervical radiculopathy 55
  cervical spondylosis 58
  corpectomy 69
  degenerative disc disease
    74–75
  discitis 77
  discogram 78
  herniated disc **118–119**
  lifting 144
  lumbar spine 154
  microdiscectomy 167
  musculoskeletal disorders 174
  osteomyelitis 199
  paraspinal muscles 215
  pregnancy, back care during
    228
  radiculitis 231
  range of motion 232
  research 234
  sciatica 251
  SED 255
  shoe choice, spinal effects of
    260
  spinal infection 268
  spinal stenosis 273
  spine 278
  spondylolysis 281

  strength training 286
  surgery 288
  synovial cyst 291
  vertebrae 303
discectomy 14, **76–77,** 119,
  166–167, 255. *See also* anterior
  cervical discectomy; selective
  endoscopic discectomy
discitis (diskitis) **77,** 147, 269
disc nucleoplasty **77–78**
discogram (discography) 56,
  78–79, 162, 255, 270
disc replacement vi, 74, 76, **79–80**
disease modifying anti-rheumatic
  drug (DMARD) 1, **80–81,** 138
DISH (diffuse idiopathic skeletal
  hyperostosis) **75**
dislocated vertebra **81–82**
DMARD. *See* disease modifying
  anti-rheumatic drug
drug interactions 116–117
dual energy X-ray absorptiometry
  (DEXA or DXA) 1–2, 43
Duchenne's muscular dystrophy
  172–173
dwarfism **82–83**
  GH disorders 112
  lordosis 147
  lumbar spine 154
  rickets 244
  scoliosis 252
  SED 279
DXA. *See* dual energy X-ray
  absorptiometry

E

eating disorders, bone loss caused
  by **84–86**
  adolescents, spinal concerns
    for 10
  bone building 39
  children, spinal concerns for
    61
  female athlete triad 99
  nutrition 187
  osteopenia 201
  osteoporosis 207
  posture 225
  rickets 244

secondary osteoporosis 254
surgery 289
vertebral compression fracture
  304
weight, effects of 314
elderly, spinal concerns of **86–88**
  activity, daily 4
  antiresorptive drug 15
  aspirin 21
  athletes, spinal concerns of
    23
  backache 28
  biofeedback 33
  bisphosphonates 38
  BMD tests 43
  calcitonin 48
  CAT scan 69
  CSM 59
  environmental influences 89
  exercise 94
  fractures 106
  herbal therapy 117
  herniated disc 119
  hydrotherapy 122
  juvenile osteoporosis 137
  kyphoplasty 140
  kyphosis 141
  lifting 144
  low back pain 148
  lumbar spine 154
  magnesium 157
  muscle relaxants 172
  musculoskeletal disorders
    175
  NSAID therapy 185, 186
  nutrition 187
  osteitis deformans **194–195**
  osteoarthritis **195–197**
  osteomyelitis 200
  osteopetrosis **201–202**
  osteophyte **202–203**
  osteoporosis **203–208**
  pain management 212
  pain relievers 213
  posture 225
  resistance training 236
  rheumatism 238
  rhomboid muscle strain 241
  risedronate sodium 244
  RSD syndrome 233

sacral vertebrae 246
SAPHO Syndrome 248
secondary osteoporosis 254
shoe choice, spinal effects of
    260
sleep 265
spinal stenosis 273
spinal tumor 277
spine 278
spondylolysis 281
strength training 286
surgery 289
thoracic spine 296
vitamin D 309
weight, effects of 314
electrolytes 226
electromyogram (EMG) **88**
    corticosteroid injection 70
    FBSS 99
    load tolerance 145
    medical tests 162
    NCV test 184
    paraspinal muscles 215
    rhabdomyolysis 237
endoscopic surgery. *See* minimally
invasive surgery
environmental influences on
spine health **88–90**
    elderly, spinal concerns of
        87
    genetic factors, genomics
        110
    infants, spinal concerns for
        130
    juvenile arthritis 135
    MBD 165
    medical tests 162
    mineral balance 168
    myeloma bone disease 176
    nutrition 187
    osteitis deformans 194
    osteoarthritis 197
    pain management 212
    paraspinal muscles 216
    post-polio syndrome 224
    rheumatoid arthritis 239
    rickets 243
    scoliosis 253
    skeletal dysplasia 262
    skeletal fluorosis 263

spinal tumor 276
    vertebrae 304
    water and spine health 311
epidural injection **90–91**
    lumbar radiculopathy 151
    nerve block 182
    pregnancy, back care during
        228
    SNRB 257
    spinal injection 269
    steroid therapy 284
Epsom salts 29, 156
ergonomic factors **91–93**
    acute back pain 9
    children, spinal concerns for
        61
    coccygeal spine 66
    elderly, spinal concerns of 87
    facet joint disorder 97
    herniated disc 119
    laminectomy 143
    low back pain 149
    musculoskeletal disorders
        175
    neck pain 180
    pain management 212
    paraspinal muscles 216
    post-polio syndrome 224
    sacral vertebrae 246
    sciatica 251
    vertebral subluxation 305
estrogen 121, 221–222
etidronate **93**
EVISTA (raloxifene) 256–257
Excedrin 3
exercise xiv, **94–96**
    resistance training 94, **236–
        237,** 242, 243
    strength training. *See* strength
        training
    weight-bearing exercise
        312–313
eyes 180–181

F

facet joint disorder 56, **97–98,**
    269–270, 281, 303
facet neurotomy (facet rhizotomy
    injection) 97, **98**

failed back surgery syndrome
    (FBSS) **98–99,** 143, 152, 184,
    212
fast food 226
FDA (U.S. Food and Drug
    Administration) 116
female athlete triad **99–100**
fever 21
feverfew 240
FEWS (Food, Exercise, Water,
    Sleep) xiv
fiber, dietary 49
fibromyalgia **100–101,** 120, 224,
    300, 307
fibrous dysplasia **101–102**
flat back **102–103**
Flexeril (cyclobenzaprine) 171–
    172
flexion-extension injury **103–
    104**
    athletes, spinal concerns of
        23
    atlantoaxial instability 25
    cervicogenic headache 60
    neck pain 180
    orthotics 192
    osteoarthritis 195
    paraspinal muscles 215
    radiculitis 231
    range of motion 232
    shaken baby syndrome **258–
        259**
    spinal stenosis 274
    spine 278
    sprain 283
    TENS unit 299
    torticollis 298
    vertebrae 303
    vertebral subluxation 305
fluoride 89, 263
fluoroscopy **104–105**
    costotransverse joint
        injections 71
    image-guided surgery 128
    medical tests 162
    myelogram 176
    sacroiliac joint pain syndrome
        247
    SED 255
    SNRB 257

fluoroscopy *(continued)*
   spinal injection 270
   surgery 288
fluorosis. *See* skeletal fluorosis
fluvoxamine (Faverin) 172
folate (folic acid; B9) 34, 51,
   105–106, 266, 307
food. *See* nutrition
food allergies 116, 135, 168, 188
food safety 188
foot. *See* shoe choice, spinal effects
   of
football 22, 23
foraminotomy **106**
Forestier's Disease. *See* diffuse
   idiopathic skeletal hyperostosis
Forteo (teriparatide) 216–217
Fosamax (alendronate) 12, 37,
   137
Fosamax Plus D 38
fractures **106–108.** *See also*
   vertebral compression fracture
      acupressure 6
      antiresorptive drug 15
      arthrodesis 20
      back injury 30
      birth injury to the spine 36
      bisphosphonates 37
      BMD tests 43
      bone graft 41
      calcitonin 48
      CAM 67
      CAT scan 69
      children, spinal concerns for
         61
      coccygeal spine 66
      disc nucleoplasty 78
      elderly, spinal concerns of 86
      exercise 94
      fibrous dysplasia 101
      hypophosphatasia 123
      juvenile osteoporosis 136
      low back pain 148
      massage therapy 161
      musculoskeletal disorders 175
      osteogenesis imperfecta 197
      osteoporosis 203, 207
      PTH 216
      QCT 230
      rib injury 242

risedronate sodium 244
RSD syndrome 233
sacral vertebrae 246
shaken baby syndrome 258
spine 278
spondylolysis **281–282**
strength training 286
strontium ranelate 287
thoracic spine 296
ultrasound therapy 302
fusion. *See* arthrodesis; lumbar
   spinal fusion

G

gastrointestinal (GI) bleeding 72
gene therapy 235
genetic factors (genomics) **109–
   110**
      adolescents, spinal concerns
         for 10
      ankylosing spondylitis 13
      dwarfism 82
      environmental influences 89
      fibrous dysplasia 102
      hypophosphatasia 123
      infants, spinal concerns for
         130
      juvenile rheumatoid arthritis
         137
      lumbar spine 154
      Marfan syndrome **159–160**
      MBD 165
      MD **172–174**
      medical tests 162
      mineral balance 168
      myeloma bone disease 177
      nutrition 187
      osteitis deformans 194
      osteoarthritis 195
      osteogenesis imperfecta
         197–199
      osteopetrosis 201–202
      osteophyte 202
      osteoporosis 206
      primary hyperparathyroidism
         229
      research 235
      resistance training 237
      rheumatoid arthritis 239

rickets 244
Scheuermann's kyphosis 249
Schmorl's node 250
scoliosis 252
SED 279
skeletal dysplasia 262
SM 292
spinal tumor 276
torticollis 298
vertebrae 304
Werdnig-Hoffman disease 315
GH disorders. *See* growth
   hormone disorders
GI (gastrointestinal) bleeding 72
gigantism 112–113
ginger 240, 290
glucocorticoids 206
glucosamine **110–111,** 188, 196–
   197, 240
glucose 223
goldenseal 117
gold salt treatment 80, 81, **111–
   112**
gold sodium thiomalate
   (Myochrysine) 112
growth hormone (GH) disorders
   112–113, 162, 198
growth hormone therapy 82

H

harpagoside. *See* devil's claw
headache, cervicogenic **60–61**
heart, effects of the spine on the
   114–115
heart disease 133
heat therapy **115–116**
      acupuncture 7
      arthritis 19
      backache 28
      back injury 30
      brachial plexus injury 47
      flexion-extension injury 103
      hydrotherapy 122
      laminectomy 143
      osteoarthritis 195
      paraspinal muscles 216
      rheumatism 239
      RICE method 243
      strain 285

heme iron 133
herbal therapy **116–118**
    arthritis 18–19
    backache 28–29
    fibromyalgia 101
    homeopathic medicine 119
    ibuprofen 126
    nutrition 188
    osteoarthritis 196
    over-the-counter products 208
    pain relievers 214
    phosphorus 220
    phytoestrogens 221
    rhabdomyolysis 237
    rheumatoid arthritis 240
    SERMs 256
    sleep 264–265
    surgery 290
herniated disc **118–119**
    acute back pain 8
    anterior cervical discectomy
        14
    back injury 30
    CAT scan 69
    degenerative disc disease 74
    discectomy 76
    FBSS 99
    foraminotomy 106
    microdiscectomy 166
    NCV test 184
    nerve block 182
    nerve compression 183
    radiculitis 231
    rib injury 242
    RSD syndrome 233
    sacroiliac joint pain syndrome
        247
    Scheuermann's kyphosis 249
    sciatica 251
    SED 255
    spinal injection 269
    spinal manipulation 272
    synovial cyst 291
Hispanics 105
homeopathic medicine 21, **119–
    121,** 208, 265
hormone replacement therapy
    (HRT) **121–122**
    absorptiometry 2
    antiresorptive drug 15

female athlete triad 100
    phytoestrogens 221
    secondary osteoporosis 254
    SERMs 256
Human Genome Project 235
hydrotherapy **122–123**
    osteoarthritis 195
    osteogenesis imperfecta 198
    paraspinal muscles 216
    pregnancy, back care during
        228
    rodding surgery 245
    RSD syndrome 234
hydroxychloroquine/chloroquine
    80, 81
hypercalcemia 177
hypophosphatasia **123–124**

I

ibandronate 37, **125,** 177
ibuprofen **125–126,** 185
IDET (intradiscal electrothermal
    therapy) **131–132**
idiopathic scoliosis 10, **126–128,**
    252
image-guided surgery **128–129**
immune system 293
infant car seats 130–131
infant massage therapy **129–130,**
    160–161
infants, spinal concerns for **130–
    131**
    birth defects of the spine
        34–35
    bone scan 46
    calcitonin 48
    cervical spine 57
    dwarfism 82
    environmental influences 89
    folate 105
    genetic factors, genomics 109
    GH disorders 112
    hypophosphatasia 123
    idiopathic scoliosis 126
    juvenile rheumatoid arthritis
        137
    kyphosis 141
    lumbar spine 154
    neurostimulation 185

nutrition 187
osteogenesis imperfecta 197
osteopetrosis **201–202**
phosphorus 219
pregnancy, back care during
    227
rodding surgery 245
sacral vertebrae 246
scoliosis 252
SED 279
shaken baby syndrome **258–
    259**
skeletal dysplasia 262
sleep 265
spina bifida 265
spinal stenosis 273
spinal tumor 277
surgery 289
thoracoplasty 296
torticollis 298
vitamin D 308
Werdnig-Hoffman disease
    315–316
inflammation v, 21, 22
intradiscal electrothermal therapy
    (IDET) **131–132**
intrathecal spinal pump **132**
iron 130, **133–134,** 158, 169, 318
isoflavones 222

J

joint 103
JRA. *See* juvenile rheumatoid
    arthritis
JSpA. *See* juvenile
    spondyloarthritis
juvenile arthritis **135–136,** 248
juvenile osteoporosis **136–137**
juvenile rheumatoid arthritis
    137–138
    DMARD 80
    gold salt treatment 111
    juvenile osteoporosis 136
    musculoskeletal disorders
        174
    rheumatoid arthritis 239
    steroid therapy 283
juvenile spondyloarthritis **138–
139**

K

kidney 168
kyphoplasty **140,** 206, 306
kyphosis **140–141**
  birth defects of the spine 35
  dwarfism 82
  flat back 102
  juvenile osteoporosis 136
  Marfan syndrome 160
  osteoporosis 203
  paraspinal muscles 215
  posture 225
  rickets 244
  Scheuermann's kyphosis
    249–250
  Schmorl's node 250
  skeletal dysplasia 262
  spinal tuberculosis 275
  spine 278
  thoracic spine 296
  vertebrae 303

L

laminaplasty. *See* cervical
  laminaplasty
laminectomy (laminotomy) vi,
  142–143
  foraminotomy 106
  herniated disc 119
  lumbar spinal fusion 152
  nerve compression 183
  osteophyte 203
  SED 255
  spinal stenosis 273
  spine 279
  surgery 288
LBD (low-back disorder) 146
lifting **144**
  acute back pain 9
  back injury 31
  discectomy 77
  elderly, spinal concerns of 87
  ergonomic factors 91
  facet joint disorder 97
  FBSS 99
  herniated disc 119
  laminectomy 143
  load tolerance 145, 146
  low back pain 148, 149

lumbar spine 154
muscle cramp/spasm 171
musculoskeletal disorders
  175
neck pain 180
osteoarthritis 197
resistance training 236
rhomboid muscle strain 241
sacral vertebrae 246
sacroiliac joint pain syndrome
  247
spine 278
strain 285
thoracic spine 296
lignans 222
LIPUS (low-intensity pulsed
  ultrasound) 302
Liquiprin 3
load tolerance **145–146**
  backache 28
  backpack safety 31
  ergonomic factors 91
  herniated disc 119
  lifting 144
  low back pain 148
  lumbar spine 154
  osteoarthritis 197
  sacral vertebrae 246
  sacroiliac joint pain syndrome
    247
  spine 278
  spondylolysis 281
lordosis **146–147**
  cervical laminaplasty 54
  dwarfism 82
  flat back 102
  lumbar spine 154
  paraspinal muscles 215
  posture 225
  spine 278
low-back disorder (LBD) 146
low back pain **147–150**
  activity, daily 4
  acupuncture 7
  athletes, spinal concerns of 22
  CES 52
  children, spinal concerns for
    62
  exercise 95
  heat therapy 115–116

herbal therapy 117
herniated disc 118
lumbar radiculopathy **151–
  152**
lumbar spinal fusion 152
lumbar spine 154
Marfan syndrome 159
massage therapy 161–162
medical tests 162–163
muscle cramp/spasm 170
muscle relaxants 171
myeloma bone disease 177
osteoarthritis 195
pain 210, 211
piriformis syndrome 223
PNT 217
posture 225
pregnancy, back care during
  227
resistance training 237
rhabdomyolysis 237
rheumatism 239
sacral vertebrae 246
sciatica 251
scoliosis 252
SNRB 257
spina bifida 266
spinal manipulation 272
spinal stenosis 273
spinal tuberculosis 275
spine 279
spondylolisthesis 280
spondylolysis 281
sprain 282–283
steroid therapy 284
strain 285
synovial cyst 291
TENS unit 300
lower back. *See* lumbar spine
low-intensity pulsed ultrasound
  (LIPUS) 302
lumbago. *See* low back pain
lumbar corset 193
lumbar laminectomy 262
lumbar puncture 104, **150–151,**
  164, 176, 259
lumbar radiculopathy **151–152,**
  251
lumbar spinal fusion 20, 41, 142,
  152–154, 232

lumbar spine **154–155**
  absorptiometry 2
  arthrodesis 20
  corpectomy 69
  DISH 75
  foraminotomy 106
  herniated disc 118
  juvenile spondyloarthritis 139
  kyphosis 141
  laminectomy 142
  lordosis 146
  low back pain 147
  lumbar radiculopathy 151
  lumbar spinal fusion 152
  microdiscectomy 166
  muscle cramp/spasm 170
  nerve block 182
  nerve compression 183
  opiates 191
  osteomyelitis 200
  osteoporosis 203
  piriformis syndrome 223
  posture 225
  pregnancy, back care during
    227
  range of motion 232
  risedronate sodium 244
  sacral vertebrae 246
  sacroiliac joint pain syndrome
    247
  Schmorl's node 250
  sciatica 251
  scoliosis 252
  SED 279
  SNRB 258
  spinal manipulation 272
  spinal stenosis 273
  spinal tuberculosis 275
  spondylolysis 281
  sprain 283
  strength training 286
  surgery 288
  synovial cyst 291
  tension 294
  vertebral subluxation 305

M

macro minerals 167–169
magnesium **156–157,** 169, 226

magnetic resonance imaging
  (MRI) vii, **157–158**
  image-guided surgery 128
  medical tests 162
  neurostimulation 185
  SED 280
  SNRB 257
magnetic therapy **158–159,** 234
manganese 169
marble bone disease. *See*
  osteopetrosis
Marfan syndrome **159–160**
Marie-Strumpell disease. *See*
  ankylosing spondylitis
massage therapy **160–162**
  acupressure 6
  arthritis 19
  brachial plexus injury 47
  children, spinal concerns for
    62
  cold therapy 66–67
  hydrotherapy 122
  infant massage therapy 129
  osteoarthritis 196
  paraspinal muscles 215, 216
  range of motion 232
  sleep 265
  spinal injury 271
  spinal manipulation 272
  trigger point therapy 300
MBD. *See* metabolic bone disease
MD. *See* muscular dystrophy
medical imaging
  fluoroscopy **104–105**
  MRI **157–158**
  PET scan **223–224**
  X-ray **317**
medical tests for conditions
  affecting the back and spine
  162–163
  discogram **78–79**
  lumbar puncture **150–151**
  MRI **157–158**
  myelogram **175–176**
  NCV test **183–184**
  PET scan **223–224**
  QCT **230**
  ultrasound therapy 302
  X-ray **317**
meningitis (meningococcal
  disease) **163–164**

meningococcal disease 150
menopause 133
metabolic bone disease (MBD)
  164–165, 187
metabolic diseases of muscle
  165–166, 187
microdiscectomy 78, 119, **166–
167**
milk 49, 220
mineral balance **167–169**
  bone building 39
  calcium 49
  juvenile osteoporosis 137
  magnesium **156–157**
  MBD 165
  MD 173
  medical tests 162
  muscle cramp/spasm 170
  nutrition 186
  osteoarthritis 196
  osteoporosis 206
  paraspinal muscles 215
  phosphorus **219–220**
  posture 225
  potassium **226–227**
  pregnancy, back care during
    228
  primary hyperparathyroidism
    229
  PTH 216
  rhabdomyolysis 237
  rickets 243
  secondary osteoporosis 254
  surgery 290
  zinc **318**
minimally invasive surgery **169–
170**
  arthrodesis 20
  discectomy 76
  disc nucleoplasty **77–78**
  image-guided surgery **128–
129**
  kyphoplasty **140**
  laminectomy 142
  lumbar spinal fusion 152
  microdiscectomy **166–167**
  osteoporosis 206
  SED **255–256**
  vertebroplasty **306**
Motrin 126

MRI. *See* magnetic resonance imaging
multiple myeloma. *See* myeloma bone disease
muscle xiii
   metabolic diseases of muscle **165–166**
   paraspinal muscles **215–216**
   rhabdomyolysis **237–238**
   rhomboid muscle strain **241–242**
muscle cramp or spasm **170–171,** 237, 282–283
muscle dilation 169
muscle mass 236
muscle relaxants 33, 58, **171–172,** 215, 240, 241
muscle stripping 169
muscular dystrophy (MD) 147, **172–174**
musculoskeletal disorders **174–175,** 181, 184, 186
mutation 109, 240
myelogram 104, 162, **175–176,** 183
myeloma bone disease **176–178**
Myochrysine (gold sodium thiomalate) 112

N
Naprosyn 179, 185
naproxen **179,** 185
National Institute for Occupational Safety and Health (NIOSH) 92
nausea 7, 290
NCV test. *See* nerve conduction study or nerve conduction velocity test
neck pain **180–181**
   athletes, spinal concerns of 22
   muscle cramp/spasm 170
   osteoarthritis 195
   sleep 265
   spinal stenosis 273
   spine 278
   spondylolysis 281
   surgery 288

tension 294
torticollis **298–299**
nerve(s) xiii, 114, 218–219, 231
nerve block 63, 98, **181–182,** 247. *See also* selective nerve root block
nerve compression 174, **182–183**
nerve conduction study or nerve conduction velocity (NCV) test 56, 162, **183–184**
nerve function test (electromyogram) 88
neural tube defects (NTDs) 105
neurostimulation 63, **184–185**
NIOSH (National Institute for Occupational Safety and Health) 92
nonheme iron 133
non-selective NSAIDS 185–186
nonsteroidal anti-inflammatory drug (NSAID) therapy **185–186**
   aspirin **21–22**
   COX-2 inhibitors **72–73**
   ibuprofen **125–126**
   naproxen **179**
NTDs (neural tube defects) 105
Nuprin 126
nutrition viii–ix, xiv, **186–190**
   activity, daily 5
   adolescents, spinal concerns for 10
   arthritis 19
   birth defects of the spine 34
   bisphosphonates 38
   bone building 39
   bone graft 42
   CAM 68
   cancer 51
   cervical spine 57
   disc, disk 76
   DISH 75
   dislocated vertebra 82
   eating disorders, bone loss caused by 84
   elderly, spinal concerns of 86
   environmental influences 90
   FBSS 99
   female athlete triad 100
   genetic factors, genomics 110

heart, effects of the spine on the 115
herbal therapy 118
homeopathic medicine 119
hydrotherapy 123
IDET 132
infants, spinal concerns for 130
iron 133
juvenile arthritis 136
juvenile osteoporosis 137
juvenile spondyloarthritis 139
laminectomy 143
lumbar spine 154
magnesium **156–157**
MBD 165
MD 173
metabolic diseases of muscle 165
microdiscectomy 167
mineral balance. *See* mineral balance
muscle cramp/spasm 171
musculoskeletal disorders 175
osteitis deformans 194
osteoarthritis 196
osteogenesis imperfecta 198
osteopenia 201
osteophyte 203
osteoporosis 205
pain management 213
paraspinal muscles 215
phosphorus 219
phytochemicals 221
phytoestrogens **221–222**
post-polio syndrome 224
potassium 226
pregnancy, back care during 228
primary hyperparathyroidism 229
rheumatism 239
rheumatoid arthritis 240
rhomboid muscle strain 241
RICE method 243
rickets 244
RSD syndrome 234
scoliosis 253

secondary osteoporosis 254
SED 280
shaken baby syndrome 259
skeletal dysplasia 262
skeletal fluorosis 263
SNRB 258
spina bifida 266
spinal infection 269
spinal tuberculosis 275
spinal tumor 277–278
spine 279
spondylolysis 282
sprain 283
steroid therapy 284
surgery 289
tension 294
vertebrae 304
vitamins. *See* specific vitamin
    entries
weight, effects of 314
weight-bearing exercise 313
zinc 318

O
Occupational Safety & Health
    Administration (OSHA) 91–92,
    144
occupational therapist (OT)
    149–150
office chairs 92
oil of wintergreen 29
omega-6 fatty acid 240
omega-3 fatty acid 240
opiates (opioids) 181, **191–192,**
    214, 304
orthotics **192–194**
    arthrodesis 21
    birth defects of the spine 35
    birth injury to the spine 36
    cervical spondylosis 58
    CSM 59
    dislocated vertebra 82
    idiopathic scoliosis 127
    juvenile spondyloarthritis 139
    kyphosis 141
    load tolerance 145
    lordosis 147
    Marfan syndrome 160
    MD 173

musculoskeletal disorders
    175
    osteitis deformans 194
    osteogenesis imperfecta 198
    over-the-counter products
    208
    paraspinal muscles 216
    posture 226
    pregnancy, back care during
    228
    rheumatoid arthritis 240
    rickets 244
    sacral vertebrae 246
    Scheuermann's kyphosis 249
    scoliosis 252–253
    shoe choice, spinal effects of
    261
    skeletal dysplasia 262
    spina bifida 266
    spinal injury 271
    spine 278
    spondylolisthesis 280
    thoracic spine 296
    vertebral compression fracture
    304
OSHA. *See* Occupational Safety &
    Health Administration
osteitis deformans 48, **194–195,**
    217
osteoarthritis **195–197**
    arthritis 18
    COX-2 inhibitors 72
    facet joint disorder 97
    glucosamine 110–111
    herbal therapy 117
    homeopathic medicine 120
    hydrotherapy 122
    ibuprofen 126
    musculoskeletal disorders
    174
    neck pain 181
    nutrition 188
    osteitis deformans 194
    research 234
    rheumatoid arthritis 239
    sacroiliac joint pain syndrome
    247
    skeletal dysplasia 262
    spondylolysis 281
    strength training 286

synovial cyst 291
TENS unit 299
osteogenesis imperfecta **197–199**
    juvenile osteoporosis 136
    lumbar spine 154
    risedronate sodium 244
    rodding surgery 245
    thoracic spine 296
    weight-bearing exercise 313
    X-ray 317
osteomalacia. *See* rickets
osteomyelitis **199–200,** 274
osteopathy ix
osteopenia **201**
    absorptiometry 2
    adolescents, spinal concerns
    for 10
    antiresorptive drug 15
    bisphosphonates 37
    eating disorders, bone loss
    caused by 84
    juvenile osteoporosis 137
    phytoestrogens 221
    PTH 216
osteopetrosis 15, **201–202**
osteophyte **202–203**
    anterior cervical discectomy
    14
    cervical spondylosis 58
    CES 52
    corpectomy 69
    degenerative disc disease 74
    DISH 75
    dwarfism 82
    facet joint disorder 97
    foraminotomy 106
    laminectomy 142
    nerve compression 183
    osteoarthritis 195
    spinal stenosis 273
osteoporosis **203–208**
    absorptiometry 1
    activity, daily 4
    adolescents, spinal concerns
    for 10
    antiresorptive drug 15
    bisphosphonates 37
    calcitonin 48
    CAM 67
    CAT scan 69

osteoporosis *(continued)*
    corticosteroid injection 70
    CSM 59
    eating disorders, bone loss
        caused by 84
    etidronate 93
    female athlete triad 100
    fractures 106
    homeopathic medicine 120
    HRT 121
    ibandronate 125
    juvenile osteoporosis **136–137**
    kyphoplasty 140
    kyphosis 141
    low back pain 148
    lumbar spine 154
    mineral balance 168
    myeloma bone disease 177
    nutrition 188, 189
    osteopetrosis 201
    phytoestrogens 221
    potassium 226
    primary hyperparathyroidism
        229
    PTH 216
    research 234
    resistance training 237
    risedronate sodium 244
    RSD syndrome 234
    sacral vertebrae 246
    secondary osteoporosis **254–
        255**
    SERMs 256
    spine 278
    strontium ranelate 287
    vertebrae 303
    vertebral compression fracture
        304
    vitamin A 307
    vitamin D 309
    weight-bearing exercise 313
    X-ray 317
OT (occupational therapist)
    149–150
over-the-counter (OTC) products
    208–209
    acetaminophen 4
    backache 29
    bisphosphonates 38
    COX-2 inhibitors 72

    naproxen **179**
    NSAID therapy 185–186
    orthotics 193
    pain relievers 213
    paraspinal muscles 216
oxalic acid 49

P

Paget's disease. *See* osteitis
    deformans
pain xiii–xiv, **210–211**. *See also
    specific forms of pain, e.g.:* acute
    back pain
pain management **211–213**
    acupuncture **7–8**
    biofeedback **33–34**
    corticosteroid injection **70–71**
    epidural injection **90–91**
    heat therapy **115–116**
    hydrotherapy **122–123**
    intrathecal spinal pump **132**
    magnetic therapy **158–159**
    massage therapy **160–162**
    nerve block **181–182**
    neurostimulation **184–185**
    NSAID therapy **185–186**
    opiates **191–192**
    pain relievers **213–215**
    PNT **217–218**
    SNRB **257–258**
    steroid therapy **283–284**
    TENS unit **299–300**
    topical analgesic **297–298**
    trigger point therapy **300–301**
pain relievers 213–215
    acetaminophen **3–4**
    naproxen **179**
    NSAID therapy **185–186**
    opiates **191–192**
    topical analgesic **297–298**
paraspinal muscles **215–216**
    acute back pain 9
    arachnoiditis 17
    arthritis 19
    athletes, spinal concerns of 22
    backache 28
    back injury 30
    children, spinal concerns for
        61

    corpectomy 70
    dislocated vertebra 81
    eating disorders, bone loss
        caused by 84
    elderly, spinal concerns of 86
    exercise 94
    facet joint disorder 97
    flexion-extension injury 104
    heat therapy 115
    hydrotherapy 122
    ibuprofen 126
    infant massage therapy 129
    iron 133
    lifting 144
    lordosis 147
    lumbar spinal fusion 153
    Marfan syndrome 159
    MD 172
    medical tests 162
    mineral balance 167
    muscle relaxants 171
    musculoskeletal disorders
        174
    orthotics 193
    posture 225
    potassium 226
    pregnancy, back care during
        228
    range of motion 232
    resistance training 236
    rhomboid muscle strain 241
    rib injury 242
    RICE method 243
    sacroiliac joint pain syndrome
        247
    Scheuermann's kyphosis 249
    Schmorl's node 250
    sciatica 251
    scoliosis 252
    spinal manipulation 272
    spinal stenosis 273
    spine 278
    spondylolisthesis 281
    sprain 283
    strength training 285
    thoracic outlet syndrome 295
    thoracic spine 296
    trigger point therapy 300
parathyroid hormone (PTH) 12,
    15, 102, **216–217,** 254

penicillamine 81
PENS (percutaneous electrical nerve stimulation). *See* percutaneous neuromodulation therapy
Percocet 3
percutaneous neuromodulation therapy (PNT) **217–218**
peripheral neuropathy **218–219**
PET (positive emission tomography) scan **223–224**
phonemics 19
phosphate salts 220
phosphorus 137, 168, 169, **219–220**
physical dependence 191–192
physical therapy v–vi
phytate 49
phytochemicals 187–188, **220–221**
phytoestrogens 188, 220, **221–222**
pinched nerve. *See* cervical radiculopathy
piriformis syndrome **222–223,** 251
pituitary gland 112
PNT (percutaneous neuromodulation therapy) **217–218**
poliomyelitis (post-polio syndrome) **224–225**
positive emission tomography (PET) scan **223–224**
post-polio syndrome 184, **224–225**
posture **225–226**
    absorptiometry 2
    acute back pain 9
    backache 28
    back injury 30–31
    backpack safety 31
    bone building 39
    CAM 68
    cervical foraminal stenosis 53
    cervical laminaplasty 54
    children, spinal concerns for 61
    dwarfism 82
    elderly, spinal concerns of 86

ergonomic factors 91
flat back 102
flexion-extension injury 104
herniated disc 119
juvenile osteoporosis 136
juvenile spondyloarthritis 139
kyphosis **140–141**
laminectomy 143
load tolerance 145
Marfan syndrome 160
MD 172
muscle cramp/spasm 170
neck pain 180
orthotics **192–194**
osteitis deformans 194
osteogenesis imperfecta 198
osteoporosis 203
peripheral neuropathy 219
post-polio syndrome 224
pregnancy, back care during 227
range of motion 232
rhomboid muscle strain 241
rickets 244
Scheuermann's kyphosis **249–250**
scoliosis 252
SED 279
shoe choice, spinal effects of 260
skeletal dysplasia 262
spina bifida 266
spinal manipulation 271
spinal tuberculosis 275
spine 278
thoracic spine 296
torticollis 298
trigger point therapy 300
vertebral subluxation 305
weight-bearing exercise 313
potassium 169, 187, 189, **226–227**
Pott's Disease 274, 275
prednisone 173, 283–284
pregnancy, back care during 34, 46, 91, 148, 225, **227–228**
pregnancy, nutrition during 266
primary hyperparathyroidism **228–229**

product labels 214
progestin 121
prostaglandins 21
PTH. *See* parathyroid hormone

Q

qi (energy) 6–8
quadriplegia 267
quantitative computed tomography (QCT) 42, **230**

R

radiation exposure 227
radiation therapy 276–277
radiculitis (radiculopathy) **231,** 291
Radiologic Vertebral Assessment (RVA) 43
raloxifene 15–16, 256–257
range of motion **232–233**
    acute back pain 9
    ankylosing spondylitis 13
    arthritis 18
    arthrodesis 21
    cervical laminaplasty 54
    cervical spine 56
    cervical spondylosis 58
    coccygeal spine 65
    degenerative disc disease 74
    elderly, spinal concerns of 87
    exercise 95
    facet joint disorder 97
    flexion-extension injury 104
    foraminotomy 106
    juvenile arthritis 135
    lumbar radiculopathy 151
    lumbar spinal fusion 153
    MD 173
    medical tests 162
    muscle cramp/spasm 170
    neck pain 180
    nerve block 182
    nerve compression 183
    orthotics 192
    osteoarthritis 197
    piriformis syndrome 223
    posture 226
    radiculitis 231

range of motion (*continued*)
    rheumatoid arthritis 239
    RSD syndrome 233
    sacroiliac joint pain syndrome
        247
    Schmorl's node 250
    sciatica 251
    spinal injury 271
    spinal manipulation 271
    spinal tuberculosis 275
    spine 278
    spondylolisthesis 280
    sprain 282
    tension 293
    thoracic outlet syndrome 295
    thoracic spine 296
    torticollis 298
    trigger point therapy 300
    ultrasound therapy 302
red pepper. *See* capsicum
reflex sympathetic dystrophy
    (RSD) syndrome **233–234**
research **234–236**
resistance training 94, **236–237,**
    242, 243
retinol 306–307
rhabdomyolysis 28, 166, **237–**
    238
rheumatism 88, 158, **238–239**
rheumatoid arthritis **239–241**
    arthritis 18
    atlantoaxial instability 26
    biofeedback 33
    COX-2 inhibitors 72
    dislocated vertebra 81
    DMARD 80
    gold salt treatment 111
    homeopathic medicine 120
    hydrotherapy 122
    ibuprofen 126
    juvenile rheumatoid arthritis
        137
    medical tests 162
    osteoarthritis 195
    osteoporosis 206
    peripheral neuropathy 218
    research 234
    spinal infection 269
    steroid therapy 283
    TENS unit 299

rheumatoid spondylitis. *See*
    ankylosing spondylitis
rheumatologist ix
rhomboid muscle strain **241–242**
rib injury 71, 81, 101, 241, **242**
RICE method 29, 53, 56, **243,**
    282, 285
rickets 102, 216, **243–244,** 308
Ridaura (auranofin) 112
risedronate sodium 37, 205,
    244–245
rodding surgery 199, **245,** 253,
    288
RSD (reflex sympathetic
    dystrophy) syndrome **233–234**
running 94–95
RVA (Radiologic Vertebral
    Assessment) 43

S

sacral obliquity 246
sacral vertebrae **246–247**
    juvenile spondyloarthritis 139
    lumbar radiculopathy 151
    lumbar spine 154
    pregnancy, back care during
        227
    sacroiliac joint pain syndrome
        247
    sciatica 251
    scoliosis 252
    shoe choice, spinal effects of
        260
    SNRB 258
    spinal tuberculosis 275
    spinal tumor 277
    spine 278
sacroiliac joint pain syndrome
    (sacroiliitis) 13, 246, **247**
safety seat 130–131
SAPHO Syndrome **247–248**
saturated fat 10
SBT (stability ball training) 303–
    304
Scheuermann's kyphosis 141,
    249–250
Schmorl's node 249, **250–251**
sciatica **251–252**
    acute back pain 8

arachnoiditis 17
back injury 30
CES 52
discectomy 76
epidural injection 90
herniated disc 118
IDET 131
lumbar spinal fusion 152
NCV test 184
piriformis syndrome **222–223**
radiculitis 231
sacroiliac joint pain syndrome
    247
SNRB 258
TENS unit 299
scoliosis **252–254**
    athletes, spinal concerns of 24
    BMD tests 43
    dwarfism 82
    idiopathic scoliosis **126–128**
    image-guided surgery 128
    load tolerance 145
    lumbar spine 154
    Marfan syndrome 160
    orthotics 192
    over-the-counter products 208
    paraspinal muscles 215
    posture 225
    rickets 244
    sacral vertebrae 246
    skeletal dysplasia 262
    spina bifida 266
    spine 278
    thoracic spine 296
    thoracoplasty 296
Scotch pine 19
secondary osteoporosis **254–255,**
    283
SED. *See* selective endoscopic
    discectomy; spondyloepiphyseal
    dysplasia
selective endoscopic discectomy
    (SED) **255–256**
selective estrogen receptor
    modulators (SERMs) 15–16,
    256–257
selective nerve root block (SNRB)
    257–258, 269, 271
SERMs. *See* selective estrogen
    receptor modulators

shaken baby syndrome, shaken infant syndrome **258–259**
shoe choice, spinal effects of **260–262**
   children, spinal concerns for 61
   exercise 94
   juvenile spondyloarthritis 139
   Marfan syndrome 160
   orthotics 192
   posture 225
   pregnancy, back care during 228
   rheumatoid arthritis 240
   spine 278
   vertebral subluxation 305
single proton absorptiometry (SPA) 1
sitting 149
skeletal dysplasia **262–263**
skeletal fluorosis **263–264**
sleep xiv, **264–265**
   arthritis 19
   backache 28
   birth defects of the spine 34
   calcium 49
   children, spinal concerns for 61
   degenerative disc disease 74
   elderly, spinal concerns of 86
   FBSS 99
   fibromyalgia 100
   genetic factors, genomics 110
   herniated disc 119
   low back pain 149
   lumbar spine 155
   magnetic therapy 159
   microdiscectomy 167
   neck pain 180
   nutrition 189
   opiates 192
   osteoarthritis 195
   pain 211
   pain management 212
   paraspinal muscles 215
   post-polio syndrome 224
   pregnancy, back care during 228

rheumatoid arthritis 240
rhomboid muscle strain 241
shaken baby syndrome 259
spinal infection 269
spinal tumor 276
spine 279
spondylolysis 282
steroid therapy 283
tension 294
weight-bearing exercise 313
SM. *See* syringomyelia
smoking 90, 307–308
SNRB. *See* selective nerve root block
sodium 168, 169, 187, 227
soft drinks 137
Solganal (aurothioglucose) 112
Soma (carisoprodol) 171
soy products 222
SPA (single proton absorptiometry) 1
Special Olympics 24
spina bifida 34, 105, 154, **265–267**
spinal cord **267–268**
   arachnoiditis 16–17
   birth injury to the spine 36
   corpectomy 69
   dwarfism 82
   medical tests 162
   MRI 157
   myelogram 175
   NCV test 184
   neck pain 181
   nerve compression 183
   QCT 230
   range of motion 232
   research 235
   rheumatoid arthritis 239
   Scheuermann's kyphosis 249
   shaken baby syndrome 258
   skeletal dysplasia 262
   skeletal fluorosis 263
   SM 292
   spinal stenosis 273
   spine 278
   surgery 288
   torticollis 298
   vertebral compression fracture 304

spinal decompression. *See* cervical laminaplasty; laminectomy
spinal fusion. *See* arthrodesis
spinal infection **268–269**
   acute back pain 8
   CAM 67
   coccydynia 65
   corticosteroid injection 70
   epidural injection 91
   exercise 94
   hydrotherapy 122
   magnetic therapy 159
   medical tests 162
   meningitis **163–164**
   meningitis, meningococcal disease **163–164**
   musculoskeletal disorders 174
   nerve block 182
   rheumatoid arthritis 239
   sacroiliac joint pain syndrome 247
   SAPHO Syndrome 248
   Scheuermann's kyphosis 249
   SED 255
   spinal tuberculosis 274
spinal injection **269–270**
   arachnoiditis 17
   flexion-extension injury 103
   fluoroscopy 104
   heart, effects of the spine on the 114
   lumbar radiculopathy 151
   sacroiliac joint pain syndrome 247
   spinal injury 271
spinal injury 41, 46, 57, **270–271**
spinal manipulation **271–273**
   arthritis 19
   birth injury to the spine 36
   brachial plexus injury 47
   cervical foraminal stenosis 53
   cervical spine 56
   cervical spondylosis 58
   cervicogenic headache 60
   degenerative disc disease 74
   heart, effects of the spine on the 114
   massage therapy 160
   rheumatoid arthritis 240

spinal manipulation *(continued)*
　rib injury 242
　Schmorl's node 250
　scoliosis 252
　spinal injury 271
　spine 279
　synovial cyst 291
　vertebral subluxation 305
Spinal-Muscular Atrophy (SMA).
　See Werdnig-Hoffman disease
spinal stenosis vi–vii, **273–274**
　cervical laminaplasty 54
　degenerative disc disease 74
　dwarfism 82
　facet joint disorder 97
　foraminotomy 106
　nerve block 182
　nerve compression 183
　orthotics 192
　paraspinal muscles 215
　SED 255
　spinal injury 271
　spinal tuberculosis 275
　spine 279
　vertebrae 303
　weight, effects of 314
spinal tap. *See* lumbar puncture
spinal tuberculosis 17, 162,
　274–276
spinal tumor **276–278**
　acute back pain 8
　cancer 50
　CAT scan 69
　children, spinal concerns for
　　61
　coccydynia 65
　CSM 59
　environmental influences 89
　epidural injection 91
　nerve compression 183
spine xii–xiii, **278–279**. *See also*
　specific regions of the spine, e.g.:
　cervical spine
spondylitis. *See* ankylosing
　spondylitis
spondyloepiphyseal dysplasia
　(SED) **279–280**
spondylolisthesis **280–281**
　backache 28
　lordosis 147

rheumatoid arthritis 239
　spinal stenosis 273
　spondylolysis 281
　synovial cyst 291
　weight, effects of 314
spondylolysis **281–282**
sports injury. *See* athletes, spinal
　concerns of
sprain **282–283**
　acupuncture 7
　exercise 94
　magnetic therapy 159
　muscle relaxants 171
　range of motion 232
　shoe choice, spinal effects of
　　260
　spine 278
　strain 285
　strength training 286
　ultrasound therapy 302
stability ball training (SBT) 303–
　304
standing 149
stem cells 268
stenosis. *See* spinal stenosis
steroid therapy v, 173, 220, 254,
　271, **283–284,** 291
strain **285**
　backache 28
　children, spinal concerns for
　　61
　exercise 94
　muscle relaxants 171
　pain management 212
　pregnancy, back care during
　　227
　range of motion 232
　rhomboid muscle strain 241
　spinal manipulation 272
　spine 278
　sprain 282
　strength training 286
　ultrasound therapy 302
strength training **285–287**
　brachial plexus injury 47
　cervical spine 57
　cervicogenic headache 60
　children, spinal concerns for
　　61
　exercise 94

flexion-extension injury 104
　metabolic diseases of muscle
　　166
　paraspinal muscles 216
　rib injury 242
　RICE method 243
stress (psychological) ix, 293–
　294. *See also* tension
strontium ranelate 15, **287–288**
substance P 214, 297
sulfasalazine 80, 81
sunscreen 308
supplements
　nutrition 187–198
　over-the-counter products 208
　phosphorus 219–220
　phytochemicals 220–221
　potassium 226
　sleep 264–265
　vitamin B-complex 307
　vitamin E 309
　zinc 318
surgery **288–291**. *See also*
minimally invasive surgery
　anterior cervical discectomy
　　14–15
　arthrodesis **20–21**
　bone graft **41–42**
　cervical laminaplasty **54**
　corpectomy **69–70**
　discectomy **76–77**
　disc nucleoplasty **77–78**
　disc replacement **79–80**
　foraminotomy **106**
　IDET **131–132**
　image-guided surgery **128–
　　129**
　kyphoplasty **140**
　laminectomy **142–143**
　lumbar spinal fusion **152–
　　154**
　microdiscectomy **166–167**
　rodding surgery **245**
　SED **255–256**
　thoracoplasty **296–297**
　vertebroplasty **306**
swayback. *See* lordosis
swimming 198
synovial cyst **291–292**
syringomyelia (SM) 59, **292**

T

tailbone 65. *See also* coccygeal
  spine
tamoxifen 256
T-cells 1
tension ix, **293–294**
  acupressure 6
  biofeedback 33
  low back pain 149
  magnesium 156
  mineral balance 168
  muscle cramp/spasm 170
  muscle relaxants 171
  neck pain 180
  nutrition 186–187
  osteoarthritis 195
  paraspinal muscles 215
  shoe choice, spinal effects of
    260
  sleep 265
  strain 285
  trigger point therapy 300
  vitamin B-complex 307
TENS unit. *See* transcutaneous
  electronic nerve stimulator unit
teriparatide 216–217, 255
testosterone 15, 122
tests. *See* medical tests for
  conditions affecting the back and
  spine
tetraplegia 267
thoracic insufficiency syndrome
  297
thoracic outlet syndrome 231,
  295
thoracic spine **296**
  arthrodesis 20
  cervical radiculopathy 55
  corpectomy 69
  DISH 75
  fractures 107
  heart, effects of the spine on
    the 114
  herniated disc 118
  infants, spinal concerns for
    131
  laminectomy 142
  lifting 144
  load tolerance 145
  nerve block 182

osteomyelitis 200
posture 225
range of motion 232
rhomboid muscle strain 241
Scheuermann's kyphosis 249
Schmorl's node 250
scoliosis 252
SED 280
spinal cord 267
spinal tuberculosis 275
spondylolysis 281
surgery 288
tension 294
thoracoplasty 296
vertebral subluxation 305
thoracoplasty **296–297**
tizanidine (Zanaflex) 172
topical analgesic 19, 29, 213,
  297–298
torticollis 23, 25, 171, **298–299**
TOS. *See* thoracic outlet syndrome
toxicity 156
trace minerals 167–169
traction 59, 118, 271, **299**
transarticular screw 25
transcutaneous electronic nerve
  stimulator (TENS) unit 19, 223,
  299–300
trigger point therapy **300–301**
T-score 201
tuberculosis. *See* spinal
  tuberculosis
turmeric 117
twisted neck. *See* torticollis
Tylenol 3

U

ultrasound therapy 8, 28, 65,
  185, **302**
ultraviolet (UV) rays 308
urinalysis 162–163
U.S. Food and Drug
  Administration (FDA) 116

V

vagus nerve 114
valerian 240, 264–265
Valium (diazepam) 171

vertebrae ix–x, **303–304**
  adolescents, spinal concerns
    for 10
  ankylosing spondylitis 13
  atlantoaxial instability 25
  cancer 50
  cervical foraminal stenosis 53
  cervical radiculopathy 55
  cervical spine 56
  cervical spondylosis 58
  ergonomic factors 92
  facet joint disorder 97
  flat back 102
  foraminotomy 106
  fractures 107
  image-guided surgery 128
  infants, spinal concerns for
    130
  juvenile osteoporosis 136
  juvenile spondyloarthritis 138
  lifting 144
  lumbar radiculopathy 151
  lumbar spinal fusion 152
  lumbar spine 154
  magnesium 156
  medical tests 162
  mineral balance 167
  musculoskeletal disorders 174
  nerve compression **182–183**
  opiates 191
  orthotics **192–194**
  osteomyelitis 200
  osteopenia 201
  peripheral neuropathy 218
  posture 225
  pregnancy, back care during
    227
  PTH 216
  range of motion 232
  research 234
  rheumatoid arthritis 239
  rib injury 242
  RICE method 243
  sacral vertebrae **246–247**
  Scheuermann's kyphosis 249
  sciatica 251
  SED **279–280**
  shaken baby syndrome 258
  spina bifida 266
  spinal cord 267

vertebrae (continued)
    spinal infection 268
    spinal manipulation 271
    spinal stenosis 273
    spinal tuberculosis 274
    spine 278
    spondylolisthesis 280
    spondylolysis 281
    steroid therapy 283
    surgery 288
    synovial cyst 291
    traction 299
    weight, effects of 314
vertebral compression fracture
    304–305
    activity, daily 4
    acute back pain 8
    antiresorptive drug 15
    bisphosphonates 38
    bone building 39
    calcitonin 48
    CAM 67
    female athlete triad 100
    fractures 107–108
    HRT 121
    kyphoplasty 140
    kyphosis 141
    low back pain 148
    lumbar spine 154
    MBD 165
    MRI 157
    musculoskeletal disorders 175
    myeloma bone disease 177
    osteitis deformans 194
    risedronate sodium 244
    sacral vertebrae 246
    SERMs 256
    thoracic spine 296
    vertebrae 303
    vertebroplasty 306
vertebral subluxation 305
    atlantoaxial instability 25
    backpack safety 32
    birth injury to the spine 36
    brachial plexus injury 47
    degenerative disc disease 74
    dislocated vertebra 81
    heart, effects of the spine on
        the 114
    nerve compression 183

paraspinal muscles 215
    rib injury 242
    spinal manipulation 271
vertebral subluxation complex
    (VSC) 36
vertebroplasty 140, 304, **306**
Vioxx 18
viral meningitis 164
vitamin A 51, 90, 133, 168,
    306–307
vitamin B-complex **307**
    birth defects of the spine 34
    CSM 59
    folate **105–106**
    magnesium 156
    mineral balance 168
    nutrition 189
    spina bifida 266
vitamin C **307–308**
    cancer 51
    elderly, spinal concerns of 86
    environmental influences 90
    herbal therapy 116
    iron 133
    mineral balance 168
    osteoarthritis 196
    secondary osteoporosis 254
    weight, effects of 314–315
vitamin D **308–309**
    calcium 49
    cervical spine 57
    coccygeal spine 66
    juvenile osteoporosis 137
    magnesium 156
    mineral balance 168
    nutrition 187
    osteitis deformans 194
    osteoarthritis 196
    osteoporosis 204, 206–207
    phosphorus 220
    rickets 243
    secondary osteoporosis 254
    SERMs 257
vitamin E 19, 51, 90, 156, 196,
    309
vitamin K 116–117, 187, 208,
    309–310
vitamin supplements 208
VSC (vertebral subluxation
    complex) 36

W
walking 4–5, 87, 143
water and spine health xiv,
    311–312
    disc, disk 75
    environmental influences 90
    rhabdomyolysis 237
    rheumatoid arthritis 240
    rhomboid muscle strain 241
    RICE method 243
    risedronate sodium 244
    secondary osteoporosis 255
    skeletal fluorosis 263
    SNRB 258
    spinal infection 269
    spinal tumor 278
    spine 279
    spondylolysis 282
    sprain 283
    steroid therapy 284
    surgery 290
    trigger point therapy 301
    vertebrae 304
    weight, effects of 315
    weight-bearing exercise 313
weight, effects of **313–315**
    athletes, spinal concerns of
        24
    birth defects of the spine 34
    cancer 51
    degenerative disc disease 74
    exercise 94
    herniated disc 119
    low back pain 148
    MD 173
    nerve compression 183
    nutrition 187
    orthotics 193
    osteoarthritis 197
    posture 225
    pregnancy, back care during
        227
weight-bearing exercise **312–
    313**
Werdnig-Hoffman disease **315–
    316**
whiplash 103
willow bark 19, 116, 214
wintergreen 29
wryneck. See torticollis

X

X-ray vii, **317**
   absorptiometry 1, 2
   ankylosing spondylitis 13
   arachnoiditis 17
   arthritis 18
   cancer 50
   CAT scan **68–69**
   discogram 78
   FBSS 99
   fluoroscopy **104–105**
   foraminotomy 106
   image-guided surgery 128
   juvenile arthritis 135
   juvenile spondyloarthritis 139
   kyphoplasty 140
   MBD 165

medical tests 162
MRI 157
myelogram **175–176**
osteoarthritis 195
osteogenesis imperfecta 198
pregnancy, back care during
   227
radiculitis 231
rheumatoid arthritis 239
rib injury 242
rickets 244
rodding surgery 245
sacroiliac joint pain syndrome
   247
Scheuermann's kyphosis 249
Schmorl's node 250
sciatica 251

scoliosis 253
SED 255
spinal injection 270
spondylolisthesis 280
spondylolysis 281
surgery 288
X STOP implant vii, 142, 274

Y

yogurt 49, 137

Z

Zanaflex (tizanidine) 172
zinc 156, 168, 169, **318**
zinc supplements 133

ABOUT THE AUTHORS

Mary Harwell Sayler is an award-winning medical writer, poet, and writing instructor with extensive publishing credits, including *The Encyclopedia of Muscle & Skeletal Systems & Disorders* released in 2005 by Facts On File.

Arya Nick Shamie, M.D., is a professor of orthopedic spine surgery and neurosurgery at UCLA with vast experience in the surgical treatment of spinal disorders. Known nationally and internationally for his frequent presentations on various topics related to spinal surgery, his published works include numerous book chapters and articles.